# Nails

Diagnosis • Therapy • Surgery

Commissioning Editor: **Belinda Kuhn**
Project Development Manager: **Shuet-Kei Cheung**
Project Manager: **Cheryl Brant**
Editorial Assistant: **Amy Lewis**
Illustration Manager: **Mick Ruddy**
Designer: **Stewart Larking**
Illustrator: **Paul Richardson**
Marketing Manager(s) (UK/USA): **Amy Hey/Megan Carr**

# Nails

## Diagnosis • Therapy • Surgery

### THIRD EDITION

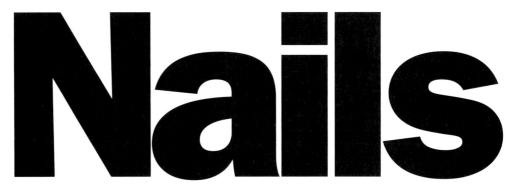

**Edited by**
**Richard K Scher MD**
Professor of Clinical Dermatology
College of Physicians and Surgeons
Columbia University
New York, NY, USA

**C Ralph Daniel III MD**
Clinical Professor of Medicine
(Dermatology)
University of Mississippi
Jackson, MS, USA
Clinical Associate Professor of
Dermatology
University of Alabama at Birmingham
Birmingham, AL, USA

**Associate Editors:**
**Antonella Tosti MD**
Professor of Dermatology
Department of Dermatology
University of Bologna
Bologna, Italy

**Boni E Elewski MD**
Professor of Dermatology
Department of Dermatology
University of Alabama at Birmingham
Birmingham, AL, USA

**Philip Fleckman MD**
Professor of Medicine (Dermatology)
University of Washington
Seattle, WA, USA

**Phoebe Rich MD**
Associate Professor of Dermatology
University of Oregon
Portland, OR, USA

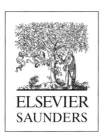

ELSEVIER
SAUNDERS

ELSEVIER
SAUNDERS

An imprint of Elsevier Inc

First edition 1990
Second edition 1997
Third edition 2005

ISBN 1-4160-2356-9

**British Library Cataloguing in Publication Data**
A catalogue record for this book is available from the British Library

**Library of Congress Cataloging in Publication Data**
A catalog record for this book is available from the Library of Congress

**Notice**
Medical knowledge is constantly changing. Standard safety precautions must be followed, but as new research and clinical experience broaden our knowledge, changes in treatment and drug therapy may become necessary or appropriate. Readers are advised to check the most current product information provided by the manufacturer of each drug to be administered to verify the recommended dose, the method and duration of administration, and contraindications. It is the responsibility of the practitioner, relying on experience and knowledge of the patient, to determine dosages and the best treatment for each individual patient. Neither the Publisher nor the editors assume any liability for any injury and/or damage to persons or property arising from this publication.
**The Publisher**

Printed in China
Last digit is the print number : 9 8 7 6 5 4 3 2 1

# Contents

# List of contributors

**Philippe Abimelec MD**
Consultant Dermatologist
Hospital Saint-Louis
Paris, France

**Philip R Cohen MD**
Clinical Associate Professor
Department of Dermatology
The University of Texas-Houston
Medical School;
Fellow
Mohs Microgaphic Surgery
Dermatologic Surgery Center of
Houston
Houston, TX, USA

**John T Crissey MD**
Emeritus Professor of Clinical
Medicine (Dermatology)
Keck School of Medicine
University of Southern California
Los Angeles, CA, USA

**C Ralph Daniel III MD**
Clinical Professor of Medicine
(Dermatology)
University of Mississippi
Mississippi, MS, USA
Clinical Associate Professor of
Dermatology
University of Alabama at Birmingham
Birmingham, AL, USA

**Christian Dumontier MD**
Associate Professor of Orthopedic
Surgery
Institut de la Main
Paris, France

**Boni E Elewski MD**
Professor of Dermatology
Department of Dermatology
University of Alabama at Birmingham
Birmingham, AL, USA

**Philip Fleckman MD**
Professor of Medicine (Dermatology)
University of Washington
Seattle, WA, USA

**Richard C Gibbs MD**
Clinical Professor of Dermatology
New York University Medical Center
New York, NY, USA

**Larry Goss DPM**
Podiatrist
Philly Foot and Ankle
Philadelphia, PA, USA

**Suthep Jerasutus MD**
Consultant
Department of Dermatology
Ramathibodi Hospital
Mahidol University
Bangkok, Thailand

**Warren S Joseph DPM**
Podiatric Consultant
Veterans Affairs Medical Center
Coatesville, PA, USA

**Monica Lawry MD**
Assistant Clinical Professor
University of California
Sacramento, CA, USA

**Harvey Lemont DPM**
Professor
Department of Podiatric Medicine
Temple University School of Podiatric
Medicine;
Laboratory of Podiatric Pathology
Philadelphia, PA, USA

**Bryan C Markinson DPM**
Chief of Podiatric Medicine and
Surgery
The Lenni and Peter W. May
Department of Orthopedic Surgery
Mount Sinai School of Medicine
New York, NY, USA

**John D Mozena DPM**
Podiatric Physician and Surgeon
Town Center Foot Clinic
Portland, OR, USA

**Lawrence Charles Parish MD**
Clinical Professor of Dermatology and
Cutaneous Biology
Thomas Jefferson University Medical
College
Philadelphia, PA, USA

**Massimiliano Pazzaglia MD**
Fellow
Department of Dermatology
University of Bologna
Bologna, Italy

**Bianca M Piraccini MD**
Researcher
Department of Dermatology
University of Bologna
Bologna, Italy

**Phoebe Rich MD**
Associate Professor of Dermatology
University of Oregon
Portland, OR, USA

**Bertrand Richert MD**
Professor of Dermatology
University of Liege
Liege, Belgium

**Richard K Scher MD**
Professor of Clinical Dermatology
College of Physicians and Surgeons
Columbia University
New York, NY, USA

**Jenny O Sobera MD**
Dermatology Resident
Department of Dermatology
University of Alabama at Birmingham
Birmingham, AL, USA

**Antonella Tosti MD**
Professor of Dermatology
Department of Dermatology
University of Bologna
Bologna, Italy

**Justin Wernick MD**
Professor and Chair
Division of Clinical Sciences
Department of Orthopedic Sciences
New York College of Podiatric Medicine
New York, NY, USA

**Martin N Zaiac MD**
Program Director
Department of Dermatology
Mount Sinai Medical Center
Miami Beach, FL, USA

# Preface to the third edition

We are very pleased to be able to produce a third edition of *Nails*. The strong positive reception of editions one and two confirms our notion that interest in nail disorders has increased at a rapidly accelerating pace. As recently as twenty years ago few texts on this subject were available. Now there are many out there! Likewise, at that time journals had infrequent articles published on nail diseases but now almost every issue of every cutaneous journal has many articles dealing with the important subject of onychology. The authors of this third edition find this very exciting.

It will be noted that the number of editors has been increased to include Dr Boni Elewski, an expert on fungal diseases, Dr Philip Fleckman, to expand basic science, Dr Phoebe Rich, prominent in nails and diabetics, and Dr Antonella Tosti to provide a European insight and view point. It is our hope that healthcare givers will find this book of value in helping patients with nail problems.

Richard K Scher and C Ralph Daniel III
2005

# Preface to the second edition

It is indeed a privilege to be able to write the second edition of a practical, easy-to-use textbook on nails that is easy to carry and not overweight. This book, like its predecessor, should be useful to virtually all health care providers because it stresses treatment after accurate diagnosis is made. The content elaborates in great detail how to identify nail disease so that subsequent therapy will be effective. The book goes significantly further than providing medical treatment protocols in its extensive development of nail surgical techniques from the simple everyday procedures to the more complex, so that both the generalist, whatever his or her field—and the trained surgeon—will find significant value in it.

The chapter on onychomycosis has been vastly expanded and rewritten in view of the breakthrough developments that have occurred since 1990. Thus a broad and complete discussion of all the new antifungal medications used for treatment of nail mycoses is presented in an easily applicable manner for everyday office implementation. A new chapter for podiatrists has been added and earlier podiatric chapters have been updated and expanded so that the podiatrist, who cares for a major segment of the onycho-dystrophies, will find this an invaluable text. Readers will also benefit from an important and unique chapter devoted to geriatric nail problems. This discussion should prove invaluable considering the huge increase in this segment of the population. The nail salon advice material is particularly appropriate considering that annually several billion dollars are spent on nail cosmetics in the United States alone. Another noteworthy portion of the book is devoted to nail disorders in the HIV-positive patient, a topic not elaborated on significantly elsewhere. All the remaining chapters have been revised and made current to keep pace with the rapidly progressive field of onychology.

The editors are grateful to all those health care practitioners who have made this book the most successful one ever devoted to nail disorders. This text has found worldwide distribution in large numbers, including translations into several languages. The authors are most appreciative of this. We look forward to this second edition as a bridge to the twenty-first century. All the authors have worked together to produce an integrated work that is not fragmented or overloaded with scores of unnecessary references.

Richard K Scher and C Ralph Daniel III

# Preface to the first edition

## What! Another book on nails?

The decade of the 1980s provided an explosive interest in the diagnosis and treatment of nail disorders. An area of dermatology long neglected by clinical and basic science-research people as well, onychology has rather suddenly become fashionable. The nail unit is no longer regarded as untouchable or an appendage to be ignored. Suddenly, investigators are peering into the chemistry, physiology, and development of the nail. Cell biology, electron microscopy, ultrasound, and numerous other sophisticated research techniques and methodologies are being applied to the study of the onychium and how it works. The geneticist and paediatrician look at the nail as a sign of inherited disease and as an aid in the assessment of syndromes seen at birth. The internist examines this structure as a window to possible systemic disease. The surgeon is devising new and advanced procedures for the repair and reconstruction of hereditary ad traumatic nail dystrophies. The podiatrist studies the toenails and alleviates painful and infected digits. The geriatrician attends to the effects of faulty biomechanics, impaired circulation, multiple drugs and abnormal gaits as well as bone and joint changes in the elderly. The osseous defects that secondarily affect the nail impact upon the orthopaedist and rheumatologist as well. The mycologist and infectious disease experts are constantly investigating patients with fungal infections and now AIDS showing nail manifestations, Finally, the dermatologist with his unique training, knowledge and expertise, more than anyone else, is exposed to all of the above facets of onychology and must therefore be thoroughly familiar with every aspect of nail diagnosis and treatment. Thus, virtually all areas of medicine are affected by the heretofore neglected and often maligned nail unit.

It is not only practitioners who need nail know-how! Another aspect of the interest in nails that emerged in the 1980s is the apparent sudden discovery of this structure by the pharmaceutical industry. Until recently, drug companies have hesitated to invest in the development of antimycotics for onychomycosis, conditioners for brittle nails, enhancers for nail growth and antipsoriatics for the psoriatic nail. This is no longer true. Millions of dollars are now being spent in an effort to find more effective medicaments for nail disease. Nor can we overlook the cosmetic industry. In 1988, $1.5 billion was spent of nail cosmetics in the United States alone. Nail salons are ubiquitous. The obsession with attractive nails is no longer limited to the female population but is expanding in an astonishing fashion among males. Consequently, the interest in nails pervades all levels and aspects of our society, and indeed it should.

## So, why another book on nails?

For the first tome to appear on the subject of nails for the 1990s, the editors have embarked on an approach differing from previous texts. The emphasis here has been on therapy and what to do – practically – for the patient with a nail problem. Common and uncommon surgical approaches have been offered by both dermatologists and hand surgeons. Diagnosis is stressed when it is needed prior to a discussion of treatment. A comprehensive treatise on histopathology of the nail is presented for the first time. The podiatrists viewpoint is offered from the view of gait and roentgenology. Cosmetic reactions, primary nail disorders, nail manifestations of systemic disease, and nail neoplasms are all offered in a very pragmatic way.

Why another nail book? Because the text of the 1990s is new, innovative, and practical. It provides important information for clinicians, pathologists, surgeons, basic scientists, cosmetitians, and the pharmaceutical industry. The authors sincerely hope that the combined efforts of all these disciplines will have one end result: relief of pain and suffering for the patient.

Richard K Scher and C Ralph Daniel III

# Dedications

RKS wishes to dedicate this book to his wife, Marlyne, as well as his children and seven grandchildren (Jacob, Shira, Jonah, Hera, Eli, Jessica, and Benjamin) and in memory of his parents, Marie and Herman Scher, to whom much gratitude is due.

CRD wishes to dedicate this book to his wife Melissa, sons Carlton and Jonathan, and to Carlton's bride, Kimberly. Also in memory of his mother Beverly and nephew David Gordon Lewis Daniel.

# 1

# Nail Signs and Symptoms

## Phoebe Rich

## Key Features

1. Important pathologic nail signs relate to nail size and shape, color, surface contour, substance texture, and growth abnormalities
2. Abnormalities of the surface of the nail plate, such as pitting and onychorrhexis, are usually due to pathology in the nail matrix or space-occupying lesions in the proximal nail fold

The accurate recognition and description of nail findings is the crucial first step in the process of correctly diagnosing a nail disorder. Pathology in any portion of the nail apparatus results in abnormal nail signs and symptoms, the recognition and identification of which allows clinicians to arrive at the appropriate differential diagnosis of a particular nail abnormality.

By definition, a nail sign is an objective, physical nail finding. It is a clinically noticeable nail feature observed by the clinician when the nail is examined, such as abnormal nail color or shape. Conversely, a nail symptom is a subjective indication of disease, pathology, or injury. Symptoms are felt or noticed by the patient and reported to the clinician, but cannot be directly observed by the physician. Examples of nail symptoms are pain, throbbing, and itching. A nail sign or symptom is not a diagnosis nor is it a pathologic process. The presence of signs and symptoms in the nail gives valuable clues that direct further workup to determine the precise diagnosis of the pathologic process.

Understanding the biology and anatomy of the nail allows the astute clinician to ascertain the location of pathology that is responsible for the nail sign. For example, pitting is a nail plate sign that indicates pathology in the nail matrix, specifically the proximal portion of the matrix from which the cells on the surface of the nail plate differentiate. Pitting is a nail plate sign, not a nail matrix sign, because there is no visible matrix change. The only true nail matrix signs are those clinically visible in the lunula, such as abnormal color or shape of the lunula.

Nail signs occur in the nail plate and the paronychial tissues including the nail bed, nail folds, and visible portion of the lunula. It is useful to think about nail signs and to categorize them by location: nail plate, nail bed, nail folds.

## NAIL PLATE SIGNS

## Nail Plate Size

### Micronychia

Small nails occur if the nail matrix is narrower than expected, resulting in a narrower nail. This can occur as a congenital disorder or resulting from a traumatic injury to the nail matrix.

*Brachyonychia* is the term used to describe a nail that is shorter than would be expected. The thumb is the digit most commonly affected, and this abnormality is often called racquet nail. This condition is often inherited as an autosomal dominant condition. Other fingers are rarely involved.

*Anonychia* is a total or partial lack of nail. This results in a thinner nail plate or even the absence of the nail plate. Anonychia occurs in congenital conditions in which the nail never forms, or could be acquired where the nail becomes atrophic secondary to disease of the matrix. Apparently the development of the nail requires underlying bone for proper development.[1] There are many congenital causes of anonychia, which might be associated with retardation, abnormal facies, and abnormal dentition. Anonychia of the thumbnail can occur in nail–patella syndrome and numerous ectodermal dysplasias (see Chapter 21).

*Onychoatrophy* can be acquired in conditions such as lichen planus (see Chapter 11) or could be a congenital anomaly. The clinical appearance of onychoatrophy is a nail that is thinner and has less volume than other nails; it might or might not have decreased length/width, resulting in a smaller surface area than normal. Congenital causes of onychoatrophy are discussed in Chapter 21.

*Hapalponychia* is defined as a thin nail. Other conditions can be associated with thinning of the nail plate, including conditions that result in the superficial layers of the nail plate disintegrating or peeling, as in onychoschizia, trachyonychia, and in aging when there are focal longitudinal groves that result in longitudinal thin weak areas of the nail that often chip and crack distally.

## Macronychia

Large nails occur when the nail plate is large, usually associated with gigantism of the corresponding digit. It has been reported in Proteus syndrome.[2]

## Increased thickness

PACHYONYCHIA Pachyonychia is characterized by thickening of the nail structure and can be due to nail plate thickening or nail bed thickening; the former is seen in pachyonychyia congenita (see Chapter 21). Thickening of the nail plate is seen when the rate of linear nail growth slows, as in elderly and yellow nail syndrome. It appears that the nail increases in thickness rather than length, and manifests parallel horizontal bands in some instances.

## Onychogryphosis

Onychogryphosis is characterized by thickened, long nails. These often curl laterally and have been described as resembling a ram's

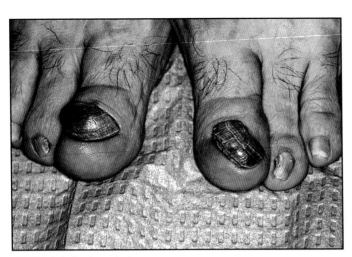

FIGURE 1–1. Onychogryphosis.

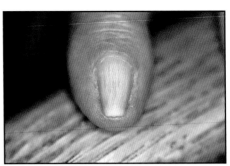

FIGURE 1–2. Pincer nail.

horn. They can result from neglect in grooming in the elderly and from poorly fitting shoes (Fig. 1.1).

## Abnormalities of Nail Shape

### Over-curvature of the nail

**CLUBBING** Clubbing of the nail is defined as over-curvature of the nail with or without hypertrophy of the soft tissues and cyanosis. Clubbing was first described by Hippocrates and is often given the eponym 'Hippocratic nails'. The classic feature of clubbing is the increase in the unguo-phalanged angle, also called the angle of Lovibond, which is the angle that is formed by the proximal nail fold and nail plate. In clubbing this angle is 180° or greater, as apposed to the normal 160°. The causes of clubbing are varied and there are many associations and several classifications;[3,4] many case reports can be found in the literature. The clinician would do well to remember a few of the more common categories but the major categories include cardiovascular, gastrointestinal, familial syndromes, and miscellaneous causes. The mechanism appears to be a vasodilatation of the vessels of the nail unit, particularly in the thickened nail bed[5] (see Chapter 15).

### Pincer nails

Over-curvature of the nail in the transverse plane can result in a pincer nail, in which the distal edges of the nail curve to the extent that they pinch the soft tissue beneath the nail. This over-curved nail plate can grow into the distal lateral nail groove, causing pain. Causes of pincer nails include trauma, pressure from tight footwear, and onychomycosis (Fig 1.2).

### Under-curvature of the nail

**KOILONYCHIA** Koilonychia is the name given to spooning of the nails where the lateral distal edges of the nail plate are elevated above a depressed center. In some cases there is peripheral hyperkeratosis under the everted edges of the nail. When koilonychia is viewed laterally the nail plate resembles the bowl of a spoon, and hence the common name 'spoon nails'. Although there are many case reports in the literature of conditions associated with koilonychia, two main categories surface: Congenital/hereditary

forms (see Chapter 15) and acquired forms. In the acquired forms, endocrinological causes such as hypothyroid and iron deficiency anemia lead the way (see Chapter 15), followed by occupational/ traumatic forms where the distal edge may be curved (see Chapter 18).

### Abnormal colors in the nail

**DYSCHROMIA** Dyschromia means abnormal color. The nail plate itself is colorless and translucent and derives its illusionary color from the underlying structures: The nail appears pink over the nail bed, white over the lunula, and there is a crisp line of demarcation between the nail bed and lunula. The free edge of the nail appears white because there is only air beneath it, which also explains why onycholysis appears white. The distal few millimeters of the nail bed in the area of the onychodermal band has a darker brownish color. The nail folds and hyponychium are normally the same color as the surrounding digital skin.

The color change in the nail might be in any or all parts of the nail unit. The most common color changes seen in the nails are leukonychia (white), melanonychia (brown), and erythronychia (red). Blue, yellow, green, and brown can appear in the nail unit.

**LEUKONYCHIA** Literally, this means 'white nail' and is a very common nail dyschromia. Leukonychia has many different and unrelated forms, depending where the pathology exists or originated. Leukonychia can be divided into several categories to make the differential diagnosis more manageable. The white color change can be complete, when the entire nail is white, or fractional (limited), when only parts of the nail are involved, as in punctate leukonychia. Authentic or absolute leukonychia occurs where the white color is present in the actual nail plate. Authentic leukonychia is seen both in vivo and in vitro. For example, in Mees lines, the nail plate clinically shows transverse white bands when the digit is examined (in vivo) and the nail plate itself exhibits the same white band after it is avulsed (in vitro). In authentic leukonychia the color change is in the substance of the nail plate. Conversely, an illusionary leukonychia derives its white appearance from the underlying structure, thus creating the illusion that the nail plate is white. In illusional leukonychia, the white color change is present only when the nail is attached to the digit because its white color comes from nail bed changes (in vivo). Muehrcke's lines are an example of illusionary leukonychia.

It is also useful to describe color changes in the nail by location of the color abnormality. For example, there might be abnormal pigmentation in the nail plate, nail bed, nail matrix, nail fold, and nail lunula. Dyschromia can also be classified by the actual color change (red, black, blue, or yellow).

# Nail Surface Morphology and Texture

The surface of the normal nail plate is smooth and has a low level of luster. Numerous nail-surface irregularities occur as a normal function of aging or as a result of a pathologic process: Pits, ridges, grooves, or flaking. Generally, such changes are due to pathology in the nail matrix, nail fold, exogenous exposure, and certain nail-bed pathology.

## Pitting

Pitting occurs in response to pathology in the nail matrix, primarily the proximal matrix. Pits are shallow depressions in the surface of the nail and can be regular, irregular, large, or small depending on the duration and extent of the pathology in the proximal matrix. Pitting is seen in psoriasis, alopecia areata, and eczematous dermatitis among other conditions (Fig. 1.3).

## Trachyonychia

Trachyonychia is characterized by fine striations of the nail that give the surface of the nail plate a rough appearance. The striations are arranged in linear longitudinal formation or very fine shallow pits. One to 20 nails can be affected, which is why it has been called 'twenty-nail dystrophy'. It is seen in alopecia areata, lichen planus, psoriasis, and eczema. Tosti biopsied 13 patients with trachyonychia and found spongiosis that was thought to be related to alopecia areata[6] in most of the cases.[7,8] Andre and Richert looked at 22 cases of trachyonychia and on biopsy found spongiotic histopathology in 10 cases and psoriasis and lichen planus in 6 cases each.[9]

## Ridges and grooves in the nail plate

Ridges and grooves in the nail occur in a longitudinal and transverse (horizontal) axis. Both types of depression in the nail plate can originate from pathology in the nail matrix or the nail fold.

**BEAU'S LINES** A growth disruption in the nail matrix results in horizontal (transverse) depressions in the nail plate. These are called Beau's lines, and were originally described in 1846. The groove usually occurs on multiple nails in the same location, parallels the distal edge of the lunula, and progresses distally as the nail plate grows out. Any systemic disease or event that is severe enough to disrupt the growth of the nail results in Beau's lines, and the timing of the event can be determined by knowing the rate of growth of the nail. The width of the line is determined by the duration of the growth arrest.

**HABIT TIC** Habit tic deformity is a common cause of parallel transverse depressions in the nail in a characteristic washboard configuration (Fig. 1.4). It is caused by repetitive self-manipulation of the proximal nail fold and lunula area. Habit tic disorders sometimes respond to the selective serotonin uptake inhibitor medications used to treat obsessive-compulsive disorders.[10]

**LONGITUDINAL DEPRESSIONS** Longitudinal depressions and ridges have several clinical presentation and causes. A common cause of a longitudinal depression in the nail plate is a space-occupying lesion such as a fibroma, wart, or digital myxoid cyst in the proximal nail fold. The lesion exerts pressure on the nail matrix and results in a longitudinal depression immediately distal to the lesion. This will disappear when the causative lesion is removed (Fig. 1.5).

**ONYCHORRHEXIS** Onychorrhexis is characterized by confluent, longitudinal, shallow grooves and ridges in the nail plate that give the surface of the nail a rough, textured appearance. A typical cause of onychorrhexis is lichen planus of the nail (Fig. 1.6).

Median nail dystrophy is a longitudinal defect of the center of the nail, usually the thumb. It results in a split in the nail that has a characteristic Christmas-tree pattern and was first described by Heller in 1928.

Parallel longitudinal ridges are seen as a normal phenomenon in aging. These ridges and grooves are thinner and weaker areas in the nail plate and are prone to distal splits.

**ONYCHOSCHIZIA** Onychoschizia – distal peeling of layers of the surface of the nail – is a common condition. It is seen in about one-third of adult women, especially those whose hands are immersed in water frequently. Distal peeling and lamellar splitting similar to fish scales, with subsequent weakening and fragility of the nail plate, are the clinical features of onychoschizia. Other

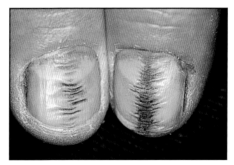

**FIGURE 1–4.** Habit tic thumbs.

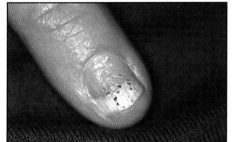

**FIGURE 1–3.** Pitting psoriasis.

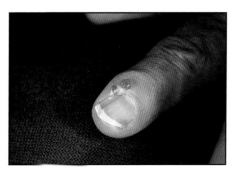

**FIGURE 1–5.** Cyst, rotated.

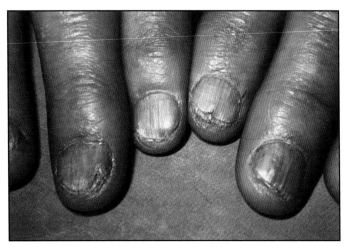

FIGURE 1–6. Onychorrhexis.

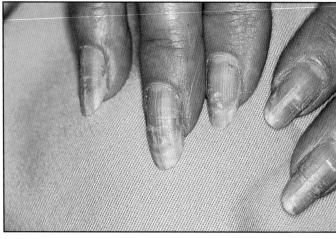

FIGURE 1–8. Keratin granulations.

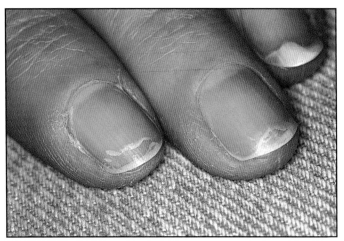

FIGURE 1–7. Onychoschizia.

exogenous factors, such as harsh solvents and nail polish remover, can cause or exacerbate onychoschizia. In vitro treatment of nails with household chemicals or even water and detergent has been found to reproduce onychoschizia after 21 days.[11] The condition can be managed by moisturizing with a heavy petrolatum-based product (Fig. 1.7).

Superficial crumbling of the nail plate is seen in two conditions of different etiology. White, superficial onychomycosis causes a white, granular, powdery, and flaky pattern on toenails and is caused by a fungal infection of the nail. A similar appearance is seen in nails subjected to lengthy applications of nail polish, resulting in a white granular surface of the nail plate (Fig. 1.8).

## Attachment and Support

Structures that support and protect the nail plate are important in preserving the overall integrity, function and structure of the nail. The nail bed and the nail folds achieve this function. Abnormality in integrity of these structures results in pathologic features, including attachment, which results in characteristic nail signs. The nail plate is firmly attached to the nail bed, and to the nail folds

and cuticle, which collectively keep it in place and protect it from the assaults of daily hand activities. The nail plate suffers when there is an abnormality of these supporting structures. Pathology in these structures (e.g. hyperkeratosis in the nail bed) prevents normal attachment of the nail plate to the nail.

## NAIL BED AND NAIL FOLD SIGNS (PERIONYCHIUM)

Attachment of the various supporting nail structures is important for healthy nail development and growth disorders of attachment of the proximal nail fold include paronychia and pterygium. Abnormality of the attachment of the nail bed results in onycholysis, with distal attachment problems, and onychomadesis, with proximal nail attachment, hyperkeratosis, and ventral pterygium.

## Pterygium

A pterygium, which is derived from the Greek word *pterygium* meaning 'wing', occurs when there is focal scarring of the nail matrix resulting in areas where the nail plate is absent. In the areas of focal nail loss the proximal nail fold attaches to the nail bed and creates the characteristic wing appearance. Lichen planus of the nail is the most common cause of pterygium but trauma and some connective tissue disorders can result in pterygium.[12] Ventral pterygium describes the change whereby the distal nail bed attaches to the ventral surface of the nail plate and grows out beyond the normal point of separation. Ventral pterygium occurs primarily in systemic sclerosis and systemic lupus erythematosus.

## Onycholysis

Separation of the nail plate from the underlying nail bed is called onycholysis. There are many different causes of onycholysis: Systemic, external, cutaneous disorders, and infections. The most common cause of onycholysis is from external contact irritants and allergens. Protective avoidance of offending substances is the cornerstone of effective treatment (Fig. 1.9 and see Chapter 9).[13]

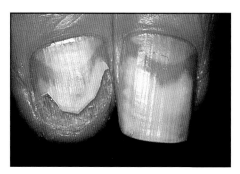

**FIGURE 1–9.**
Onycholysis, thumbs.

## Onychomadesis

Onychomadesis is characterized by separation of the nail plate from the proximal side with subsequent shedding of the nail as a new nail grows in beneath the old loose one. A number of systemic illnesses, drug reactions, bullous diseases, and drug reactions have been reported to cause onychomadesis. In some cases it is idiopathic, as in periodic shedding of the nails. A severe paronychia in which there is acute infection and pus under the proximal nail plate can account for onychomadesis of the diseased nails. Onychomadesis can appear as a wide Beau's line that subsequently sheds the entire nail.

## Nail Bed Hyperkeratosis

Nail bed hyperkeratosis is characterized by thickening of the nail bed. This hyperproliferative state occurs in a variety of nail conditions. There are inflammatory causes of hyperkeratosis (e.g. psoriasis and eczema), infectious causes (e.g. onychomycosis), and genetic causes (e.g. pachyonychia congenital).

## Nail Fold Pathology

Many conditions affect the proximal and lateral nail folds, the most common of which are infections, tumors, and inflammatory skin diseases such as psoriasis. Many skin conditions that affect the nail folds appear to behave similarly to the condition elsewhere on the skin. Tumors in the proximal nail fold often cause a groove in the corresponding portion of the nail plate.

## Paronychia

Paronychia is defined as inflammation or infection of the nail folds. It is a multifactorial condition with several etiologies and presentations but the primary event is a breach in the seal that the cuticle makes where it attaches to the nail plate. This gap or breach in the seal that protects the nail acts as a portal for infection. A bacterial infection of the nail folds results in an acute paronychia that is red, tender, swollen, and often purulent. This is usually caused by staphylococcal organisms and is treated with systemic antibiotics.

The more common form of paronychia is a chronic indolent process that begins with loss of the cuticle attachment to the nail plate. This loss of cuticle occurs for a variety of reasons, mostly external, and results in a space under the nail fold that then becomes irritated, red, tender, and puffy. It is sometimes secondarily infected with yeast, staphylococcus aureus or *Pseudomonas.* Excessive exposure to water and detergents, and trauma to the cuticle are common causes of chronic paronychia (see Chapter 10). Paronychia can be associated with other cutaneous conditions that affect the nail folds, such as psoriasis and eczema.

## NAIL LUNULA SIGNS

### Lunula Color

*Red lunula*

A diffuse, red color in the lunula can be caused by many systemic and cutaneous disorders or can be idiopathic. Cardiovascular disorders, carbon monoxide poisoning, systemic lupus erythematosus, and alopecia areata are a few of the many reported associations with red lunula (see Chapter 7).

Small red dots in the lunula can be seen in a variety of skin conditions such as psoriasis, alopecia areata, eczema, ichthyosis, and in IgA diseases.

### Lunula Shape

Normally, the shape of the distal lunula corresponds to the shape of the free edge of the nail plate. Triangular lunula is seen in nail–patella syndrome (hereditary osteo-onychodysplasia (see Chapter 21).

### Nail Unit Symptoms

Symptoms of the nail unit include pain, throbbing, and pressure usually due to trauma, infection, edema, or pressure in the nail unit. Sensory nerves populate the nail bed, matrix and folds allow for the sensation of pain. Pressure under the nail plate from a tumor or hemorrhage is experienced as pain, throbbing and pressure. Injuries and tumors in the nail unit or the underlying bone often result in pain.

## REFERENCES

1. Baran R, Juhlin L. Bone dependent nail formation. Br J Dermatol 1986; 114:371–375
2. Child FJ, Werring AB, Vivier AWP. Proteus syndrome: diagnosis in adulthood. Br J Dermatol 1998; 139;132–136
3. Daniel R, Sams WM, Scher RK. Nails in systemic disease. In Scher RK, Daniel CR (eds). Nail: therapy, diagnosis, surgery. 2nd edn. WB Saunders, 1997:219–225
4. Baran R, Dawber R. Diseases of the nails and their management. Blackwell Science, 2001:51
5. Currie AE, Galligher PJ. The pathology of clubbing: vascular changes in the nail bed. Br J Dis Chest 1988; 82:382–385
6. Tosti A, Fanti PA, Morelli R et al. Spongiotic trachyonychia. Arch Dermatol 1991; 127:584–585
7. Tosti A, Bardazzi F, Piraccini BM, Fanti PA. Idiopathic trachyonychia (twenty-nail dystrophy): a pathological study of 23 patients. Br J Dermatol 1994; 131:6866–6872
8. Tosti A, Bardazzi F, Piraccini BM et al. Is trachyonychia, a variety of alopecia areata, limited to the nails? J Invest Dermatol 1995; 104 (5 Suppl):27S–28S
9. Richert B, Andre J. Trachyonychia: a clinical and histological study.
10. Vittorio CC, Phillips KA. Treatment of habit tic disorders with fluoxetine. Arch Dermatol 1997; 133:1203–1204
11. Wallis MS, Bowen WR, Guin JR. Pathogenesis of onychoschizia lamaller dystrophy. J Am Acad Dermatol 1991; 24:44–48

12. Caputp R, Cappio F, Rigorri C. Pterygium inversum unguis. Arch Dermatol 1993; 129:1307

13. Daniel CR, Daniel MP, Daniel J et al. Managing simple chronic paronychia and onycholysis with ciclopirox 0.77% lotion and an irritant avoidance regimen. Cutis 2004; 73:81–85

# 2

# Historic Aspects of Nail Disease

John Thorne Crissey and Lawrence Charles Parish

Nails fit awkwardly into the dermatologic scheme of things. They are altered by internal disturbances and by skin diseases as well. They are subject to the effects of environment and the whims and cosmetic manipulations of their owners and have, in addition, a set of diseases all their own. In dealing with nails, authors of dermatologic texts for 200 years have had to compromise with the tenets of orderliness and sound organizational procedures to distribute information concerning nails here and there in the body of their works, wherever it seemed appropriate. Yet they have still found it necessary to create large, elastic, catch-all categories in which to stow whatever is left. These problems are brought into particularly sharp focus when one attempts, as we have here, to track the development of our knowledge of nail structure, function, and disease. The accumulation of facts was painfully slow. It followed no discernible pattern and was recorded in the literature of a variety of disciplines that communicated poorly with one another.

Nails also present clinical problems. They are capable of no more than a narrowly limited number of morphologic responses to a very large number of pathologic stimuli, and nail dystrophies, therefore, tax the diagnostic abilities of even the most experienced clinicians. Moreover, the nail complex, unlike the skin, does not readily lend itself to biopsy. Patient resistance, and the ever-present risk of producing permanent damage with biopsy procedures involving the nail, more often than not deprived dermatologists of their favorite diagnostic aid.

Anatomic and physiologic difficulties also confront the examiner. In accordance with medical wisdom, the intelligent management of nail disease requires a thorough understanding of normal structure, growth, and function. Authors face a maximum challenge to their ingenuity and literary skills to lay these matters out for their readers in a manner that is both interesting and easily understood. This challenge has not been successfully met in the past. An examination of the older dermatologic texts, which were originally issued in paper covers and later bound in cloth, shows that the sections on nail anatomy and physiology are often uncut and thus were never read. Nor do we see many finger marks, or underlining, or dog-ears on the analogous pages of similar sections in more modern works.

If it is difficult to splice together a coherent and useful picture of the nail and its diseases, even equipped as we now are with all the advantages, techniques, and accumulated knowledge – imagine the obstacles faced by interested physicians in the days before the simple fact was known that tissue is made up of cells. This extract from an 1827 paper by London's renowned surgeon–anatomist Sir Astley Patson Cooper illustrates the thinking behind the pre-cellular approach:[1]

*Opposite the hollow at the root of the nail is placed a highly vascular and villous surface, which I call the ungual gland,*

*and the portion of the nail over this surface is thinner than the rest. Beyond this secreting surface appear a number of laminae, like the underpart of the mushroom, which are parallel with those placed in the inner part of the nail, and which pass in the direction of the axis of the finger. The parts of the nail usually cut project beyond these laminae.*

*The ungual gland is a very vascular surface, and its use is to secrete the nail, which proceeds from it between the laminae placed before it, so that the nail grows from its root, as may be easily seen by cutting a notch there, which grows gradually out in about three months, advancing until it reaches the extremity of the nail.*

The first investigator to consider nail structure in any detail after the acceptance of the cellular theories of Schwann was Rudolph Albert von Kölliker, of Würzburg, whose *Manual of Human Histology* (1852) ranks as one of the most important works in 19th-century medicine. The 15-page description of the nail complex, which appears in the first edition of Kölliker's manual, is rich in detail and reads very smoothly even now.[2]

The transfer of cellular anatomic concepts to the study of nail diseases was accomplished in the same era by Gustav Simon, of Berlin, whose *Hautkrankheiten Durch Anatomische Untersuchungen Erlaütert*, published in 1848, was the earliest textbook devoted entirely to dermatohistopathology.[3] Virchow's 1854 essay on the subject was also a contribution of considerable importance.[4]

Studies on nail growth rates were mentioned as early as 1684, in the work of the remarkable British investigator Robert Boyle, whose *Experiments and Considerations About the Porosity of Bodies* also marked the beginning of investigations into the transfer of substances across the natural barrier of the skin.[5] Actual data on nail growth appeared first in 1741 in Albrecht Haller's addition to Boerhave's *Predilectiones Academicae*. Haller estimated, from the movement of gold salt stains on nails, that transit from cuticle to free edge took place in 3 months.

Nail growth and its corollaries have long intrigued individuals in a broad spectrum of disciplines – for example, in the biological sciences, anthropology, and sociology. The subject also has been of interest to Asian princesses, Siamese actresses, Brazilian zither virtuosos, the compilers of the *Guinness Book of World Records*, and certainly Herr Otto Kellner, whose 25-year collection of his own nail clippings (Fig. 2.1) was considered impressive enough to be placed on display in the Royal Anatomical Museum in Berlin. However, in the more prosaic world of science, the measurement and study of nail growth were placed on a modern footing in 1850 by the assiduous and detailed research carried out by Arnold Berthold of Göttingen.[6]

In the early years of the 19th century, tissues belonging to the 'horny substance' class were regarded as among the simplest in the

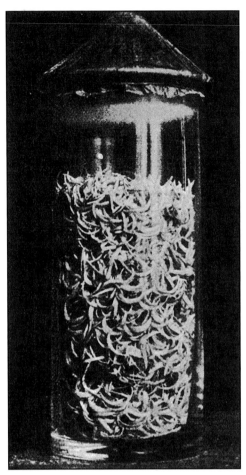

FIGURE 2–1. Herr Otto Kellner's personal nail clippings, collected over a 25-year period and placed on display in the Royal Anatomical Museum in Berlin. Total weight, 51.5 g.

Caroline Institute in Stockholm, whose enormous paper on sulfur–protein combinations (1902) is now considered a classic, noted the surprisingly high content of sulfur in hair, mostly in the form of cystine.[11] In 1907, Hans Buchtala of Graz used Mörner's techniques to demonstrate that such was also the case for nails.[12] It is one of history's many little quirks that cystine, the first of the amino acids to be discovered (in 1810) was the last to be identified in horny tissues;[13] extraction methods used throughout the 19th century unfortunately ensured denaturation of cystine before it could be detected. From this point on, the elucidation of the nature of nail protein merges with the study of molecular structure of keratin in general, our knowledge of which owes so much to experiments on wool fibers conducted in the 1930s by W.T. Astbury, H.J. Woods, and J.B. Speakman, all of whom worked at the University of Leeds in England.[14]

Paul Unna and L. Golodetz published the first detailed analysis of the fatty substances associated with the nail matrix in 1905,[15] although the presence of fat had been duly noted in the 1837 thesis of Matecki.

That disturbances in the nails can be secondary to larger problems in the organism is an ancient idea. Indeed, the earliest reference of any sort to nails in the medical literature is a one-liner included in the *Prognostics* of Hippocrates as one of the symptoms of empyema: 'The nails of the hand are bent', which is to say curved over the tips of the fingers. The association with clubbing to complete the picture of the 'Hippocratic fingers' was later described, from time to time, in a large number of pulmonary diseases.

The Parisian doctor Joseph Honoré Simon Beau described his famous transverse line in 1846 as a part of an in-depth study of nail growth in general.[16] His suspicions that the temporary interference in keratin formation represented by the lines could follow innumerable disturbances in the body economy have been confirmed many times over in the perpetual rediscovery of his sign, which, because it is so easily demonstrated, continues to interest clinicians to a degree beyond its practical worth.

The association of nail changes with specific skin diseases is a 19th-century phenomenon made possible by the successful separation of these clinical entities one from another by Robert Willan in England, and by his energetic disciples in France. Willan himself was the first to describe the nail changes in psoriasis. In his chef d'oeuvre *On Cutaneous Diseases* (1808) he set up a special category, Psoriasis unguium, to accommodate the condition:[17]

*The Psoriasis unguium sometimes occurs alone, but it is usually connected with scaly patches on the arms, hands, etc. In some cases, the nails from the middle appear brown or yellowish; they bend upwards and are ragged at the ends and rough on the surface. In other cases they are thickened, deeply indented, and bent downwards over the ends of the fingers.*

The association of nail dystrophy with eczematous eruptions is first described in the 1835 treatise of Pierre Rayer (Fig. 2.2). The clinical *verismo* that characterizes all of the work of this Parisian master is evident again in his account of the condition as it occurred in an 80-year-old man under his care:[18]

*For the last 12 years he has been subject to eczema, at one time in the squamous, at another in the humid state, between the buttocks and about the margin of the anus. Two years ago*

animal organism and considered merely as different forms of the same matrix, which, as C.G. Lehmann (one of the era's leading authorities on chemistry) said in 1854: 'certain chemists were ready enough to discover and to designate by the name Keratin'. 'The zealous labours of recent histologists,' he added, 'have, however, shown us that even these apparently homogeneous tissues have a complicated and, in many respects, a variable structure'.[7] He was referring, of course, to the work of Kölliker, Simon, and Virchow.

The first biochemical study of nails with any claim to modernity is to be found in the 1837 inaugural dissertation of Theodore Theophil Matecki of Breslau, *De ungue humano*.[8] Destined later to become one of Poland's most prominent citizens, in this early work Matecki outlined the results of distillation, alcohol extraction, and residual ash experiments, along with investigations into acid and base solubilities and the like; however, real progress along these lines was not possible until the publication in 1838 of the classic papers on the nature of protein by Gerardus Mulder,[9] an associate at the time of the renowned Julius Liebig of Giessen, who trained most of the important biochemists of the era. In 1840, Johann Joseph Scherer, another associate of Liebig, followed the lead of Mulder and calculated for the first time the C, H, N, O, and S percentages for nails, hair, horn, and feathers.[10] By the end of the 19th century, individual amino acid constituents of various proteins were routinely being reported, and K.A.H. Mörner of the

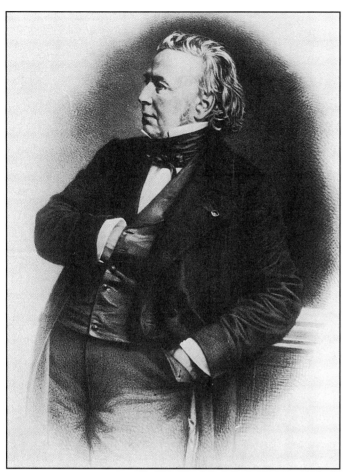

FIGURE 2-2. Pierre François Olive Rayer (1793-1867). Rayer was the leading authority on nail diseases (among many other things) in the early decades of the 19th century.

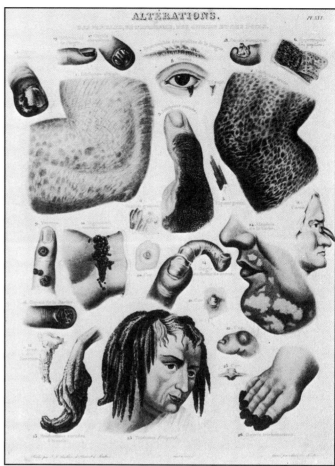

FIGURE 2-3. Plate XXI from Rayer's *Traité Théorique et Pratique des Maladies de la Peau* (1835) This treatise was the first in which nail diseases were considered in any detail. A number of nail problems were illustrated in Plate XXI for the very first time.

*an aggregation of the same kind made its appearance about the nails of the toes, and subsequently about those of the fingers. The nails of the toes are particularly remarkable for their deformity; they are of a greenish-yellow color, and are detached from their matrices, being raised upon a mass of solid matter of the same color, and of a faint and sickly smell, three or four lines in thickness, which even extends beyond their ends and edges. The nails are painful when cut, the action of the knife or scissors jarring the roots. A yellowish liquid matter occasionally exudes from under the lateral parts of the nails, which are then more than usually painful.*

The Rayer treatise is by far the best source of information on nails and nail diseases in the early part of the 19th century. It is in fact the first publication in which these structures were considered in any detail at all and also the first to feature illustrations of nail problems. Indeed, plate XXI (Fig. 2.3) in the atlas that accompanied the magnificent second edition of the treatise no doubt set some sort of record in the annals of medical illustration.[19] Onychomycosis, onychogryphosis, acute paronychia, traumatic onychia, subungual wart, and congenital deformities of the nail all make their initial appearance there in picture form, along with the first illustrations of verruca vulgaris, verruca filiformis, black hairy tongue, and alopecia of the beard. Nail changes associated with

eczema, psoriasis, tuberculosis, and syphilis are also illustrated, again for the first time, in other plates. Paul Gerson Unna regarded the Rayer treatise as one of the finest works ever written on skin diseases, and certainly we concur with his opinion.

Pityriasis rubra pilaris can also affect the nails. The original descriptions of the disease appear in the works of Rayer[20] and Alphonse Devergie,[21] but the disease was distinguished from psoriasis and lichen planus only after an incredible amount of clinical bickering in print. The matter was settled late in the 19th century when case presentations at various international dermatologic meetings demonstrated the disease to be a clinically distinct entity. The nail changes were first noted by Jonathan Hutchinson in 1878 in a review paper on nail problems that was much admired at the time:[22]

*Pityriasis rubra [pilaris] is a rare and very peculiar malady. We know nothing of its causes, and most of which we know of its course can be summed up in the following statements: In certain adult persons a state of persistent congestion of the whole integument with exfoliation of epidermis may occur, the patient becoming everywhere of vivid red colour, and the epidermis peeling off in large flakes. Where the skin is thick, as in the palms and soles, the epidermis may accumulate in layers like the leaves in a book, sometimes making up a thickness of half an inch, or even more. The disease is chronic, prone to relapse, and often attended by great debility. For our present purpose we are concerned with this malady only because in it there is usually much disease of the nails. The changes consist in opacity of the nail, with deposit of epidermis between it and its bed. When the skin disease subsides, the nails participate in the benefit. In these cases the nails are implicated as parts of the general integument, the whole skin being affected. It is, however, remarkable that they should suffer so severely. I have rarely seen nails so much thickened and deformed as in some of these cases.*

The earliest pictures of pityriasis rubra pilaris, including the nail changes (Fig. 2.4), were also prepared under the direction of Hutchinson for the New Sydenham Society Atlas (1860–1875).

We note in passing that Hutchinson was fascinated by nail diseases throughout his life, as he was by all disturbances in the integument and its accessory structures, and he was always on the lookout for new ways of looking at dermatologic problems. 'It is convenient,' he wrote, 'to think of a nail as a gigantic flattened hair, the walls of the follicle of which are flattened on one side.'[22] This idea helped explain to the clinicians of the time the simultaneous involvement of hair and nails in so many conditions and even now remains valid, if one takes into account the obvious difference that hair growth is cyclic, whereas nails grow continuously.

Lichen planus affects the nails in some 5 to 10% of cases, and yet the nail changes were not noticed until 1901, four decades after

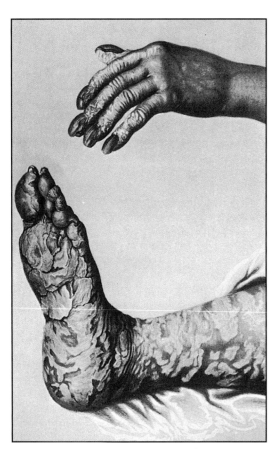

FIGURE 2–4. Pityriasis rubra pilaris. Section of a lithograph prepared under the direction of Jonathan Hutchinson for the New Sydenham Society Atlas (1860–1884).

Erasmus Wilson's original description of the disease itself. The association was made by the remarkable William Dubreuilh of Bordeaux, clinician extraordinaire and restless experimenter, who could also claim among his many accomplishments the first description of plantar warts. The heart of his 'lichen plan des ongles' report reads like this:[23]

*The nails are profoundly altered. They show very fine longitudinal striations. These striations are perfectly parallel and occupy the entire length of the nail; they are at least a third of a millimeter in width, are deep and contiguous, and at some points are clearly formed by longitudinal splitting in narrow elevated grooves. The nail appears uneven, as though roughened by a rasp or coarse grit. In short, the appearance corresponds exactly to the changes I have previously described under the name onychorrhexis. The general shape of the nails is preserved; they do not appear to be reduced in thickness, but according to the patient, they are fragile and often break; they are adherent to the bed, which is normal, and the external surface alone is altered. However, both little fingers show a cornified pad under the free edge of the nail, brownish in color, and attributable to hyperkeratosis of the bed.*

Syphilis of the nails received a great deal of attention in the dermatologic and venereologic literature of the 18th and 19th centuries. The first description of any length is to be found in John Hunter's *Treatise on Venereal Diseases* (1786), the same great compendium in which the hunterian chancre description appears, along with the account of the author's celebrated and unlucky self-inoculation experiment. Hunter described the nail changes as follows:[24]

*The disease on its first appearance often attacks that part of the fingers upon which the nail is formed, making that surface red which is seen shining through the nail, and if allowed to continue, a separation of the nail takes place, similar to the cuticle in the before described symptoms; but here there cannot be that regular succession of nails as there is of cuticle.*

That simple account gave way to more and more elaborate descriptions as the disease became the subject of intense investigation in the middle and later decades of the 19th century. By 1879, for example, the handsome and eminently successful New York venereologist Freeman J. Bumstead, America's first authentic genitourinary expert, was able in his textbook to spin out several thousand words on the subject.[25] It had become clear by this time that nail involvement was more likely to be associated with relapsing or late syphilis than with the early stages, as well as with the congenital form of the disease. Until the 20th century, syphilis of the nails was often called onychia maligna. The name, which finally succumbed to its obvious disadvantages, was coined by James Wardrop of London in a famous and much-quoted review of the diseases of fingers and toes published in 1814.[26] It is a measure of the distance we have come that today's busy dermatologists or even venereologists might spend a lifetime without ever seeing such a case.

The earliest references to diseases originating in the nail complex itself are also ancient. Celsus (53 BCE to CE 7) considered both acute paronychia and the swollen flap of skin, with or without granulation tissue, that often extends over the nail plate in these cases.[27] He recommended surgical intervention when conservative methods failed. No doubt his clinical material included ingrown toenails, although he did not mention that condition specifically. Paulus Aeginita, a 7th-century Greek physician, dealt with similar problems.[28] He also made recommendations for the treatment of subungual hemorrhages and furnished several prescriptions containing sulfur, arsenic, and cantharides for the removal of diseased nails, especially those that were 'leprous', whatever that might have meant.

Chiropodists would have us believe that Lewis Durlacher of London was the first to delineate accurately the lowly ingrown toenail and the troubles that surround it.[29] Durlacher, who was by far the best-known practitioner of his profession in England in the middle decades of the 19th century, was the first to emphasize, or perhaps even to mention, that incorrect cutting of the nail was usually the cause of the problem; however, in every other aspect of precedence, he was far down on the list. Paulus Aeginita gave an easily recognizable description of the condition,[28] as did most of the ancients. Indeed, along with paronychia, the ubiquitous ingrown toenail must have been a common cause of limping about in the caves of the Cro-Magnons and Neanderthals, contributing in a small way to the natural surliness of the species.

In 1726, Daniel Turner described ingrown nails in his remarkable treatise on skin diseases[30] but it was not until the beginning of the 19th century that the condition was considered in any detail. Diseases sometimes become fashionable subjects for medical writing for mysterious reasons that have little to do with new discoveries or with perceived alterations in the course or demography of the conditions, and such would appear to be the case with unguis incarnatus at that time. Baron Dupuytren, then the leading surgeon, supplied the most influential of the many accounts available. He managed the condition as follows:[31]

*I pass one blade of a pair of straight, strong, sharp scissors rapidly under the middle of the nail almost to its base, and divide it at a single stroke into two nearly equal halves. With a pair of pliers I then grasp the half that lies over the ulceration and pull it off by turning it back upon itself. If the other side is also diseased, I remove it in the same way. In those cases in which the fungoid tissue adjacent to the wound is considerably elevated I apply the hot cautery to destroy it and to ensure, in so far as possible, a cure for the disease.*

Dupuytren claimed that the procedure was not particularly painful but Pierre Prosper Baumès, the notable dermatologist from Lyons, was more honest about it when he admitted that even the most stoic of his patients 'suffered horribly' and cried out in agony when the operation began.[32] It is of course possible that in those days before the advent of anesthesia, the pain of so trivial an operation failed to impress a general surgeon like the Baron, who had to inflict great suffering every working day of his life.

The original description of subungual malignant melanoma is attributed to Dubourg, who called the lesion 'melanic subungual cancer' and described it as a large, black, spherical tumor more than 4 inches in diameter, with a knobby surface, growing steadily for 3 years at the site of a preexisting thin, black line beneath the nail. The line had persisted unchanged for 27 years.[33] The tumor 'creaked' when cut across with the knife, a sign considered indicative of cancer at the time. Melanotic whitlow was redescribed, and named, by Jonathan Hutchinson in 1857.[34] Three decades and half

a dozen disastrous cases later, in 1886 he warned his colleagues that these lesions were extraordinarily dangerous, always malignant, and in need of prompt, effective intervention.[35]

Descriptions of mycotic infections of the nail, identifiable as such, appear first in the 1829 treatise on scalp ringworm by the Parisian empiric Mahon the younger.[36] Mahon was the most prominent member of a family that contracted to take care of favus and allied scalp conditions at l'Hôpital St Louis in Paris in the early and middle decades of the 19th century. The family, no member of which was a physician, used 'secret' remedies in their scalp treatment station, mostly depilatories consisting of sulfur and sodium carbonate. In his treatise, Mahon extolled the virtues of his secret pomades and advertised his skills in an unconscionable manner. Despite its commercial approach, the book contained much of value – for example, the earliest description of 'gray patch', or microsporum tinea capitis, which was new to Europe at the time. Mahon also used his treatise as a forum from which to attack some of the dangerous and brutal methods then used for the treatment of favus, and his efforts led to much-needed therapeutic reforms. In this remarkable work the first description of favus of the nails appears:[36]

*The nails of the toes and fingers showed to the highest degree those changes attributable to the favic influence; they were very thick and split into layers at the tips, as it were, reminding the observer of the statue of Daphne changing into the laurel tree, in which the transformation of human into ligneous material is depicted–although there is, to be sure, a considerable distance between the graceful aspect of that artistic production and the appearance of this unfortunate individual who was reduced to that deplorable state which some would leave to nature alone to cure.*

*The alterations in the nails caused by favus would appear to result from a disturbance and an increase in the corneous secretion of which they are composed, because they increase in thickness and grow outward to an unusual degree. The regularity and polish of the normal state gives way to a longitudinal rugosity; they become frayed at the ends; they do not fall off, but become more sensitive than normal; they take on the yellow color characteristic of favus.*

The metaphor was labored – Daphne changed into a laurel tree to escape from the amorous advances of Apollo – but the clinical description, the first of onychomycosis, was perfectly satisfactory. In a later section, Mahon noted similar nail changes in a case of gray patch ringworm but observed that the yellow color was lacking.

Credit for the discovery of the dermatophyte itself in nail substance belongs to George Meissner (the discoverer of the corpuscles that go by his name), who in 1853 observed hyphae in a potassium hydroxide preparation of a 'thick finger nail, bent claw-like', taken from an 80-year-old man.[37] The term 'onychomycosis' appears to have been coined by Virchow 3 years later in 1856.[38]

*Candida albicans* infection of nails was first reported by Dübendorfer in 1904.[39]

Finally, for those who wish to pursue the subject further, we offer a helpful suggestion. As Rayer was the most knowledgeable authority on nails in the early decades of the 19th century, so Julius Heller (1864–1931) of Berlin was the Herr Nägel – the 'Mr Nails' – at the beginning of the 20th century. His *Krankheiten der Nägel*[40] (Fig. 2.5), a 300-page *Meisterstück*, appeared in print in 1900.

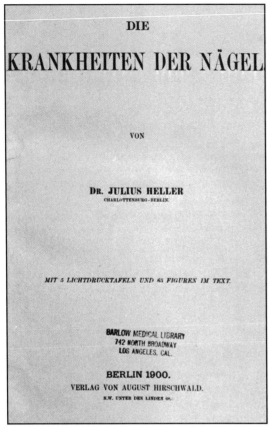

DIE

KRANKHEITEN DER NÄGEL

VON

Dr. JULIUS HELLER
CHARLOTTENBURG-BERLIN.

MIT 5 LICHTDRUCKTAFELN UND 65 FIGUREN IM TEXT.

BARLOW MEDICAL LIBRARY
742 NORTH BROADWAY
LOS ANGELES, CAL.

BERLIN 1900.
VERLAG VON AUGUST HIRSCHWALD.
N.W. UNTER DEN LINDEN 68.

FIGURE 2-5. Title page of Heller's *Krankheiten der Nägel* (Diseases of the nails), which was published in 1900. Julius Heller (1864-1931) was the 'Mr Nails' of the medical world in the early decades of the 20th century. The exhaustive treatment of the subject in his treatise far exceeded anything that had gone before.

Thoroughly Teutonic in its treatment, organization, and detail, this work contains many original observations and references to almost everything worth knowing about nails in the literature of the time. Heller's lifelong preoccupation with nails culminated in an exhaustive essay on the subject in the Jadassohn *Handbuch* of 1927. Serious reviews of the older literature should begin with these two works.

# REFERENCES

1. Cooper A. Diseases of the nails. Lond Med Phys J 1827; 57:289
2. Kölliker RA. Manual of human histology. London: Sydenham Society; 1853:153–168
3. Simon G. Hautkrankheiten durch anatomische Untersuchungen erläutert. Berlin: G. Reimer; 1848:366–375
4. Virchow R. Zur normalen und pathologischen Anatomie der Nägel. Verhandl Med Phys Gesellschft Würzburg 1854; 5(B):83
5. Boyle R. Experiments and considerations about the porosity of bodies. London: Samuel Smith; 1684
6. Berthold A. Beobactungen über das quantative Verhältniss der Nägel-und Haarbildung beim Menschen. Müller's Arch 1850
7. Lehmann CG. Physiological chemistry. London: Cavendish Society; 1854:53
8. Matecki TT. De ungue humano. Inaugural dissertation, Wratislaviae; 1837
9. Mulder GJ. Guzammensetzung von Fibrin, Albumin, Leimzucker, Leucin, usw. Ann Pharm 1838; 28:73
10. Scherer JJ. Animal chemistry of organic chemistry. London: Taylor and Walton; 1842
11. Mörner KAH. Zur Kentniss der Bindung des Schwefels in den Proteinstoffen. Hoppe-Seyler's Z Physiol Chem 1902; 34:207
12. Buchtala H. Ueber das Mengenverhältnis des Cystins in Hornsubstanzen. Hoppe-Seyler's Z Physiol Chem 1907; 52:474
13. Vickery HB, Schmidt CL. History of the discovery of the amino acids. Chem Rev 1931; 9:169
14. Fraser RDB, Gillespie JM. Wool structure and biosynthesis. Nature 1976; 261:650
15. Unna PG, Golodetz L. Die Hautfette. Biochem Z 1909; 20:469
16. Beau JHS. Note sur certains charactères de séméologie rétrospective présentés par les ongles. Arch Gen Méd 1846; 11:447
17. Willan R. On cutaneous diseases, vol. VI. London: J Johnson; 1808:169
18. Rayer P. Theoretical and practical treatise on the diseases of the skin. Philadelphia: Carey and Hart; 1845:383
19. Rayer P. Traité des maladies de la peau, atlas. Paris: JB Baillière; Paris, 1835
20. Rayer P. Traité des maladies de la peau, vol. 2. Paris: JB Baillière; 1835:158
21. Devergie A. Pityriasis pilaris. Traité pratique des maladies de la peau, 2nd edn. Paris: Libraire de Victor Masson; 1857:454–455
22. Hutchinson J. On the nails and the diseases to which they are liable. Medical Times Gazette 1878; April 20:423–426
23. Dubreuilh W. Lichen plan des ongles. Ann Dermatol Syphilig 1901; 2:606
24. Hunter J. Treatise on the venereal disease. 13 Castle Street, London; 1786:321
25. Bumstead FJ, Taylor RW. Pathology and treatment of venereal diseases, 4th edn. Philadelphia: Henry C Lea; 1879:578–582
26. Wardrop J. An account of some diseases of the toes and fingers, with observations on their treatment. Med Clin Trans 1814; 5:129
27. Celsus. Of medicine, in eight books [lib VI, chap XIX]. London: H Renshaw; 1838:335–336
28. Paulus Aeginita. The seven books of Paulus Aeginita, vol. 6 (679–683), vol. 2 (414–416). London: Sydenham Society; 1844
29. Dagnall JC. Durlacher and 'the nail growing into the flesh'. Br Chirop J 1962; 27:263
30. Turner D. De Morbis Cutaneis, 3rd edn. London: R and J Bonwicke; 1726:267–273
31. Dupuytren G. Leçons Orales de Clinique Chirurgicale de Dupuytren, vol. 4. Paris; 1834:392
32. Baumès PP. Nouvelle dermatologie, vol 2. Paris: JB Baillière; 1842:381–387
33. Dubourg NI. Cancer mélané du petit doigt de la main droite. J Hébdom Méd 1830; 7:73
34. Hutchinson J. Melanotic whitlow. Trans Pathol Soc 1857; 8:404
35. Hutchinson J. Melanosis often not black; melanotic whitlow. Br Med J 1886; 1:491
36. Mahon M Jr. Recherches sur la siège et la nature des teignes. Paris: JB Baillière; 1829:59–61, 139
37. Meissner G. Pilzbildung in den Nägeln. Arch Phys Heilkünde 1853; 12:193
38. Virchow R. Beitrage zur Lehre von den beim Menschen vorkommenden pflan zlichen Parasiten. Virchows Arch 1856; 9:557
39. Dübendorfer E. Ein Fall von Onchomycosis blasomycetica. Dermatol Zentralbl 1904; 7:290
40. Heller J. Krankheiten der Nägel. Berlin: August Hirschwald; 1900

# 3

# Structure and Function of the Nail Unit

## Philip Fleckman

## Key Features

1. The nail unit consists of the proximal and lateral nail folds, nail matrix, nail bed, and hyponychium. These structures form what is commonly called the nail

2. The nail unit develops between the 10th and 17th week in utero by a complex series of mesenchymal–ectodermal interactions

3. The cuticle seals the proximal nail fold to the dorsal surface of the nail plate. Disruption of this seal results in production of a real space from the potential space between the ventral surface of the proximal nail fold and the dorsal surface of the nail plate, and may result in chronic paronychia

4. Active melanocytes are more numerous in distal than in proximal matrix; most pigmented bands originate from this area

5. Splinter hemorrhages form when blood from vessels in the nail bed or hyponychium extravasates into the unique, longitudinal, tongue-in-groove spatial arrangement of papillary dermal papillae and epidermal rete ridges of the nail bed

6. The hyponychium seals the area where the nail plate lifts off the nail bed. The hyponychium is usually the initial site of injury in onycholysis and the site of invasion by dermatophytes in distal subungual onychomycosis

7. The distal phalanx lies immediately below the structures of the nail unit. Pressure from tumors lying in the nail unit may erode the bone; likewise, bony tumors of the distal phalanx often manifest as nail abnormalities. Even simple surgical procedures in the nail unit, such as punch biopsy, extend to the periosteum; therefore careful attention to sterile technique is indicated

8. Fingernails grow an average of 0.1-0.15 mm/day (3 mm/month). A normal fingernail therefore grows out completely in about 6 months. Toenails grow at half to one-third the rate of fingernails and take 12 to 18 months to grow out

9. The nail plate is formed almost exclusively by the nail matrix. The proximal matrix makes the dorsal nail plate and the distal matrix makes the ventral portion of the nail plate. The nail bed contributes a few cells to the undersurface of the nail plate

10. A combination of the small contribution of cells by the nail bed to the undersurface of the plate and the interdigitating, tongue-in-groove spatial arrangement of the nail bed rete and dermal papillae probably hold the plate to the bed

1. How does the nail unit form and what controls this process? What does this tell us about congenital nail disorders and regeneration of the nail unit?

2. What is the basic anatomy of the nail unit and how does this apply to disorders of the nail and to surgical procedures involving the nail unit?

3. What seals the proximal nail fold to the nail plate, and how is this affected by pathologic processes that produce chronic paronychia?

4. What is the source of pigment in the nail unit? How can this information be used to understand and treat leukonychia and abnormalities of nail pigmentation?

5. What explains the optical properties of the nail? Why is the lunula white?

6. What holds the nail down and how is this affected by pathologic processes that produce onycholysis?

7. What makes the nail plate? How does this affect one's ability to diagnose and treat nail disorders?

8. What factors control the rate of nail growth? Can these factors explain pathologic processes such as the decreased rate of growth in the yellow nail syndrome and increased rate of growth in psoriasis?

9. What holds the nail together? Why is the nail hard? What causes brittle, thin, or split nails?

10. What controls the penetration of substances into the nail? How can effective topical therapies be designed for treatment of nail bed and nail matrix diseases?

## EMBRYOLOGY AND DEVELOPMENT

The embryology of the nail unit was investigated as early as the late nineteenth century (reviewed in refs 5 and 6). Lewis,[5] Zaias,[6] Hashimoto and colleagues,[7] and Holbrook[8] have studied the embryology of the human nail. Their work has been reviewed recently.[9,10]

Fingers are first recognized in the sixth week in utero, toes the following week. By the eighth week, digits are separated, but the earliest visible external changes defining the nail unit are appreciated only in the 10th week. A smooth, shiny, quadrangular surface – the primary nail field – is at this time delineated on the dorsum of the distal digit by shallow grooves. The distal groove, the most distal of these shallow grooves, delineates the distal edge of the primary nail field. By the 11th week, well-formed fingers with joints are seen. At the tip of the finger in the distal part of the primary nail field just proximal to the distal groove, the distal ridge appears as an area of thickened epidermis. This distal ridge is the first area in the embryo to become keratinized (develop a granular layer and an orthokeratotic stratum corneum). The distal ridge

Published interest in the nails began in the nineteenth century[1–3] (see also Chapter 2). This chapter reviews the embryology and development, anatomy and cell biology, physiology, biochemistry, biophysics, and pharmacology of the nail unit. Where appropriate, clinical correlations with basic science are discussed. The term 'nail unit', defined by Zaias as the four structures that together form what is commonly called the nail[4] will be used throughout this review. The terms 'nail plate' and 'nail' will be used interchangeably.

In a book devoted to the diagnosis and treatment of nail disorders, it is appropriate to focus what is known about the basic science of nails by asking the following questions:

becomes the hyponychium, the area first invaded by dermatophytes in distal subungual onychomycosis.[11] At the same time, an area in the proximal primary nail field – the matrix primordium – grows into the substance of the distal phalanx. The matrix primordium grows proximally and ventrally, isolating a wedge of dermis dorsally that becomes the proximal nail fold. Beginning at its distal end and proceeding proximally, the matrix primordium differentiates into the matrix. By the 14th week, a recognizable nail plate can be seen emerging from beneath the proximal nail fold. The entire nail bed is covered by a stratum corneum. By the 16th week, the nail plate covers half the nail bed. The plate initially forms via keratohyalin granules. Only later, after the nail plate has grown over the matrix, does the nail plate form via the process seen in the adult. By the 17th week, the nail plate covers almost the entire nail bed. From this time on, changes in the nail unit are mainly those of growth. As the nail plate grows over the distal ridge the distal ridge progressively flattens, forming the hyponychium.

Nail unit development is integrally tied to limb bud development. Both involve communication between mesenchymal and ectodermal structures by way of signaling molecules, transcriptional regulators, and growth factors.[12] Nail unit development is integrally tied to dorsal–ventral determination, controlled by at least three factors: Wnt-7a (a secreted glycoprotein), en-1 (a homeobox-containing transcription factor), and lmx1-b (another transcription factor).[13] Mutations in lmx-1b underlie the nail–patella syndrome.[14]

# ANATOMY AND CELL BIOLOGY

The topography of the nail unit was described by Zaias (Fig. 3.1).[6] The nail unit consists of the proximal nail fold, the matrix, the nail bed, and the hyponychium (Figs 3.1 to 3.4). These structures together form the nail plate – the flat, rectangular, convex, translucent, hard structure sitting on top of the digits and extending past their free edge.

The nail plate consists of close-packed, adherent, interdigitating cells that lack nuclei or organelles. Cells in the plate are very flat, lying with the smallest diameter perpendicular to the plane of the

nail plate surface. There is a progression from the top (dorsal surface) of the plate, where cell borders are straight, to the middle of the plate, where cell borders are much more 'meandering'.[15] Many intercellular links are present, including tight, intermediate, and desmosomal junctions.[16] The cells at the surface of the nail plate overlap, slanting from 'proximal–dorsal to distal–volar'.[17] Scanning electron microscopy reveals that the dorsal surface of the nail plate is smooth but the palmar surface is irregular.[18] The nail plate is approximately 0.5 mm thick in women and 0.6 mm thick in men.[19] In normal nails, distal plate thickness can be ranked thumb > index > middle > ring > little finger.[20] Based on autoradiographic data, the length of the matrix determines the thickness of the nail plate.[4] The progressive increase in nail plate thickness with age may be due to the decreased growth rate and the increasing size of the cells in the plate.[19] This view is supported by cytologic study

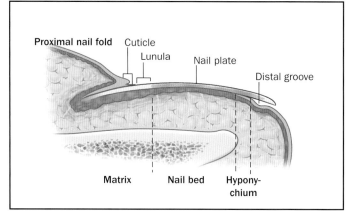

FIGURE 3–2. Diagram of a sagittal section through the nail unit. The nail unit consists of the proximal nail fold, the matrix, the nail bed, and the hyponychium. Together, these structures form and support the nail plate (from Zaias N. The embryology of the human nail. Arch Dermatol 1963; 87:39. Copyright 1963, American Medical Association, with permission of the author and publisher).

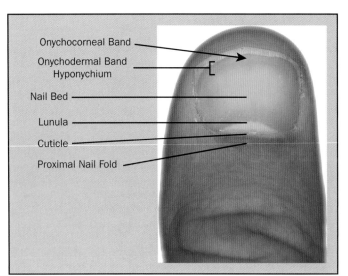

FIGURE 3–1. The topography of the nail unit. The surface landmarks of the nail unit, viewed from the top.

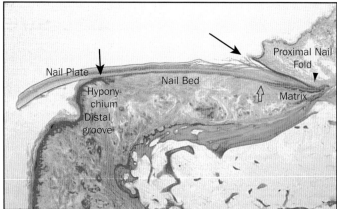

FIGURE 3–3. Photomicrograph of a sagittal section through the nail unit (newborn). In this nail unit no lunula would be seen, as the junction of the matrix and nail bed (open arrow) is beneath the proximal nail fold. Note the cuticle (large arrow) growing out on the nail plate from the distal tip and undersurface (roof) of the proximal nail fold. Arrowhead indicates the transition in the roof (ventral surface) of the proximal nail fold from normal epithelium to nail matrix, with loss of keratohyalin granules. Note how thin the epithelium of the nail bed is compared with that of the matrix. Neither epithelium contains keratohyalin granules. The junction of the nail bed and the hyponychium is marked by the small arrow. Note the abrupt appearance of keratohyalin granules and a normal, keratinized (orthokeratotic) stratum corneum (figure courtesy of Dr Karen A. Holbrook).

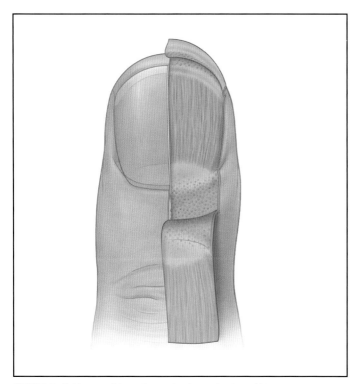

FIGURE 3–4. Diagram of the nail unit with the proximal nail fold, matrix, nail bed, and hyponychium reflected. The epidermis of the proximal nail fold, matrix, and nail bed is reflected back, and the epidermis of the hyponychium is reflected forward to expose the underlying dermal papillae. Note the parallel, tongue-in-groove spatial arrangement of the epidermal rete and dermal papillae of the nail bed, compared with the conventional rete of the papillary dermis seen in the matrix and hyponychium (from Zaias N, Ackerman AB. The nail in Darier–White disease. Arch Dermatol 1973; 107:193. Copyright 1973, American Medical Association, with permission of the author and editor).

If the nail plate were removed, three potential spaces would become apparent, the proximal nail groove (see Figs 3.2 and 3.3) and the two lateral nail grooves. Folds of skin – the proximal and lateral nail folds – overlap the nail plate to form these grooves. The proximal nail fold (PNF) (see Figs 3.1 to 3.4) is an invaginating, wedge-shaped fold of skin on the dorsum of the distal digit. The nail plate arises from under this fold. The dorsum of the PNF consists of a continuation of the epidermis and dermis of the dorsal digit with sweat glands but no follicles or sebaceous glands. At the distal tip of the PNF, the skin reflects proximally and ventrally, traveling about 5–8 mm toward the distal interphalangeal joint. The skin of the ventral surface of the PNF is quite thin, has no appendages, and is closely applied to the dorsal surface of the nail plate. The epithelium of the ventral surface of the PNF has also been called the eponychium.[27] The stratum corneum of the tip and the ventral surface of the PNF grows out a short way on the dorsal surface of the nail plate as the cuticle (see Figs 3.1 to 3.3) before being shed. The cuticle seals the proximal nail fold to the dorsal surface of the nail plate. Disruption of this seal results in production of a real space from the potential space between the ventral surface of the proximal nail fold and the dorsal surface of the nail plate and may result in chronic paronychia.

The ventral surface of the PNF forms the roof of the proximal nail groove; the nail matrix (see Figs 3.2 to 3.4) forms its floor; the nail plate lies between the two. In fact, the matrix begins just before the roof of the proximal nail groove makes its distal bend towards the tip of the digit. The matrix is a thick epithelium and has no granular layer. Because of the abrupt loss of the granular layer, the transition from the ventral surface of the PNF to matrix is easily appreciated (see Fig. 3.3). Nail matrix cells have been cultured and shown to express both epithelial ('soft') and 'hard' keratins (see p. 24).[28,29] The basal surface of the matrix cells interdigitates in fingerlike projections.[23] Despite this interdigitation, one can undermine and move the matrix surgically with ease.

The matrix of Caucasians contains sparse, poorly developed melanocytes.[30] Active (dopa-positive) melanocytes are more numerous in distal than in proximal matrix; the cells are located both in the basal layer and suprabasally, as single cells and in small clusters of three to four cells.[31] In contrast, dormant melanocytes recognized by other markers are more numerous in the proximal matrix.[32] The distal matrix of people of color is thought to contain more active melanocytes than are seen in Caucasians; this is in contrast to interfollicular skin, where pigment formation is increased, but the number of melanocytes is the same. For example, the distal matrix of Japanese people contains several hundred well-developed, active melanocytes per square millimeter.[33] As with Caucasians, the number of active melanocytes (and the intensity of the dopa reaction in those melanocytes) is much greater in distal than in proximal (Japanese) matrix. Investigators have speculated that the proximal–distal difference is because those melanocytes in the proximal matrix are protected by the PNF from stimulation by ultraviolet light and other exogenous agents.[33] The location of active melanocytes in the matrix is directly related to the location of pigmented bands, most of which originate in the distal matrix and do not involve the proximal matrix.[33] Langerhans cells have also been identified in matrix,[30] and Merkel's cells have been found in the matrix and nail bed epithelium.[34,35]

When the matrix extends beyond the edge of the PNF, it is seen as the lunula (see Figs 3.1 to 3.4). The lunula is the white, half moon-shaped area seen on some, but not all nails. The shape of the lunula determines the shape of the nail plate.[36] Several

of the cells of the dorsal nail plate, which shows that the area of the cells correlates with growth rate, increasing with decreasing growth rate and with the age of the subject.[21]

The nail plate is formed by a progressive broadening and flattening of cells in the matrix as they mature to form nail plate, with fragmentation and lysis of nuclei and retention of nuclear membranes in nail plate cells.[5,6] There is an increase in intermediate (tono)filaments, with clumping, lateral accretion, and the eventual formation of the keratin pattern (a morphologic pattern seen with the electron microscope in stratum corneum)[22] as basal cells differentiate and rise to form the nail plate. Lamellar granules are observed extruding contents into the extracellular space, and marginal band formation is seen. With the exception of second-trimester embryonic nail formation, the matrix keratinocytes form nail plate by a process in which no keratohyalin granules are produced. This process is similar to formation of hair, although trichohyalin granules are seen in that appendage. Although both profilaggrin and trichohyalin are found in the nail unit, neither keratohyalin granules nor trichohyalin granules are seen in the nail matrix or nail bed (see Fig. 3.3).[23,24] Because of the analogy to hair, this process is known as onycholemmal keratinization.[25] Frequent gap junctions are observed near the area where lamellar granules are discharging their contents, and it has been suggested that a substance with the size of lanthanum complex might be able to pass through the nail plate through such intercellular channels. Perhaps such channels explain why the nail plate is more permeable to polar solvents than is skin.[26]

hypotheses have been proposed to explain why the lunula is white. Burrows suggested that the matrix was not firmly adherent to the underlying connective tissue, became separated, and produced a reflecting surface that appeared white.[37] Lewin[38] stated that the flat, shiny surface (in contrast to the rougher, distal part of the nail), the opacity of the proximal nail plate, the relative avascularity of the subepidermal layer, and the loose texture of the dermal collagen contributed to the color of the lunula. Zaias commented that the nail plate is thinner over the lunula than over the nail bed and that the area of the lunula corresponds with that of the keratogenous zone, the zone of cytoplasmic condensation in the matrix just before cells form the nail plate.[4] Samman pointed out that the lunula remains apparent in both the nail plate and the underlying nail bed after nail avulsion and stated that the color is likely due to a combination of incomplete keratinization in the nail plate and loose connective tissue in the underlying dermis.[39] This hypothesis is supported by high-resolution MRI, which reveals a well-defined area beneath the nail matrix that histologically is composed of loose connective tissue.[40] The area is supplied by large regular meshes of vascular networks.[41] Zaias suggested that the color is the same as that seen in leukonychia, in which nucleated cells are often found in the nail plate.[42]

The nail bed begins where the lunula or distal matrix ends (see Figs 3.1 to 3.4). Like the lunula, the nail bed has no granular layer, but unlike the lunula, the nail bed is an extremely thin epithelium. Thus, the end of the matrix and beginning of the nail bed is easily appreciated histologically (Figs 3.2 and 3.3). The nail bed has a unique, longitudinal, tongue-in-groove spatial arrangement of papillary dermal papillae and epidermal rete ridges (see Fig. 3.4). In transverse section, this arrangement is appreciated as a serrated interdigitation of papillae and rete (Fig. 3.5). When spirally coiled vessels in the hyponychium rupture,[43] the blood extravasates into these longitudinal grooves to form splinter hemorrhages. If one avulses the plate and studies the undersurface by scanning electron microscopy, one sees grooves.[44] Rand and Baden speculated that the nail plate adheres to the nail bed by way of these grooves.[45] It is unclear whether the ridges seen belong to the nail bed epithelium that remains attached to the nail plate after avulsion[46,47] or are actually etched into the undersurface of the plate, although they are not seen at the free edge of the plate and avulsed epidermis was not removed from the undersurface of the nail plate before it was studied by scanning electron microscopy (Montagna W, personal communication, 10 June 1988). A combination of the deep interdigitation of the nail bed epithelium with underlying papillary dermis and the thin epithelium of the nail bed probably makes moving the nail bed difficult surgically.

The nail bed ends beneath the nail plate at the beginning of the hyponychium (see Figs 3.2 to 3.4). The hyponychium marks the beginning of normal volar epidermis. As with the dorsal skin of the PNF, a granular layer and eccrine glands begin to appear, and this epithelium undergoes normal keratinization. The hyponychium is the first site of keratinization in the nail unit[5,6] and of all epidermis in the embryo.[8] The hyponychium is said to make waterproof the area where the nail plate lifts off the nail bed.[17] The hyponychium is the initial site of invasion by dermatophytes in the most common type of onychomycosis, distal subungual onychomycosis.[11]

Beneath the distal nail plate, just proximal to the white line that marks the separation of the nail plate from the hyponychium, lies the onychodermal band[48] (see Fig. 3.1). This narrow band, normally from 0.5 to 1.5 mm wide, was described by Terry as paler than the pink nail bed, with a slightly amber tinge and a trans-

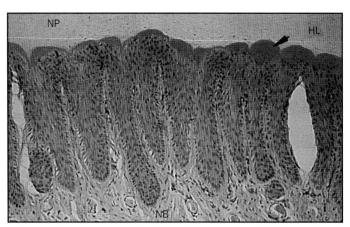

FIGURE 3–5. Photomicrograph of a coronal (transverse) section through the midline of the nail bed. Note the serrated, interdigitating nail bed epidermal rete ridges (arrow down) and dermal papillae (arrows up). NP, nail plate; HL, horny layer of the nail plate. Hematoxylin and eosin, X 450 (from Zaias N. Psoriasis of the nail. Arch Dermatol 1969, 99:569. Copyright 1969, American Medical Association, with permission of the author and editor).

lucent quality. However, Stewart and Raffle commented that 'many normal onychodermal bands are actually a *deeper* (their emphasis) pink' than the adjacent distal nail bed;[49] I agree. The band may be pigmented in black skin. Terry speculated that this area had a blood supply different from the remainder of the nail bed; this is supported by the work of Martin and Platts.[43] The area of the onychodermal band can become prominent in chronic renal failure, cirrhosis, and other chronic disease.[48,50–52] Sonnex and coworkers[53] described the onychocorneal band, which they pointed out was originally described by Pinkus[1] (see Fig. 3.1). This is a thin, transverse, white line, 0.1–1 mm wide, which transects the accentuated pink band at the distal edge of the nail bed that is the onychodermal band. The authors described this as the point of attachment of the epidermis of the skin of the fingertip to the undersurface of the nail plate and proposed that the area was necessary for 'maintaining the integrity of nail attachment'. They stated that this was the site of resistance to a probe passed proximally from beneath the undersurface of the free edge of the nail plate, although Terry stated that the site of resistance was at the proximal edge of the onychodermal band. How can all this be interpreted? The onychodermal band and the onychocorneal band are easily observed when one extends the finger. The point of attachment of the undersurface of the nail plate to the volar epidermis of the fingertip is obviously vital in sealing the nail plate to the nail bed and preventing onycholysis. If the observations of Sonnex and colleagues withstand the scrutiny of others, the onychocorneal band marks this site.

The most distal boundary of the nail unit is marked by the distal groove (see Figs 3.2 to 3.4). This indentation of the volar epidermal skin marks the distal site of demarcation of the primary nail field, the earliest external change in the embryonic development of the nail.[6]

The basement membrane zone of the nail unit resembles that of interfollicular epidermis and expresses target antigens in an identical manner.[54]

The distal phalanx lies immediately below the structures of the nail unit. An extensor tendon runs over the ventral surface of the distal interphalangeal joint and attaches to the distal phalanx, proximal to the reflection of the proximal nail groove. Lateral

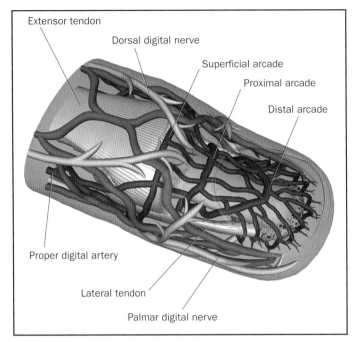

Extensor tendon
Dorsal digital nerve
Superficial arcade
Proximal arcade
Distal arcade
Proper digital artery
Lateral tendon
Palmar digital nerve

**FIGURE 3–6.** Diagram of the arterial and venous blood supply and tendons of the nail unit.

ligaments extend from the ungual processes of the distal phalanx to the base of the distal phalanx (Fig. 3.6). The importance of the phalanx in normal development of the nail unit has been emphasized by Kelikian and others.[55,56] Because the dermis is quite thin and there is no subcutis in this area, pressure from tumors lying in the nail unit may erode the bone; likewise, bony tumors of the distal phalanx often manifest as nail abnormalities. Even simple surgical procedures in the nail unit, such as punch biopsy, extend to the periosteum; therefore careful attention to sterile technique is indicated.

## BLOOD AND NERVE SUPPLY OF THE NAIL UNIT

The blood supply of the nail unit derives from the lateral digital arteries[57–59] (see Fig. 3.6). These arteries give off medium-sized branches that cross over the dorsal surface of the distal interphalangeal joint to supply a superficial arcade, which supplies the PNF and matrix. The lateral digital arteries then enter the distal digit adjacent to the volar surface of the bone and give off branches to the bone and the superficial arcade.[5,59] The digital arteries then course dorsally around the 'waist' of the distal phalanx in the confined space between the bone and the lateral ligament and perforate the septum of the pulp space. Here they divide to form proximal and distal arcades, which supply the matrix and nail bed. Thus, the matrix has two sources of blood supply, the superficial and the proximal arcades.[57,59] This is beneficial when disease (e.g., scleroderma) affects the vessels in the pulp.

The digital arterial system manifests two characteristic anatomic features, arched anastomotic arteries in the deep dermis and more superficial terminal arteries that branch to supply the rete.[58] The arteries possess inner longitudinal and outer circular

coats of smooth muscle, but no internal elastic lamina. The vasculature of the nail bed is unique in that it must supply a vascular structure between two hard surfaces, the nail plate and the bone. Venous drainage follows arterial vasculature but combines proximally, forming two veins, one on each side of the plate in the PNF.[58]

Beneath the hyponychium, where the longitudinal rete ridges are replaced by conventional papillary dermis, long, thin-walled, spirally wound, looped vessels of wide caliber are found.[43] These vessels rupture, filling the longitudinal troughs formed by the rete and papillae in the nail bed with blood to form splinter hemorrhages. Large arteriovenous (AV) anastomoses are found at the level of the anastomotic arteries and the deep venous circulation in all areas of the nail unit except the PNF. These AV anastomoses vary morphologically, from simple, unmodified anastomoses to a complex association of vessels.[58] The simple structures probably function as AV shunts. The more complex structures are confined to the nail bed and volar areas; their function is speculative. It is unclear whether the occurrence of glomus tumors is restricted to either structure.

The innervation of the nail unit roughly parallels the blood supply. Distal to the distal interphalangeal joint, the palmar digital nerve trifurcates to supply the nail unit, the tip, and the pulp of the distal digit.[60]

## NAIL PLATE GROWTH

The rate of nail growth has been studied extensively.[61,62] A consensus about these numbers has evolved despite failure to assess variation within or between subjects, inconsistent statistical analysis, and the use of many different techniques to measure growth.[63] Normal fingernail growth varies from less than 1.8 to more than 4.5 mm/month and varies markedly between individuals, but is more constant among members of the same family.[19] The average rate of growth of 0.1 mm/day (3 mm/month)[4] is useful for determining the approximate time of trauma to a nail and for predicting future events. For example, a nail that has a rim of polish 3 mm distal to the PNF was last painted about 1 month previously. It takes a normal fingernail about 2 months to grow the 5–8 mm out from under the PNF. A normal fingernail therefore grows out completely in about 6 months. Toenails grow at half to one-third the rate of fingernails, so a normal toenail takes 12–18 months to grow out.[39] Approximately 3 g of fingernail plate is produced annually.[64]

Nails grow faster when regenerating after avulsion in squirrel monkey[46] and in humans (personal observation). In any individual, nail growth is proportional to the length of the finger.[65,66] Nail growth is faster in the dominant hand and faster in males than in females.[19] Nail growth is faster than normal during pregnancy,[67,68] in nail biters,[66] in warm climates,[66,69] and in persons with psoriasis[65] and onycholysis (psoriatic and idiopathic).[70] The rate of nail growth peaks between the ages of 10 and 14 and begins an inexorable decrease with age after the second decade.[19,62,65,71] The rate of nail growth is less than normal in persons who are immobilized or paralyzed;[62,72] those with decreased circulation,[62] malnutrition,[73] or the yellow nail syndrome;[74] at night;[75] during lactation;[62] in acute infection;[76,77] and during therapy with antimitotic drugs.[65]

The question of where the nail plate is formed is disputed.[4,39,78,79] Unna[3] and Pinkus[1] believed that the nail plate was formed by the matrix. Based on staining of the nail plate with a silver protein stain and on morphology of keratinizing cells, Lewis concluded that the nail plate was the product of three different matrices.[5] He postulated the dorsal matrix in the roof of the PNF, which made the dorsal part of the nail plate; the conventional matrix, which made the intermediate nail; and the ventral matrix on the nail bed, which made the ventral part of the nail plate. The ventral and dorsal parts of the nail were produced by an 'inflation–deflation cycle,' while the intermediate nail was made by 'gradient parakeratosis.' The dorsal nail was thin, compared with the intermediate nail, while the ventral nail varied from absent to one-third the thickness of the intermediate nail. Lewis' hypothesis was supported by differential staining of the nail plate,[80] by Zeiss–Nomarski differential interference contrast microscopy,[23] by ultrastructural observation of keratohyalin granules in embryonic nail,[24] by physical properties of dissected nail clippings,[15] and by synchrotron X-ray microdiffraction.[81] Johnson and colleagues suggested approximately 20% of normal nail plate is contributed by the nail bed.[82,83] However, Zaias and Alvarez used radio-autography to show that the nail plate is formed exclusively by the matrix in squirrel monkey.[84] They showed that the most proximal part of the matrix makes the dorsal nail plate while the distal matrix makes the ventral portion of the nail plate. This work was criticized by Hashimoto.[23] These criticisms were answered when Norton confirmed Zaias's work by following the incorporation of 3H-labeled glycine and thymidine in human toenails.[79] Samman reported other evidence supporting the exclusive formation of the nail plate by the matrix;[59] Caputo and Dadati[16] and Forslind[15] reported that ultrastructurally the nail plate was an homogeneous structure with no evidence of formation from three different matrices; Forslind and colleagues[85,86] and Robson and Brooks[87] used electron probe microanalysis (analytic electron microscopy) to show that there was no difference between dorsal and intermediate nail plate in dry mass, sulfur content, calcium, or potassium levels; and Hashimoto[23] reported that all parts of the adult nail plate keratinized similarly. Monoclonal antibody staining of nail-associated keratin proteins also supports exclusive formation of the nail plate by the (conventional) matrix[28,88] (see p. 22). To add one final bit of confusion, Samman suggested that although under normal conditions the nail plate is made exclusively by the matrix, in certain pathologic conditions the nail bed adds a ventral nail to the undersurface of the nail plate.[39,89]

Why has there been so much effort to complicate the matrix, and where *is* the nail plate formed? Lewis seized on his histochemical findings to explain the nail plate dystrophy one observes in paronychia (ventral matrix inflammation) and in diseases of the nail bed (e.g., psoriasis and distal subungual onychomycosis). Samman could not confirm the dorsal nail findings but supported the idea of a ventral nail in disease. The data of Zaias and Norton are irrefutable; the nail plate is formed predominantly by the matrix under normal conditions, with a small contribution of cells to the undersurface of the nail plate by the nail bed. Rather than postulate a dorsal matrix, dorsal nail plate dystrophy produced by PNF disease (e.g., paronychia) is best explained by an effect of inflammation on the underlying proximal matrix, which produces the dorsal surface of the nail plate.[84] Whether a ventral nail exists under pathologic conditions remains to be proved.

Why do nails grow out instead of up? Kligman postulated that the cul-de-sac of the proximal nail groove forced the cells of the matrix to grow out.[90] He showed that nail matrix transplanted to forearm produced a vertical cylinder of hard keratin that had

histologic characteristics of nail. Hashimoto stated that the long axis of the matrix cells in embryonic nail was directed upward and distally.[7] Baran disputed Kligman's findings on the basis of observations of surgically excised proximal nail folds and the lack of bone under the forearm graft.[91] Kikuchi's examination of a congenital ectopic nail supports Kligman's hypothesis.[92] Dawber and Baran summarize the literature and conclude that all hypotheses are partially correct.[63] One can only agree with Kligman in his assessment of the problem, 'the subject of nail growth … is worthy of further consideration.'[93]

How the nail plate grows out and the relationship between the nail plate and the nail bed in nail growth are questions directly related to the clinical problems of onycholysis and nail growth. Pinkus is quoted by Silver in discussing the observation that splinter hemorrhage, which occurs between the plate and bed, grows forward with the plate.[94] If the plate merely moved over the bed, the extravasated blood would not move; therefore, the upper part of the bed must move out with the plate. Krantz removed the distal two-thirds of one side of the plate, marked the underlying nail bed, and observed these marks moving forward.[95] From this he concluded that there is no 'gliding' of the nail plate over the bed; rather, the two grow forward together. Kligman removed a transverse strip of nail plate distal to the lunula so that there was a strip of plate on the distal nail bed not connected to the more proximal plate.[96] He observed the distal strip of plate move forward and shed before the gap was closed and concluded that 'the hyponychium is dragging the nail plate'. Zaias observed the crust produced after nail avulsion was pushed off by regrowing nail instead of growing forward with the nail bed.[46] Zaias repeated the experiment of Kligman but did not find that the distal strip of nail plate moved forward.[97] He suggested that Kligman's observations were based on the result of trauma. He also repeated the experiment of Krantz, with the exception of removing the entire side of a nail plate instead of the distal two-thirds of one side. Zaias observed that although the proximal nail bed marks moved out as Krantz reported, the distal marks did not. He concluded that the proximal nail bed moves out, either by 'pressures by the advancing [regrowing] plate' or because of trauma, but that the distal nail bed and hyponychium do not move. Norton's findings support the movement of cells from the distal matrix to the proximal nail bed.[79] More recently, Zaias reported data clarifying the mechanism of nail plate growth and its relationship to the nail bed.[4] From the data he concluded that 'basal cells labeled at the nail bed origin [proximal nail bed] move distally and differentiate to the [under-] surface [of the plate] along the entire length of the nail bed. The growth rate or movement of the matrix and nail bed cells is identical.' At the Council for Nail Disorders' annual meeting on 5 February 2004, Zaias proposed a compartment of cells located at the distal matrix that populate the nail bed.

What attaches the nail plate to the nail unit? The nail bed contributes significantly to the attachment of the nail plate to its underlying structures. When one avulses a nail plate, most of the resistance is encountered in the nail bed (personal observation, supported by Samman).[39] Zaias and others have observed that most of the epithelium of the nail bed remains attached to the undersurface of the avulsed plate.[46,47] Zaias comments that although the nail bed contributes nothing to the mass of the plate, it does contribute a few cells to the undersurface of the plate.[4] The hyponychium contributes cells to the undersurface of the free edge of the nail plate.[17,96] A combination of the small contribution of cells by the nail bed to the undersurface of the plate and the interdigitating, tongue-in-groove spatial arrangement of the nail bed rete and dermal papillae probably hold the plate to the bed.[45] The area is sealed distally by the hyponychium/onychocorneal band. The question remains, if the nail bed contributes directly to the undersurface of the nail plate and the nail plate is firmly attached to the nail bed, how does the plate move out? Does the plate slide over the bed? To quote Hashimoto, 'It is difficult to conceive that the nail bed provides just a sliding floor for the nail plate produced more proximally.'[23] Does the nail bed grow out with the plate or is there some other mechanism of attachment and release, akin to the making and breaking of desmosomal contacts between keratinocytes as the cells differentiate and rise in the epidermis? Does the nail bed 'pull' the overlying, attached nail plate out, or is the plate 'pushed' out as the matrix makes new plate? How does the unique spatial arrangement of the nail bed rete and dermal papillae contribute to the attachment and movement of the nail plate? The answers to these questions remain to be clarified.

# BIOCHEMISTRY OF THE NAIL UNIT

What is the nail plate composed of? Many investigators have studied the composition of the nail plate with the idea that nail plate, as an epithelial product, will reflect body mineral metabolism. A second assumption is that the slow growth of nail plate will temper transient factors that may perturb serum mineral levels and confuse understanding of overall mineral metabolism. More recently investigators have applied molecular techniques to expand understanding of the proteins of the nail plate. Their findings are summarized in Table 3.1 and highlighted below.

Components of the nail plate can be divided into inorganic and organic. Inorganic elements can be divided into trace metals and electrolytes (circulating ions in the plasma and other body fluids). Serious technical difficulties arise in measuring inorganic elements in nail plates. External (environmental) contamination and the accuracy of the technique employed probably account for both the wide range of values reported by individual investigators and the differences reported between investigators. Variability between investigators may be compounded by different washing procedures aimed at removing environmental contaminants but resulting in differential extraction of the elements from the nail plate being studied.[98] Large variations between subjects,[99] twofold variation between fingers of the same individual,[100] 25% variation between sections of one nail plate and great variations between successive segments of the same nail over time[101] have been reported in measurement of one element. Unfortunately, despite such large variation in measured results, statistical evaluation of data is often not reported. Therefore, the significance of the reported observations can be questioned. Some methods (e.g., emission spectroscopy and spark source mass spectrometry) are useful for the detection of several metals on small samples of one specimen (including toxic metals such as arsenic) but are too insensitive to detect small variations occurring in metabolic disease. More sensitive techniques, such as chemical methods, flame photometry, and atomic absorption spectroscopy, are better suited for smaller changes.[99,100,102]

In spite of technical difficulties in the measurement of inorganic elements in nail plates, many interesting observations have been reported: calcium and zinc are higher and magnesium is lower in nail plates from males than in those from females,[102] magnesium and sodium are higher in the nails of children than in the nails of adults,[95,101] and copper is increased in the nail plates of patients with Wilson's disease.[103] Iron has been reported to be decreased in the nail plates of adolescents and either decreased[104] or unchanged[105] in patients with iron-deficiency anemia. Magnesium was increased in the nails of two patients undergoing chronic dialysis,[100] and sodium and calcium are higher and magnesium is lower in the nail plates of children with kwashiorkor than in normal children.[87,106] The concentration of sodium is increased in nail plates from patients with cystic fibrosis and may be useful in diagnosis of the disease where sweat test results are inconclusive and in subjects living in remote areas.[107,108] Fluoride content of nail plate reflects fluoride intake.[109] The level of arsenic in the nail plate increases within hours of exposure and can be useful for demonstrating acute and chronic arsenic intoxication.[110–112]

Organic elements are less difficult to quantify. Although carbon is technically the only organic element, sulfur and nitrogen are included because in the nail plate they are found almost exclusively in amino acids.[113] Nitrogen content of nails is reduced in neonates,[114] slightly higher in Caucasian than in black adolescents, but unaffected by nutritional status.[115] In the nail plate, sulfur is found almost exclusively in the amino acid cystine,[113] the oxidative, disulfide-bonded product of two cysteine residues. Hess detected lower concentrations of cystine in nails from patients with arthritis.[116] Klauder and Brown showed that the sulfur content of nails was reduced in a number of cutaneous and systemic diseases, but concluded that determination of the concentration of sulfur in diseased nails or in nails of patients with systemic disease was of no value.[113] Reduced nail plate cystine has been reported in uranium mine workers.[117] Cystine content does not vary as a function of ethnic group, differing dietary habits, or pregnancy[118] but may be reduced in nails when koilonychia is present.[119]

Nail plates, like hair and epidermis, contain a group of tough, fibrous proteins called keratins (from the Greek word for horn).[120] Early studies of wool revealed two components, fibrous proteins and less-structured, globular matrix proteins that surround the fibrous proteins. These proteins were collectively called keratins. Subsequently investigators determined that the fibrous proteins were part of a large family of structural proteins that contribute to the integrity of all cells, called intermediate filaments,[121] and began to restrict the term keratin to the fibrous proteins. The globular matrix proteins are now known as keratin associated proteins. Compared with the fibrous keratin proteins, matrix proteins contain high levels of the sulfur-containing amino acid cystine. Wool chemists speculate that the matrix proteins hold the fibrous proteins together, with the disulfide bonds of cystine acting as a glue. The proteins of nail are similar to those of wool and can be divided into fibrous keratins and globular (nonfibrous), keratin associated proteins on the basis of solubility, amino acid composition, electrophoretic mobility, and X-ray diffraction pattern.[122] Compared with stratum corneum of epidermis, the proteins of nail plate are quite different. Not only is the pattern of the keratin expression distinct[122–125] but also no high-sulfur matrix component has been found in stratum corneum.

The fibrous proteins, the keratins, belong to the group of intermediate filament proteins that contribute to the cytoskeleton of the cell.[126] Approximately 50 keratin proteins have been described.[127] Keratins can be divided into two groups of acidic and neutral-basic proteins; they are expressed as a pair, one from each group. The keratin pairs expressed vary with both the tissue and the stage of differentiation, e.g. the pair expressed in suprabasal

**TABLE 3-1. Summary of findings on nail composition***

| | N | Ca | Mg | Na | K | Fe | Cu | Zn | Au | Mn | P | S[a] | Cys[a] |
|---|---|---|---|---|---|---|---|---|---|---|---|---|---|
| Baden et al.[122] (4)[o,c] | | | | | | | | | | | | 3.2%[n]<br>5.5%[n]<br>20.3%[n]<br>3.8%[c,o] | 10.6%[n]<br>α-helix<br>'matrix'<br>24.0%[c,o] |
| Block[159,f(?)] | 14.9%[d,o] | | | | | | | | | | | | |
| Cotzias et al.[160] (4)[b,e] | | | | | | | | | | 0.2–0.8 | | | |
| Djaldetti et al.[105] (17)[h] | | 18.74 ± 0.68% | | | | 0.80 ± 0.84% | 0.78 ± 0.52% | 1.26 ± 0.80% | | | | 78.24 ± 3.08% | |
| Forslind[15,86] | | 1060[f,g] [720–1880] | | | | | | | | | | 3–6%[h] | |
| Goldblum et al.[99] (18)[b,i] | | 940–5900 | 23–110 | | | 18–65 | 9.4–81 | 116–3080 | | | 82–278 | 138 | |
| Grozdanovic et al.[117] (40)[c,f] | | | | | | | | | | <1 | | | |
| Harrison et al.[100,102] | | | | | | | | | | | | | |
| Female (7)[b,g] | | 821 [701–982] | 111 [68–152] | | | 38 [14–90] | 44 [28–53] | 222 [130–360] | | | | | |
| Male (10)[b,g] | | 904 | 106 | | | 41 | 62 | 178 | | | | | |
| Both (17)[b,i] | | [687–1270] | [68–140] | | | [28–109] | [45–102] | [135–391] | | | | | |
| Hein et al.[115,b,d] | | | | | | | | | | | | | |
| White (49) | 141 × 10³ | [450–1600] | [11–380] | | | [16–200] | [17–64] | [62–360] | | | | | |
| Black (127) | 137 × 10³ | | | | | | | | | | | | |
| Hess[116,f(?),c] | | | | | | | | | | | | | |
| Normal | | | | | | | | | | | | | 12.0%[o] |
| Arthritic | | | | | | | | | | | | | 9.8%[o] |
| Jacobs et al.[104] (50 adults)[b,c] | | | | | | 129–227 | | | | | | | |
| Jalili et al.[119,c,f,o] | | | | | | | | | | | | | |
| Normal (29) | | | | | | | | | | | | 8.12 ± 1.17% | |
| Koilonychia (6) | | | | | | | | | | | | 2.54 ± 0.83% | |
| Anemia (17) | | | | | | | | | | | | 6.32 ± 1.4% | |
| Kanabrocki et al.[1C1,e,k] | | | | | | | | | | | | | |
| Adults (13) | | | | 900 ± 538 | | 51 ± 23 | | 0.5 ± 0.6 | 0.9 ± 0.3 | | | | |
| Children (6) | | | | 2370 ± 1836 | | 86 ± 45 | | 0.4 ± 0.6 | 1.9 ± 1.4 | | | | |
| Kile[145] (5)[b,c] | | 725 | | | | | | | | | 310 | 3.2% | 12.0%[o] |
| Klauder & Brown[113] (11)[f(?),c] | | | | | | | | | | | | | |
| Kopito et al.[108,b,i] | | | | | | | | | | | | | |
| Children with CF (149) | | | | 3220 ± 1220 | 1680 ± 1060 | | | | | | | | |
| Healthy children (44) | | | | 1060 ± 550 | 700 ± 390 | | | | | | | | |
| Parents of CF (87) | | | | 800 ± 600 | 550 ± 740 | | | | | | | | |
| Healthy adults (32) | | | | 670 ± 480 | 430 ± 430 | | | | | | | | |
| Sibs of CF (64) | | | | 1450 ± 740 | 1020 ± 630 | | | | | | | | |

**TABLE 3-1. (Cont'd) Summary of findings on nail composition***

| | N | Ca | Mg | Na | K | Fe | Cu | Zn | Au | Mn | P | S^a | Cys^a |
|---|---|---|---|---|---|---|---|---|---|---|---|---|---|
| Leonard et al.[106] (25)^b | | $3070 \pm 2010^m$ | $2480 \pm 1660^m$ | $3010 \pm 970^l$ | $2400 \pm 1150^l$ | | | | | | | | |
| Lockard et al.[114] | | | | | | | | | | | | | |
| Adult (24)^k,d | $146 \pm 6 \times 10^3$ | | | | | | | | | | | | |
| Neonates (67) | $131 \pm 14 \times 10^3$ | | | | | | | | | | | | |
| Normal (40) | $136 \pm 10 \times 10^3$ | | | | | | | | | | | | |
| III (27) | $123 \pm 17 \times 10^3$ | | | | | | | | | | | | |
| Martin[103],b,c | | | | | | | | | | | | | |
| Normal male (6) | | | | | | | $14.8 \pm 3.8$ | | | | | | |
| Normal female (7) | | | | | | | $10.6 \pm 2.8$ | | | | | | |
| Wilson's disease male (2) | | | | | | | 21.1,32.2 | | | | | | |
| Wilson's disease female (1) | | | | | | | 11.4 | | | | | | |
| Pascher[161],b,c | | | | | | | | | | | | | 9.4% |
| Petushkov et al.[162] (3)^f(?),e | | | | | [240–3900] | | – | [1200–2700] | [0.006–0.085] | – | | | |
| Pruzanski et al.[118] c,f(?) | | | | | | | | | | | | | |
| Males (67) | | | | | | | | | | | | | $8.8 \pm 0.9\%$ |
| Females (52) | | | | | | | | | | | | | $8.9 \pm 1.3\%$ |
| Sobdewski et al.[163],b,g | | | | | | | | | | | | | |
| Healthy adult (40) | | | | | | 12.5 [6–26] | | | | | | | |
| Iron deficient (5) | | | | | | 1.6 [4–3] | | | | | | | |
| Iron deficient under treatment (4) | | | | | | 10 [8–16] | | | | | | | |
| Cadaver (15) | $148 \pm$ | | | | | 8.9 [<1–21] | | | | | | | |
| Vellar[64] (10)^f(?) | $1g \times 10^{-3d}$ 14.7–17.6% | | $368 \pm 53^g$ | $440 \pm 92^g$ | $357 \pm 72^g$ | $27 \pm 4^c$ | $21 \pm 8^g$ | $73 \pm 8^g$ | | –^g | | | |
| Way (discussion in Kile[145]) | | | | | | | | | | | | 2.47–3.12% | |

*Values are in μg/gm unless otherwise specified. Numbers in parentheses indicate number of patients studied. Numbers in square brackets indicate range. Numbers following ± indicate standard deviation. –, failed to detect; blank, not determined; CF, cystic fibrosis. ^aCystine contains 26.7% sulfur. ^bDry weight. ^cChemical. ^dKjeldahl. ^eNeutron activation. ^fWet weight. ^gAtomic absorption. ^hFigures for quantitative X-ray microradiography reported as percentage of the total weight of the elements examined. ^iSpectrography. ^jSpark source mass spectrometry. ^kAir dried. ^lFlame photometry. ^mFluorometric. ^nResidues/100 residues; ^og/100 g.

epidermis is different from that expressed in suprabasal esophagus, or from that expressed in the basal layer of epidermis. A number of 'hard' keratins have been identified in hair and nail. The nail unit expresses both hard keratins and keratins seen in other epithelia[28,88,124,128,129] (Fig. 3.7). Mutations in at least four of these keratins have been demonstrated in individuals with pachyonychia congenita.[130,131] Mouse models for this (these) disease(s) offer the potential for understanding the role of the keratins in the normal and diseased nail unit.

Baden studied the proteins of normal nail plates and showed a genetic variant in the (low-sulfur) keratins.[132] The variant appeared in approximately 5% of the population studied and appeared to be inherited as an autosomal dominant trait. This likely reflects keratin polymorphisms.[133] Gillespie and Marshall confirmed the presence of high- and low-sulfur-containing proteins in nail plate and showed that among species there were considerable differences among the fibrous proteins but that the electrophoretic pattern of the high-sulfur matrix proteins was preserved.[134] Marshall defined the keratin and matrix proteins of nail using two-dimensional electrophoresis and showed that there are genetic variants not only in the keratin proteins but also in the matrix proteins.[135] When the variant keratin proteins are present, the variant matrix proteins are also found; however, the variant matrix proteins can be found in the absence of the variant keratins. No differences in the physical properties of the nail plate have been associated with the variant proteins. Data from the human genome project reveal the presence of many, as yet uncharacterized, keratin associated proteins in hair;[136] there is every reason to assume similar proteins will be found associated with keratins of the nail unit. Expression of microtubule associated protein 2, another cytoskeletal-associated protein, is uniquely restricted to the upper layers of the nail matrix, along with the companion layer of the hair follicle.[137] The significance of this observation is unclear.

The cornified cell envelope is a chemically resistant structure found in the stratum corneum of the epidermis[138] and in the nail plate.[24] A cornified cellular envelope-enriched fraction of protein from nail plates has been prepared and shown to contain relatively high levels of proline.[139]

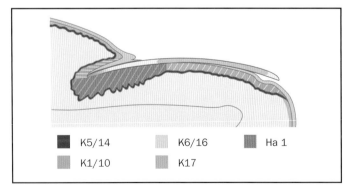

FIGURE 3–7. Pattern of keratin expression in the nail unit. Red, keratins 5 and 14 expressed in the basal layer; green, keratins 1 and 10 expressed in the suprabasal layers of the proximal nail fold and the volar epidermis of the finger tip; purple, hard keratins (including Ha1) expressed sporadically in the upper parts of the suprabasal layers of the nail matrix; blue, keratins 6, 16, and 17, expressed in the suprabasal layers of the nail bed epithelium. The thickness of the nail bed epithelium is artifactually thickened to demonstrate the limited expression of keratins 6, 16, and 17 (based on refs 28 and 88).

# BIOPHYSICAL PROPERTIES OF THE NAIL PLATE

X-ray diffraction studies of the nail plate have shown that the fibrous proteins (the keratins) are oriented in the plane of the plate, perpendicular to the axis (longitudinal) of growth.[140–143] There is no specific axis of fiber orientation in newly formed plate other than in the plane of the plate; as the plate grows out fibers develop this directional orientation parallel to the free edge of the plate.[141]

Nail-plates of normal thickness transmit approximately 30% of grenz rays and 85% of X-rays.[144] Transmission of grenz rays is directly correlated with the thickness of the nail plate. Attempts to treat the nail bed through thick nails with grenz ray are futile; superficial X-ray should be used.

The water content of nails varies between 10 and 30%[122,145] and is directly related to relative humidity.[122] At high humidity, much less water is held by nail plate than by stratum corneum.[122] The physical properties of hydrated nails are altered.[146,147] The rate of water diffusion through a nail plate is approximately 10 times greater than through abdominal skin.[122,148,149] Therefore considering that stratum corneum thickness is about $\frac{1}{100}$ that of nail plate, the diffusion constant of water through nail is several hundred times that through most skin. Although in stratum corneum the water-holding capacity is decreased and the diffusion of water through skin is increased by extraction of lipids, water-holding capacity and diffusion of water through nail plate are unaffected by lipid extraction.[141] The loss of water through the nail plate can be stopped by applying a layer of petroleum jelly or nail polish on the plate.[150,151]

# PHARMACOLOGY OF THE NAIL UNIT

As with water diffusion out of the nail plate, nail plate permeability to water is greater than stratum corneum.[26] N-alkanols have been used as model compounds with varying polarity. Unlike stratum corneum, the permeability coefficient of nail to N-alkanols decreases as the compound becomes increasingly hydrophobic. If the alkanol permeabilities could be extrapolated to other low-molecular-weight organics, 'then very polar compounds might be surprisingly easily delivered through the nail plate to underlying tissues.'[152] Pharmacodynamic studies of systemic drugs have shown rapid delivery of drug to the entire nail plate.[153–156] Data from new agents being developed to enhance absorption of topical drugs for treatment of subungual diseases such as psoriasis of the nail bed and distal subungual onychomycosis are encouraging.[157,158]

# ACKNOWLEDGEMENTS

Robert Underwood and Marcia Usui assisted in the creation of Figures 3.1 and 3.3.

# REFERENCES

1. Pinkus F. Der Nagel. In: Jadassohn J, ed. Handbuch. New York, Springer-Verlag, 1927:266–289
2. Rainey E. On the structure and formation of the nails of the fingers and toes. Trans Microscop Soc London 1849; 2:105–109

3. Unna PG. Entwichtlungsgeschichte und anatomy. In: Ziemessen, ed. Leipzig, Vogel FCW, 1883:38–51
4. Zaias N. The nail in health and disease. 2nd ed. Norwalk, CT, Appleton & Lange, 1990
5. Lewis BL. Microscopic studies of fetal and mature nail and surrounding soft tissue. AMA Arch Dermatol Syph 1954; 70:732–747
6. Zaias N. Embryology of the human nail. Arch Dermatol 1963; 87:77–93
7. Hashimoto K, Gross BG, Nelson R, et al. The ultrastructure of the skin of human embryos: III. The formation of the nail in 16–18-weeks-old embryos. J Invest Dermatol 1966; 47:205–217
8. Holbrook KA. Human epidermal embryogenesis. Int J Dermatol 1979; 18:329–356
9. Holbrook KA. Structural abnormalities of the epidermally derived appendaages in skin from patients with ectodermal dysplasia: insight into developmental errors. Recent Adv Ectodermal Dysplasia. Birth Defects Orig Artic Ser 1988; 24:15–44
10. Holbrook KA. Structure and function of the developing human skin. In: Physiology, biochemistry, and molecular biology of the skin. 2nd ed. Goldsmith LA, ed. New York, Oxford University Press, 1991:63–110
11. Zaias N. Onychomycosis. Arch Dermatol 1972; 105:263–274
12. Tickle C. Molecular basis of vertebrate limb patterning. Am J Med Genet 2002; 112:250–255
13. Chen H, Johnson RL. Dorsoventral patterning of the vertebrate limb: a process governed by multiple events. Cell Tissue Res 1999; 296:67–73
14. Clough MV, Hamlington JD, McIntosh I. Restricted distribution of loss-of-function mutations within the LMX1B genes of nail–patella syndrome patients. Hum Mutat 1999; 14:459–465
15. Forslind B. Biophysical studies of the normal nail. Acta Dermatovener 1970; 50:161–168
16. Caputo R, Dadati E. Preliminary observations about the ultrastructure of the human nail plate treated with thioglycolic acid. Archiv Klin Exp Dermatol 1968; 231:344–354
17. Runne U, Orfanos CE. The human nail. Curr Probl Derm 1981; 9:102–149
18. Forslind B, Thyresson N. On the structure of the normal nail: a scanning electron microscopic study. Arch Derm Forsch 1975; 251:199–204
19. Hamilton JB, Terada H, Mestler GE. Studies of growth throughout the lifespan in Japanese: growth and size of nails and their relationship to age, heredity and other factors. J Gerontology 1955; 10:401–415
20. Finlay AY, Moseley H, Duggan TC. Ultrasound transmission time: an in vivo guide to nail thickness. Br J Derm 1987; 117:765–770
21. Germann H, Barran W, Plewig G. Morphology of corneocytes from human nail plates. J Invest Dermatol 1980; 74:115–118
22. Brody I. The keratinization of epidermal cells of normal guinea pig skin as revealed by electron microscopy. J Ultrastruct Res 1959; 2:482–511
23. Hashimoto K. Ultrastructure of the human toenail. Cell migration, keratinization, and formation of the intercellular cement. Arch Derm Forsch 1971; 240:1–22
24. Hashimoto K. Ultrastructure of the human toenail. II. Keratinization and formation of the marginal band. J Ultrastr Res 1971; 36:391–410
25. Stenn K, Fleckman P. Hair and nail physiology. In: Hordinsky MK, Scher RK, eds. Atlas of hair and nails. Philadelphia, Churchill Livingstone, 2000:3–8
26. Walters KA, Flynn GL, Marvel JR. Physiocochemical characterization of the human nail: I. Pressure sealed apparatus for measuring nail plate permeabilities. J Invest Dermatol 1981; 76:76–79
27. Le Gros Clark WE. Nails. In: Press C, ed. Tissues of the body. Oxford, Clarendon Press, 1965:315–319
28. Kitahara T, Ogawa H. Cultured nail keratinocytes express hard keratins characteristic of nail and hair in vivo. Arch Dermatol Res 1992; 284:253–256
29. Picardo M, Tosti A, Marchese, et al. Characterization of cultured nail matrix cells. J Am Acad Dermatol 1994; 30:434–440
30. Hashimoto K. Ultrastructure of the human toenail. I. Proximal nail matrix. J Invest Dermatol 1971; 56:235–246
31. Tosti A, Cameli N, Piraccini BM, et al. Characterization of nail matrix melanocytes with anti-PEP1, anti-PEP8, TMH-1, and HMB-45 antibodies. J Am Acad Dermatol 1994; 31:193–196
32. Perrin C, Michiels JF, Pisani A, et al. Anatomic distribution of melanocytes in normal nail unit: an immunohistochemical investigation. Am J Dermatopathol 1997; 19:462–467
33. Higashi N, Saito T. Horizontal distribution of the dopa-positive melanocytes in the nail matrix. J Invest Dermatol 1969; 53:163–165
34. Hashimoto K. The ultrastructure of the skin of human embryos. X. Merkel tactile cells in the finger and nail. J Anat 1972; 111:99–120
35. Cameli N, Ortonne JP, Picardo M, et al. Distribution of Merkel cells in adult human nail matrix [letter]. Br J Dermatol 1998; 139:541
36. Le Gros Clark WE. The problem of the claw in primates. Proc Zool Soc 1936; 1:1–24
37. Burrows MT. The significance of the lunula of the nail. Johns Hopkins Hosp Rep 1919; 18:357–361
38. Lewin K. The normal finger nail. Br J Dermatol 1965; 77:421–430
39. Samman PD, Fenton DA. Samman's the nails in disease. 5th ed. London, Butterworth-Heinemann, 1995
40. Drape JL, Wolfram-Gabel R, Idy-Peretti I, et al. The lunula: a magnetic resonance imaging approach to the subnail matrix area. J Invest Dermatol 1996; 106:1081–1085
41. Wolfram-Gabel R, Sick H. Vascular networks of the periphery of the fingernail. J Hand Surg 1995; 20B:488–492
42. Mitchell JC. A clinical study of leukonychia. Br J Dermatol 1953; 65:121–130
43. Martin BF, Platts MM. A histological study of the nail region in normal human subjects and in those showing splinter hemorrhages of the nail. J Anat 1959; 93:323
44. Montagna W, Parakkal PF. The structure and function of skin. 3rd edn. New York, Academic Press, 1974
45. Rand R, Baden HP. Pathophysiology of nails-onychopathophysiology. In: Soter NA, Baden HP, eds. Pathophysiology of dermatologic diseases. New York, McGraw-Hill, 1991:209
46. Zaias N. The regeneration of the primate nail studies of the squirrel monkey, Saimiri. J Invest Dermatol 1965; 44:107–117
47. Fleckman P, Omura EF. Histopathology of the nail. Adv Dermatol 2001; 17:385–406
48. Terry RB. The onychodermal band in health and disease. Lancet 1955; i:179–181
49. Stewart WK, Raffle EJ. Brown nail-bed arcs and chronic renal disease. Br Med J 1972; 1:784–786
50. Holzberg M, Walker HK. Terry's nails revisited: revised definition and new correlations. Lancet 1984; i:896–899
51. Lindsay PG. The half-and-half nail. Arch Intern Med 1967; 119:583–586
52. Raffle EJ. Terry's nails. Lancet 1984; i:1131
53. Sonnex TS, Griffiths WAD, Nicol WJ. The nature and significance of the transverse white band of human nails. Semin Dermatol 1991; 10:12–16
54. Sinclair RD, Wojnarowska F, Leigh IM, et al. The basement membrane zone of the nail. Br J Dermatol 1994; 131:499–505
55. Kelikian H. Congenital deformities of the hand. Philadelphia, WB Saunders, 1974
56. Baran R, Juhlin L. Bone dependent nail formation. Br J Dermatol 1986; 114:371
57. Flint MH. Some observations on the vascular supply of the nail bed and terminal segments of the finger. Br J Plast Surg 1955; 8:186–195
58. Hale AR, Burch GE. The arteriovenous anastomoses and blood vessels of the human finger. Medicine 1960; 39:191–240
59. Samman PD. The human toenail: its genesis and blood supply. Br J Dermatol 1959; 71:296–302
60. Fleckman P, Allan C. Surgical anatomy of the nail unit. Dermatol Surg 2001; 27:257–260
61. Bean WB. A note on fingernail growth. J Invest Dermatol 1953; 20:27–31
62. Bean WB. Nail growth: 30 years of observation. Arch Intern Med 1974; 134:497–502
63. Dawber R, Baran R. Nail growth. Cutis 1987; 39:99–103
64. Vellar OD. Composition of human nail substance. Am J Clin Nutr 1970; 23:1272–1274

65. Dawber R. Fingernail growth in normal and psoriatic subjects. Br J Dermatol 1970; 82:454–457

66. Le Gros Clark WE, Buxton LHD. Studies in nail growth. Br J Dermatol 1938; 50:221–235

67. Halban J, Spitzer MZ. Uber das gesteigerte wachstum der nagel in der schwangerschaft. Monatsschrift fur Geburtshulfe und Gynakologie 1929; 82:25–31

68. Hillman RW. Fingernail growth in pregnancy relations to some common parameters of the reproductive process. Human Biology 1960; 323:119–134

69. Geoghegan B, Roberts DF, Sampford MR. Possible climatic effect on nail growth. J Appl Physiol 1958; 13:135–138

70. Dawber RPR, Samman PD, Bottoms E. Fingernail growth in idiopathic and psoriatic onycholysis. Br J Dermatol 1971; 85:558–560

71. Orentreich N, Markofsky J, Vogelman JH. The effect of aging on the rate of linear nail growth. J Invest Dermatol 1979; 73:126–130

72. Head H, Sherren J. The consequence of injury to the peripheral nerves in man. Brain 1919; 28:263–275

73. Gilchrist ML, Buxton LHD. The relation of finger-nail growth to nutritional status. J Anat 1939; 73:575–582

74. Samman PD, White WF. The 'yellow nail' syndrome. Br J Dermatol 1964; 76:153–157

75. Basler VA. Wachstumsvorgange am vollentwickelten organismus (Growth processes in fully developed organisms). Med Klin 1937; 33:1664–1666

76. Bean WB. Nail growth: twenty-five years' observation. Arch Intern Med 1968; 122:359–361

77. Sibinga MS. Observations on growth of fingernails in health and disease. Pediatrics 1959; 24:225–233

78. Baran R, Dawber RPR, De Berker DAR, et al. Diseases of the nails and their management. 3rd ed. Oxford, Blackwell Scientific Publications, 2001

79. Norton LA. Incorporation of thymidine-methyl-H3 and glycine-2-H3 in the nail matrix and bed of humans. J Invest Dermatol 1971; 56:61–68

80. Jarrett A, Spearman RIC. The histochemistry of the human nail. Arch Dermatol 1966; 94:652–657

81. Garson JC, Baltenneck F, Leroy F, et al. Histological structure of human nail as studied by synchrotron X-ray microdiffraction. Cell Mol Biol (Noisy -le-grand) 2000; 46:1025–1034

82. Johnson M, Comaish JS, Shuster S. Nail is produced by the normal nail bed: a controversy resolved. Br J Dermatol 1991; 125:27–29

83. Johnson M, Shuster S. Continuous formation of nail along the bed. Br J Dermatol 1993; 128:277–280

84. Zaias N, Alvarez J. The formation of the primate nail plate. An autoradiographic study in squirrel monkey. J Invest Dermatol 1968; 51:120–136

85. Forslind B, Lindstrom B, Philipson B. Quantitative microradiography of normal human nail. Acta Dermatovener 1971; 51:89–92

86. Forslind B, Wroblewski R, Afzelius BA. Calcium and sulfur location in human nail. J Invest Dermatol 1976; 67:273–275

87. Robson JRK, Brooks GJ. The distribution of calcium in fingernails from healthy and malnourished children. Clin Chim Acta 1974; 55:255–257

88. De Berker D, Wojnarowska F, Sviland L, et al. Keratin expression in the normal nail unit: markers of regional differentiation. Br J Dermatol 2000; 142:89–96

89. Samman PD. The ventral nail. Arch Dermatol 1961; 84:192–195

90. Kligman AM. Why do nails grow out instead of up? Arch Dermatol 1961; 84:181–183

91. Baran R. Nail growth direction revisited. J Am Acad Dermatol 1981; 4:78–83

92. Kikuchi I, Ogata K, Idemori M. Vertically growing ectopic nail. J Am Acad Dermatol 1984; 10:114–116

93. Kligman AM. Response. J Am Acad Dermatol 1981; 4:82–83

94. Silver H, Chiego B. Nails and nail changes. II. Modern concepts of anatomy and biochemistry of the nails. J Invest Dermatol 1940; 3:133–142

95. Krantz W. Beitrag zur anatomie des nagels. Dermatol Zeitschrift 1932; 64:239–242

96. Kligman AM. Nails. In: Pillsbury DM, editor. Dermatology. Philadelphia, WB Saunders, 1956:32–39

97. Zaias N. The movement of the nail bed. J Invest Dermatol 1967; 48:402–403

98. Bank HL, Robson J, Bigelow JB, et al. Preparation of fingernails for trace element analysis. Clinica Chimica Acta 1981; 116:179–190

99. Goldblum RW, Derby S, Lerner AB. The metal content of skin, nails and hair. J Invest Dermatol 1953; 20:13–18

100. Harrison WW, Clemena GG. Survey analysis of trace elements in human fingernails by spark source mass spectrometry. Clin Chim Acta 1972; 36:485–492

101. Kanabrocki E, Case LF, Graham LA, et al. Neutron-activation studies of trace elements in human fingernail. J Nucl Med 1968; 9:478–481

102. Harrison WW, Tyree AB. The determination of trace elements in human fingernails by atomic absorption spectroscopy. Clin Chim Acta 1971; 31:63–73

103. Martin GM. Copper content of hair and nails of normal individuals and of patients with hepatolenticular degeneration. Nature 1964; 202:903–904

104. Jacobs A, Jenkins DJ. The iron content of finger nails. Br J Dermatol 1970; 72:145–148

105. Djaldetti M, Fishman P, Hart J. The iron content of finger-nails in iron deficient patients. Clinical Sicence 1987; 72:669–672

106. Leonard PJ, Morris WP, Brown R. Sodium, potassium, calcium and magnesium contents in nails of children with kwashiorkor. Biochem J 1968; 110:22P–23P

107. Bock H, Koch E, Stephan U, et al. Investigations on electrolyte concentrations in the nails of cystic fibrosis patients and controls. Mod Probl Pediat 1967; 10:279–283

108. Kopito L, Mahmoodian A, Townley RRW, et al. Studies in cystic fibrosis. New Engl J Med 1965; 272:504–509

109. Whitford GM, Sampaio FC, Arneberg P, et al. Fingernail fluoride: a method for monitoring fluoride exposure. Caries Res 1999; 33:462–467

110. Lander H, Hodge PR, Crisp CS. Arsenic in the hair and nails. J Forensic Med 1965; 12:52–67

111. Shapiro HA. Arsenic content of human hair and nails: its interpretation. J Forensic Med 1967; 14:65–71

112. Mandal BK, Ogra Y, Suzuki KT. Speciation of arsenic in human nail and hair from arsenic-affected area by HPLC-inductively coupled argon plasma mass spectrometry. Toxicol Appl Pharmacol 2003; 189:73–83

113. Klauder JV, Brown H. Sulphur content of hair and of nails in abnormal states. II. Nails. Arch Dermatol Syphil 1935; 31:26–34

114. Lockard D, Pass R, Cassady G. Fingernail nitrogen content in neonates. Pediatrics 1972; 49:618–620

115. Hein K, Cohen MI, McNamara H. Racial differences in nitrogen content of nails among adolescents. Am J Clin Nutr 1977; 30:496–498

116. Hess WC. Variations in amino acid content of finger nails of normal and arthritic individuals. J Biol Chem 1935; 109:xiii

117. Grozdanovic J, Ulbert K. Oscillopolarographic determination of cysteic acid level in the fingernails followed chronic irradiation in humans. Strahlentherapie 1970; 139:735–737

118. Pruzanski W, Arnon R. Determination of cystine and other amino acids in the fingernails of members of various ethnic groups in Israel. Israel J Med Sci 1966; 2:465–467

119. Jalili MA, Al-Kassab S. Koilonychia and cystine content of nails. Lancet 1959; iii:108–110

120. Fraser RDB. Keratins. Sci Amer 1969; 221:86–96

121. Coulombe PA, Ma L, Yamada S, et al. Intermediate filaments at a glance. J Cell Sci 2001; 114:4345–4347

122. Baden HP, Goldsmith LA, Fleming B. A comparative study of the physiocochemical proterties of human keratinized tissues. Biochem Biophys Acta 1973; 322:269–278

123. Baden HP, Kubilus J. A comparative study of the immunologic properties of hoof and nail fibrous proteins. J Invest Dermatol 1984; 83:327–331

124. Powell BC, Rogers GE. Differentiation in hard keratin tissues: hair and related structures. In: Leigh IM, Lane EB, Watt FM, editors. The

keratinocyte handbook. Cambridge, Cambridge University Press, 1994:401–436

125. Lynch MH, O'Guinn WM, Hardy C, et al. Acidic and basic hair/nail ("hard") keratins: Their colocalization in upper cortical and cuticle cells of the human hair follicle and their relationship to 'soft' keratins. J Cell Biol 1986; 103:2593–2606

126. Fuchs E. Keratins: mechanical integrators in the epidermis and hair and their role in disease. Prog Dermatol 1996; 30:1–12

127. Hesse M, Magin TM, Weber K. Genes for intermediate filament proteins and the draft sequence of the human genome: novel keratin genes and a surprisingly high number of pseudogenes related to keratin genes 8 and 18. J Cell Sci 2001; 114:2569–2575

128. Wang Z, Wong P, Langbein L, et al. Type II epithelial keratin 6hf (K6hf) is expressed in the companion layer, matrix, and medulla in anagen-stage hair follicles. J Invest Dermatol 2003; 121:1276–1282

129. Wojcik SM, Longley MA, Roop DR. Discovery of a novel murine keratin 6 (K6) isoform explains the absence of hair and nail defects in mice deficient for K6a and K6b. J Cell Biol 2001; 154:619–630

130. Bowden PE, Jaley JL, Kansky A, et al. Mutation of a type II keratin gene (K6a) in pachyonychia congenita. Nat Genet 1995; 10:363–365

131. McLean WH, Rugg EL, Lunny DP, et al. Keratin 16 and keratin 17 mutations cause pachyonychia congenita. Nat Genet 1995; 9:273–278

132. Baden HP, Lee LD, Kubilus J. A genetic electrophoretic variant of human hair α polypeptides. Am J Hum Genet 1975; 27:472–477

133. Mischke D, Wild G. Polymorphic keratins in human epidermis. J Invest Dermatol 1987; 88:191–197

134. Gillespie JM, Marshall RC. Proteins of the hard keratins of echidna, hedgehog, rabbit, ox and man. Aust J Biol Sci 1977; 30:401–409

135. Marshall RC. Genetic variation in the proteins of human nail. J Invest Dermatol 1980; 75:264–269

136. Shimomura Y, Aoki N, Rogers MA, et al. Characterization of human keratin-associated protein 1 family members. J Investig Dermatol Symp Proc 2003; 8:96–99

137. Hallman JR, Fang D, Setaluri V, et al. Microtubule associated protein (MAP-2) expression defines the companion layer of the anagen hair follicle and an analogous zone in the nail unit. J Cutan Pathol 2002; 29:549–556

138. Kalinin AE, Kajava AV, Steinert PM. Epithelial barrier function: assembly and structural features of the cornified cell envelope. Bioessays 2002; 24:789–800

139. Shono S, Toda K. The structure proteins of the human nail. Curr Prob Dermatol 1983; 11:317–326

140. Astbury WT, Sisson WA. X-ray studies of the structure of hair, wool, and related fibres. Proc Royal Soc 1935; 150:533–551

141. Baden HP. The physical properties of nail. J Invest Dermatol 1970; 55:115–122

142. Derksen JD, Heringa GC, Weidinger A. On keratin and cornification. Acta Neerlandica Morph 1937; 1:31–37

143. Forslind B, Nordstrom G, Toijer D, et al. The rigidity of human fingernails: a biophysical investigation on influencing physical parameters. Acta Dermatovener 1980; 60:217–222

144. Gammeltoft M, Wulf HC. Transmission of 12 kv grenz rays and 29 kv X-rays through normal and diseased nails. Acta Dermatovener 1980; 60:431–462

145. Kile RL. Some mineral constituents of fingernails. AMA Arch Dermatol Syphil 1954; 70:75–83

146. Finlay AY, Frost P, Keith AD, et al. An assessment of factors influencing flexibility of human fingernails. Br J Dermatol 1980; 103:357–365

147. Wessel S, Gniadecka M, Jemec GB, et al. Hydration of human nails investigated by NIR-FT-Raman spectroscopy. Biochim Biophys Acta 1999; 1433:210–216

148. Burch GE, Winsor T. Diffusion of water through dead plantar palmar and torsal human skin and through toe nails. Arch Dermatol Syphil 1946; 53:39–41

149. Spruit D. Measurement of water vapor loss through human nail in vivo. J Invest Dermatol 1971; 56:359–361

150. Jacobi O. Die nagel des lebenden menschen und die perspiratio insensibilis. Arch Klin Exp Dermatol 1962; 214:559–572

151. Spruit D. Effect of nail polish on the hydration of the fingernail. American Cosmetics and Perfumery 1972; 87:57–58

152. Walters KA, Flynn GL, Marvel JR. Physicochemical characterization of the human nail: permeation pattern for water and the homologous alcohols and differences with respect to the stratum corneum. J Pharm Pharmacol 1983; 35:28–33

153. Cauwenbergh G, Degreef H, Heykants J, et al. Pharmacokinetic profile of orally administered itraconazole in human skin. J Am Acad Dermatol 1988; 18:263–268

154. Faergemann J, Zehender H, Denouel J, et al. Levels of terbinafine in plasma, stratum corneum, dermis-epidermis (without stratum corneum), sebum, hair, and nails during and after 250 mg terbinafine orally once per day for four weeks. Acta Derm Venereol (Stockh) 1993; 73:305–309

155. Finlay AY. Pharmacokinetics of terbinafine in the nail. Br J Dermatol 1992; 126 (Suppl 39):28–32

156. Matthieu L, De Doncker P, Cauwenbergh G, et al. Itraconazole penetrates into the nail matrix and the nail bed - an investigation in onychomycosis. Clin Exp Dermatol 1991; 16:374–376

157. Ceschin-Roques CG, Hanel H, Pruja-Bougaret SM, et al. Ciclopirox nail lacquer 8%: in vivo penetration into and through nails and in vitro effect on pig skin. Skin Pharmacol 1991; 4:89–94

158. Hui X, Chan TC, Barbadillo S, et al. Enhanced econazole penetration into human nail by 2-n-nonyl-1,3-dioxolane. J Pharm Sci 2003; 92:142–148

159. Block RJ. The composition of keratins: the amino acid composition of hair, wool, horn, and other eukeratins. J Biol Chem 1939; 128:181–186

160. Cotzias GC, Papavasiliou PS, Miller ST. Manganese in melanin. Nature 1964; 201:1228–1229

161. Pascher G. Bestandteile der menschlichen hornschict. Archiv Klinische Exper Dermatol 1964; 218:111–125

162. Petushkov AA, Linekin DM, Balcius JF, et al. High-resolution gamma-ray spectrometry in the determination of trace elements in human fingernails. J Nucl Med 1969; 10:730–731

163. Sobolewski S, Lawrence ACK, Bagshaw P. Human nails and body iron. J Clin Path 1978; 31:1068–1072

# 4 An Approach to Initial Examination of the Nail

C Ralph Daniel III

## Key Features

1. All polish, socks, shoes, etc. are removed before examining all 20 nails
2. Nail questionnaire is filled out before the doctor sees the patient
3. When making an appointment, the patient is asked to bring all nail cosmetics and instruments to the exam as well as a list of medications and medical problems
4. Inform the patient that nails often grow slowly thus treatment may be slow to show positive results

Examination of the nails is often quite revealing. At a glance, well-kept nails versus bitten, dirty or unkept nails can give a significant first impression. On closer examination, the nails may act as a window into the body. To maximize proper examination, there are a number of important suggestions.

When the patient first calls for the appointment, he or she should be reminded that all 20 nails need to be examined, so that nail polish, lacquer (or other topical substances), pantyhose, etc. must be removed prior to examination. Furthermore, at this time inform the patient to bring all nail-care products to the appointment, whether cosmetic or instruments. A nail questionnaire may be mailed to the patient at this time. Before the doctor enters the examination room, the doctor's assistant should ensure that socks, shoes, etc. have been removed and that the nail questionnaire has been completed.

Adequate lighting without glare, natural sunlight being the preferred source, is a necessity when examining nails. All nail polish, lacquer, or other topical substances should be removed before examination. At times, the surface of the nail plate should be cleansed with a solvent such as alcohol or acetone, especially if a subtle change of the nail is being investigated. This may remove substances superficially adhering to the nail plate and will diminish glare. If this procedure or scraping the nail surface with a sharp object does not remove or diminish an apparently superficial nail plate abnormality, the examiner should suspect a deeper or more inherent process.

Be sure to examine all of the nails. The pattern of nail involvement must be considered in each patient. Frequently, if only one or very few nails are affected, local factors such as fungus, trauma, tumors, circulation, and so forth are to blame for the abnormality. Keep in mind, however, that this is not always the case and that there are few hard-and-fast rules governing examination of the nails. In addition, note the portion of the nail unit manifesting the abnormality. Periungual location, nail bed, matrix, and plate all have certain disorders more common to each area. Yet certain conditions, for example, trauma, psoriasis, or lichen planus, can affect only one or all parts of the nail unit concomitantly. Furthermore, as is discussed in later chapters, remember that the portion of the matrix affected often governs the site of clinical disease in different levels of the nail plate. The proximal portion of the matrix contributes mostly to the superficial nail plate and the distal portion mainly to the deeper nail plate.

When examining the nails, the patient's digits should be relaxed and not pressed against any surface. Failure to ensure this may alter the hemodynamics of the nail bed and change the appearance of the nails. If a subtle change in pigmentation is being examined, squeeze the tip of the digit to see if the appearance of the abnormality changes. In pigmented nail abnormalities, if a subtle vascular alteration is causative, it may be less visible with pressure on the nail unit.

Another clinical aid is a penlight. Shining a penlight up from distal digital pulp through the nail plate may be helpful. One should then observe the illuminated digit from all sides. This may help to localize an abnormality.

There are helpful rules to follow when examining nails for the effects of systemic disease or drugs and ingestants (see Chapter 16). Physical examination of the nail is sometimes all that is required to make the proper diagnosis. Most of the time, however, other information is needed and simple physical examination alone is not adequate. A thorough history with particular attention to disease chronology, occupation, topical substance exposure, medical history, family history, drug history, and so forth will usually aid in obtaining the proper diagnosis. A screening questionnaire given to the patient prior to examination is often helpful and may aid in pinpointing your investigation (Fig. 4.1).

If the history and physical examination have not revealed the diagnosis, other measures are available. Some of these include X-ray films, MRI, potassium hydroxide preparation, fungal cultures, bacterial cultures, nail biopsy with appropriate stains and microscopy, fluorescence with a black light if porphyria or tetracyclines are suspected as factors, exfoliative cytology, nail composition studies (as when looking for arsenic content), and immunological testing (for certain fungi).

After completing a proper history and physical examination, one should have a basic method of categorizing the problem. Again, there are no firm rules, and numerous classifications may overlap. Two general divisions separate conditions acquired after birth and familial or congenital problems. Here, too, there is some overlap because many dermatologic conditions, such as psoriasis, have associated hereditary factors. When assessing an acquired nail abnormality, mentally classify the problem according to the following categories:

1. predominantly dermatologic conditions
2. predominantly systemic disorders
3. systemic drugs
4. organisms (bacterial, fungal, viral, and so forth)
5. local or topical agents in the vicinity of the nail

**6.** tumors, either benign or malignant

**7.** physical agents

**8.** other.

Once this is done, proceed with the investigation.

YOUR NAME: _____ AGE: _____ SEX: _____ DATE: _____

NAIL QUESTIONNAIRE

1. Were you born with this problem?

   When did you first ever have a problem like this?

2. Which nails were affected first? (Place a * by these)

   Which are affected now? (Place a √ a by these)

3. How has this changed from beginning to now?

4. Describe your nails in general (hard, brittle, soft, etc.).

5. Have you ever traumatized any of the involved nails (stubbed your toe, hit the nail with a hammer, caught it in a door, etc.)?

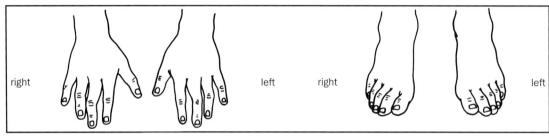

**FIGURE 4–1.** Screening questionnaire.

6. What kind of work do you do? Do you do anything to affect your nails or the tips of your fingers or toes?

   Contact with chemicals or irritants, such as strong soaps, hair straightener, lye, etc.?

   Hands or feet in water a lot?

   Hands or feet moist because of sweating or other reasons?

7. List hobbies in which you might traumatize or otherwise affect your nails (tennis, jogging, basketball, racquetball, painting, playing the piano, etc.).

8. Did you in the past or have you recently

   a. Pick at your nails?

   b. Bite or suck on your nails?

   c. Tear your nails off?

   d. Have ingrown nails?

   e. Wear tight or pointed-toe shoes?

   f. Push the cuticle back (how often?)

   g. Remember "runarounds" or swelling around cuticles?

9. Personal nail care

   a. List any nail cosmetics or conditioners that you use:

      1. Base coat

      2. Top coat

      3. Enamel

      4. Nail strengtheners

      5. Nail hardeners

      6. Cuticle treatment

      7. Gloss

      8. Nail conditioners

      9. Other

      10. Please bring any of these products with you on your next office visit, along with list of ingredients, if possible.

   b. List any instruments that you use to care for your nails.

      What do you do with these instruments?

      How often do you do this?

    c.   Do you go to a manicurist?

        How often?

        What is usually done to your nails?

    d.   Have you ever had the following? (If so, how often and when was the last time?)

        1.   Sculptured nails

        2.   False or artificial nails or "gel" nails or nail tips

        3.   Nail "wraps"

        4.   Acrylic nails

        5.   Other.

10.   Do you have any other skin or hair problems, or have you ever had any in the past?

    Lichen planus

    Psoriasis

    Ringworm

    "Jock itch"

    Athlete's foot

    Vaginal yeast infection or other yeast infection

    Other.

11.   List any medical problems that you have had in the past or have now (diabetes, heart trouble, thyroid problem, etc.).

12.   List any medications - prescription and non-prescription - that you have taken during the last year (sulfa, water pills, tetracycline, high-blood-pressure medicines, constipation medicine, chemotherapy, pain pills, vitamins, supplements, oral contraceptives, oral pills to help you tan, eye drops for glaucoma, pills for psoriasis therapy, retinoic acid, Neo-Synephrine, steroids, HIV treatment, etc.).

13.   What treatment (self and professional) have you had for your nail problem (past and present)?

    a.   List pills and dates used.

    b.   List topical treatments and dates used.

    c.   List surgical treatment and dates performed.

14.   Does anyone in your family have

    a.   Nail problems

    b.   Diabetes

    c.   Hair and skin problems (psoriasis, lichen planus, fungus, etc.)

    d.   Thyroid problems.

15.   What do you think is the cause of your nail problem?

# 5 Subungual Exostosis, Nail Disease and Radiologic Considerations

Harvey Lemont and Larry Goss

## Key Features

Subungual osteochondroma:
1. Seen in young females with chronic big toe paronychia, medial border usually involved
2. Order lateral and medial oblique radiographs of the toe to demonstrate flat-topped exostosis
3. Treatment of the paronychia requires either excision of exostosis or removal of border
4. Histology shows hyaline cartilage cap undergoing ossification

Subungual osteoarthritic exostosis:
1. Affects adults between 40 and 60 years old with dorsiflexed big toes
2. Patients exhibit pincer-shaped nails, which cause nail groove and subungual nail bed discomfort due to focal callus build-up
3. Order lateral radiographs to demonstrate pointed central exostosis
4. Conservative therapy is indicated, consisting of cutting the incurvated portions of the nail pate and debridement of subungual nail groove and subungual callus

By far the most common osseous lesion associated with nail disease is the subungual exostosis. Two distinct varieties exist, each making their appearance at different ages and exhibiting different clinical presentations. We have divided these lesions into two clinical–pathologic types: type 1 (subungual osteochondroma) and type 2 (subungual osteoarthritic spur) (Table 5.1).

## TYPE 1 (SUBUNGUAL OSTEOCHONDROMA)

These poorly understood bony proliferations are found most notably in the hallux and rarely in the fingers[1–3] and lesser toes.[4,5]

Described as early as 1847 by Dupuytren,[6] discrepancies regarding the pathology and natural history of these growths have appeared in the literature. Cytogenetic investigation of Dupuytren subungual exostosis has found a clonal abnormality suggesting that this particular heterotopic ossification may be neoplastic in nature rather than a purely reactive process or an exuberant growth in response to trauma. G-banded karyotypes showed four translocations involving a total of seven chromosomes.[7] An absolute consensus does not exist concerning whether this neoplasm originates from the bone itself or elsewhere, such as the reticular dermis. Some consider the lesion to represent a heterotopic ossification of soft tissue with a marked predilection to involve the great toe.[8] The term 'exostosis' in their opinion is a misnomer. It is their feeling that this lesion has nothing to do with osteochondroma as described in other bones of the body, which are true exostoses that exhibit continuity to the underlying bone. In possible support of that argument of heterotopic formation of the lesion, one can at times see signs of chondroid metaplasia to fibrous tissue within the reticular dermis above the hyaline cap in some cross sections of excised specimens (Figs 5.1 and 5.2).

Subungual osteochondroma is a cartilage capped osseous lesion, located usually at the medial mid-diaphyseal of the distal phalanx of the hallux (Fig. 5.3). Characteristically the clinical profile consists of a teenager or young adult who seeks care for a chronic parenchia. Commonly, the medial nail border is ingrown exhibiting granulation tissue (Fig. 5.4) or a pyogenic granuloma (Fig. 5.10). A common history is that the child has had this problem for months but either did not bring the problem to the parents' attention, or repeated removal of the ingrown toenail by a physician did occur, but the ingrown nail and infection consistently recurred. In this situation, radiographs usually establish the presence of an underlying subungual osteochondroma. While, an increased rounded density on dorso-plantar views provides a

TABLE 5–1. Comparison of type 1 (genetic subungual exostosis) and type 2 (acquired subungual exostosis)

| FACTOR | TYPE 1: GENETIC SUBUNGUAL EXOSTOSIS | TYPE 2: ACQUIRED SUBUNGUAL EXOSTOSIS |
|---|---|---|
| Paronychia | Frequent | Usually absent |
| Nail bed hypertrophy | Medial aspect of nail bed | Entire nail bed |
| Nail shape | Elevation of nail plate medially | Incurvation of medial and lateral aspects of nail plate |
| Accentuation of interphalangeal skin crease | Absent | Present |
| Age | Second and third decades of life | Fourth through to sixth decade of life |
| Location | Dorsomedial diaphysis | Distal dorsal and central ungual tuberosity |
| Histology | Hyaline or fibrous cartilage covering | No cartilage covering |
| Radiographic findings | Plateau or dome-shaped exostosis | Blunted or sharp protuberance |

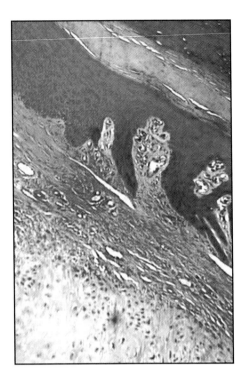

FIGURE 5-1. Cross-section of skin demonstrating the roof of an underlying osteochondroma within the dermis. H&E 20×.

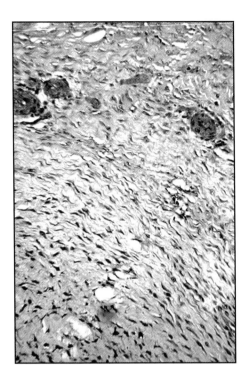

FIGURE 5-2. Skin section demonstrating chondroid metaplasia of fibrous tissue. H&E 40×.

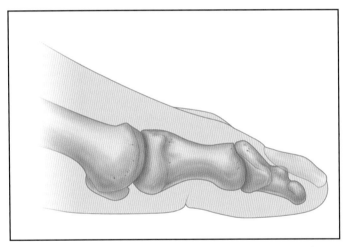

FIGURE 5-3. Diagram of lateral toe demonstrating mid-diaphyseal location of osteochondroma.

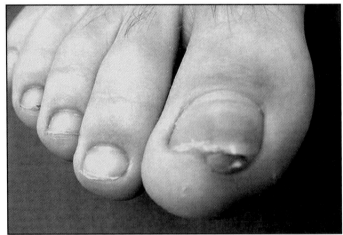

FIGURE 5-4. Child exhibiting paronychia with granulation tissue affecting the medial nail groove.

subtle radiologic clue suggesting subungual osteochondroma (Fig. 5.5), lateral radiographs of the toe are diagnostic demonstrating a characteristic plateau-shaped exostosis (Fig. 5.16, Fig. 5.17 and Fig. 5.18). Lesser digits may also be involved but lack this feature on radiographs (Fig. 5.14 and Fig. 5.15).

When these lesions are removed they tend to be smooth-surfaced and hard (Fig. 5.6). Most commonly, physicians preoperatively believe these lesions to be an epidermoid cyst and are often shocked when a pathology report of osteochondroma is received. Microscopic findings in an early osteochondroma consist of a circumscribed cap of large, immature chondrocytes (Fig. 5.7) Beneath this cartilaginous zone, gradual ossification of cartilage can be seen, characterized by immature, thin, elongated bone trabeculae situated within a vascular, loosely fibrous marrow.

While granulation tissue located at the medial nail border is common, it is not unusual to note the presence of granulation tissue or the presence of a pyogenic granuloma located centrally within the nail bed (Figs 5.8 and 5.9).

In older patients between the ages of 20 and 30, definite histologic confirmation of a subungual osteochondroma may not be easy because hyaline cartilage may already have undergone ossification with only fibrocartilage being seen (Figs 5.11 and 5.12). Alternatively, it might not be present at all because of prior complete ossification of cartilage to bone, with only fibrous tissue being noted (Fig. 5.13). Differentiation from an osteoarthritic spur at that stage may be difficult. In the absence of hyaline cartilage, the overall shape of the growth and the presence of immature bone is suggestive of an ossified osteochondroma.

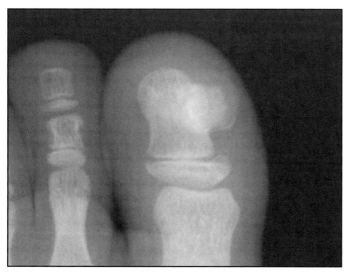

FIGURE 5–5. Radiographs of toe demonstrating medially located osseous tumor.

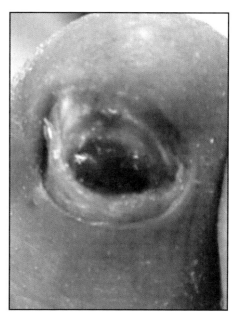

FIGURE 5–8. Pyogenic granuloma located in central nail bed.

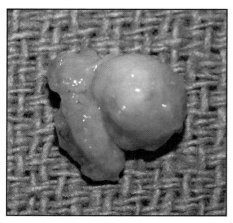

FIGURE 5–6. Circumscribed smooth-surfaced osteochondroma covered by nail bed epithelium.

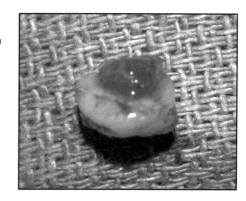

FIGURE 5–9. Pyogenic granuloma removed *en toto*.

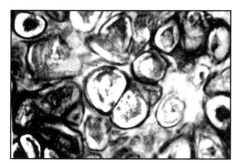

FIGURE 5–7. Note hyaline cartilage cap. Note large plump immature chondrocytes characteristic of a young osteochondroma. H&E 40×.

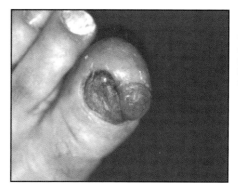

FIGURE 5–10. A red nodule around the nail unit in a child or young adult should alert the physican to the possibility of an underlying exostosis.

33

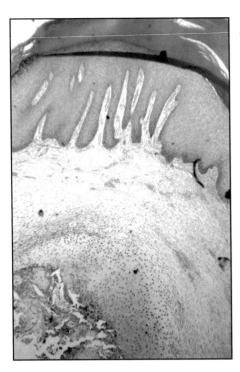

FIGURE 5-11. Mature osteochondroma noted to be extending up into the dermis capped primarily by fibrocartilage. H&E 10×.

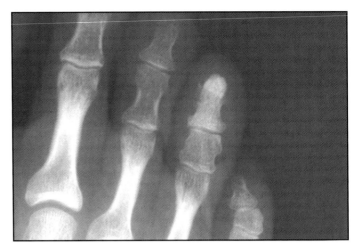

FIGURE 5-14. Third toe subungual osteochondroma exhibiting a sclerotic appearance on dorsal-plantar projection.

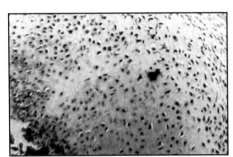

FIGURE 5-12. Cartilage capped by a zone of fibrocartilage. H&E 40×.

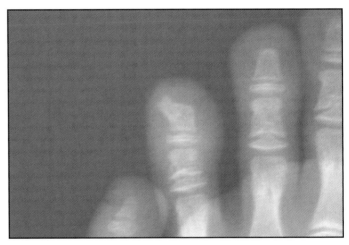

FIGURE 5-15. Fourth toe osteochondroma in a child.

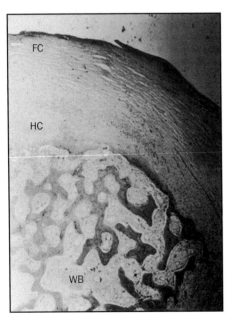

FIGURE 5.13. Osteochondroma demonstrating complete ossification with only fibrous tissue covering of bone surface. FC, fibrous cap, HC, hyaline cartilage; WB, woven bone. H&E 10×

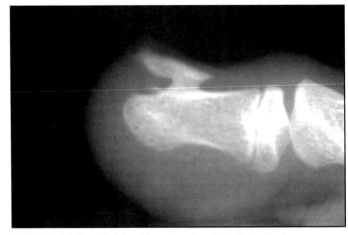

FIGURE 5-16. Characteristic, plateau-shaped exostosis diagnostic of osteochondroma. The tumor is seen extending up into the nail bed.

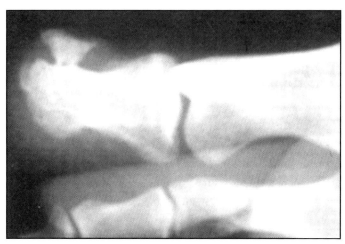

FIGURE 5–17. Subungual exostosis. Plateau-shaped exostosis is diagnostic of osteochondroma.

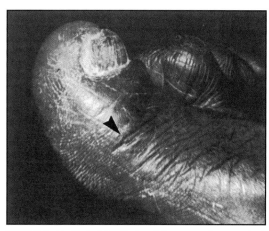

FIGURE 5–19. Marked dorsiflexion of the toe contributes to the formation of ungual osteoarthritic remodeling. Note accentuation of the dorsal–interphalangeal joint crease (arrowhead): a cutaneous skin marker for osteoarthritis of the first metatarsal–phalangeal joint, a contributing factor for toe extension.

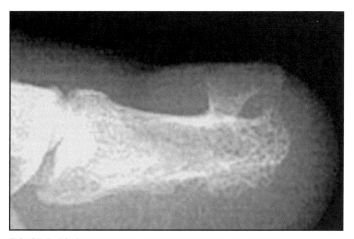

FIGURE 5–18. Osteochondroma on lateral view exhibiting plateau-shaped configuration.

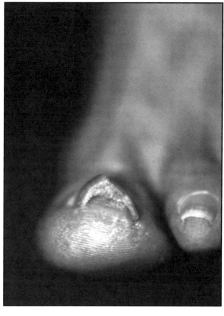

FIGURE 5–20. Pincer-type nail deformity due to nail plate and nail bed remodeling around an ungual tuft spur.

# TYPE 2 (SUBUNGUAL OSTEOARTHRITIC EXOSTOSIS)

Unlike type 1 subungual osteochondroma, type 2 osteoarthritic exostoses are seen later in life, between the fourth and sixth decades. The exostosis located at the distal, dorsal, and central aspect of the tuft of the distal phalanx results from excessive distal interphalangeal dorsiflexion and jamming of the big toe against the shoe. In our opinion, these exostoses commonly develop as a result of an abnormal positional relationship between the first metatarsal head and proximal phalanx of the hallux, resulting in loss of motion at that joint. In order to compensate for this lack of motion, the distal phalanx at the interphalangeal joint tends to compensate with excess dorsiflexion (Fig. 5.19). Remodeling of the ungual tuberosity and surrounding nail bed (Figs 5.20 and 5.21) creates the appearance of a pincer-type nail. Nail groove discomfort due to this incurvation is a common presenting complaint. Nail bed hypertrophy is also characteristic, with a build-up of focal painful hyperkeratosis occasionally being seen beneath the nail plate distally. Lateral radiographs reveal a sharp distal projection at the distal ungual tuft (Fig. 5.22). Microscopic evaluation of the spur reveals remodeling of the distal phalanx ungual tuft with extrusion of phalangeal bone noted distally and dorsally. The spur is covered by fibrous tissue and fibrocartilage, which represents an enthesis attachment site (Fig. 5.23).

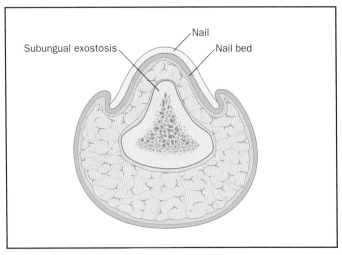

**FIGURE 5-21.** Diagram demonstrating mechanism for nail plate and nail bed remodeling around dorsal subungual exostosis.

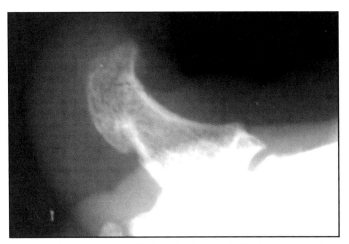

**FIGURE 5-22.** Extended toe exhibiting pointed osteoarthritic subungual exostosis.

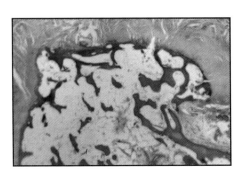

**FIGURE 5-23.** Photomicrograph of osteoarthritic spur covered by fibrocartilage, which represents an enthesis attachment site.

# REFERENCES

1. Matthewson MH. Subungual exostosis of the fingers. Are they really uncommon? Br J Dermatol 1978; 98:187
2. Bennett RG, Gammer S. Painful callus of the thumb due to phalangeal exostoses. Arch Dermatol 1973; 108: 826,1973
3. Lowenthal K. Subungual exostosis on a forefinger NY State J Med 1964; 64:2691
4. Chester SM, Balser RSW. Subungual exostosis. Am Podiatr Assoc 1978; 68:733
5. Cohen HJ, Frank SB, Minkin W, et al. Subungual exostosis. Arch Dermatol 1973; 107:431
6. Dupuytren G. On the injuries and diseases of the bones. London, Publications of the Sydenham Society, 1847; 20:408, cited by Zimmerman EH. Subungual exostosis. Cutis 1977; 19:185
7. Dal Cin P, Pauwels P, Poldermans LJ, et al. Clonal chromosome abnormalities in a so-called Dupuytren's subungual exostosis. Genes Chromosomes Cancer 1977; 24:162–164
8. Kilpatrick SE, Koplyay P, Pope TL, Ward WG. Clinical, radiologic, and pathologic spectrum of myositis ossificans and related lesions: a unifying concept. Adv Anat Pathol 1997; 5:277–282

# 6 Histopathology

## Suthep Jerasutus

A variety of skin diseases may involve the nails or the area around nails in the absence of cutaneous lesions. Nail biopsy is one investigation that not only provides etiologic, diagnostic, and prognostic information but also aids in improving understanding of the pathogenesis of nail diseases.

Knowledge of the histopathology of nail disease is much more limited than that of skin disease, not only because of its small number of biopsy specimens but also because of its distinct anatomic structures, which are more complex than those of the skin. Thus, close communication between the clinician and the pathologist is required regarding orientation and handling of the specimen for proper interpretation. The main problem with a small specimen, as is usually obtained from a nail unit biopsy, is the same as for a skin biopsy: proper orientation may be lost. Therefore, the clinician must mark the specimen and request the pathologist to cut it in a particular orientation; orientation can be important in histologic diagnosis.

Understanding pathologic processes in the nail, as in any organ, requires a thorough grounding in normal structure and function.

## HISTOLOGY OF THE NAIL UNIT

The nail unit consists of the nail plate and the four epithelial structures around and beneath it. Beginning proximally, the epithelial structures that can be seen on longitudinal section are the proximal nail fold, nail matrix, nail bed, and hyponychium. The proximal nail fold consists of both dorsal and ventral surface epithelia (Fig. 6.1). The dorsal surface is a continuation of the dorsal skin of the digit, containing sweat glands but no pilosebaceous units. The epidermis includes all four layers found in normal skin with its undulating rete ridge–dermal papilla pattern (Fig. 6.2). The ventral surface epithelium is also cornified and includes all four layers of the normal epidermis; however, it is quite thin and has neither a rete ridge–dermal papilla pattern nor epidermal appendages. The epithelium of the ventral surface of the proximal nail fold has also been called the 'eponychium'. The cornified layer at the ventral surface and at the tip of the proximal nail fold grows over the dorsal surface of the nail plate to constitute the cuticle (Fig. 6.3).

The nail matrix, the germinative epithelium, has no granular cell layer and consists mostly of matrix cells. The matrix epithelium is thick and has broad, club-shaped rete ridges that point downward and proximally (Figs 6.4 and 6.5). The proximal margin of the nail matrix is the ventral surface of the proximal nail fold; the distal margin is the nail bed. Melanocytes are present in the normal nail matrix and nail bed, although they differ from those elsewhere in the skin. They are poorly developed and fewer in number, whereas the proximal matrix contains a lower density of melanocytes

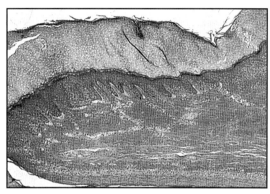

FIGURE 6-1. The proximal nail fold consists of two surfaces of epidermis: dorsal and ventral.

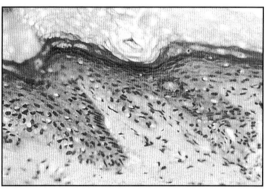

FIGURE 6-2. The dorsal surface of the proximal nail fold. Four layers can be recognized: (1) basal, (2) spinous, (3) granular, and (4) cornified. Note the presence of an intraepidermal eccrine duct.

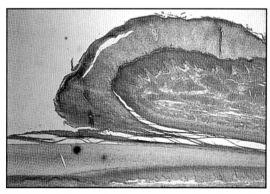

FIGURE 6-3. The ventral surface of the proximal nail fold cornifies by forming the cuticle, which extends over the dorsal surface of the nail plate.

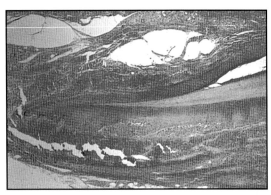

FIGURE 6-4. Junction between the nail matrix and the ventral proximal nail fold. The latter shows flat epithelium with a granular layer.

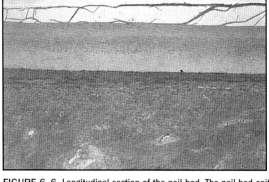

FIGURE 6-6. Longitudinal section of the nail bed. The nail bed epithelium is relatively thin, lies beneath the nail plate, and weakly stains with eosin.

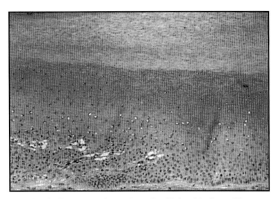

FIGURE 6-5. Nail matrix consists of a thick epithelium with no granular layer. Note the keratogenous zone, lined by keratinocytes with dark, small nuclei and eosinophilic cytoplasm, between the nail matrix and the nail plate.

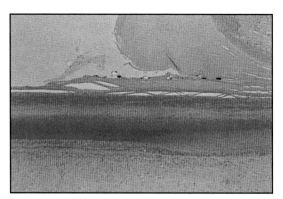

FIGURE 6-7. The nail plate is strongly positive with acid-fast stains.

than the distal matrix.[1,2] The difference in number of melanocytes probably exists because these melanocytes are protected from ultraviolet stimulation by the proximal nail fold. The nail plate contains melanin by melanosome transfer from these melanocytes to the differentiating matrix cells.[1] Nail pigment is quite common in Blacks and quite rare in Whites. Langerhans' cells and rare Merkel cells have also been identified in the matrix.[1] The lunula – the white, halfmoon area – corresponds with the keratogenous zone, which consists of epithelial cells with flattened nuclei and eosinophilic cytoplasm[3] (see Fig. 6.5). These keratogenous zone cells lose their nuclei and form the nail plate cells, or onychocytes.

The nail plate consists of closely packed cornified cells arranged in lamellae that stain weakly with eosin and strongly with acid-fast stains (Figs 6.6 and 6.7). The dorsal surface of the nail plate is smooth but the ventral surface is irregular, as demonstrated by electron microscopy. The nail plate is approximately 0.5 mm thick; the nail plate over the lunula is thinner than that over the nail bed.

The nail bed epithelium lies beneath the nail plate and is bordered proximally by the nail matrix and distally by the hyponychium. The epithelium of the nail bed has no granular cell layer, relatively thin epithelium, in sagittal section, and few parakeratotic cells (Figs 6.6 and 6.8). The parakeratotic cells of the nail bed tightly adhere to the undersurface of the nail plate and move forward as the nail plate grows toward the distal groove. The nail bed, in transverse sections, is firmly attached to the underlying dermis by long, narrow epithelial rete ridges that are interlocked

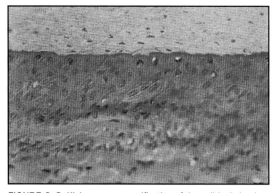

FIGURE 6-8. Higher power magnification of the nail bed showing a thin layer of parakeratotic cells and no granular layer.

with dermal papilla, forming regular longitudinal folds along the nail bed (Fig. 6.9).

The hyponychium is a narrow zone of epidermis beneath the free edge of the nail plate and between the nail bed and distal nail groove. The hyponychium cornifies like volar skin (i.e. it produces a granular cell layer and a thick, compact cornified layer) (Fig. 6.10).

The dermis of the nail unit is highly vascular and is supplied by digital arteries. In addition, there are numerous glomus bodies, which function as special arteriovenous shunts to regulate the temperature of the digits (Figs 6.11 to 6.13). Nerve endings and

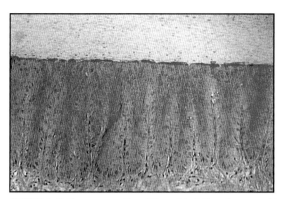

FIGURE 6–9. Transverse section of the nail bed. Note the serrated interdigitating nail bed epithelium and dermal papillae.

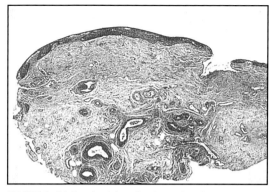

FIGURE 6–11. Dermis of the nail unit, a region characterized by prominent blood vessels and neural structures devoid of epithelial adnexa.

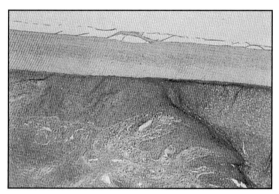

FIGURE 6–10. Hyponychium. It is composed of all four layers of the epidermis, with a thick, compact, cornified layer as volar skin.

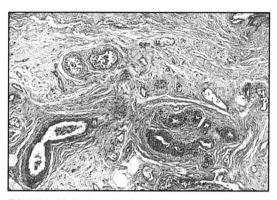

FIGURE 6–12. The lower dermis, which is composed of thin, loosely arranged collagen fibers in contrast to superficial dermis. Note the abundant blood vessels and glomus bodies.

nerve trunks are also numerous, with special nerve structures such as Meissner's corpuscles and Vater–Pacini corpuscles. There are no adnexal epithelial structures in the ventral surface of the proximal nail fold, nail matrix, nail bed, and hyponychium. **The dermis of the nail unit lies directly on the phalanx without subcutaneous fat tissue.** The upper reticular dermis is composed of thick collagen bundles primarily arranged parallel to the skin surface, whereas in the lower reticular dermis the collagen fibers are thin and loosely arranged. Proportionally, there are more plump fibroblasts and ground substance in the lower reticular dermis. Infrequently, lipocytes can be found within the deep dermis.

# EMBRYOLOGY: HISTOLOGIC ASPECTS

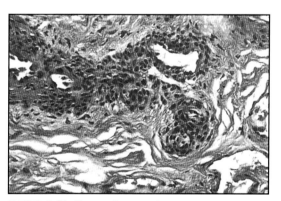

FIGURE 6–13. Glomus cells surrounding arterioles and venules of special shunts; known as glomus bodies.

At the gestational age of 7 to 8 weeks, the epidermis of the digits consists of a single layer of epithelium, whereas the dermis is composed of abundant undifferentiated mesenchymal cells (Fig. 6.14). Numerous mitotic figures are present in both the epithelial and mesenchymal components. Fetal cartilage is also present at this stage (Fig. 6.15).

The nail unit first appears at about 9 weeks gestation. The invagination of the surface epithelium forms the proximal, lateral, and distal grooves. The area outlined by these grooves is termed the nail field (Fig. 6.16A). The surface epithelium of the nail field is more developed than the surrounding epithelium and consists of

multiple epithelial cell layers, including a granular cell layer (Fig. 6.16B). Along the proximal groove, there is a wedge of epithelial cells – the matrix primordium – growing downward proximally to form the precursor of the nail matrix and the ventral surface of the proximal nail fold. Endochondral ossification and cartilage are present at this stage (Fig. 6.17).

At 15 weeks gestation, the matrix primordium differentiates and separates into two components. The upper component forms the ventral surface of the proximal nail fold, whereas the lower component forms the nail matrix. The rete ridges and eccrine sweat

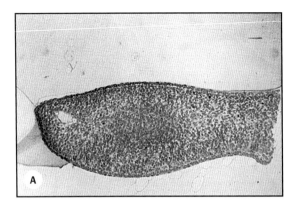

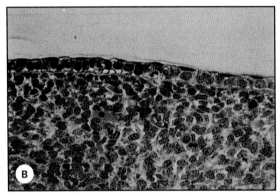

FIGURE 6-14. A and B, Longitudinal section of finger at 7 weeks gestation consisting of a single layer of epithelium and dermis with abundant undifferentiated mesenchymal cells.

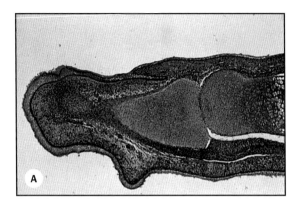

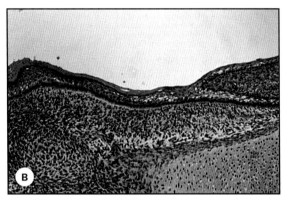

FIGURE 6-16. A and B, Longitudinal section of finger at 9 weeks gestation. Note the matrix primordium, which grows downward proximally at the nail field.

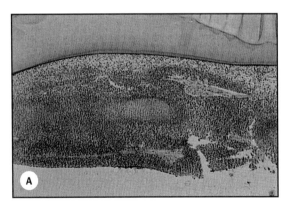

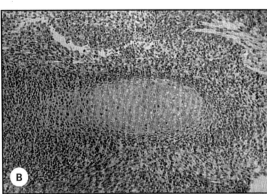

FIGURE 6-15. A and B, Longitudinal section of finger at 8 weeks gestation. In this stage, formation of fetal cartilage appears in the mesenchymal tissues.

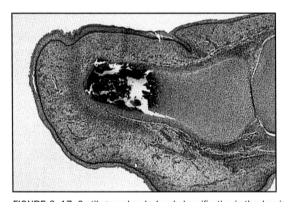

FIGURE 6-17. Cartilage and endochondral ossification in the dermis at 10 weeks gestation.

primordial are also developed in the dermis of volar epithelium at this stage (Fig. 6.18).

When the fetus reaches 20 weeks of gestational age, the nail unit is virtually complete. The nail matrix produces mature onychocytes, which can be demonstrated with sulfhydryl stains. The nail plate grows along the surface of the nail bed from the proximal nail fold toward the distal groove, whereas its lateral surfaces are bordered by the lateral nail folds. The nail unit of the toes develops in the same manner as the nail unit of the fingers, but the development occurs more slowly.

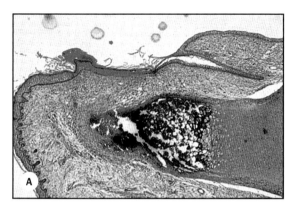

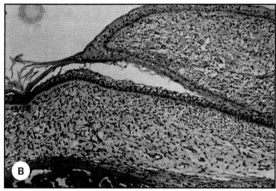

FIGURE 6–18. A and B, Longitudinal section of finger at 15 weeks gestation. Formation of nail matrix and ventral portion of the proximal nail fold occurs by separation of the matrix primordium.

## HISTOPATHOLOGY OF NAIL DISEASES

A number of diseases affect the skin and nail unit. Some of them may occur only as changes in the nails; therefore, a nail biopsy is often required for diagnosis. The histologic changes in the nail unit are usually similar to those in the skin, but some findings are rather specific to the nail.

When doing nail biopsies when one suspects an inflammatory disorder, do not remove the nail plate beforehand as this may remove diagnostic structures.

## Psoriasis

Nail involvement in psoriasis is quite common; varying from 10 to 50% of cases.[4,5] Psoriasis involving only the nail unit is not uncommon. However, it is slightly more difficult to diagnose

clinically on the basis of the nail changes alone. The histologic study may, therefore, be necessary to confirm the clinical diagnosis.

Nail psoriasis has the same pathogenesis as skin psoriasis, but the clinical manifestations are quite different from the skin lesions, namely pitting and other nail plate abnormalities, discoloration of the nail bed, subungual hypekeratosis, onycholysis, and splinter hemorrhages (Table 6.1).

Psoriasis can involve any part of the nail unit and cause a variety of clinical and pathologic manifestations. The majority of changes can be observed in and under the nail plates.

Psoriatic involvement of the proximal nail matrix causes pitting and a rough-surfaced nail plate. The histology of nail pitting reveals foci of parakeratotic cells in the upper portion of the nail plate. When the parakeratotic cells fall off, they produce pits on the dorsal nail plates (Fig. 6.19). Psoriatic involvement of the middle and distal nail matrix produces a smooth-surfaced leukonychia that histologically reveals foci of parakeratotic cells in the deeper portion of the nail plates. It may also produce focal onycholysis.

Psoriasis of the nail bed results in a discoloration of the nail bed, subungual hyperkeratosis, onycholysis, and splinter hemorrhages. The nail biopsy in psoriasis is usually taken from the nail bed and nail plate. Psoriasis of the nail bed and skin has many histologic features in common, among them neutrophils in the epidermis, psoriasiform hyperplasia, and a superficial infiltrate of lymphocytes and neutrophils around widely dilated capillaries and venules (Figs 6.20 and 6.21). However, some features of psoriasis of the nail bed differ from those of psoriasis of the skin (see Table 6.1). Nail bed psoriasis shows more spongiosis and hyperplasia in the epidermis and more serum accumulation in the cornified layer than does skin psoriasis. The prominent granular cell layer, a feature not usually

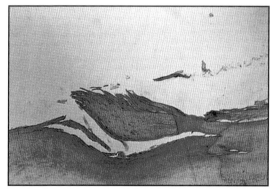

FIGURE 6–19. Pitting nail, evolving lesion. Small clusters of parakeratotic cells are shed from the surface of nail plate. This lesion has evolved into pitting nail.

| TABLE 6–1. Manifestations of psoriasis in the nails and skin | |
| --- | --- |
| **NAIL PSORIASIS** | **SKIN PSORIASIS** |
| Mild to moderate hyperkeratosis | Marked hyperkeratosis |
| Hypergranulosis not unusual | Hypergranulosis unusual |
| Serum globules in cornified layer usual | Serum globules in cornified layer unusual |
| Hemorrhage in the cornified layer usual | Hemorrhage in the cornified layer unusual |
| Papillomatous epidermal hyperplasia common (transverse section) | Papillomatous epidermal hyperplasia uncommon |
| Spongiosis common | Spongiosis uncommon |

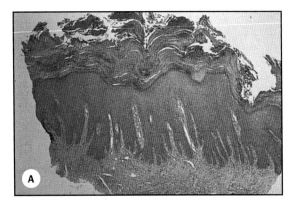

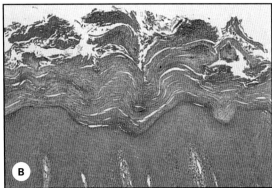

FIGURE 6–20. A and B, Nail psoriasis. The diagnostic features are focal parakeratosis admixed with neutrophils, psoriasiform epidermal hyperplasia, superficial perivascular lymphocytic infiltrate, and dilated tortuous capillaries in the papillary dermis.

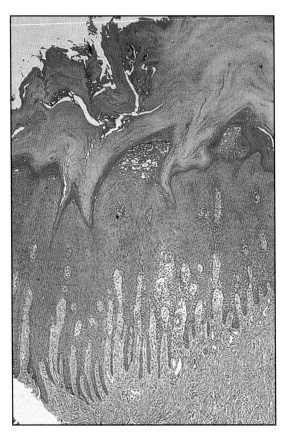

FIGURE 6–22. Nail psoriasis (low-power magnification). One observes hyperkeratosis, spongiosis, acanthosis, and papillomatosis.

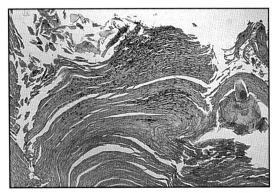

FIGURE 6–21. Nail psoriasis (high-power magnification of Figure 6.20). Tiers of neutrophils within mounds of parakeratosis are diagnostic of active lesions.

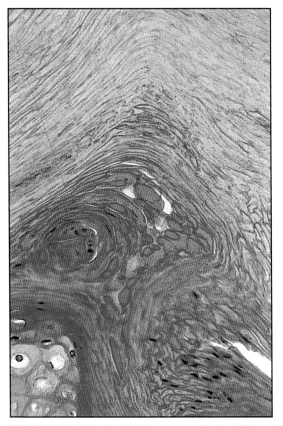

FIGURE 6–23. Nail psoriasis (high-power magnification of Figure 6.22). Scaly crusts lie in the thickened cornified layer.

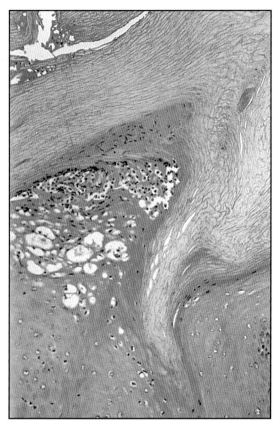

FIGURE 6–24. Nail psoriasis (high-power magnification of Figure 6.22). Neutrophils within epidermis in spongiform are important diagnostic features of acute stage. Note a small area of hemorrhage in the thickened, cornified layers.

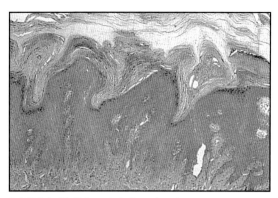

FIGURE 6–26. Nail psoriasis. Foci of parakeratosis, acanthosis, papillomatosis, and dilated tortuous capillaries are features of chronic lesion.

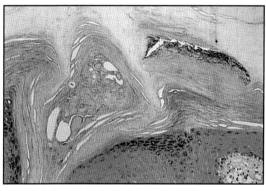

FIGURE 6–27. Nail psoriasis (high-power magnification of Figure 6.26). Neutrophils within mounds of parakeratosis, scaly crusts, and hypergranulosis are common features in nail psoriasis.

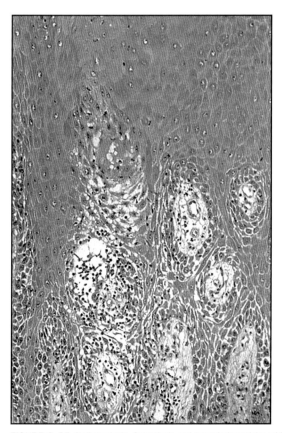

FIGURE 6–25. Nail psoriasis. Spongiosis and spongiotic vesicles within epidermis are common features in nail psoriasis.

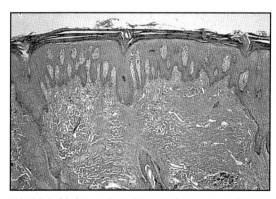

FIGURE 6–28. Skin psoriasis. Diagnostic features are confluent parakeratosis, hypogranulosis, psoriasiform epidermal hyperplasia, dilated tortuous capillaries, and perivascular lymphocytic infiltrate.

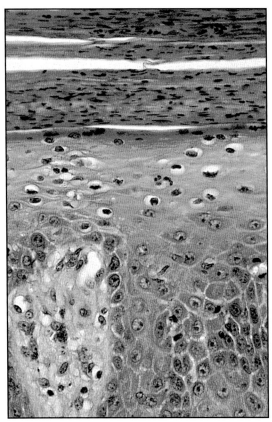

FIGURE 6–29. Skin psoriasis (high-power magnification of Figure 6.28). Note the neutrophils within confluent parakeratosis and epidermis with absence of granular layer.

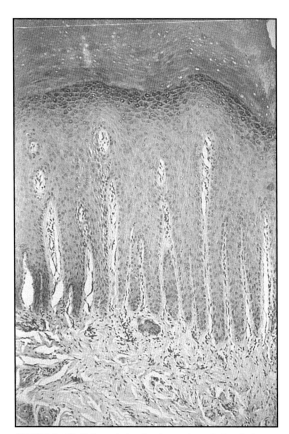

FIGURE 6–30. Nail psoriasis; chronic, persistent lesion. It shows compact hyperkeratosis, hypergranulosis, psoriasiform epidermal hyperplasia with thin, elongated rete ridges and dilated tortuous capillaries.

seen in normal nail bed or skin psoriasis, is usually present in nail psoriasis (Figs 6.22 to 6.29).

In late lesions of psoriatic nails, there is an absence of neutrophils in the cornified layer. However, these lesions can be diagnosed as psoriasis because of the psoriasiform hyperplasia with thin, elongated rete ridges, thin suprapapillary plates, and dilated, tortuous capillaries in the papillary dermis. Lichen simplex chronicus is often superimposed on old lesions of psoriatic nails, especially when there is partial or complete absence of the nail plate secondary to persistent rubbing and picking of the nail bed and hyponychium. These lesions are also characterized by compact orthokeratosis, hypergranulosis, and coarse collagen in vertical streaks in a thickened papillary dermis (Figs 6.30 and 6.31).

Onycholysis results from psoriatic involvement of the nail bed and hyponychium. Histologic study of the nail plate of onycholytic nails shows mounds of parakeratosis containing neutrophils in the subungual cornified layer, and the separation is actually between the layer of neutrophils containing the parakeratotic horn of the nail bed and hyponychium, not between the nail bed and nail plate (Figs 6.32 and 6.33).

Reiter's syndrome and psoriasis have the same histologic changes.

## Lichen Planus

Nail involvement occurs in approximately 10% of lichen planus cases and may occur without skin or mucous membrane involvement.[6] The nail changes in lichen planus are not necessarily pathognomonic for the disease. Severe involvement of the nail unit

can produce permanent damage; therefore, early nail biopsy is necessary to make a specific diagnosis and institute appropriate therapy to prevent sequelae.

Lichen planus of the nail unit has many features in common with that of the skin, among them hyperkeratosis, hypergranulosis, irregular epidermal hyperplasia, necrotic keratinocytes (Civatte bodies – round, homogeneous eosinophilic bodies resulting from necrotic keratinocytes), vacuolar alteration, dense lichenoid lymphohistiocytic infiltrate with melanophages in the upper dermis that obscures the dermal-epidermal interface, and coarse collagen bundles in a thickened papillary dermis (Figs 6.34 and 6.35). By contrast, lichen planus of the nail unit has certain histologic features that differentiate it from lichen planus of the skin (Table 6.2). The compact hyperkeratosis of the cornified layer in nail lichen planus is usually associated with focal parakeratosis or scaly crust, but the same is not true of skin lichen planus. Hypergranulosis of skin lichen planus is situated focally in an otherwise normal granular cell layer, whereas that of nail lichen planus tends to be diffuse (Figs 6.34 to 6.41). In addition, in the late lesion of nail lichen planus, fibrosis occurs more prominently in the upper dermis, and may result in permanent atrophy and scarring (Figs 6.43 to 6.47). In contrast, in skin lichen planus, postinflammatory pigmentary alteration and slight fibrosis result (Fig 6.42).

## Onychomycosis

The nail changes in onychomycosis sometimes cannot be distinguished clinically or histologically from other nail diseases; therefore, potassium hydroxide (KOH) preparation and fungus

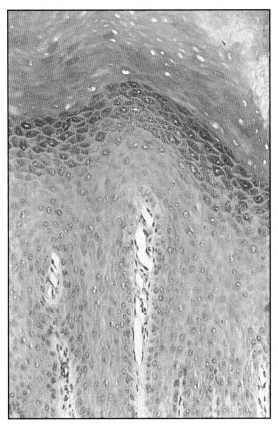

FIGURE 6–31. Nail psoriasis (high-power magnification of Figure 6.30). Note the compact orthokeratosis, hypergranulosis, thin suprapapillary plates and dilated tortuous capillaries, and absence of neutrophils within the epidermis.

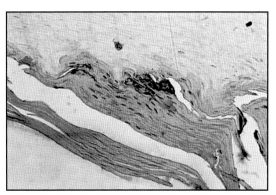

FIGURE 6–33. Psoriatic onycholysis (high-power magnification of Figure 6.32) demonstrates neutrophils within mounds of parakeratosis. Separation occurs between cells in the parakeratotic nail bed.

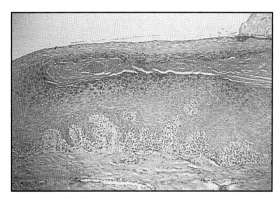

FIGURE 6–34. Nail lichen planus. Diagnostic features seen in this photomicrograph include orthokeratosis, hypergranulosis, epidermal hyperplasia, and lichenoid infiltrate of lymphocytes that obscure the dermoepidermal junction.

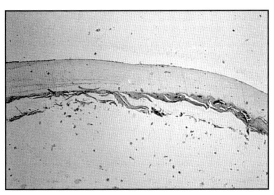

FIGURE 6–32. Psoriatic onycholysis. It demonstrates mounds of parakeratosis in the undersurface of the nail plate.

culture are often used to confirm the clinical diagnosis. Scrapings of the nail specimen are usually too superficial because the spores and hyphae of fungi are characteristically located in the cornified layer of the nail bed or the deep portion of the nail plate, resulting in negative cultures and KOH preparations (Fig. 6.48A and B). Norton found 50% of infected nails to have negative results on KOH preparation and fungus culture.[7] Hence, nail biopsy is warranted to demonstrate fungus in such culture-negative cases. Furthermore, a biopsy can also be helpful in the decision as to whether a nondermatophytic fungus cultured from an abnormal nail is a pathogen or merely a contaminant.

The histologic diagnosis of onychomycosis is based on the clinical types of distal and proximal subungual onychomycosis, necessitating the presence of spores and hyphae in the cornified

| TABLE 6–2. Histologic features of lichen planus in nails and skin | |
| --- | --- |
| **NAIL LICHEN PLANUS** | **SKIN LICHEN PLANUS** |
| Marked compact orthokeratosis and focal parakeratosis | Slight to moderate compact orthokeratosis |
| Scaly crust in cornified layer common | Scaly crust in cornified layer uncommon |
| Diffuse hypergranulosis | Wedge-shaped hypergranulosis |
| Marked fibrosis in the papillary and reticular dermis | Slight fibrosis in the papillary dermis |
| May resolve with scar | Usually resolves without scar |

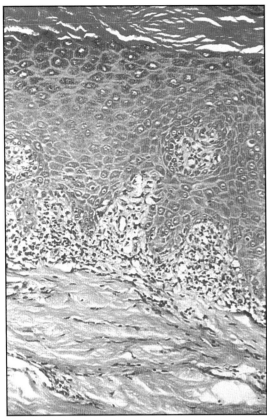

FIGURE 6–35. Nail lichen planus (high-power magnification of Figure 6.34). Several features are evident: compact orthokeratosis; diffuse hypergranulosis, irregular epidermal hyperplasia, with jagged sawtooth appearance of the rete; vacuolar alteration; and lichenoid infiltrate of lymphocytes.

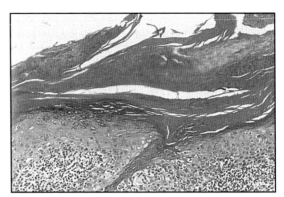

FIGURE 6–38. Nail lichen planus. Note the presence of scaly crusts in the cornified layer.

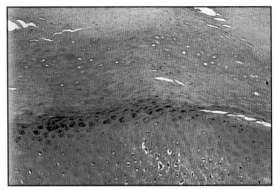

FIGURE 6–37. Nail lichen planus (high-power magnification of Figure 6.41). Note the presence of focal parakeratosis in the thickened, cornified layer and diffuse hypergranulosis.

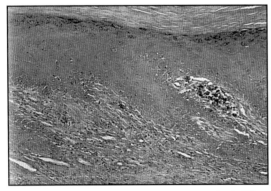

FIGURE 6–36. Nail lichen planus, old lesion. This lesion is differentiated from the early ones by less lichenoid infiltrate of lymphocytes with numerous melanophages in the thickened papillary dermis in addition to hyperkeratosis and hypergranulosis.

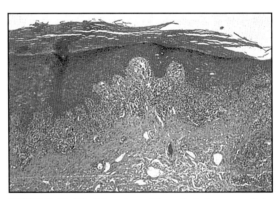

FIGURE 6–39. Skin lichen planus. Diagnostic features are orthokeratosis, focal hypergranulosis, irregular epidermal hyperplasia, and lichenoid infiltrate of lymphocytes that obscure the dermoepidermal junction.

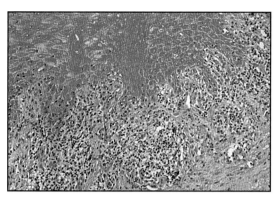

FIGURE 6–40. Skin lichen planus (high-power magnification of Figure 6.39). Irregular epidermal hyperplasia with jagged sawtooth appearance of the rete, lichenoid infiltrate of lymphocytes, and melanophages are evident.

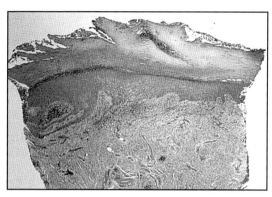

FIGURE 6–43. Nail lichen planus, resolving lesion. This lesion is differentiated from a fully developed lesion by having flattened rete ridges, sparse rather than dense band-like infiltrate of lymphocytes, and considerable fibrosis of the upper dermis.

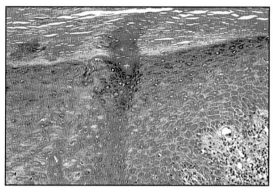

FIGURE 6–41. Skin lichen planus (high-power magnification of Figure 6.40). Compact orthokeratosis and wedge-shaped hypergranulosis are evident.

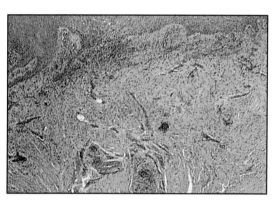

FIGURE 6–44. Nail lichen planus, resolving lesion (high-power magnification of Figure 6.43). A sparse, band-like infiltrate of lymphocytes with marked fibrosis in the thickened papillary dermis and upper reticular dermis is evident.

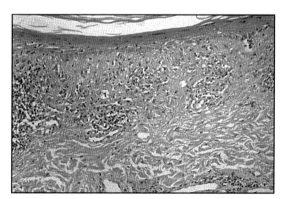

FIGURE 6–42. Skin lichen planus, resolving lesion. Note thinned epidermis, mild lichenoid lymphocytic infiltrate, and fibrosis in the thickened papillary dermis.

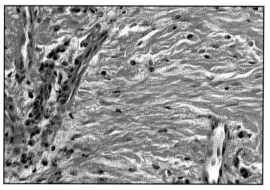

FIGURE 6–45. Nail lichen planus, resolving lesion (high-power magnification of Figure 6.44). Note that fibroblasts and collagen fibers are oriented parallel to the skin surface, whereas thick-walled vessels run perpendicular to it.

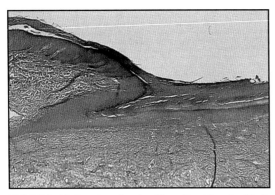

FIGURE 6–46. Pterygium. Atrophy of the nail matrix and nail bed epithelium devoid of rete ridges and scar in the underlying dermis is evident.

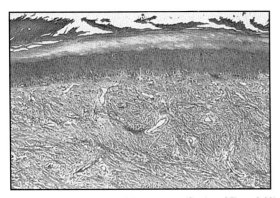

FIGURE 6–47. Pterygium (high-power magnification of Figure 6.46). Scar in the dermis is composed of scattered fibroblasts, altered collagen, and blood vessels.

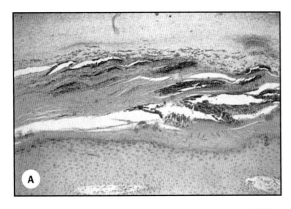

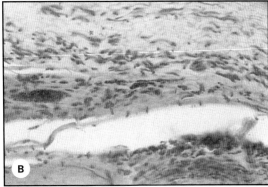

FIGURE 6–48. A and B, Subungual onychomycosis. Section demonstrates numerous hyphae in the thickened, cornified layer of the nail bed and lower nail plate.

layer of the nail bed, the deep portion of the nail plate, or the hyponychium for accurate diagnosis. In the absence of fungal elements, the diagnosis of psoriasis must be considered.

Dermatophyosis and subungual onychomycosis have many histologic features in common, namely hyperkeratosis containing neutrophils, spongiosis, epidermal hyperplasia, and a lymphocytic infiltrate with occasional neutrophils in the papillary dermis (Figs 6.49 to 6.58). However, some features of subungual onychomycosis differ from those of dermatophytosis. In contrast to dermatophytosis, onychomycosis tends to have marked hyperkeratosis often associated with plasma in scaly crust and small collections of blood clots (Table 6.3).

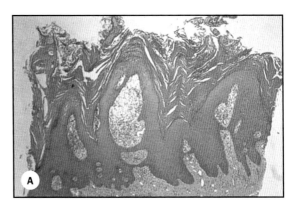

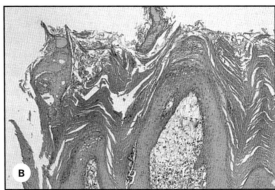

FIGURE 6–49. A and B, Subungual onychomycosis, acute lesion. Histologic changes show hyperkeratosis, spongiosis, acanthosis, papillomatosis, edema of the papillary dermis, and dense superficial perivascular infiltrate of lymphocytes and neutrophils that cannot be differentiated from nail psoriasis.

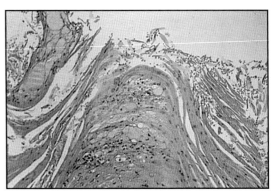

FIGURE 6–50. Subungual onychomycosis (high-power magnification of Figure 6.49). Scaly crusts and neutrophils within epidermis in spongiform are evident.

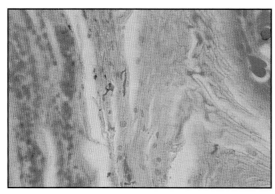

FIGURE 6-51. Subungual onychomycosis. Periodic acid-Schiff stain reveals hyphae that may not be easily discerned with hematoxylin and eosin stain.

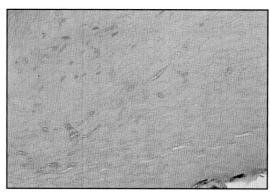

FIGURE 6-54. Subungual onychomycosis (high-power magnification of Figure 6.53). Numerous hyphae can be seen in orthokeratotic portion of cornified layer.

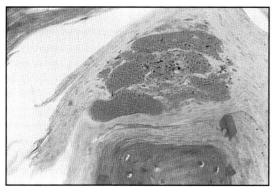

FIGURE 6-52. Subungual onychomycosis. Note the area of hemorrhage in the thickened, cornified layer that is not uncommon in onychomycosis.

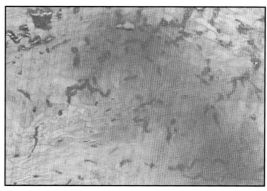

FIGURE 6-55. Subungual onychomycosis. Numerous hyphae are easily discerned with periodic acid-Schiff stain.

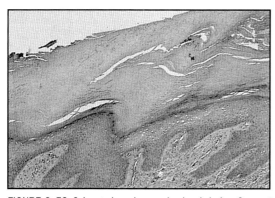

FIGURE 6-53. Subungual onychomycosis, chronic lesion. Compact hyperkeratosis, hypergranulosis, acanthosis, papillomatosis, and a sparse superficial perivascular infiltrate of lymphocytes are characteristic features.

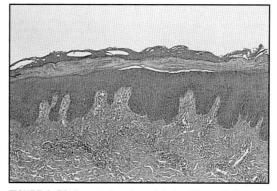

FIGURE 6-56. Dermatophytosis, scaly lesion. Diagnostic features are confluent parakeratosis beneath normal orthokeratosis, acanthosis, and dense perivascular infiltrate of lymphocytes and neutrophils.

| TABLE 6-3. Subungual onychomycosis versus dermatophytosis | |
| --- | --- |
| **ONYCHOMYCOSIS** | **DERMATOPHYTOSIS** |
| Marked hyperkeratosis | Slight to moderate hyperkeratosis |
| Hyphae present in compact horn | Hyphae present between basketweave horn and compact horn or between orthokeratosis and parakeratosis (sandwich sign) |
| Scaly crust common | Scaly crust uncommon |
| Papillomatous epidermal hyperplasia common (transverse section) | Papillomatous epidermal hyperplasia uncommon |
| Extravasated erythrocytes usually in cornified layer | Extravasated erythrocytes usually in papillary dermis |

The nondermatophytic fungi are often causative agents of distal subungual onychomyosis of the toenails. Histologically, nondermatophytic onychomycosis is diagnosed when it shows invasion of fungal elements in the nail plate, with the typical histologic picture of onychomycosis in the nail bed and nail plate.

The histologic findings of superficial white onychomycosis reveal hyphae of dermatophytes or nondermatophytic fungi in the superficial portion of the nail plate, whereas the underlying nail bed is normal (Figs. 6.59 to 6.61). Furthermore, *Candida albicans* is a common cause of onycholysis and can be distinguished from psoriasis. The separation in candidal onycholysis occurs between the lytic nail plate and the nail bed, with organisms present in the fragment of the lytic nail plate and the cornified layer of the nail bed (Fig. 6.62).

Since onychomycosis is responsible for about 50% of nail visits to the doctor, if enough tissue is available an biopsy PAS stains should be done on all nail biopsies.

## Pityriasis Rubra Pilaris

Nail changes are seen in many of the disorders in the differential diagnosis of type I pityriasis rubra pilaris and include distal

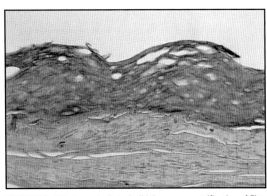

FIGURE 6-57. Dermatophytosis (high-power magnification of Figure 6.56). Hyphae at the junction between orthokeratosis and parakeratosis (sandwich sign) are evident.

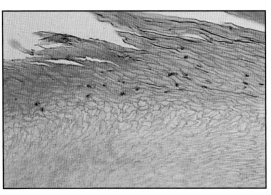

FIGURE 6-60. White superficial onychomycosis (high-power magnification of Figure 6.59). Hyphae of dermatophytes within the dorsal nail plate (periodic acid-Schiff stain) are evident.

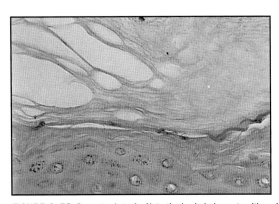

FIGURE 6-58. Dermatophytosis. Note the hyphal elements with periodic acid-Schiff stain.

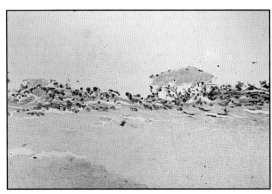

FIGURE 6-61. White superficial onychomycosis. Fungus consists of round, eroding bodies and hyphae of nondermatophytic fungi seen in the dorsal nail plate.

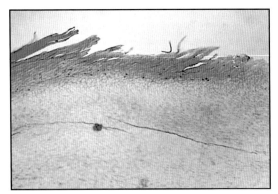

FIGURE 6-59. White superficial onychomycosis. Note the rough and irregular surface of the dorsal nail plate.

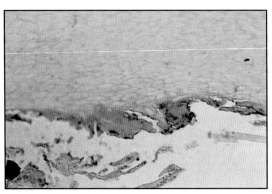

FIGURE 6-62. Candida onycholysis. Note hyphae and yeast within lytic nail plate and clusters of cornified cells at the undersurface of the nail plate.

yellow–brown discoloration, subungual hyperkeratosis, nail plate thickening, and splinter hemorrhages. Histology from a nail biopsy demonstrates patchy parakeratosis in the nail plate and cornified layers of nail bed. The epithelium of the nail bed is slightly thickened. Granular cell layers are intermittently present. The dermal vessels are dilated in some areas but are not abnormally tortuous. A sparse perivascular infiltrate of lymphocytes is seen in the papillary dermis. These changes are more prominent in the nail bed than in the nail matrix. Orthokeratosis and parakeratosis are present at the hyponychium.[8]

## Nail clippings

When dermatologists are reluctant to perform a nail biopsy because of fear of causing permanent nail dystrophy, a nail plate clipping should be obtained. This technique is simple, noninvasive, and effective for the diagnosis of distal subungual onychomycosis and psoriatic nail. The histologic findings of psoriatic nails from nail plate clippings include thick and confluent or mounds of parakeratosis with the nuclei of cells showing thin, elongated pyknosis arranged in dense aggregates. The parakeratotic cells are admixed with neutrophils (Fig. 6.63). Small pustules with a well-circumscribed collection of degenerated neutrophils and their exudate might be observed (Fig. 6.64). The histology of onycho-mycosis is indistinguishable from that of psoriasis except for the presence of a fungal element within the cornified layer of the nail bed or lower portion of the nail plate (Figs 6.65 and 6.66). The nail change of pityriasis rubra pilaris is focal parakeratosis and

orthokeratosis, horizontally and vertically, in the thick cornified layer of the nail bed (Fig. 6.67A and B). Idiopathic onycholysis usually shows a jagged sawtooth appearance of the undersurface of the nail plate when clusters of cornified cells have been shed (see Fig. 6.68).

## Spongiotic Trachyonychia

Trachyonychia is a morphologic manifestation that can occur in different conditions. Definitive diagnosis of the specific disease that causes trachyonychia requires a pathologic examination of the nail and cannot be determined clinically.

This clinicopathologic entity is characterized by thin, rough, friable, and opalescent nail plates, with excessive longitudinal

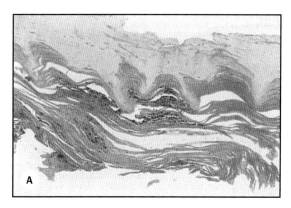

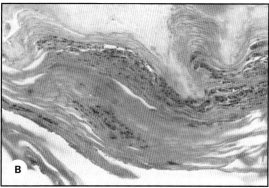

FIGURE 6–65. A and B, Onychomycosis. Mounds of parakeratosis containing neutrophils should prompt a search for fungi.

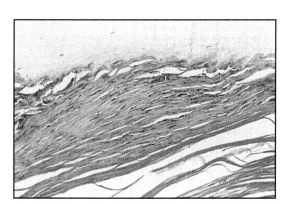

FIGURE 6–63. Psoriatic nail. Characteristic features are mounds of parakeratosis containing neutrophils and absence of hyphae beneath the nail plate.

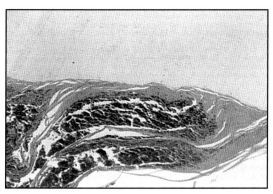

FIGURE 6–64. Psoriatic nail. Well-circumscribed intracorneal pustules are not uncommon findings in psoriasis.

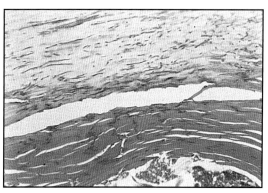

FIGURE 6–66. Onychomycosis. Periodic acid-Schiff stain demonstrates numerous hyphae in the cornified layer of the nail bed and the ventral nail plate.

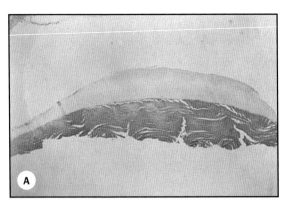

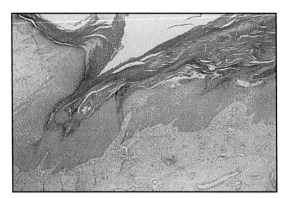

FIGURE 6–69. Spongiotic trachyonychia. Mounds of parakeratosis and scaly crust, spongiotic epidermal hyperplasia, and superficial perivascular inflammatory cell infiltrate are typical features. Note that the cornified layer stains pink with hematoxylin and eosin as does normal skin.

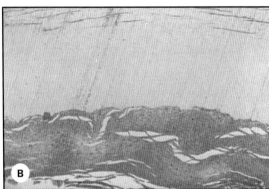

FIGURE 6–67. A and B, Pityriasis rubra pilaris. Nail plate clipping shows parakeratosis that alternates with orthokeratosis, both vertically and horizontally, in the cornified layer beneath the nail plate.

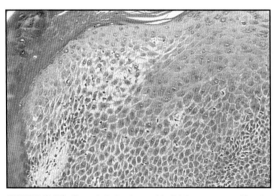

FIGURE 6–70. Spongiotic trachyonychia (high-power magnification of Figure 6.69). Foci of spongiosis associated with epidermal hyperplasia and hypergranulosis are evident.

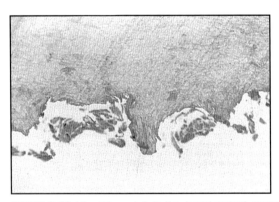

FIGURE 6–68. Idiopathic onycholysis. Note jagged sawtooth appearance with clusters of cornified cells shed at the undersurface of the nail plate.

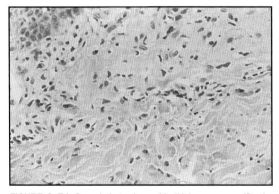

FIGURE 6–71. Spongiotic trachyonychia (high-power magnification of Figure 6.69). Inflammatory cell infiltrate of lymphocytes and eosinophils is evident.

striation and distal splitting (Fig. 6.68). There is no pterygium formation as a rule in spongiotic trachyonychia. It may involve a few nails or all 20 nails and present with the clinical features of twenty-nail dystrophy.[9] This condition may be seen in patients with alopecia areata or atopy or may be apparently idiopathic.[9–11] The histologic changes of spongiotic trachyonychia show an inflammatory response confined to the epithelial component and superficial dermis of the nail matrix. Epithelial hyperplasia and spongiosis can occur, with an inflammatory infiltrate under and within the matrix epithelium. The degree of spongiosis varies from mild changes (Figs 6.69 to 6.71) to most severe changes with intraepidermal microvesicles (Figs 6.72 and 6.73). The inflammatory cells are composed of lymphocytes with a variable number of eosinophils. The nail plate overlying these inflamed areas shows focal parakeratosis with inflammatory cells. The nail plates stain pink with hematoxylin and eosin stain and are similar in appearance to the adjacent stratum corneum of the volar skin. The prominent granular cell layer is usually observed.[9]

## Lichen Striatus

Lichen striatus is a self-limited linear eruption occurring in childhood. It may extend along a finger or a toe as far as the proximal

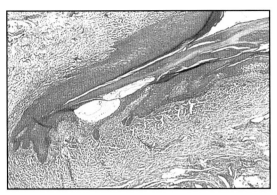

FIGURE 6–72. Spongiotic trachyonychia. Varying degrees of spongiosis, including spongiotic vesicles, can be seen in the severe lesion.

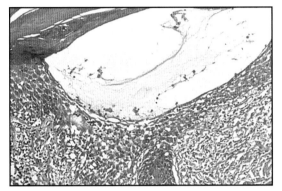

FIGURE 6–73. Spongiotic trachyonychia (high-power magnification of Figure 6.72). Evolution from spongiosis to spongiotic vesiculation within the nail matrix can be seen.

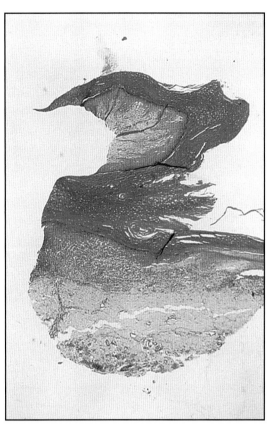

FIGURE 6–74. Lichen striatus. Diagnostic findings are foci of both spongiosis and vacuolar alteration in association with superficial perivascular and focal lichenoid infiltrate containing lymphohistiocytes.

nail fold and affect the nail plate. There are several types of onychodystrophy, including longitudinal splitting, punctate or transverse leukonychia, onycholysis, shredding, and total nail loss.[12] Histology shows a superficial perivascular and focal lichenoid infiltrate of lymphocytes and histiocytes. Lymphocytes may also be present at the dermal–epidermal junction, where there is vacuolar alteration. Lymphocytes usually predominate at the interface, especially in early lesions, but in the dermal papillae there may be a predominance of histiocytes, among them melanophages. The inflammatory infiltrate is usually also seen in and around some of the deeper vessels. The epidermal changes consist of spongiosis, dyskeratotic cells, and parakeratosis. In the old lesions, the infiltrate shows a focal lichenoid pattern under the spongiotic foci (Figs 6.74 to 6.76). The same histologic changes are also observed in the dorsal surface of the proximal nail fold.

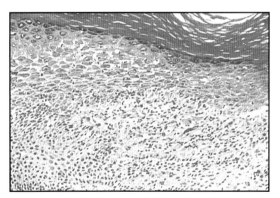

FIGURE 6–75. Lichen striatus (high-power magnification of Figure 6.74). Foci of both spongiosis and vacuolar alteration in association with dense lichenoid infiltrate of lymphocytes and histiocytes are evident.

## Histiocytosis X

Nail changes in histiocytosis X can be observed in both fingernails and toenails and include longitudinal grooves, purpuric striae, subungual hyperkeratosis, subungual pustules, onycholysis, chronic paronychia, deformation, and pitting of the nail plate.[13–15] Histologic study shows superficial perivascular and lichenoid infiltrate of atypical histiocytes (Figs 6.77 and 6.78). The histiocytes possess large, kidney-shaped, eccentrically placed nuclei and well-defined eosinophilic cytoplasm (Fig. 6.79). Some histiocytes are usually present focally within the epidermis. The upper dermis is markedly edematous. A few scattered lymphocytes and varying numbers of eosinophils may be present. Extravasated erythrocytes frequently lie within the infiltrate of histiocytes. Electron microscopy confirms that these are Langerhans' cells, which possess Birbeck granules, and immunohistochemical investigations show that these cells are s-100 protein and CD1 positive.

In persistent lesions, extensive aggregates of Langerhans' cells may be found extending deep into the dermis. Multinucleated giant cells are seen frequently. In addition, some eosinophils, neutrophils, lymphocytes, and plasma cells may be present (Figs 6.80 and 6.81).

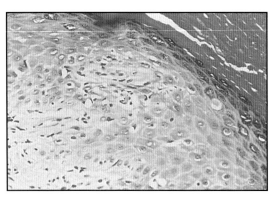

FIGURE 6–76. Lichen striatus. The subtle changes of both focal spongiosis and vacuolar alteration are also seen in the proximal nail fold.

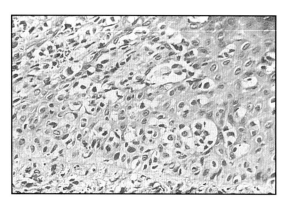

FIGURE 6–79. Histiocytosis X, proliferative lesion (high-power magnification of Figure 6.78). The histocytes show bean-or kidney-shaped nuclei and abundant, well-demarcated cytoplasm.

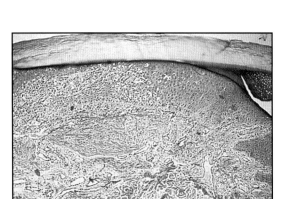

FIGURE 6–77. Histiocytosis X, proliferative lesion. The lesion shows dense lichenoid infiltrate of atypical histiocytes in the papillary dermis with epidermotropism.

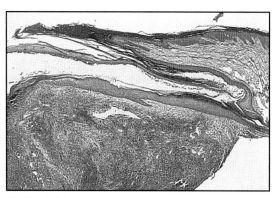

FIGURE 6–80. Histiocytosis X, granulomatous lesion. The lesion shows extensive aggregates of predominantly histiocytes in the dermis of the nail bed.

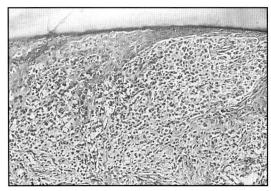

FIGURE 6–78. Histiocytosis X, proliferative lesion (high-power magnification of Figure 6.77). Dense infiltrate of atypical histiocytes in the papillary dermis and epidermis of the nail bed is evident.

## Darier–White Disease

The clinical nail manifestations of Darier–White disease include longitudinal, subungual red and white streaks associated with distal wedge-shaped subungual hyperkeratosis. Rarely, Darier–White disease is limited to the nails. The histologic picture may show suprabasilar clefts containing acantholytic cells on the dorsal surface of the proximal nail fold, nail matrix, and epidermis of the volar skin. Additionally, the presence of numerous multinucleated epithelial cells with abundant eosinophilic cytoplasm throughout

the length of the nail bed, the nail matrix, and the nail plate has been described.[16]

## Pachyonychia Congenita

Pachyonychia congenita is characterized by three major features: subungual hyperkeratosis, keratosis palmaris et plantaris, and leukokeratosis of the oral mucosa. The abnormalities of the nail unit are mostly confined to the nail bed, whereas the nail plate itself is actually normal. The nail bed shows marked hyperkeratosis, papillomatous epidermal hyperplasia, and the presence of a granular cell layer. The hyperplastic nail bed and subungual hyperkeratosis push up the plate so that it grows out, angled away from the axis of the fingers (Fig. 6.82). The distal matrix is also hyperplastic and papillomatous, producing large quantities of cornified material mixed with plasma.[17]

## Keratosis Punctata

Nail involvement has occasionally been described in keratosis punctata. The presenting symptoms include onychogryphosis, nail thickening, subungual hyperkeratosis, longitudinal fissures, and onychomadesis.[18] Pathologic studies of the nail bed reveal a sharply limited column of parakeratosis associated with hyper-granulosis and depression of the underlying nail bed epithelium. Similar changes may be seen in the distal nail matrix. No inflammatory infiltrate is observed.[19]

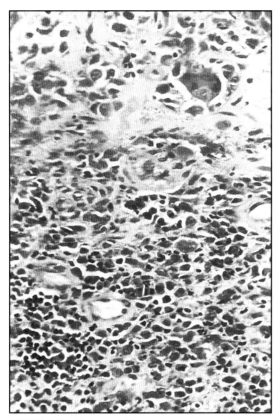

FIGURE 6–81. Histiocytosis X, granulomatous lesion (high-power magnification of Figure 6.80). Multinucleated giant cells, eosinophils, and plasma cells also lie within the aggregates of histiocytes.

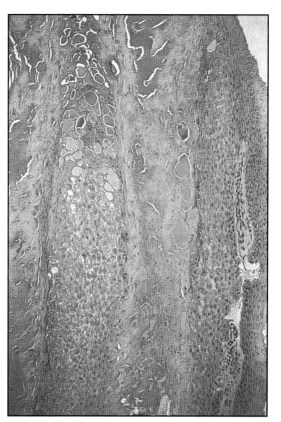

FIGURE 6–82. Pachyonychia congenita. There is pronounced hyperkeratosis with scaly crusts, hypegranulosis, and digitated epidermal hyperplasia of the nail bed epithelium.

## Leukonychia

Leukonychia is the most common chromatic nail abnormality of the nail plate. The clinical spectrum of leukonychia ranges from the variable presence of discrete white punctata or striae to complete nail whitening. Hereditary leukonychia has been observed to have an autosomal dominant pattern of inheritance with variable penetrance. Acquired leukonychia may arise after local trauma or in association with a wide range of systemic conditions. Microscopically, the nail bed shows parakeratosis and hypergranulosis with large nuclei and keratohyaline granules, beneath the normal nail plate.[20]

## Keratotic Scabies

The nail unit is not usually involved in scabies infestation, except in keratotic scabies (Norwegian scabies). The persistence of mites subungually is generally due to resistance to treatment, unless the nails are cut short and the scabicide is vigorously brushed beneath them. Microscopically, the nail bed shows marked hyperkeratosis with focal parakeratosis. Ascarides can be seen in the cornified layer of the nail bed[21] (Figs 6.83 and 6.84).

## Yellow Nail Syndrome

In patients with yellow nail syndrome, results of light microscopy of the nail plate are normal, but electron microscopy reveals keratohyalin granules, which are not normally seen in the nail

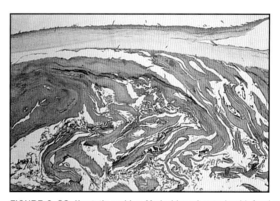

FIGURE 6–83. Keratotic scabies. Marked hyperkeratosis with focal parakeratosis beneath the nail plate is evident.

matrix and are postulated to be associated with the slowed nail growth.[22]

## Pyogenic Granuloma

Pyogenic granuloma of the nail unit occurs primarily along the lateral nail fold and can result from an ingrown nail. Histologic examination reveals a well-circumscribed lobular lesion characterized by a markedly increased number of widely dilated capillaries associated with edematous stroma, a scattered mixed inflammatory cell infiltrate, and an eroded surface (Figs 6.85 and 6.86). In old lesions, the stroma is fibrotic, with thickened collagen bundles,

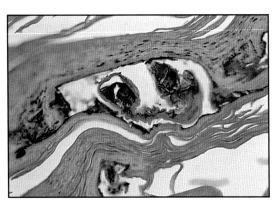

FIGURE 6–84. Keratotic scabies (high-power magnification of Figure 6.83). Ascarides in the thickened, cornified layer are evident.

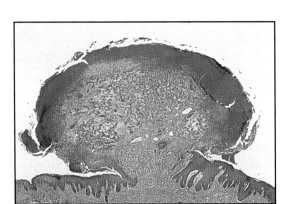

FIGURE 6–85. Pyogenic granuloma, acute stage. The lesion shows ulcerated exophytic granulation tissue. Note the characteristic collarettes of elongated epidermal rete ridges on both sides that point toward the center of the lesion.

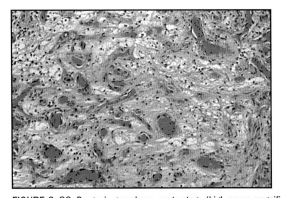

FIGURE 6–86. Pyogenic granuloma, acute stage (high-power magnification of Figure 6.85). One observes considerable proliferation of capillaries and venules lined by plump endothelial cells. The stroma is edematous and contains a mixed inflammatory cell infiltrate.

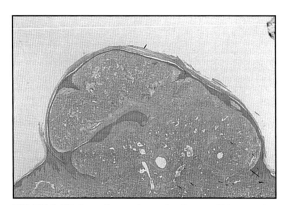

FIGURE 6–87. Pyogenic granuloma, chronic stage. This stage shows an exophytic angiomatous mass with fibrous trabeculae intersecting the angiomatous elements and prominent epidermal rete ridges.

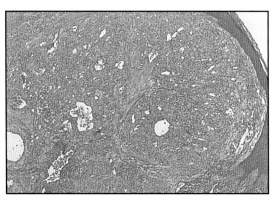

FIGURE 6–88. Pyogenic granuloma, chronic stage (high-power magnification of Figure 6.87). Note trabeculation by fibrous septum.

increased numbers of fibroblasts, and prominent interlobular septa (Figs 6.87 and 6.88). The overlying epidermis has flattened rete ridges and a collarette of epithelium at the base of the lesion.

## Epithelial Neoplasma

Most of the neoplasms of the epidermis that affect the skin may also occur in the nail unit. Solar keratosis and basal cell carcinoma

seldom occur in the nail unit except on the proximal nail fold because this particular area is not protected by the nail plate against solar damage.

## Subungual Basal Cell Carcinoma

Although basal cell carcinoma is the most common skin malignancy, usually occurring in actinically damaged skin, subungual basal cell carcinoma is extremely rare.[23,24] It usually presents as a chronic paronychia or periungual eczematous lesion often associated with ulceration, granulation tissue, and pain. Histologic findings include aggregations of atypical basal cells with large hyperchromatic pleomorphic and palisading nuclei protruding from the surface epithelium of the nail bed or nail matrix and extending into the subadjacent dermis. An abundance of melanin and melanin-producing cells may be observed in some nests of tumor cells.

## Squamous Cell Carcinoma

Squamous cell carcinoma is the most common malignant tumor found in the nail bed. The presenting symptoms of squamous cell carcinoma of the nail bed include paronychia, ingrown nail, nail separation, nail deformity, dyschromia of the nail plate, bleeding, and pain.[25,26] Histologically, squamous cell carcinoma in situ, or Bowen's disease, is diagnosed when there is a proliferation of

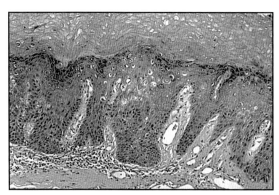

FIGURE 6–89. Bowen's disease. There are atypical keratinocytes with large hyperchromatic nuclei at all levels of the epidermis.

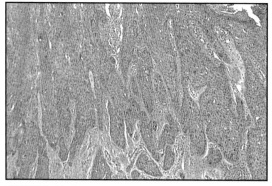

FIGURE 6–91. Squamous cell carcinoma. The lesion shows irregularly shaped aggregations of atypical squamous epithelium extending into the reticular dermis.

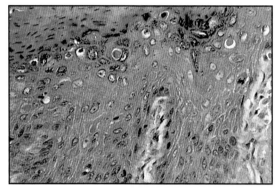

FIGURE 6–90. Bowen's disease (high-power magnification of Figure 6.89). Atypical keratinocytes, dyskeratotic cells, and mitotic figures in the thickened epidermis are evident.

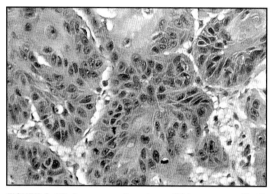

FIGURE 6–92. Squamous cell carcinoma (high-power magnification of Figure 6.91). Nuclear atypia and mitotic figures of squamous cells are evident.

atypical keratinocytes consisting of large, hyperchromatic, pleomorphic nuclei with eosinophilic cytoplasm involving the full thickness of the epidermis (Figs 6.89 and 6.90). When the neoplasm extends into the reticular dermis, the diagnosis of squamous cell carcinoma can be rendered (Figs 6.91 and 6.92). The features of preexisting verrucae, including large parakeratotic cells, papillomatosis, hypergranulosis, and perinuclear vacuoles of keratinocytes, may be found in some lesions.[26]

## Carcinoma Cuniculatum (Verrucous Carcinoma)

Carcinoma cuniculatum (verrucous carcinoma on volar skin) is a rare, low-grade variant of squamous cell carcinoma characterized by a local aggressive clinical behavior but a low potential of metastasis. The sole of the foot is the typical site of tumor development; however, reports in the literature of nail apparatus involvement are uncommon.[27] Histologically, carcinoma cuniculatum exhibits both exophytic and endophytic growth patterns. The tumor is characterized by an invaginated proliferation of well-differentiated keratinocytes, some of which have central crypts containing keratinous debris. The surface of the neoplasm shows diffuse parakeratosis and hypogranulosis with a papillated surface. The base of the neoplasm consists of bulbous islands of well-differentiated squamous epithelium infiltrating the dermis and deeper structure. The squamous cells may have scant or no atypia.

Mitotic figures are minimal and are usually confined to the basal cell layer (Figs 6.93 to 6.95). The tumor may grow to involve the phalangeal bone.

## Subungual Keratoacanthoma

Subungual keratoacanthoma is an uncommon distinctive tumor of the nail bed. It can easily be confused with well-differentiated squamous cell carcinoma and verrucous carcinoma. Distinctive features of subungual keratoacanthoma include pain, rapid growth, and early underlying bony destruction. Unlike keratoacanthoma arising on other parts of the skin, subungual keratoacanthoma seldom resolves spontaneously and is more locally destructive. Histologically,[28,29] the neoplasm is characterized by bulbous aggregations of squamous epithelium involving the dermis and underlying structures, with epithelial lips at the periphery and a central crater filled with cornified debris. Keratinization is abrupt and without an intervening granular layer. Numerous eosinophilic dyskeratotic cells are scattered throughout the cell layers. There are infrequent mitoses in the basal cell layer and atypia is minimal. The base of the neoplasm is somewhat wedge shaped, with a sparse lymphocytic infiltrate in the underlying stroma (Figs 6.96 to 6.99). The tumor and associated inflammatory infiltrate are adjacent to the bone at the site of the cortical erosion. The bone marrow may show reactive fibrosis and increased osteoclastic activity. The major histologic feature that distinguishes subungual keratoacanthoma from squamous cell carcinoma or verrucous carcinoma is the

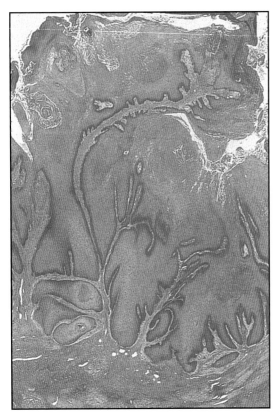

FIGURE 6-93. Carcinoma cuniculatum (verrucous carcinoma on volar skin). There is a papillated proliferation of well-differentiated squamous cells. The base extends into the deep reticular dermis.

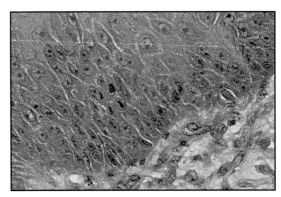

FIGURE 6-95. Carcinoma cuniculatum (high-power magnification of Figure 6.94). Nuclear atypia and mitotic figures at the base of the neoplastic epithelium are evident.

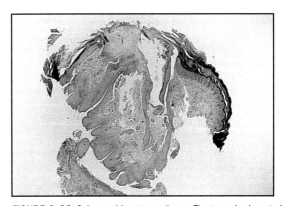

FIGURE 6-96. Subungual keratoacanthoma. The tumor is characterized by an endophytic growth of squamous epithelium with a central keratin-filled crater.

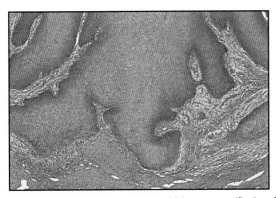

FIGURE 6-94. Carcinoma cuniculatum (high-power magnification of Figure 6.93). At the base of the neoplastic epithelium, there are bulbous aggregations in association with a dense mixed inflammatory cell infiltrate.

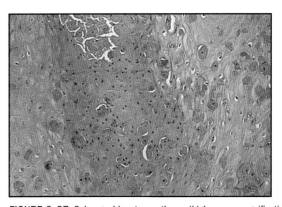

FIGURE 6-97. Subungual keratoacanthoma (high-power magnification of Figure 6.96). The central crater is filled with cornified debris and parakeratotic cells. The keratinization is abrupt, and there is no intervening granular layer.

different and distinctive architectural pattern. Subungual keratoacanthoma differs from typical keratoacanthoma in that it occurs on non-hair-bearing skin and has more vertical orientation, less or no cytologic atypia, less associated inflammation, and many more dyskeratotic cells[28] (Figs 6.100 to 6.102).

## Wart

Common warts on the nail unit usually involve the proximal and lateral nail folds, so-called periungual warts. The warts that initially affect the hyponychium may grow toward the nail bed and eventuate into subungual warts. The histopathology of periungual and subungual warts is indistinguishable from that of volar skin. The early lesion shows hyperkeratosis, hypergranulosis, papillomatous epidermal hyperplasia, and elongated and inward bending of the peripheral rete ridges with widely dilated capillaries in the papillary dermis (Fig. 6.103). There are perinuclear halos and coarse keratohyalin granules in the granular cell and upper spinous cell layers (Fig. 6.104). In old warts, in contrast to new warts, the surface is less papillated and more endophytic, with epidermal

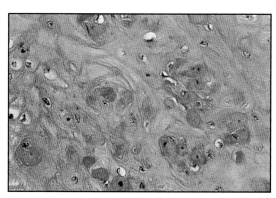

FIGURE 6–98. Subungual keratoacanthoma (high-power magnification of Figure 6.96). The neoplastic epithelium consists of keratinocytes with dark, small nuclei; glassy, pale eosinophilic cytoplasm, and numerous dyskeratotic cells.

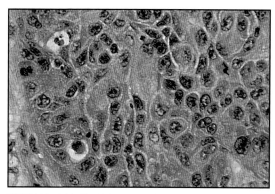

FIGURE 6–101. Classic keratoacanthoma (high-power magnification of Figure 6.100). A greater degree of nuclear atypia is seen than in subungual keratoacanthoma.

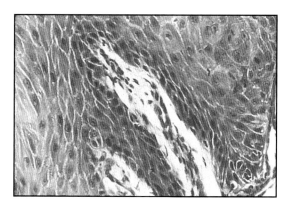

FIGURE 6–99. Subungual keratoacanthoma (high-power magnification of Figure 6.96). There is a sparse inflammatory cell infiltrate at the base of the neoplastic epithelium.

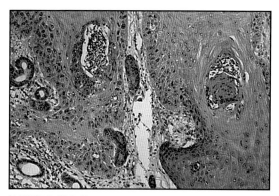

FIGURE 6–102. Classic keratoacanthoma (high-power magnification of Figure 6.100). Dense mixed inflammatory cell infiltrate with intraepithelial abscess within the neoplasm is evident.

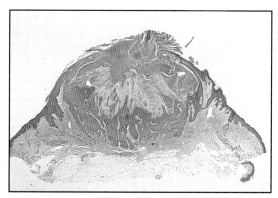

FIGURE 6–100. Classic keratoacanthoma. There is an exophytic–endophytic neoplasm with a central keratin-filled crater surrounded by overhanging lips of epithelium.

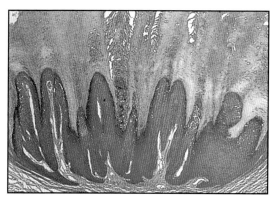

FIGURE 6–103. Verruca vulgaris, early lesion. There is thick, compact hyperkeratosis, acanthosis, and papillomatosis with collarettes of epithelium at the periphery of the lesion.

hyperplasia and hypergranulosis (Figs 6.105 and 6.106). The changes in resolved lesions are characterized by hyperkeratosis above a cup-shaped hyperplastic epidermis with hypergranulosis and a collarette of epithelium at the periphery. The papillary dermis contains widely dilated capillaries, thickened collagen bundles, and plump fibroblasts (Fig. 6.107).

Deep palmoplantar warts occur not only on the palms and soles but also on the lateral aspects and tips of the fingers and toes. Unlike the common wart, palmoplantar warts usually appear as deeply seated keratotic papules covered with a thick callus. When the callus is removed, the wart appears as soft, granular, white, or yellow tissue.

Histologically, deep palmoplantar warts are characterized by endophytic growth of epidermis with hyperkeratosis, hypergranulosis, papillomatosis, and elongated and inward bending of the peripheral rete ridges (Figs 6.108 and 6.109). There are numerous homogeneous eosinophilic bodies within the cytoplasm of keratinocytes in the upper malpighian layer. In addition to these

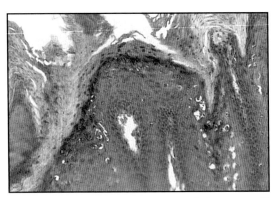

FIGURE 6-104. Verruca vulgaris, early lesion (high-power magnification of Figure 6.103). Focal parakeratosis at the tips of the epidermal digitations, hypergranulosis, perinuclear halos in the granular layer, and dilated blood vessels in the dermal papillae are evident.

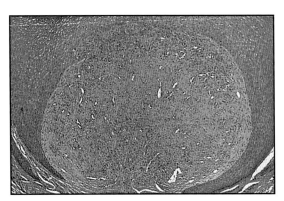

FIGURE 6-107. Verruca vulgaris, resolving lesion. The epidermis shows endophytic, club-shaped hyperplasia and epidermal collarettes; the papillary dermis is filled with dilated blood vessels, coarse collagen fibers, and fibroblasts.

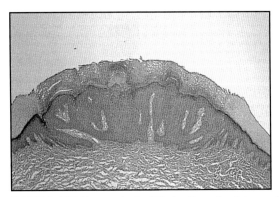

FIGURE 6-105. Verruca vulgaris, old lesion. The surface is less papillated. Note epithelial collarettes at the periphery.

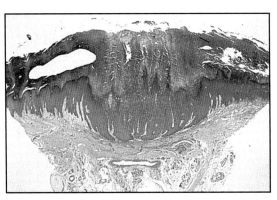

FIGURE 6-108. Deep palmoplantar wart. The lesion is characterized by endophytic growth of epidermis with hyperkeratosis, papillated epidermal hyperplasia, and collarettes of the rete ridges at the periphery.

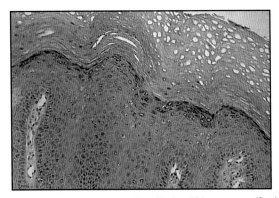

FIGURE 6-106. Verruca vulgaris, old lesion (high-power magnification of Figure 6.105). Focal parakeratosis, perinuclear halos, and coarse keratohyaline granules in the hyperplastic granular layer are evident.

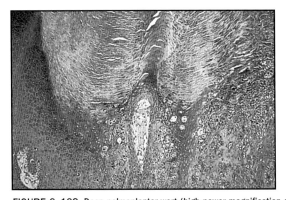

FIGURE 6-109. Deep palmoplantar wart (high-power magnification of Figure 6.108). Hypergranulosis with coarse keratohyaline granules and perinuclear halos in the upper malpighian layer are evident.

bodies, some of the cells in the upper malpighian layer with vacuolar nuclei show a small intranuclear eosinophilic inclusion body. The keratinocytes in the granular layer show coarse keratohyalin granules and perinuclear vacuolization. The nuclei in the cornified layer persist, appearing as deeply basophilic round bodies surrounded by a clear zone (Fig. 6.110).

## Subungual Epidermoid Cyst

Two types of subungual epidermoid cysts have been reported in the literature. The common variety is bone-located pidermoid cysts associated with osteolysis.[30,31] The usual symptoms are redness, pain, tenderness, and swelling of the terminal phalanx, resulting in clubbing or pincer nails. It is better referred to as an epidermoid

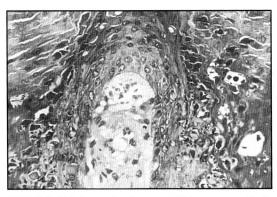

FIGURE 6–110. Deep palmoplantar wart (high-power magnification of Figure 6.109). Numerous homogeneous purplish inclusions within the cytoplasm and the nuclei in the upper malpighian layer are evident.

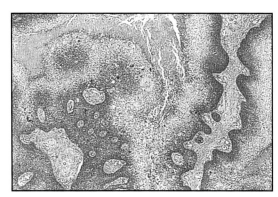

FIGURE 6–112. Malignant proliferating onycholemmal cyst. The tumor is cornposed of irregularly shaped lobules of squamous epithelium undergoing abrupt change into amorphous, cornified material.

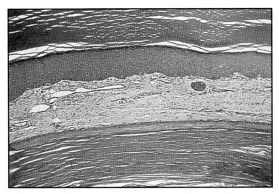

FIGURE 6–111. Subungual epidermal cyst. The wall of the cyst is a squamous epithelium resembling epidermis and is filled with compact, cornified layer.

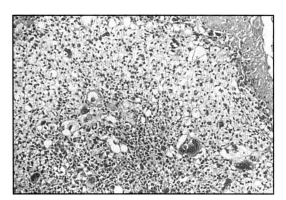

FIGURE 6–113. Malignant proliferating onycholemmal cyst (high-power magnification of Figure 6.112). Atypical squamous epithelium consisting of atypical nuclei and clear abundant cytoplasm is seen. Note the absence of the intervening granular layer.

implantation cyst. The other type of subungual epidermoid cyst is simply a cystic lesion with no bone involvement (Fig. 6.111). The clinical features are subungual hyperkeratosis associated with a shortened and dystrophic nail plate.[32] The pathologic features of epidermoid implantation cyst include a round epidermal inclusion cyst in the bone filled with laminated cornified material and lined by stratified squamous epithelium with a granular layer[30,31] whereas the histologic findings of subungual epidermoid cysts include a small keratinous cyst. The wall of the cysts is formed by nail bed epithelium[33] or nail matrix,[32] giving rise to a compact cornified material generally without a granular layer.[32] These histologic features resemble trichilemmal features of the hair follicle; therefore, they should also be defined as onycholemmal cysts. The overlying nail bed usually shows hyperkeratosis and acanthosis.

## Malignant Proliferating Onycholemmal Cyst

The malignant proliferating onycholemmal cyst is a slow-growing tumor of the nail unit that is regarded as the malignant analogue of the onycholemmal cysts arising from the nail bed epithelium[33] or nail matrix.[32] The growth of the tumor is infiltrative and it may destroy the phalangeal bone. Histologically, the tumor is composed of cornified cysts and solid nests and strands of atypical keratinocytes. The cystic structure is filled with eosinophilic, amorphous cornified material and lined by atypical squamous epithelium devoid of a granular layer[34] (Figs 6.112 and 6.113). Periodic acid-

Schiff (PAS) stains reveal small amounts of glycogen in the epithelial nests associated with clear cell change. The histology is homologous to that of a follicular cyst, being comparable to the malignant proliferating trichilemmal cyst.

## Eccrine Porocarcinoma

Eccrine porocarcinoma is a rare malignant neoplasm. Its most common localization is on the extremities, especially the lower limbs. Few cases of periungual porocarcinoma have been described, suggesting an origin at the proximal or lateral nail folds.[35,36] Histologic studies show irregular nests of epithelial cells that vary from a monomorphous poroid cell type that predominates in eccrin eporoma to a highly pleomorphic large cell component (Figs 6.114 to 6.117). In the solid tumor, there are small ductal cavities surrounded by cuticular cells. Some areas show en masse necrosis of neoplastic cells. Many cells are in mitosis. Some accumulation of acid mucopolysaccharides is observed between tumor cells and in small cystic spaces. The neoplasm shows a strongly infiltrative growth that even penetrates into the bone of the distal phalanx.

## Onychomatrixoma

Onychomatrixoma, a hamartomatous lesion of the nail matrix described by Baran and Kint, is characterized clinically by a yellow discoloration along the entire length of the nail plate with splinter

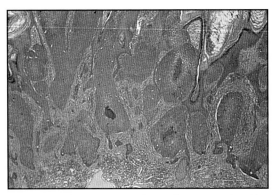

FIGURE 6–114. Eccrine porocarcinoma. The tumor consists of irregular bands and nests of neoplastic cells protruding into the deep reticular dermis.

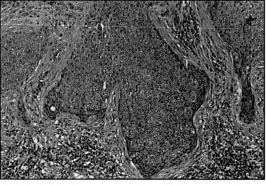

FIGURE 6–116. Eccrine porocarcinoma (high-power magnification of Figure 6.114). In some foci, the neoplastic aggregates consist of large, atypical cuboidal cells. A dense inflammatory infiltrate is present at the base of the lesion.

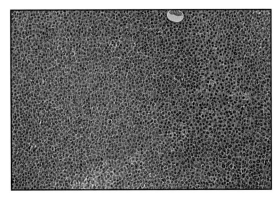

FIGURE 6–115. Eccrine porocarcinoma (high-power magnification of Figure 6.114). In some foci, the tumor has an appearance similar to that of eccrine poroma consisting of uniformly small, cuboidal cells. Note the ductal lumina at the top of this photomicrograph.

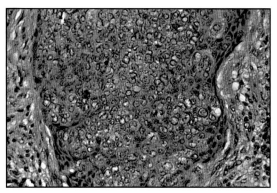

FIGURE 6–117. Eccrine porocarcinoma (high-power magnification of Figure 6.116). The malignant cells have large, hyperchromatic, irregularly shaped nuclei and may be multinucleated.

hemorrhage in its proximal portion, a tendency toward transverse over-curvature of the affected nails, and exposure of a matrix tumor after the nail has been avulsed and the proximal nail fold turned back.[37] Histologically, the tumor consists of epithelial cell strands emanating from the nail matrix and penetrating vertically into the dermis. In the central parts of the strands, the epithelial cells evolve to the parakeratotic cell layer, oriented along the long axis of the strands. Lacunae are observed in the center of some of these epithelial strands after elimination of the parakeratotic cells. The peritumoral stroma is sharply delineated from the underlying dermis and is composed of loose connective tissue with numerous fibroblasts and thin collagen bundles. The elastic fibers are sparse and thin. No mucin or inflammatory cell infiltrates are found.[37]

## Mucinous Syringometaplasia

Mucinous syringometaplasia is a distinct pathologic entity that demonstrates mucin-laden cells in the eccrine duct epithelium. Most cases of mucinous syringometaplasia are solitary lesions on the plantar surface,[38,39] but it may present with verrucous lesions beneath the nail.[40] Histologic examination shows focal invagination of the epidermis lined by squamous epithelium, with some eccrine ducts leading into the invagination. The eccrine ductal epithelium contains mucin-laden goblet cells. There is also mucinous syringometaplasia of the underlying eccrine coils.

## Pigmented Lesions

The pigmented lesions of the nail unit are similar to those elsewhere on the skin, except for the lesions within the nail matrix that cause longitudinal pigmented streaks or melanonychia striata in the longitudinum. The histologic spectrum ranges from epithelial hyperpigmentation to benign or malignant neoplasms, namely epithelial hyperpigmentations, simple lentigines, melanocytic nevi, or malignant melanomas.

Epithelial hyperpigmentation may occur secondary to inflammation, trauma, irradiation, drugs, and endocrine diseases. The histologic change of epithelial hyperpigmentation is characterized by increased melanin in the basal cell layer with or without the presence of melanophages in the papillary dermis (Fig. 6.118A and B). Microscopically, simple lentigine has a slightly increased number of melanocytes, some of them dendritic, and increased melanin in the basal cell layer with or without corresponding elongated rete ridges (Fig. 6.119A and B). Junctional nevi consist of melanocytes in both nests and solitary units at the dermal–epidermal junction (Fig. 6.120A and B), whereas malignant melanoma of the nail matrix has the same histologic picture as malignant melanoma of the skin, namely an asymmetric, poorly circumscribed lesion characterized by a proliferation of atypical melanocytes arranged both as solitary units and nests at all levels of the nail matrix (Fig. 6.121A and B). In addition to a melanocytic

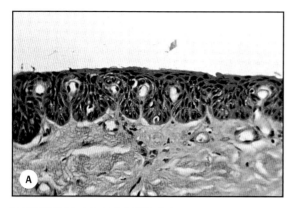

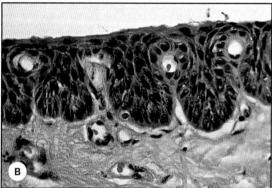

FIGURE 6–118. A and B, Epithelial hyperpigmentation. The lesion shows an increase in epidermal melanin in the nail matrix, most prominent in the basal layer. Note a solitary melanocyte at the basal layer.

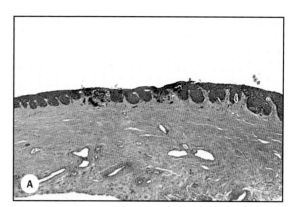

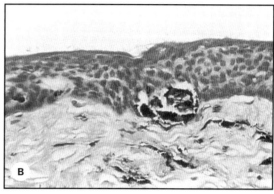

FIGURE 6–120. A and B, Junctional nevus. In contrast to simple lentigines, this lesion consists of melanocytes arranged both as solitary units and nests in the basal layer of the nail matrix.

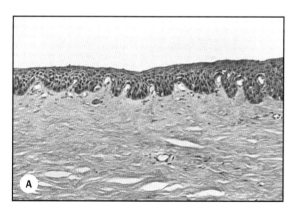

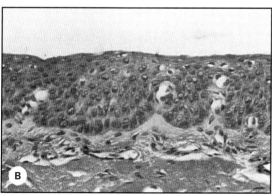

FIGURE 6–119. A and B, Simple lentigines. There is a marked increase in the number of typical melanocytes arranged as a solitary unit at the basal layer.

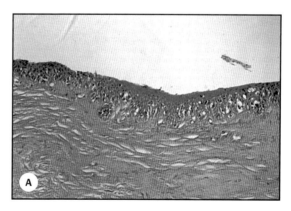

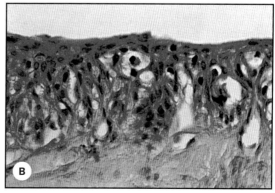

FIGURE 6–121. A and B, Malignant melanoma in situ. Many solitary melanocytes and nests of melanocytes are present at all layers of the nail matrix.

proliferation, epidermal hyperplasia, including subungual hyper-keratosis, hypergranulosis, and acanthosis of the nail bed and matrix, may be observed (Fig. 6.122 A and B). Once in the dermis, however, atypical melanocytes tend to continue to descend progressively. The amount of inflammatory infiltrate in malignant melanoma varies. In malignant melanoma in situ and early invasive lesion, the papillary dermis shows a band-like infiltrate of lymphocytes, often intermingled with melanophages, at the base of the tumor (Fig. 6.123). In more advanced lesions, the inflammatory infiltrate is quite variable, but it is often only slight to moderate rather than pronounced. In addition, the epidermal component is less prominent or even absent, in contrast to that of early lesions or malignant melanoma in situ (Figs 6.124 and 6.125).

## Subungual Hemorrhage

Subungual hemorrhage is often seen in nail biopsy specimens because clinically it looks like a melanocytic lesion. Histologic findings show collections of homogeneous eosinophilic and yellow–brown masses under the nail plate or within it (Figs 6.126 and 6.127). These yellow–brown masses, consisting of lysed red blood cell hemoglobin, remain negative with Prussian blue stain used

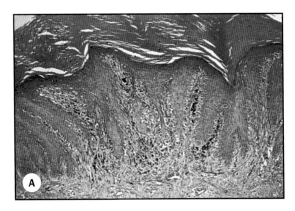

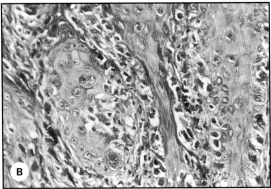

FIGURE 6–122. A and B, Malignant melanoma in situ. In addition to a proliferation of atypical melanocytes, the nail bed shows hyperkeratosis, hypergranulosis, and acanthosis.

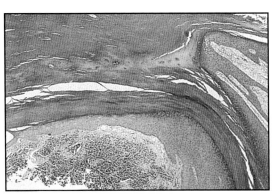

FIGURE 6–124. Malignant melanoma, nodular lesion. The upper dermis of the nail unit contains dense aggregates of atypical melanocytes.

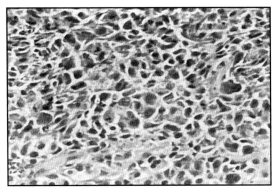

FIGURE 6–125. Malignant melanoma (high-power magnification of Figure 6.124). The tumor cells possess atypical nuclei and eosinophilic cytoplasm.

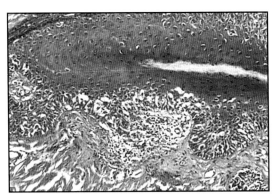

FIGURE 6–123. Malignant melanoma in situ. Atypical melanocytes are seen in the nail matrix epithelium. The upper dermis contains dense inflammatory infiltrate intermingled with melanophages.

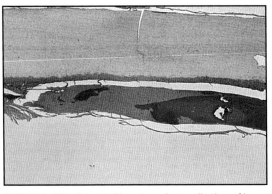

FIGURE 6–126. Subungual hematoma. Large collections of homogeneous eosinophilic and yellow–brown material beneath the nail plate are evident.

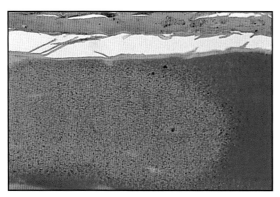

FIGURE 6–127. Subungual hematoma (high-power magnification of Figure 6.126). Homogeneous yellow–brown mass representing lysed red blood cells is evident.

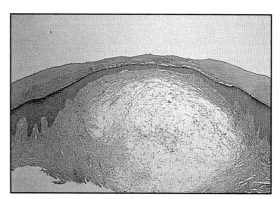

FIGURE 6–129. Myxoid cyst. The dermis contains a relatively well-defined collection of mucinous material.

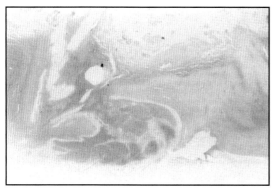

FIGURE 6–128. Subungual hematoma. The Perl stain for iron is negative.

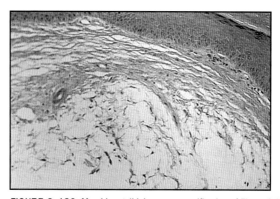

FIGURE 6–130. Myxoid cyst (high-power magnification of Figure 6.129). Scattered fibroblasts in the mucinous material are evident.

for the demonstration of hemosiderin (Fig. 6.128) but positive (brown) with benzidine stain for hemoglobin.[41]

# Soft Tissue Tumors

## Focal mucinosis (myxoid cyst)

Histologically, focal mucinosis does not show an epithelial lining[42] and therefore should not be termed a cyst. Microscopic change reveals a relatively well-circumscribed area of mucin in the upper dermis (Fig. 6.129). Spindle-shaped fibroblasts are usually seen interspersed among mucinous material. A large cavity forms, with marginal compression of the surrounding collagen (Fig. 6.130). In addition, the overlying surface epithelium shows compact hyperkeratosis with a collarette of hyperplastic epidermis. The mucinous material stains pale basophilic with hematoxylin and eosin and stains positive with alcian blue or colloid iron for acid mucopolysaccharides.

## Ganglion

This occurs as a cystic or myxoid mass on the dorsum surface of the wrist in young persons. In about half of the cases the lesion is associated with tenderness or pain. They frequently attach to the joint capsule and tendon sheath. The genesis of this lesion is obscure. It is postulated that most arise as herniations through a defect in the wall of the joint capsule or tendon sheath. However, the

difficulty in demonstrating such a connection raises the possibility that these may arise in displaced rests of synovial tissue or by the transformation of primary connective tissue into synovial cells that then secrete mucin to create the cystic space. Microscopically, the cyst frequently shows synovial cell lining around mucoid mass.[43]

## Glomus tumor

The solitary type of glomus tumor is an extremely tender nodule usually located in the nail bed. Microscopic examination reveals a well-circumscribed vascular neoplasm characterized by a slightly increased number of dilated vascular spaces lined by a single layer of flattened, often elongated endothelial cells (Figs. 6.131 and 6.132). Peripheral to the endothelial cells is a row of cells with uniform round to oval nuclei and pale eosinophilic cytoplasm (glomus cells) (Fig. 6.133). The neoplasm is outlined by compressed collagen at the periphery. The stroma is edematous and rich in unmyelinated neural elements.[44]

## Acquired digital fibrokeratoma

Histologically, acquired digital fibrokeratoma appears as a dense fibrous core with a surrounding epithelial envelope (Fig. 6.134). The central core is characterized by interlacing fascicles of thick collagen bundles predominantly oriented along the longitudinal axis and associated with an increased number of plump fibroblasts and capillaries (Figs 6.135 and 6.136). The tumor is devoid of

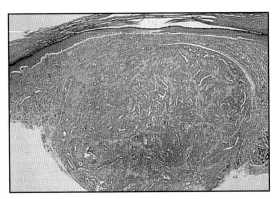

FIGURE 6–131. Glomus tumor. The tumor appears as well-circumscribed cellular aggregates compressing the surrounding collagen.

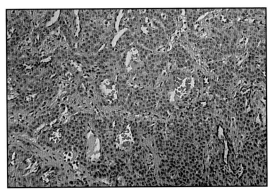

FIGURE 6–132. Glomus tumor (high-power magnification of Figure 6.131). Anastomosing aggregations of the cells around dilated, thick-walled blood vessels are evident.

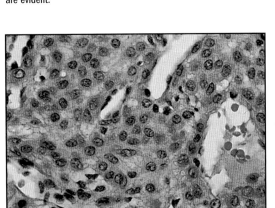

FIGURE 6–133. Glomus tumor (high-power magnification). The tumor cells are composed of round or oval nuclei and pale cytoplasma.

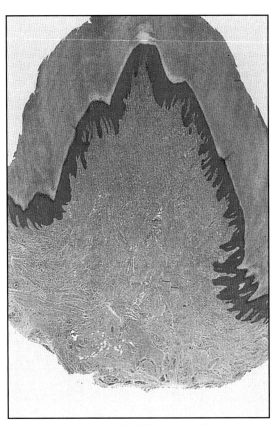

FIGURE 6–134. Acquired digital fibrokeratoma. The tumor is characterized by exophytic growth of fibrous tissues, which are covered by hyperkeratotic and hyperplastic epidermis.

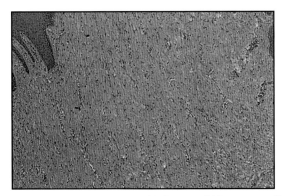

FIGURE 6–135. Acquired digital fibrokeratoma (high-power magnification of Figure 6.134). The central core is composed of interlacing fascicles of collagen bundles and plump fibroblasts.

epithelial adnexal structures, and elastic tissue is diminished. The paucity or absence of neural elements has also been described. The overlying epidermis is acanthotic and hyperkeratotic.[45]

### Infantile digital fibromatosis (recurrent infantile digital fibroma)

Infantile digital fibromatosis is a smooth, dome-shaped, dermal nodule that is usually located on the dorsal surface of the fingers and toes. The lesion develops at birth or during infancy. On reaching the nail unit, the lesion may elevate the nail plate, leading to dystrophy. Histologically, the lesion is composed of interlacing fascicles of spindle-shaped fibroblasts and collagen bundles (Fig. 6.137). A characteristic diagnostic feature is the presence of paranuclear eosinophilic inclusion bodies within some fibroblasts (Fig. 6.138). These inclusion bodies measure from 3 to 10 μm in diameter.[46] The inclusion bodies stain deep red with phosphotungstic acid-hematoxylin and purple with Masson trichrome. Electron microscopic study shows that the tumor cells are typical myofibroblasts containing inclusion bodies and bundles of microfilaments. Immunohistochemistry shows the paranuclear inclusion consisting of actin fibers.

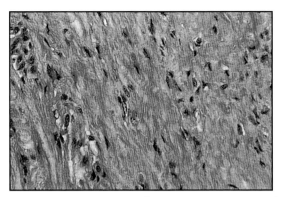

FIGURE 6–136. Acquired digital fibrokeratoma (high-power magnification). Fibroblasts markedly increasing in number are large and stellate.

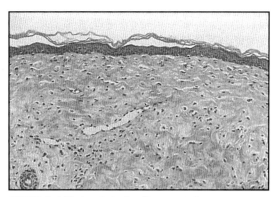

FIGURE 6–139. Juvenile hyaline fibromatosis. The nodule is composed of scattered fibroblasts among homogeneous eosinophilic ground substance.

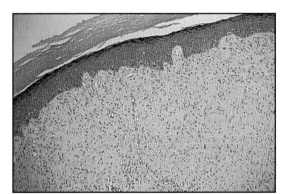

FIGURE 6–137. Infantile digital fibromatosis. The upper dermis shows numerous fibroblasts and collagen bundles arranged in interlacing fascicles.

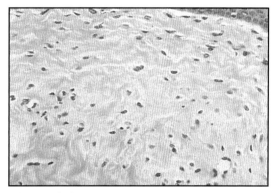

FIGURE 6–140. Juvenile hyaline fibromatosis (high-power magnification of Figure 6.139). Note clefts around the fibroblasts with the appearance of chondroid cells.

## Periungual fibroma (Koenen's tumor)

Periungual fibroma is a rare benign fibrous tumor occurring around a nail plate and may be acquired or associated with tuberous sclerosis. The tumor usually develops underneath the proximal or lateral nail fold and rests on the nail plate. The lesion may develop at the nail bed (subungual) and lift the nail plate distally. Histologically, the fibroma is similar to acquired digital fibrokeratoma, but areas of fibromatosis may have the large size and stellate shape of fibroblasts. The distal part of the tumor contains coarse collagen fibers, arranged haphazardly, and prominent capillaries (Figs. 6.141 and 6.142), whereas the proximal part is composed of thinner collagen fibers and seemingly arranged mostly parallel to the skin surface, fading into the contiguous dermis of the nail fold (Fig. 6.143). The lesion is usually elongated and covered with a slightly acanthotic epidermis, hyperkeratosis, and an epidermal collarette (see Fig. 6.141). No elastic fibers or neural structures are observed in the tumor.[48]

Invaginated fibrokeratoma, a histologic variant of periungual fibroma with matrix differentiation,[49] usually occurs as a keratotic lesion simulating a rudimentary nail plate and fuses with the normal nail. The tumor is cone-shaped, thickened proximally, and tapered distally. Histologically, it is characterized by a downward growth of a well-demarcated fibrous nodule lined between the ventral surface of the proximal nail fold and nail matrix. The fibrous mass consists of bundles of collagen densely packed with fibroblasts predominantly parallel to the longitudinal axis. The

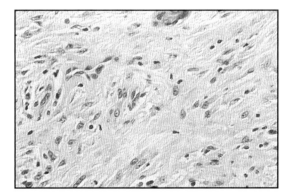

FIGURE 6–138. Infantile digital fibromatosis (high-power magnification of Figure 6.137). The presence of eosinophilic intracytoplasmic inclusion bodies within some fibroblasts is evident.

## Juvenile hyaline fibromatosis

Juvenile hyaline fibromatosis is characterized by skin nodules, muscle weakness, flexion contractures of large joints, and gingival hypertrophy. The nodules are found in the head and neck region, on the trunk, and at the tip of the digits, where acro-osteolysis and clubbing may be seen.[47] The histology of the skin nodules includes fibroblasts in homogeneous eosinophilic ground substance that are strongly PAS positive and diastase resistant (Fig. 6.139). Clefts are seen between the fibroblast and the ground substance that give rise to the appearance of chondroid cells (Fig. 6.140).

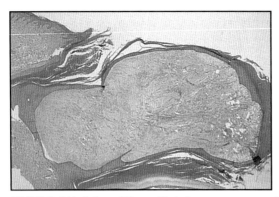

FIGURE 6–141. Periungual fibroma. The lesion appears as an exophytic mass protruding from the proximal portion of the ventral proximal nail fold.

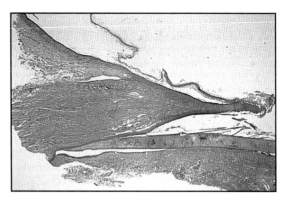

FIGURE 6–144. Invaginated fibrokeratoma. The lesion shows endophytic growth of the fibrous tissue at the junction of the ventral proximal nail fold and proximal nail matrix.

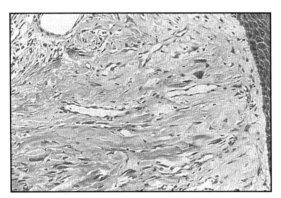

FIGURE 6–142. Periungual fibroma (high-power magnification of Figure 6.141). The distal portion of the tumor is composed of large stellate fibroblasts, coarse collagen bundles, and dilated, thick-walled blood vessels arranged haphazardly.

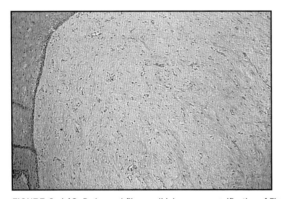
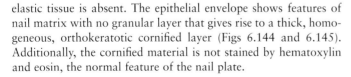

FIGURE 6–143. Periungual fibroma (high-power magnification of Figure 6.141). The proximal portion is composed of thinner collagen bundles and spindle-shaped fibroblasts.

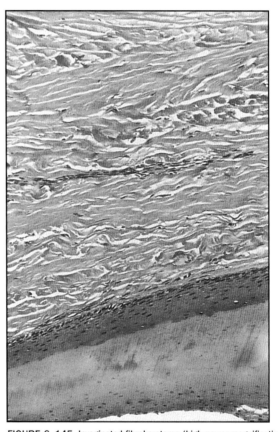

FIGURE 6–145. Invaginated fibrokeratoma (high-power magnification of Figure 6.144). The lower portion of the tumor is covered by nail matrix epithelium.

elastic tissue is absent. The epithelial envelope shows features of nail matrix with no granular layer that gives rise to a thick, homogeneous, orthokeratotic cornified layer (Figs 6.144 and 6.145). Additionally, the cornified material is not stained by hematoxylin and eosin, the normal feature of the nail plate.

## Giant cell tumor of tendon sheath

Giant cell tumor of tendon sheath most commonly occurs on the hands and fingers, typically adjacent to the interphalangeal joints. Less common sites include the foot, ankle, knee, and hip. It may

occur adjacent to the nail fold and produce wide longitudinal grooving of the adjacent nail that clinically mimics myxoid cyst.[50]

Its origin does not represent a component of the skin or nail unit, but it arises from the tendon sheath, joint ligament, or joint synovium, forming a firm nodule fixed deeply to the fibrous tissue of origin and there is often a history of preceding trauma. Histologically, giant cell tumors of the tendon sheath are characterized by a circumscribed, lobulated mass surrounded by dense collagen. The appearance of the tumor varies depending on the proportion of mononuclear cells, giant cells, and collagen. The cellular area is composed of a sheet of round or polygonal cells that blend with hypocellular collagenized zones. Most cells in the cellular areas have the appearance of histiocytes and synovial cells (Figs 6.146 and 6.147). Xanthoma cells are also frequent and often contain fine hemosiderin granules. Hypocellular areas show fibroblasts within a fibrous or homogenized stroma (Fig. 6.148). The characteristic multinucleated giant cells are found scattered randomly throughout both cellular and fibrous areas. Their cytoplasm is deeply eosinophilic and irregularly demarcated and contains a variable number of haphazardly distributed nuclei (see Fig. 6.149). They resemble normal osteoclasts.

## Fibroma of the tendon sheath

Fibroma of the tendon sheath is a slow-growing fibrous tumor firmly attached to the tendon sheath. It is found most frequently in the hands and feet; the thumb is the most common single site. Microscopically, it is characterized by a well-circumscribed lobular mass composed of scattered fibroblasts in a hyalinized collagenous stroma (Figs 6.149 and 6.150). A gradual transition between the hyalinized hypocellular collagenous areas and more cellular areas is occasionally found. In contrast to giant cell tumor of the tendon sheath, fibroma of the tendon sheath has no xanthoma cells or

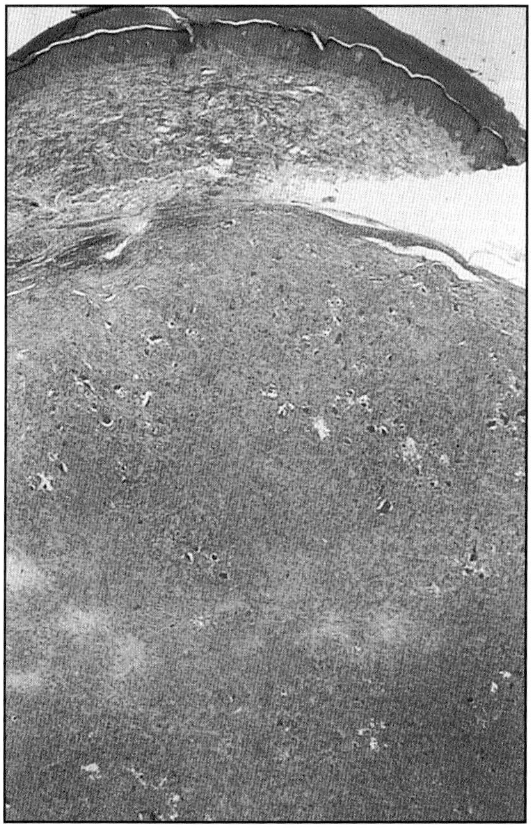

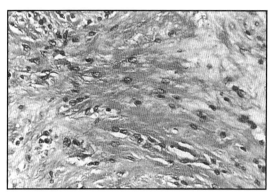

FIGURE 6–148. Giant cell tumor of tendon sheath (high-power magnification of Figure 6.146). In the hypocellular area, most of the cells are fibroblasts that are embedded in a hyalinized stroma.

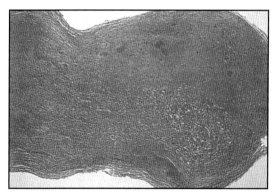

FIGURE 6–149. Fibroma of tendon sheath. The lesion appears as a well-circumscribed, lobular mass.

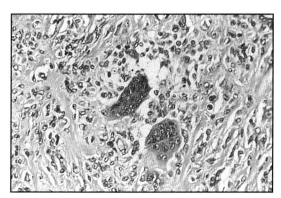

FIGURE 6–146. Giant cell tumor of tendon sheath. The lesion is characterized by a circumscribed cellular mass surrounded by dense collagen.

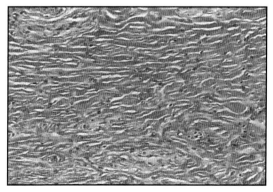

FIGURE 6–150. Fibroma of tendon sheath (high-power magnification of Figure 6.149). Scattered fibroblasts in a hyalinized collagenous stroma are evident.

FIGURE 6–147. Giant cell tumor of tendon sheath (high-power magnification of Figure 6.146). In the cellular area, the cells are composed of histiocytes and multinucleated giant cells.

multinucleated giant cells. Foci of myxoid changes, rarely osseous or chondroid metaplasia, may occur in a small portion of the lesions.

## Osteochondroma

Osteochondroma is a benign, painful neoplasm that occurs on the terminal digit and nail unit. The tumor is loosely attached to bone and rarely may be soft tissue tumor with bony attachment.[51] Histologically, in the dermis there are islands of hyaline cartilage (Fig. 6.151). The mature cartilaginous cell is characterized by a dark, small, and uniform nucleus and is surrounded by a halo as a result of shrinkage of the cytoplasm (Fig. 6.152). Along the margin of the hyaline cartilage, the cells flatten, simulating spindle-shaped fibroblasts so that there is no well-defined transition between the cartilage cells and surrounding connective tissue. Bone formation is seen in the center of the lesion, characterized by spicules of bone containing osteocytes (Fig. 6.153).

## Subungual exostosis

Subungual exostosis is not a true neoplasm but rather an outgrowth of normal bone that is usually caused by antecedent trauma. The lesions mainly arise in the distal aspect of the terminal phalanx and radiologically are continuous with the tuft of the terminal phalanx. The histologic picture is similar to that of osteochondroma (i.e. proliferation of bone spicules extending into the dermis[52] (Fig. 6.154). The ossification or calcification in the lesion

is relatively minimal. Its distal portion, however, is covered by fibrocartilage instead of hyaline cartilage (Fig. 6.155).

## Subungual metastatic tumor

Cutaneous metastases are not uncommon and are most often found on the head, neck, chest, and abdomen. Metastasis to the digits and nail units is rare; the most common site of metastasis is the thumb. The lung is probably the most common site of primary lesions that metastasize to this region. Most metastatic lesions in the fingers initially involve the bone and subsequently spread to the

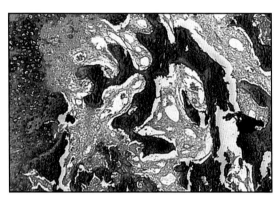
FIGURE 6–153. Osteochondroma (high-power magnification of Figure 6.151). Bone formation is seen in the center of the lesion.

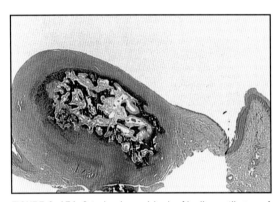
FIGURE 6–151. Ostochondroma. Islands of hyaline cartilage are found in the dermis.

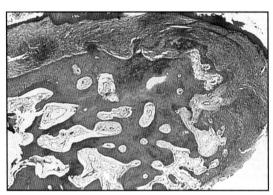
FIGURE 6–154. Subungual exostosis. The tumor appears as an outgrowth of bone spicules in the upper dermis.

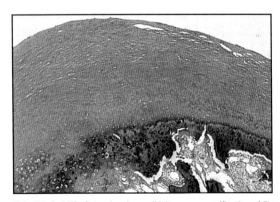
FIGURE 6–152. Osteochondroma (high-power magnification of Figure 6.151). The mature cartilaginous cells show dark, small nuclei and clefts around the cytoplasm.

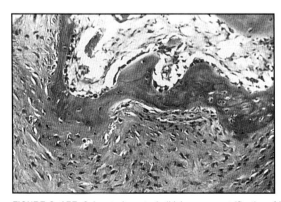
FIGURE 6–155. Subungual exostosis (high-power magnification of Figure 6.154). The bone is lined by osteoblasts and contains blood vessels and connective tissue.

skin and nails. Metastatic tumors to the digits frequently appear swollen, tender, and red, and fluctuate as acute inflammatory lesions. The lesion is often mistaken for an infection or inflammation such as a felon, whitlow, paronychia, or osteomyelitis[53,54] because these lesions suffer injury easily. Cutaneous metastases should therefore be considered in the differential diagnosis of inflammatory process of the digits and histopathology should be performed in every doubtful case. The histologic features consist of solid islands, nests, and cords of atypical tumor cells in the dermis. The cells appear irregularly shaped and large, and contain hyperchromatic nuclei.

# REFERENCES

1. Hashimoto K. Ultrastructure of the human toenail: Proximal nail matrix. J Invest Dermatol 1971; 56:235

2. Higashi N, Saito T. Horizontal distribution of the dopa-positive melanocytes in the nail matrix. J Invest Dermatol 1969; 53:163

3. Zaias N. The nail in health and disease. New York, SP Medical, 1980

4. Crawford GM. Psoriasis of the nails. Arch Dermatol Syphilology 1938; 38:583

5. Alkiewicz J. Psoriasis of the nail. Br J Dermatol 1948; 60:195

6. Samman PD. The nails in lichen planus. Br J Dermatol 1961; 73:288

7. Norton LA. Nail disorders: a review. J Am Acad Dermatol 1980; 2:451

8. Sonnex TS, Douber RPR, Zachary CB, et al. The nail in adult type I pityriasis rubra pilaris: a comparison with Sezary syndrome and psoriasis. J Am Acad Dermatol 1986; 15:956

9. Jerasutus S, Suvanprakorn P, Kitchawengkul O. Twenty nail dystrophy: a clinical manifestation of spongiotic inflammation of the nail matrix. Arch Dermatol 1990; 126:1068

10. Wilkinson JD, Dowber RPR, Fleming K, et al. Twenty nail dystrophy. Arch Dermatol 1979; 115:369

11. Tosti A, Fanti PA, Morelli R, et al. Trachyonychia associated with alopecia areata: a clinical and pathologic study. J Am Acad Dermatol 1991; 25:266

12. Baran R, Dawber RPR. Diseases of the nail and their management. Oxford, Blackwell Scientific, 1994

13. Holzberg M, Wade TR, Buchanan ID, et al. Nail pathology in histocytosis X. J Am Acad Dermatol 1985; 13:522

14. Diestel Meier MR, Soden CE, Rodman OG. Histiocytosis X: a case of nail involvement. Cutis 1982; 30:483

15. Timpatanapong P, Hathirat P, Isarangkura P. Nail involvement in histiocytosis X. Arch Dermatol 1984; 120:1052

16. Zaias N, Ackerman AB. The nail in Darier–White disease. Arch Dermatol 1973; 107:193

17. Su DWP, Chun S II, Hammond DE, et al. Pachyonychia congenita: a clinical study of 12 cases and review of the literature. Pediatr Dermatol 1990; 7:33

18. Stone OJ, Mullin JF. Nail changes in keratoses punctata. Arch Dermatol 1965; 92:557

19. Tosti A, Morelli R, Fanti PA, et al. Nail changes of punctate keratoderma: a clinical and pathological punctate keratoderma. A clinical and pathological study of two patients. Acta Derm Venereol (Stockh) 1993; 73:66

20. Stevens KR, Leis PF, Peters S, et al. Congenital leukonychia. J Am Acad Dermatol 1998; 39:509

21. Scher RK. Subungual scabies. Am J Dermatopathol 1983; 5:187

22. Pavlidaky GP, Hashimoto K, Blum D. Yellow nail syndrome. J Am Acad Dermatol 1984; 11:509

23. Alpert LI, Zak FG, Werthamer S. Subungual basal cell epithelioma. Arch Dermatol 1972; 106:599

24. Hoffman S. Basal cell carcinoma of the nail bed. Arch Dermatol 1973; 108:828

25. Kouskoukis CE, Scher RK, Kopf AW. Squamous cell carcinoma of the nail bed. J Dermatol Surg Oncol 1982; 8:853

26. Guitart J, Bergfeld WF, Tuthill RJ, et al. Squamous cell carcinoma of the nail bed: a clinicopathologic study of 12 cases. Br J Dermatol 1990; 123:215

27. Tosti A, Morelli R, Fanti PA, et al. Carcinoma cuniculatum of the nail apparatus: report of three cases. Dermatology 1993; 186:217

28. Stoll DM, Ackerman AB. Subungual keratoacanthoma. Am J Dermatopathol 1980; 2:265

29. Oliwiecki S, Peachey RDG, Bradfield JWB, et al. Subungual keratoacanthoma: a report of four cases and review of the literature. Clin Exp Dermatol 1994; 19:230

30. Byers P, Mantle J, Salm R. Epidermal cyst of phalanges. J Bone Joint Surg 1966; 488:577

31. Baran R, Broutart JC. Epidermal cyst of the thumb presenting as pincer nail. J Am Acad Dermatol 1988; 9:143

32. Fanti PA, Tosti A. Subungual epidermoid inclusions: report of 8 cases. Dermatologica 1989; 178:209

33. Lewin K. Subungual epidermoid inclusion. Br J Dermatol 1969; 81:671

34. Alessi E, Zorzi F, Gianotti R, et al. Malignant proliferating onycholemmal cyst. J Cutan Pathol 1994; 183

35. Requena L, Sanchez M, Aguilar A, et al. Periungual porocarcinoma. Dermatologica 1990; 180:177

36. Van Gorp J, Van der Putte SCJ. Periungual eccrine porocarcinoma. Dermatology 1993; 187:67

37. Baran R, Kint A. Onychomatrixoma: filamentous tufted tumor in the matrix of a funnel-shaped nail. A new entity (report of three cases). Br J Dermatol 1992; 126:510

38. King DT, Barr RJ. Syringometaplasia: mucinous and squamous variants. J Cutan Pathol 1979; 6:284

39. Mehregan AH. Mucinous syringometaplasia. Arch Dermatol 1980; 116:988

40. Scally K, Assad D. Mucinous syringometaplasia. J Am Acad Dermatol 1984; 11:503

41. Hafner J, Hacnseler E, Ossent P, et al. Benzidine stain for the histochemical detection of hemoglobin in splinter hemorrhage (subungual hematoma) and black heel. Am J Dermatopathol 1995; 17:362

42. Goldman JA, Goldman L, Jaffe MS, et al. Digital mucinous pseudocysts. Arthritis Rheumatol 1997; 20:997

43. Salasche SJ. Myxoid cysts of the proximal nail fold. J Dermatol Surg Oncol 1984; 10:35

44. Shuguart RRR, Soule BH, Johnson EW Jr. Glomus tumor. Surg Gynecol Obstet 1963; 117:334

45. Bart RS, Andrade R, Kopf AW, et al. Acquired digital fibrokeratomas. Arch Dermatol 1968; 97:120

46. Shapiro L. Infantile digital fibromatosis and aponeurotic fibroma. Arch Dermatol 1969; 99:37

47. Camarosa JG, Moreno A. Juvenile hyaline fibromatosis. J Am Acad Dermatol 1987; 16:881

48. Kint A, Baran R. Histopathologic study of Koenen tumors. J Am Acad Dermatol 1988; 12:816

49. Perrin C, Baran R. Invaginated fibrokeratoma with matrix differentiation: a new histologic variant of acquired fibrokeratoma. Br J Dermatol 1994; 130:654

50. Atta KB, Tan CY. Giant cell tumor of tendon sheath producing a groove deformity of the nail plate and mimicking a myxoid cyst. Br J Dermatol 1999; 140:780

51. Cahlin DC, Salvador AH. Cartilagenous tumors of the soft tissues of the hand and feet. Mayo Clin Proc 1974; 49:721

52. Cohen HJ, Frank SB, Minkin W, et al. Subungual exostoses. Arch Dermatol 1973; 107:431

53. Baran R, Tosti A. Metastatic carcinoma to the terminal phalanx of the big toe. J Am Acad Dermatol 1994; 31:259

54. Kagel MF, Scher RK. Metastasis of pulmonary carcinoma to the nail unit. Cutis 1985; 35:121

# 7

# Pigmentation Abnormalities

## Martin N Zaiac and C Ralph Daniel III

## Key Features

1. Nail pigmentation is a diagnostic challenge and needs to be addressed to differentiate benign from malignant processes
2. Single nail involvement with dark brown or black pigmentataion may suggest a neoplastic process
3. Many systemic diseases can be associated with nail pigmentation
4. Drugs taken systemically or applied topically are often implicated in nail pigmentation
5. Many agents in our daily activities when in contact with the nail unit can cause nail pigmentation

A pigmented nail can present a diagnostic challenge for any physician. The differential diagnosis can be as simple as a topical agent in contact with the nail plate or as serious as a life-threatening malignant melanoma. To evaluate pigmentation abnormalities in the nail unit one should have a clear picture of what the normal nail unit should look like; there will be variations in this picture based on ethnic differences. The normal nail unit anatomy has already been discussed (see Chapter 3); however, from a nail pigmentation point of view we must have a clear understanding of how pigment can affect the nail unit so as to have a baseline starting point.

The normal nail unit, regardless of ethnic background, will have a translucent nail plate through which can be seen the pink to reddish nail bed. Proximally, one should see a crescent-shaped whitish to opaque pattern, which is referred to as the lunula; this is the distal matrix. Distally, the nail plate overlies the hyponychium and extends onto normal skin. The surrounding proximal and lateral nail folds should match the adjacent skin color of your patient. Any variation in the above description, whether it be color; opaqueness; loss of the translucent quality of the nail plate;

change in the color of the lunula (matrix), nail bed, or surrounding proximal or lateral nail folds is considered to be a pigment abnormality of the nail unit.

Color changes or pigment abnormalities in the nail unit make up a significant portion of onychopathology. The ability to examine the abnormality properly, and identify which portion or portions of the nail unit are involved is needed to pursue a cause.

One should study all 20 nails. If polish or lacquer is on the nails, it should be removed before examination. One should examine the nails with the digits relaxed and not pressed against any surface.[1,2] Failure to do so may alter nail hemodynamics and obscure subtle changes. The observer should squeeze the digit tip to see whether the color change is altered substantially. This may help to differentiate discoloration of the nail plate from that caused by a vascular alteration. Pressing on the distal digit often grossly changes the latter. In addition, unless the digit is too thick, it is frequently possible to transilluminate a digit by shining a strong penlight upward through the pulp. This procedure may aid in pinpointing more closely the location of the color change or possibly the etiologic agent.

Another tool that can be used to assist the clinician is a dermatoscope. This is a noninvasive instrument in which, through a drop of oil, the nail unit can be illuminated and seen through a magnifying lens. The anatomy of the nail unit can make the use of the dermatoscope difficult but the instrument allows visualization of some pathologic characteristics that are not visible to the naked eye. Dermatoscopic changes that might help distinguish causes of nail pigmentation are in the process of being described; much work is still needed to perfect the diagnostic criteria.

Examination of the nail plate looking at it straight on or at cross-section can help identify where in the matrix the pigmentation is being produced (Fig. 7.1). If the pigment is seen on the dorsal side of the nail plate then the pigment is being produced in

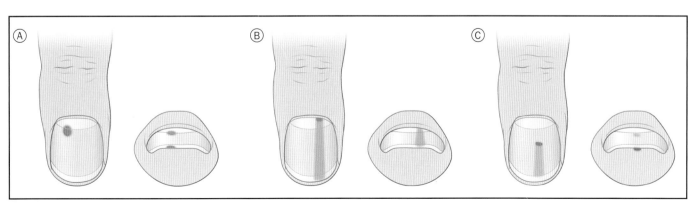

FIGURE 7–1. Views of pigment in the nail plate that correspond to lesions in the nail unit.

the proximal matrix; if the pigment is located on the ventral surface then it is being deposited in the distal matrix; if the pigment is in the mid-nail plate then its source is the mid-matrix; if the entire nail plate is involved then it is being produced by the entire matrix; finally, if no pigment is seen in the nail plate then the lesion is located in the nail bed. Figure 7.2 shows a benign pigmented lesion located in the distal matrix based on the observation of pigment seen in the ventral aspect of the nail plate.

A thorough history may be necessary if no obvious external cause is determined. The review of systems, occupational and recreational activities, medications, topical contactants, and a physical examination may provide valuable information.

Various causes of nail pigmentation abnormalities have been compiled and presented previously, with proven cause relationship and most with anecdotal case reports in the literature.[1–6] Trying to find an easy classification to list these reports is difficult because of the many pigmentation abnormalities which have been described. Subdivision according to the reported cause by major categories yields tables listed as abnormal nail pigmentation attributable to: (i) systemic disorders, (ii) predominantly dermatologic conditions, (iii) inherited or congenital diseases, (iv) systemic drugs or ingestants, (v) local agents, and (vi) miscellaneous named nail entities.[1] Various nail pigmentation abnormalities with eponymic or specific descriptions are also tabulated. The cause, discoloring agent, color description, and site of discoloration in the nail complex are given in many instances when data are available.[1,4]

Most of the nail disorders associated with systemic diseases are not diagnostic of a condition when they are considered alone; however, specific diseases have been associated with certain nail unit findings. One example is yellow nail syndrome (Fig. 7.3).[1] Zaias appropriately stated that if nail discoloration follows the shape of the lunula, it is likely to be caused by internal factors because the discoloration is being deposited in the matrix, whereas if it corresponds to the shape of the proximal nail fold, external factors predominate.[8,9] Many of the inherent pigment abnormalities seen in nails are the result of increased melanogenesis in the matrix. This can be induced by disease states or by oral medications and ingestants;[9] the mechanism is unclear. Other mechanisms include alterations in keratinization, infection, by-products of metabolism, ischemia, genetic abnormalities, and lack of nutrients. Table 7.1 lists some systemic disorders that may cause changes in nail pigmentation.

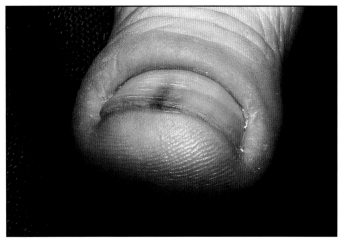

FIGURE 7-2. Pigment in the ventral nail plate corresponds to the junctional nevus in the distal matrix.

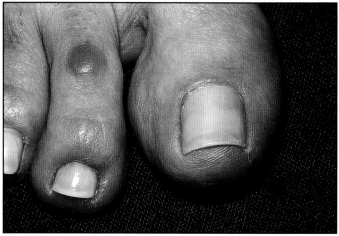

FIGURE 7-3. Yellow nail syndrome: yellowish pigment in the nail plate.

TABLE 7-1. Abnormal nail pigmentation attributable to some systemic disorders

| DISORDERS | DISCOLORING OR CAUSAL AGENT | COLOR | SITE |
|---|---|---|---|
| Adrenal insufficiency[17] | Melanin | Longitudinal brown lines or diffusely brown | Nail plate |
| Alkaline metabolic diseases[18] | ? | Variable white | ? |
| Anemia | Vascular | Pallor | Vascular bed |
| Vitamin B$_{12}$ deficiency[19–22] | Melanin | Variable brown–black | Nail plate, nail bed |
| Bazex's syndrome[23] | ? | Yellow | Nail plate |
| Breast cancer[24] (versus postirradiation) | Melanin | Diffuse hyperpigmentation | Nail plate (?) |
| Bronchiectasis (with hapalonychia)[a] | ? | Light blue tinge or yellowish | Nail plate |
| Carbon monoxide poisoning | Hemoglobin | Cherry red, especially lunula | Vascular bed |
| Cardiac decompensation[17] | ? | Yellow | Distal nail plate |

**TABLE 7–1.** (*Cont'd*) Abnormal nail pigmentation attributable to some systemic disorders

| DISORDERS | DISCOLORING OR CAUSAL AGENT | COLOR | SITE |
|---|---|---|---|
| Cardiac failure[b] | Abnormal adhesion of nail bed to nail | Red lunula | Lunula |
| Carpal tunnel syndrome[25] | Melanin | Longitudinal brown band | Nail plate |
| Cirrhosis[18,26,27] | Probable vascular alteration, a vasodilator polypeptide | Distal red band, white proximal nail; red lunula alone | Vascular bed (?) |
| Cronkhite-Canada syndrome[28] | ? | Yellowish | ? |
| Cushing's syndrome[a] | Melanin | Black | Nail bed, matrix |
| Cyanotic disease | Hemoglobin | Diffuse bluish | Vascular bed |
| Diabetes mellitus[29] | ? | Yellow | Toenails with distal accentuation |
| Fogo selvagem[a] | ? | Yellow canalized lines | ? |
| Fucosidosis[30] | ? | Purple nail bands | ? |
| Gangrene[31] | Necrosis | Black | Probable nail bed |
| Hemochromatosis[32] | Iron or melanin (?) | Diffuse gray, brown, white | Nail plate |
| Hyperbilirubinemia[32] | Melanin | Diffuse brownish | Nail plate |
| Hyperthyroidism[33,34] | Dirt (?) melanin | Variable brown | Nail plate |
| Hypoalbuminemia[35] (e.g., nephrotic syndrome, cirrhosis) | See Muehrcke's lines, Table 7.4 | | |
| Hypocalcemia[18] | ? | Variable white | ? |
| Hypopituitarism[18] | ? | Diffuse brown | Nail plate |
| Hypocalcemia[18] | ? | Variable white | ? |
| Impaired peripheral blood supply[36] | ? | Variable brownish discoloration | ? |
| Leprosy[37] | ? | Diffuse white | Nail plate |
| Lichen planus[20,38] | Melanin | Variable brownish discoloration, longitudinal pigmented band[c]; bluish or reddish color (early change)[c] | Nail plate, nail bed |
| Lupus erythematosus (discoid)[39] | ? | Red–blue longitudinal striae | Nail plate |
| Lymphogranuloma venereum[18] | Vascular | Red lunula | Lunula |
| Malabsorption[18] | ? | Variable white | Lunula |
| Malaria[18,37] | Vascular (?) | Variable gray (?) | Vascular bed |
| Malnutrition[40] | Melanin | Diffuse brown or brown bands | Nail plate (?) |
| Melanosis (postinflammatory)[41] | Melanin | Diffuse brown–black | Nail plate |
| Menstruation[42] | ? | Leukonychia striata | Nail plate |
| Multiple myeloma[43] | ? | Absent lunula | Lunula |
| Pellagra[18] | ? | Diffuse milky white | ? |
| Pinta[21,22] | Melanin | Diffuse brown-black | Nail bed |
| Pregnancy[30,44] | ? | Brown longitudinal pigmented bands | Nail plate |
| Reiter's syndrome | ? | Diffuse brown | ? |
| Renal failure (chronic)[9,45–49] | Melanin | Distal brownish portion | Nail plate |
| Reticulohistiocytosis (multicentric)[50] | ? | Periungual red nodules, 'hyperpigmented' | Periungual |
| Reticulosarcoma[18] | Vascular | Red lunula | Lunula |
| Rheumatoid arthritis[18] | ? | Lilac line of Milan (as in syphilis) | Nail bed or lunula area (?) |
| Sarcoid[51] | ? | Yellowish | Nail plate |
| Syphilis with hypertrophic onychauxis[52] | ? | Diffuse grayish brown | ? |
| Visceral leishmaniasis[43] | ? | Diffuse gray | ? |
| Yellow nail syndrome (acquired)[22,53] | Serum | Diffuse yellow | Nail plate |

See Chapter 15 for additional entries.

[a]D. Swinehart, personal communication, 1979.
[b]C.R. Daniel III, personal observation, 1982.
[c]R. Baran, personal communication, December 1982.
Data from Cutis.[1–4]

TABLE 7–2. Abnormal nail pigmentation attributable to some predominantly dermatologic conditions

| DISORDER | CAUSAL AGENT | COLOR | SITE |
|---|---|---|---|
| Acantholytic epidermolysis bullosa[17] | ? | Longitudinal red and white bands | Nail plate |
| Acanthosis nigricans[41] | ? | Variable brownish discoloration | Nail plate |
| Alopecia areata[23] | ? | Pale yellow leukonychia[42] | Lunula |
| Dyshidrosis[11] | ? | White | Plate |
| Keratosis lichenoides chronica (possible variant of lichen planus)[54] | ? | Yellow–brown | Nail plate |
| Laugier's essential melanotic pigmentation | Melanin | Brownish | Plate |
| Frictional melanonychia[11] | Melanin | Longitudinal brown streaks | Plate |
| Pityriasis rubra pilaris (may be familial)[24] | ? | Diffuse gray or brownish | ? |
| Prurigo vulgaris[18] | ? | Longitudinal yellow–brown lines | Nail plate |
| Psoriasis[9,43,55] | Blood glycoprotein | Brown–yellow | Nail plate |
| Psoriasis[a] | Green nail syndrome (?) | Greenish | ? |
| Senile nails[18] | ? | Absent lunula and opaque | Lunula |
| Vitiligo[9] | Lack of melanin | Variable brown | Nail bed |

[a]R. Baran, personal communication, 1981.

Tables 7.2 and 7.3 list some abnormalities resulting from predominantly dermatologic disorders and inherited or congenital disorders, respectively.

Table 7.4 lists the numerous color changes caused by systemic drugs. For the most part, these changes are simple asymptomatic side effects of treatment, which affect all or multiple nails. Drug-induced nail pigmentation abnormalities may result from toxicity to the matrix, nail bed, or periungual tissues. Phototoxic, photo-allergic, other allergic reactions, and simply the metabolism of the product may cause discolorations, pain, nail shedding, and other symptoms. Depending on the pattern of pigmentation and the historic time reference of any ingested medication, changes can occur to help determine a cause – effect relationship. The most common drug-induced nail changes are those seen with chemotherapeutic agents and the changes seen correspond directly to the dosing cycles. Large numbers of drugs have been reported to produce nail abnormalities; most reports, though, are anecdotal, and reversible once the medication has been stopped. Some examples are: the development of Mee's lines as clues of ingestion of arsenic and the development of nail pigmentation after taking azidethymidine (AZT) for over 8 months (Fig. 7.4). See Chapters 15 and 16 for further information and examples of nail unit changes.

Table 7.5 lists numerous local agents that may affect the nails. Examples of cosmetics, medications, fungi, bacteria, neoplasms, and occupational and physical agents are listed. Numerous topical agents affect the nail plate through adsorption of the substance directly into the plate.[1,10] Various mechanisms are present for other categories. If the substance is impregnated more deeply into the nail or is subungual, specific diagnostic studies such as potassium hydroxide (KOH) preparations, nail composition studies, a biopsy specimen examined with a light microscope, special stains, or possibly an electron microscopic study may be indicated to help analyze the culprit coloration.[1] If scraping the nail plate surface, local cleansing, or use of a solvent such as acetone removes the discoloration, a topical agent is suggested as the cause. Figures 7.5, 7.6 and 7.7 are examples of nail pigmentation in this category.[1]

The initial presenting symptom of malignant melanoma of the nail complex is often a discolored nail. This is the single most important distinction we as nail experts must make to make a proper diagnosis when dealing with a nail pigment abnormality. Failure to diagnose could have fatal consequences for the patient. If one cannot rule out malignant melanoma as a case of benign longitudinal nail pigmentation (Table 7.6), if Hutchinson's sign is noted (leaching of pigment from the nail to a nail fold), or if for whatever reason there is suspicion, a biopsy is mandatory.

Longitudinal pigmented bands (LPB) can be seen in individuals with skin types 1 to 6, although they are seen most commonly in skin types 3 to 6. In these individuals, this is commonly seen in multiple nails. Baran[11,12] gave some helpful suggestions when trying to differentiate benign LPB from those associated with subungual melanoma (SM):[12]

*The clinician should be suspicious when LPB: (1) begins in a single digit of a person during the sixth decade of life or later; (2) develops abruptly in a previously normal nail plate; (3) becomes suddenly darker or wider; (4) occurs in either the thumb, index finger, or great toe; (5) occurs in a person who gives a history of digital trauma; (6) occurs as a single band in the digit of a dark-skinned patient, particularly if the thumb or great toe is affected; (7) demonstrates blurred, rather than sharp, lateral borders; (8) occurs in a person who gives a history of malignant melanoma; (9) occurs in a person in whom the risk for melanoma is increased (e.g., dysplastic nevus syndrome, or family history of melanoma); (10) is accompanied by nail dystrophy, such as partial nail destruction or disappearance.*

Other signs besides the ones listed above have been reported and are noteworthy[11,12] but not necessarily helpful in establishing the likelihood of malignancy. We must take note of these reports and develop personal criteria for diagnosing longitudinal pigmented bands.

1. Lightly pigmented bands are less likely to represent SM; although, a lightly melanotic SM has been reported, the pathologist may have difficulty visualizing the melanin and melanocytes that constitute light pigmented bands.

TABLE 7–3. Abnormal nail pigmentation attributable to some inherited or congenital diseases

| DISORDER | DISCOLORING OR CAUSAL AGENT | COLOR | SITE |
| --- | --- | --- | --- |
| Pili torti[4,56] | ? | Leukonychia | Nail plate |
| Pernicious anemia[57] | ? | Blue | ? |
| Acquired immunodeficiency syndrome[58,59] | ? | Yellowish | ? |
| Vitamin $B_{12}$ deficiency[60] | ? | Bluish–black | ? |
| Acrodermatitis enteropathica[43] | ? | Variable brownish discoloration | ? |
| Amyloidosis with polyneuropathy (familial)[29] | ? | Yellow | Toenails with distal accentuation |
| Bart–Gorlin–Anderson syndrome[42] | ? | Gray–yellow | ? |
| Coat's syndrome[30] | ? | Red | Nail bed |
| Darier's disease[61,62] | ? | Brown or white, and red streaks | Nail bed, matrix |
| Great toenail dystrophy[23] | ? | Dark colored | Great toenails |
| Ectodermal defect (congenital)[41] | ? | Diffuse brownish | Nail plate |
| Erythropoietic protoporphyria[63] | ? | No lunula, grayish | Absent lunula (?) |
| Genetic tendency for nail pigmentation after chemotherapy?[64] | ? | Brown | ? |
| Hidrotic ectodermal defect[43] | ? | Diffuse yellow | ? |
| Hutchinson–Gilford syndrome[9] | ? | Variable yellow | ? |
| Ichthyosiform syndrome (congenital) with keratitis and deafness[65] | ? | Diffuse white | ? |
| Incontinentia pigmenti[52,66] | ? | Diffuse yellowish | ? |
| Leukonychia, knuckle pads, deafness[67] | ? | Partial white | Nail plate |
| Leukonychia totalis (congenital)[68] | ? | Diffuse white | Nail plate |
| Nevi (familial congenital pigmented)[69] | Melanin | Punctate or longitudinal brownish | Nail plate, matrix |
| Ochronosis[70] | Hemogenistic acid (?) | Diffuse grayish | Nail bed (?) |
| Pachyonychia congenita[9] | ? | Diffuse brownish | Nail plate |
| Peutz–Jeghers syndrome[71,72] | Melanin | Punctate brown | Nail plate, nail bed |
| Phenytoin effects (congenital)[73] | ? | Brown (ocher) | Nail plate |
| Porphyria (congenital erythropoietic) | Porphyrin | Red fluorescence with Wood's light | Nail plate |
| Progeria[9] | ? | Yellowish | ? |
| Racket nail (congenital)[18] | ? | Diffuse white | Lunula (?) |
| Soft nail disease[74] | ? | Absent lunula | Matrix |
| Telangiectasia (hereditary acrolabial)[75] | ? | Diffuse blue | Nail bed |
| Telangiectasia (hereditary hemorrhagic)[76] | Vascular components | Punctate red | Vascular bed |
| Trichothiodystrophy[77] | ? | Yellow | Toenails |
| Yellow nail syndrome (congenital)[9,53] | Thickened nail plate (?) | Diffuse yellow | Nail plate |
| Wilson's disease[9,78] | Copper | Blue, especially lunula | Nail plate pigmentation abnormalities |

Data from Cutis.[1–4]

2. Darker shades of brown do not necessarily represent melanoma. Nevi and melanoma may manifest identical shades of brown. In White persons, black bands may be an important clue to melanoma; in African–Americans, however, jet-black bands are not unusual. Theoretically, color variegation suggests melanoma; however, variegation is common in persons with multiple benign bands.

3. Theoretically, wide bands suggest melanoma; however, the critical width that determines melanoma has yet to be established.

4. Bands that do not extend distally to the free edge of the nail are unlikely to represent melanoma because they do not take their origin from the nail matrix. However, they may represent metastatic melanoma or LPB arising from the nail bed.

The management of African–American patients or any patient with pigmented bands – singular or multiple – can be difficult. Although multiple nail involvement suggests benign LPB, there may be substantial variability in the color and width of bands within a single nail plate and or among different nails in the same patient, making the decision to biopsy or not difficult. Reports of malignant melanoma occurring in both African–American and Caucasian patients with multiple nail LPB have been reported.[13] Whether a LPB in a thumb or great toe represents malignant melanoma or racial variation is not necessarily easily determined

TABLE 7–4. Abnormal nail pigmentation caused by some systemic drugs or ingestants

| DRUG | DISCOLORING AGENT | COLOR | SITE |
|---|---|---|---|
| Acetanilid[52] | ? | Variable purple | ? |
| Acetylsalicylic acid[42] | ? | Purpura | Nail bed |
| Acridine derivations[11] (acriflavine, trypaflavine) | | Whitish | Distal bed |
| Androgen[79] | ? | Half-and-half nail–like changes | ? |
| Aniline poisoning[52] | ? | Variable blue-violet | ? |
| Antimalarials[9,21,22,79,80] | Melanin, antimalarial | Diffuse blue, brown, variable | Nail plate, nail bed |
| Antimony[11] | ? | Leukonychia | ? |
| Arsenic[81] | Melanin (?) | Transverse white lines, diffuse brown | Nail plate |
| Azidothymidine[82,83] | | Dark, bluish, brownish | |
| Beta carotene[29,42] | Beta carotene | Yellow | Nail bed |
| Brome[30] | Hemorrhage | Reddish | Nail bed |
| Canthaxantine[11] | ? | Yellow | Bed |
| Caustic soda[30] | ? | Yellow | Nail plate |
| Chromium salts[11] | | Yellow | Plate |
| Corticotropin[11] | | Longitudinal diffuse brown | Plate |
| Dichromates[42] | ? | Yellow ocher | ? |
| Dicyanidamide[a] | ? | Brownish | ? |
| Dinitrophenol[11] | ? | Yellow or long streaks | Bed |
| Emetine chlorate[18] | ? | Variable white | ? |
| Fluoride (fluorosis)[40] | Melanin (?) | Brown bands | Nail plate, matrix |
| Gold (allergic reaction)[41] | ? | Variable brown | ? |
| Heparin[30] | Acute poisoning | Red band | Nail bed |
| Ibuprofen[85] | ? | Longitudinal pigmented bands | Nail plate |
| Ketoconazole[30] | ? | Longitudinal band splinter hemorrhage | Nail plate, nail bed |
| Lead[86] | Lead | Hyperpigmentation | ? |
| Lithium carbonate[87] | ? | Change from golden to normal | Probably nail plate |
| Mepacrine[23] | ? | Variable brown | ? |
| Mercury[9] | Mercury (?) | Variable brown | Nail bed[88] |
| Methoxsalen[84] | ? | Diffuse brown | Nail plate |
| Minocycline[89] | ? | Blue-gray | ? |
| Mitoxantrone | ? | Blue | ? |
| Melanoyte-stimulating hormone[11] | ? | Brown | Plate |
| Neo-Synephrine (phenylephrine)[52] | ? | Nail bed purpura | Nail bed |
| Para-aminosalicylic acid[11] | ? | Cyanosis | Bed |
| Picric acid[11] | ? | Yellow | Bed |
| Phosphorus[11] | ? | Hemorrhage | Bed |
| Polychlorinated biphenyls[30] | ? | Brown to gray line | Nail plate and nail bed |
| D-Penicillamine[90] | ? | Yellow nail syndrome | ? |
| Penicillamine[91] | ? | Absence of lunula | Lunula |
| Penicillamine[11] | ? | Yellow | Plates |
| Phenindione | ? | Diffuse brown–yellow,[70] orange[92] | ? |
| Phenolphthalein[43] | ? | Diffuse gray | ? |
| Phenothiazine (photoreaction)[93] | ? | Variable brown | ? |
| Phenytoin[73] | ? | Brown (ocher) | Nail plate |
| Pilocarpine poisoning[42] | ? | Leukonychia or plate | Nail bed (?) |
| Practolol[7] | ? | Subungual blotchy erythema | Nail bed |
| Santonin[29] | ? | Yellow | Nail plate (?) |
| Silver (argyria)[22,94] | Silver | Diffuse azure, dark gray | Lunula, nail plate, matrix |
| Sulfonamide (allergic reaction)[18] | ? | Variable brown with drug reaction | ? |
| Sulphydrilic acid[18] | ? | Variable blue | ? |
| Tetracycline[22,56,95,96] | Photoonycholysis splinter hemorrhages | Variable brown, red | Nail plate, nail bed |
| Tetryl[30] | Nitramine | Yellow | Nail bed |
| Thallium[37] | ? | Variable white | ? |
| Timolol[97] | ? | Brown | Probably nail plate |
| Trinitrotoluene (absorption)[52] | ? | Nail bed purpura | Nail bed |
| Warfarin sodium[98,99] | ? | Purplish | Nail bed |

TABLE 7–4. (*Cont'd*) Abnormal nail pigmentation caused by some systemic drugs or ingestants

| DRUG | DISCOLORING AGENT | COLOR | SITE |
|---|---|---|---|
| **Cancer chemotherapeutic agents** | | | |
| Bleomycin[100,101] | Melanin | Variable brown, blue | Nail plate |
| Busulfan[32] | ? | Variable brown | Lunula, nail plate |
| Cyclophosphamide[32,102] | ? | Variable black | Nail plate |
| Daunorubicin[88] | ? | Transverse brown-black bands | Nail plate |
| Dinitrochlorobenzene[b] | ? | Brownish | Nail plate (?) |
| Doxorubicin[102–105] | Melanin | Variable brown–blue | Nail plate, bed |
| 5-Fluorouracil[79] | ? | Half-and-half nail-like changes, variable brown | ? |
| Hydroxyurea[34,103] | ? | Variable brownish | Nail plate, bed |
| Melphalan[32] | ? | Variable brown | Nail plate, bed |

See Table 7.6
[a]R. Baran, personal communication, 1980.
[b]R. Baran, personal communication, 1981.
Data from Cutis.[1–4]

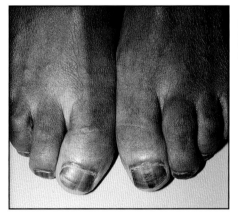

FIGURE 7–4. Patient's nails after 8 months of azidethymidine (AZT) treatment. Pigment in the nail plate.

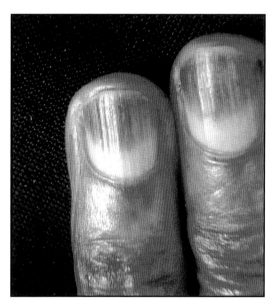

FIGURE 7–5. Hydroquinone pigmentation from a 'fade' cream.

by history and inspection alone. Change in the morphology of LPB is the most important clue to the possibility of melanoma in these patients and is a significant reason for concern, and a biopsy. Multiple bands in multiple nails are not usually neoplastic in origin, although multiple subungual melanomas have been observed. A thorough examination of the skin and nails, complete review of systems, drug history, culture for a possible nail infection and a biopsy will usually reveal the underlying cause of multiple LPB.[12] Pseudo-Hutchinson's sign may be caused by drugs such as minocycline, by the acquired immunodeficiency syndrome, Peutz–Jegher's syndrome, and frictional melanonychia (R. Baran, personal communication, 4 December 1993). A subungual hematoma from trauma, which extends to the proximal nail matrix, may also cause this sign to occur. These causes can be determined by a complete history, and examination as described previously. One must develop personal criteria by which to determine how to handle longitudinal bands. Following the above personal and reported tips will be helpful.

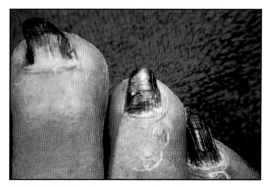

FIGURE 7–6. Potassium permanganate soaks.

**TABLE 7–5. Abnormal nail pigmentation attributable to some local agents**

| CAUSE | DISCOLORING AGENT | COLOR | SITE |
|---|---|---|---|
| Ammoniated mercury[106] | Mercury | Gray | Nail plate |
| Amphotericin B[23] | Amphotericin B | Yellow | Nail plate |
| Anthralin[41] | Anthralin | Variable brown | Nail plate surface |
| Arning's tincture[28] | Tincture | Brownish | Nail plate |
| Burnt sugar[52,107] | Burnt sugar | Variable brown | Nail plate surface |
| Chlorophyll derivations[2] | Same | Green | Plate |
| Chlorophyllin copper complex and sodium propionate (Prophyllin) | Sodium propionate | Variable green | Nail plate surface |
| Chloroxine[30] | ? | Different colors | ? |
| Chromium salts[32] | Chromium salts | Variable ocherous | Nail plate (?) |
| Chrysarobin[41] | Chrysarobin | Variable brown | Nail plate surface |
| Coffee (roasted)[52,107] | Coffee | Variable brown | Nail plate surface |
| Copper sulfate[a] | Copper sulfate | Greenish | Nail plate |
| Derifil (chlorophyllin copper complex) | Chlorophyll | Green | Nail plate |
| Dinitrochlorobenzene[11] | ? | Yellow | Plate |
| Dinitroorthocresol[108] | Dinitroorthocresol | Variable yellow | Nail matrix |
| Dinubuton[32] | ? | Variable yellow | ? |
| Diquat[68,109] | ? | Variable brown | ? |
| Dirt | Dirt | Variable brown | Nail plate surface subungual |
| Dynap insecticide[b] | Insecticide | Yellow | Nail plate |
| Ebony workers[52] | Ebony | Dark yellow or blackish | Nail bed region |
| Eosin[11] | Same | Red | Plate |
| 5-Fluorouracil[11] | ? | Brown | Plate |
| Fluorescein[29] | Fluorescein | Yellow | Nail plate |
| Formaldehyde[106] | Formaldehyde | Variable brown | Nail plate surface |
| Fuchsin[11] | Same | Purple | Plate |
| Galvanizer's (silver and cyanide)[107] | Silver and cyanide | Diffuse dark blue | ? |
| Gentian violet | Gentian violet | Variable purple | Nail plate surface |
| Glutaraldehyde[110] | Glutaraldehyde | Golden brown | Nail plate |
| Hatter's chemicals[52] | ? | Variable yellow | Nail plate surface |
| Henna[52] | ? | Variable brown | ? |
| Hydrofluoric acid[20] | Hydrofluoric acid | Yellow | Nail plate |
| Hydroquinone[7,c] | Hydroquinone | Orange-brown | Nail plate |
| Ink | Ink (variable) | Variable | Nail plate surface |
| Iodine | Same | Yellowish brown | Plate |
| Iodochlorohydroxyquin (Vioform) | Iodochlorhydroxyquin | Brownish | Nail plate |
| Iron (elemental)[111] | Iron | Orange-brown | Nail plate |
| Mahogany[112] | ? | Brownish | Nail plate |
| Merbromin (mercurochrome) | Same | Reddish-purple | Plate |
| Mercury | Same | Blackish | Plate |
| Mercury bichloride plus sun exposure[94] | Mercury bichloride | Gray–blue | Probable nail plate |
| Methylenedianiline[29a] | ? | ? | ? |
| Methyl green[11] | Same | Green | Plate |
| Methylene blue[11] | Same | Blue | Plate |
| Nail enamel | ? | Variable brown | Nail plate surface |
| Nicotine, tar | Nicotine, tar | Variable brown | Nail plate surface |
| Nitric acid[11] | Same | Yellow | Plate |
| Nitrocellulose reacting with resorcin and toluene sulfonamide[94] | ? | Variable brown | Nail plate surface |
| Oxalic acid in radiators[106,107] | Oxalic acid | Variable blue | ? |
| Paraquat[68,109] | ? | Variable brown | ? |
| Pecans | Pecans | Diffuse brown | Nail plate surface |
| Photographic developer[22,43,52] | Methol or *p*-methyl-aminophenol sulfate hydroquinone | Variable black | Nail plate |

**TABLE 7–5. (Cont'd) Abnormal nail pigmentation attributable to some local agents**

| CAUSE | DISCOLORING AGENT | COLOR | SITE |
|---|---|---|---|
| Picric acid[43] | ? | Variable brown | Nail plate surface (?) |
| Potassium permanganate[41] | Potassium permanganate | Variable brown or yellow | Nail plate surface |
| Pyrogallol[28] | Pyrogallol (?) | Brownish | Nail plate |
| Radiotherapy (local)[42] | Irradiation | Brown transverse or longitudinal pigmented bands | ? |
| Resorcinol[22,41,43,95] | Resorcinol | Variable brown | Nail plate surface |
| Rivanol[28] | Rivanol (?) | Brownish | Nail plate |
| Rhus dermatitis[30] | ? | Yellow | ? |
| Shoe polish | Shoe polish | Variable | Nail plate surface |
| Silver nitrate | Silver | Variable black | Nail plate surface |
| Sodium hypochlorite[11] | Same | Whitish | Onycholysis |
| Sublimate[28] | Sublimate | Brownish | Nail plate |
| Tar | Same | Yellowish brown | Plate |
| Tartrazine[11] | Same | Yellow | Plate |
| Tetracycline (topical)[11] | Same | Yellowish | Plate |
| Thermal injury[a] | ? | Yellow-brown | ? |
| Triamcinolone (intradermal)[113] | Steroid | Hypopigmented | Periungual |
| Walnuts[52,107] | Walnuts | Variable brown | Nail plate surface |
| Wine (red)[107] | Wine components | Variable black | Nail plate surface |

## Fungi (partial listing)

| | | | |
|---|---|---|---|
| Alternaria tenuis[52] | ? | Black lateral edges | ? |
| Aspergillus flavus[52] | Fungus | Peripheral green or punctate white | Nail plate |
| Aspergillus terreus[11] | Same | Longitudinal pigmented brownish bands | Plate |
| Blastomycetes[32,52] | Fungus | Variable blue-green, black | ? |
| Botryodiplodia theobromae[114] | Fungus | Variable brown | Nail plate |
| Candida albicans[115] | Fungus | Longitudinal white streaks | Nail plate |
| Candida species | Fungus (?) | Variable yellow | Nail plate |
| Cephalosporium[43] | Fungus | Punctate white | Superficial nail plate |
| Chaetomium perpulchrum[11] | Same | Longitudinal pigmented brownish bands | Plate |
| Cladosporium carrionii[11] | Same | Longitudinal pigmented brownish bands | Plate |
| Curvularia lunata[11] | Same | Longitudinal pigmented brownish bands | Plate |
| Favus (Trichophyton schoenleinii)[32] | Fungus | Variable grayish yellow | ? |
| Fusarium oxysporum[32,116] | Fungus (?) | Variable black, whitish, or white | Superficial nail plate |
| Hendersonula toruloidea[117] | Fungus | Variable brown | "Nail tissue" |
| Homodendrum species[32] | ? | Variable black | ? |
| Microsporum persicolor[15] | Same | Longitudinal pigmented brownish bands | Plate |
| Scopulariopsis brevicaulis | ? | Peripheral yellowish | ? |
| Tinea imbricata[52] | Fungus | Variable ash gray | Nail plate |
| Numerous trichophytons (proximal subungual onychomycosis)[43] | Fungus | White areas proceeding distally from proximal nail fold | Nail plate |
| Pyrenochaeta unguius-hominis[11] | Same | Longitudinal pigmented brownish bands | Plate |
| Scytalidium dimidiatum[11] | Same | Longitudinal pigmented brownish bands | Plate |
| Trichophyton mentagrophytes[9] | ? | Punctate white | Superficial nail plate |
| Trichophyton rubrum[118] | Fungus | Variable white | Nail plate |
| Trichophyton tonsurans[15] | Same | Longitudinal pigmented brownish bands | Plate |
| Wangiella dermatitidis[11] | Same | Longitudinal pigmented brownish bands | Plate |

**TABLE 7–5. (*Cont'd*) Abnormal nail pigmentation attributable to some local agents**

| CAUSE | DISCOLORING AGENT | COLOR | SITE |
|---|---|---|---|
| **Bacteria** | | | |
| Concomitant with dermatophytes[32] | ? | Variable brown, gray, green | ? |
| Various other causes of paronychia[43] | Variable | Variable | Variable |
| *Proteus mirabilis*[32] | Bacteria (?) | Variable black | Nail plate |
| *Pseudomonas*[22] | Pyocyanin, fluorescein | Variable green | Nail plate |
| **Nevi and tumors** | | | |
| Angioma | Vascular | Variable red | Vascular bed |
| Enchondroma | Tumor | Bluish | Subungual, nail bed[d] |
| Exostosis[11] | Same | Brown | Bed |
| Glomus tumor | Vascular | Localized red | Vascular bed |
| Mucous cyst[e] | ? | Longitudinal brownish band | ? |
| Nevi (junctional)[68,119,120] | Melanin | Punctate brown | Nail plate |
| Pigmented cutaneous horn[8] | Cutaneous horn | Pigmented | Matrix – nail bed |
| Subungual epidermal cysts[121] | ? | Yellowish white | Nail bed |
| Subungual epidermoid inclusions[122] | Subungual epidermoid inclusions | Black | Nail bed |
| Subungual melanoma or Hutchinson's melanotic whitlow[21,22] | Melanin | Variable black | Nail plate, nail bed periungual |
| **Physical agents** | | | |
| Hemorrhage | Blood components | Variable red–brown | Nail bed |
| Ionizing radiation[8] | ? | Longitudinal red | Lunula – nail bed |
| Irradiation[22,123] | Melanin | Variable brown–black | Nail plate |
| Microwaves[30] | ? | Whitish | Nail bed |
| Trauma | Variable | Variable | Variable |
| Vibrating power tools[30] longitudinal bands | ? | Yellow–white | ? |
| Yellow staining in molded plastic workers | 4,4-methylenedianiline | Yellow | Nail plate |

See further additions in Table 7.6 (longitudinal pigmented bands).
[a]R. Baran, personal communication, 1981.
[b]C.R. Daniel III, unpublished data, 1980.
[c]C.R. Daniel III, unpublished observation, 1981.
[d]D. Swinehart, personal communication, 1979.
[e]S. Salasche, personal communication, December 1982.
Data from Cutis.[1–4]

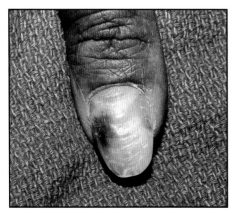

FIGURE 7–7. Green pigmentation under the nail plate: *Pseudomonas* species.

Table 7.6 lists several named nail entities with abnormal pigment nail changes. Much of this information can be found scattered throughout the other chapters in this book. It is helpful to have many of the causes compiled in one location for the purpose of cross-referencing and differential diagnosis.

The term 'leukonychia' has various meanings to different physicians. I evaluate a patient with leukonychia by asking myself the following questions:[14,15]

1. Is it congenital or acquired?
2. Is the color change caused by an aberration mainly of the nail plate (parakeratosis) or elsewhere?
3. Is it endogenously induced or idiopathic (more often multiple nails) or caused by exogenous or nonsystemic factors (more often fewer nails)?
4. What is the pattern (partial, total, striate, punctate, location, number of nails, and so forth)?

**TABLE 7–6. Abnormal nail pigmentation attributable to some named nail entities** 83

| ENTITY | CAUSE OR ASSOCIATION | DISCOLORING AGENT | COLOR | SITE |
|---|---|---|---|---|
| Arcs (brown)[32,46] | Chronic renal failure | Melanin | Distal brown arc | Nail plate |
| Bissell's lines[17,124] | Adrenal insufficiency | Melanin | Longitudinal brown lines | Nail plate |
| Crescents[46,47,125] | Systemic illness | Probable vascular alteration | Distal red band | Vascular bed |
| Great toenail dystrophy[23] | Inherited | ? | Dark colored | ? |
| Expedition nails[23] | Possible protein deficiency | ? | Transverse white bands | Nail plate (?) |
| Half-and-half nails[45,46,48,49,69] | Chronic renal failure – stimulation of matrix melanocytes | Melanin | Proximal white or proximal normal brown distal nail | Nail plate |
| Idiopathic azure nails[26] | ? | ? | Diffuse azure | ? |
| Laugier's essential melanotic pigmentation[32,64a] | ? | Melanin | Diffuse brownish or patterned | Nail plate |
| Leukonychia (white discoloration) | Acrokeratosis verruciformis,[126] acute rejection of renal allograft,[127] alkaline metabolic disease,[18] alopecia antimony,[127] areata,[42] anemia, cachectic state,[18] carbon monoxide,[128] carcinoid syndrome,[127] cirrhosis,[27] congenital leukonychia,[68] cortisone,[127] cryoglobulinemia,[128] Darier's disease,[62,68] diquat,[18] dyshidrosis,[42] emetine chlorhydrate,[18] endemic,[127] erythema multiforme,[11] exfoliative dermatitis,[8] fluorosis,[8] formaldehyde (nail hardener),[129,130] fungi,[9,43] gout,[11] half-and-half nail,[46,47] herpes zoster,[11] Hodgkin's disease,[35] hypoalbuminemia,[35] hypocalcemia,[18] Kawasaki syndrome,[127] kidney transplantation,[127] lead poisoning,[52,127] LEOPARD syndrome,[42,127] leprosy,[127] leukonychia striata semilunaris,[52] malaria,[8] manic-depressive illness,[18] Mees' lines,[37,131] Muehrcke's lines[35,132] (see previous tables), pachyonychia congenita (autosomal recessive),[127] paraquat,[18] pellagra,[18] pilitorti,[49a] pilocarpine,[127] pneumonia,[8] rickettsial infection,[127] sickle-cell anemia,[8] some diseases with fever,[18] sulfonamides,[18] sympathetic symmetric punctate leukonychia[133] (syndrome of leukonychia, knuckle pads, deafness),[67] syphilis,[11] tuberculosis,[11] trauma,[68,134] trichinosis,[18] ulcerative colitis,[18] zinc deficiency (see other tables as well as Chapter 15) | | | | |

TABLE 7–6. (*Cont'd*) Abnormal nail pigmentation attributable to some named nail entities

| ENTITY | CAUSE OR ASSOCIATION | DISCOLORING AGENT | COLOR | SITE |
|---|---|---|---|---|
| Leukonychia (longitudinal) | Erythema multiforme,[30] gout,[30] herpes zoster,[30] leuko-onycholysis paradentotica,[30] microwaves,[110] nevoid matrix changes,[28] Darier's disease | | | |
| Longitudinal brownish pigmented bands | Acrodermatitis Variable enteropathica,[135] *Acrotherium niger*,[69] adrenal insufficiency,[17] doxorubicin (Adriamycin),[12,88,136] acquired immunodeficiency syndrome,[137] *Alternaria tenuis*,[138] antimalarials,[23,135] arsenic poisoning,[18] blastomycetes,[12] bleomycin,[7] *Botryodiplodia theobromae*,[135] Bowen's[16a] disease,[139] busulfan,[135] bullous primary amyloidosis,[42] *Candida* species,[71] carpal tunnel syndrome,[25] cyclophosphamide,[136] daunorubicin,[135] diquat,[12] exostosis,[135] fluorosis,[40] foreign body,[12] Fusarium,[12] gangrene,[135] gold therapy,[18] hematoma,[12] hemosiderosis,[12] *Hendersonula toruloidea*,[12] *Homodendrum elatum*,[12] hydroxyurea,[140] hyperbilirubinemia,[137] hyptherthyroidism,[137] hypopituitarism,[135] idiopathic,[118,124,141] ketoconazole,[30] Laugier–Hunziker syndrome, lichen planus,[32] local radiotherapy,[42] gemfibrozil (Lopid),[142] malnutrition,[54] melphalan,[7] mepacrine,[12,135] mercury,[135] methotrexate,[135] minocycline,[143] mucous cyst,[a] nevi,[69] nitrogen mustard,[12] nitrosourea,[12] ochronosis,[135] onychophagia,[144] osteomyelitis,[135] Peutz–Jegher's syndrome,[71,72] phenolphthalein, phenol, regressing nevoid melanosis in childhood,[170] phthalein poisoning,[18] phenothiazine,[135] phenytoin, pinta,[12] porphyria,[145] postinflammatory hyperpigmentation,[12] pregnancy,[30] *Proteus mirabilis*,[12] prurigo vulgaris,[18] psoralen,[12] subungual epidermal inclusions,[146] subungual fibrous histiocytoma,[12] sulfonamide,[12] syphilis (secondary),[30,135] tetracycline,[12] thermal injury,[135] 3'azidodeoxythymidine,[147] timolol,[12] trauma,[115,148] *Trichophyton soudanese*,[12] verucca vulgaris,[135] vitamin $B_{12}$ deficiency,[94a] Bowen's disease of nail unit,[60,108] basal cell carcinoma,[111a,149] melanoma,[6] azidothymidine,[83] ibuprofen[85] (see Chapter 15) | | | |

**TABLE 7–6.** (*Cont'd*) Abnormal nail pigmentation attributable to some named nail entities

| ENTITY | CAUSE OR ASSOCIATION | DISCOLORING AGENT | COLOR | SITE |
|---|---|---|---|---|
| Mees' lines[37] | Arsenic, cardiac insufficiency, Hodgkin's disease, leprosy, malaria, myocardial infarction, pellagra, pneumonia, psoriasis, renal failure, sickle-cell anemia, thallium, other serious systemic diseases | Variable | Single or multiple white transverse | Nail bed |
| Muehrcke's lines | Hypoalbuminemia | Alteration of nail bed– plate attachment (?) | Usually double white transverse | Vascular bed versus nail bed plate attachment |
| Senile nails[18,41] | Age, solar, refractile (?) | ? | No lunula and/or brown or opaque | Matrix or nail plate |
| Splinter hemorrhages | Bacterial endocarditis,[93,134] Darier's disease,[62] dialysis,[150,151] drug reaction,[93] methoxsalen,[152] fungi,[68] general illness,[150,153] mycosis fungoides,[28] Osler–Weber–Rendu disease,[18] peptic ulcer,[68] psoriasis,[93] radiodermatitis,[128] rheumatoid arthritis,[68] scurvy,[93] 10 to 20% of normal population,[70,153] tetracycline,[96] thyrotoxicosis,[93,153,154] trauma,[150,154] trichinosis,[68,93,153] vasculitis[93] | | | |
| Terry's nails[27] | Cirrhosis | Probable vascular alteration | Prominent onychodermal band, white proximal nails | Vascular bed |
| Yellow nail syndrome | Bronchiectasis,[155] carcinoma larynx,[155] chronic bronchitis,[155] chronic lymphedema,[155] rheumatoid arthritis,[156] sinusitis,[155] thyroid disease[155] | | | |
| Miscellaneous changes of lunula (see also other tables) | | | | |
| All pigmented individuals[18] | ? | Smaller lunula | Lunula change | Lunula |
| Blue lunulae | Argyria,[94] hereditary acrolabial telangiectasia,[30] paronychia (bacterial, probably *Pseudomonas*),[94] quinacrine,[94] topical bichloride or mercury followed by sunlight (see Wilson's disease, Table 7–1), zidovudine | | | |
| Diffusion of lunula | Ischemia[157] | ? | Whitish | Lunula |

**TABLE 7–6. (*Cont'd*) Abnormal nail pigmentation attributable to some named nail entities**

| ENTITY | CAUSE OR ASSOCIATION | DISCOLORING AGENT | COLOR | SITE |
|---|---|---|---|---|
| Diminished or absent abnormal lunula | Acromegaly,[18] adiposogenital syndrome,[18] atherosclerosis,[171] chronic obstructive pulmonary disease,[171] chronic polyarthritis,[18] brachyonychia,[171] congenital onychodysplasia of the index fingers (ISO and Kikuchi syndrome),[160] erythropoietic protoporphyria,[171] hereditary osteoungual dysplasia,[18] hyperthyroidism,[171] hypothyroidism,[171] hypopituitarism,[18] Goltz's syndrome,[42] malnutrition,[171] lymphedema,[171] iron deficiency anemia,[171] leprosy,[18] multiple myeloma,[158] HIV,[171] pachyonychia congenita,[171] penicillamine,[91] renal failure,[171] rheumatoid arthritis,[171] porphyria cutanea tarda,[171] porphyria,[42] nail patella syndrome,[171] nerve injury,[171] soft nail disease,[171] monosomy 4p,[42] scleroderma,[159] trisomy 21[171] | | | |
| Indians (India)[18] | ? | Extended lunula | Lunula | Lunula |
| Large lunulas | Habit tic,[42] hydrocortisone on cuticle,[161] median nail dystrophy[23] | ? | Large lunulas | Lunula |
| Multiple myeloma[43] | ? | No lunula | Lunula change | Lunula |
| Pseudo-Hutchinson's sign[170] | Ethnic pigmentation,[170] Laugier–Hunziker syndrome,[170] Peutz–Jeghers syndrome,[170] radiation therapy,[170] malnutrition,[170] menopause,[170] patients with AIDS,[170] trauma induced,[170] congenital nevus,[170] after biopsy of longitudinal melanonychia,[170] regressing nevoid melanosis in childhood,[170] subungual hematoma,[170] | | | |
| Punctate red spots | Alopecia areata,[28,162] psoriasis[b] | ? | | Lunula |

Miscellaneous changes of lunula (see also other tables in Chapter 7)

| ENTITY | CAUSE OR ASSOCIATION | DISCOLORING AGENT | COLOR | SITE |
|---|---|---|---|---|
| Reddish lunula (see Table 7.1 for the following: cardiac failure, cirrhosis, lymphogranuloma venereum, reticulosarcoma, rheumatoid arthritis [iliac]),[116] systemic lupus erythematosus, possibly chronic obstructive pulmonary disease,[163] carbon monoxide | | | | |
| Dark red lunulae[42] | Sometimes seen in twenty-nail dystrophy | ? | Reddish lunula | Lunula |

**TABLE 7-6. (Cont'd) Abnormal nail pigmentation attributable to some named nail entities**

| ENTITY | CAUSE OR ASSOCIATION | DISCOLORING AGENT | COLOR | SITE |
|---|---|---|---|---|
| Alopecia areata[164,165] | ? | ? | Reddish lunula | Lunula |
| Psoriasis[c] | ? | ? Serum glycoprotein | Reddish lunula often spotted | Lunula |
| Dermatomyositis[116] | ? | ? | Reddish lunula | Lunula |
| Soft nail disease[74] | ? | No lunula | Lunula change | Lunula |
| Triangular lunulae[9,166] | Nail–patella syndrome, trauma,[171] trisomy 21,[171] idiopathic | Matrix damage (?) | Triangular white lunula | Lunula |
| Yellow lunulae[20] Trisomy 21[167] | Tetracycline | Tetracycline | Yellow | Lunula |

[a]S. Salasche, personal communication, December 1982.
[b]C.R. Daniel III, unpublished observation, 1982.
[c]C.R. Daniel III, unpublished data, 1980.
Data from Cutis.[1-4]

Various modifiers of the term leukonychia may be added as a result of the answers to these questions and may help the clinician describe leukonychia, so that more readers may know exactly the disease process.

As one may conclude from perusing the tables, among the causes of acquired leukonychia are trauma, drugs and ingestants, systemic disease, and other disorders. The majority of cases of acquired partial leukonychia seem to result from trauma to the matrix. Thus, dyskeratinization, often resulting in parakeratotic foci, imparts a whitish color to the nail plate. The nail unit may appear white with a normal nail plate because of vascular changes, among other causes. In some cases of traumatic leukonychia, airspaces may be found instead of dyskeratosis.[16]

In various cases, a pigmentary abnormality was arbitrarily placed in one category rather than in multiple listings to refrain from repeating identical information.[1] Furthermore, some material may have been listed several times to ensure that readers can locate their objective in a short period of time without having to use too many cross-references. In some situations, personal experience was noted without the use of a reference.[1,4] In numerous instances in the tables, an exact entry could not be assigned. The uncertainties are indicated by a question mark.[1,4] Abnormal nail pigmentation is an important facet of onychopathology. The differentiaton between benign and malignant causes is critical to the course of treatment. These tables and guidelines will hopefully be helpful in making those decisions and in stimulating further study to improve our diagnostic capabilities.

# REFERENCES

1. Daniel CR III, Osment LS. Nail pigmentation abnormalities: Their importance and proper examination. Cutis 1980; 25:595
2. Daniel CR III, Osment LS. Nail pigmentation abnormalities: Their importance and proper examination. Cutis 1982; 30:348
3. Daniel CR III. Nail pigmentation abnormalities, updated entries. Cutis 1982; 30:627
4. Daniel CR III. Nail pigmentation abnormalities, an addendum. Cutis 1982; 30:364
5. Daniel CR III. Nail pigmentation abnormalities. Dermatol Clin 1985; 3:431
6. Daniel CR III, Zaias N. Pigmentation abnormalities of the nails with emphasis on systemic diseases. Dermatol Clin 1988; 6:305, 313
7. Norton LA. Nail disorders. J Am Acad Dermatol 1980; 6:451
8. Zaias N. The nail in health and disease. New York, SP Medical Books, 1980
9. Zaias N. Disease of the nails. In: Demis J, Dobson RL, Crounse RG, eds. Clinical dermatology. New York, Harper & Row, 1974
10. Scher RK. Cosmetics and ancillary preparations for the care of nails. J Am Acad Dermatol 1980; 6:523
11. Baran R, Dawber RPR. Physical signs. In: Diseases of the nails and their management, 2nd edn. Oxford, Blackwell Scientific, 1994:35–80
12. Baran R, Kechijian P. Longitudinal melanonychia (melanonychia striata): diagnosis and management. J Am Acad Dermatol 1989; 21:1165
13. Beltrani VP, Scher RK. Evaluation and management of melanonychia striata in a patient receiving phototherapy. Arch Dermatol 1991; 127:319
14. Daniel CR III. Leukonychia (letter). J Am Acad Dermatol 1985; 13:158
15. Zaias N. The nail in health and disease, 2nd edn. Norwalk, CT, Appleton & Lange, 1990:93
16. Hudson JA, Cockrell CJ. Traumatic leukonychia striata: an electron microscopic and morphologic study. Poster presented at the annual meeting of the American Academy of Dermatology, Dallas, TX, December 1991
16a. Baran R, Simon CI. Longitudinal melanonychia: A symptom of Bowen's disease. J Am Acad Dermatol 1988; 18:1359
17. Bissell GW, Surakomol K, Greenslit F. Longitudinal banded pigmentation of nails in primary adrenal insufficiency. JAMA 1971; 215:1666
18. DeNicola P, Morsiana M, Zavagli G. Nail diseases in internal medicine. Springfield, IL, Charles C Thomas, 1974
19. Baker SJ, Ignatius M, Johnson S, et al. Hyperpigmentation of skin. Br Med J 1963; 1:1713
20. Localized hyperpigmentation: signs and symptoms of the skin. In: Roche handbook of differential diagnosis. New York, Roche Laboratories, 1976:9
21. Nail discoloration: signs and symptoms of the skin. In: Roche handbook of differential diagnosis. New York, Roche Laboratories, 1978:3, 7, 9
22. Zaias N, Boden HP. Disorders of nails. In: Fitzpatrick TB, Arndt KA, Clark WH Jr, et al. (eds). Dermatology in general medicine. New York, McGraw-Hill, 1971
23. Samman PD. The nails in disease. 3rd edn. Chicago, William Heinemann, 1978

24. Krutchik AN, Toshima CK, Buzdar AU, et al. Longitudinal nail banding associated with breast carcinoma unrelated to chemotherapy. Arch Intern Med 1978; 138:1302

25. Aratari E, Regesta G, Rebora A. Carpal tunnel syndrome appearing with prominent skin symptoms. Arch Dermatol 1984; 120:517

26. Baran R, Gioanni T, Holla D. Nail dyschromias. Cutis 1972; 9:307

27. Terry RB. The onychodermal band in health and disease. Lancet 1955; i:179

28. Runne U, Orfanos CE. The human nail. Curr Prob Dermatol 1981; 9:102

29. Hendricks AA. Yellow lunulae with fluorescence after tetracycline therapy. Arch Dermatol 1980; 116:438

29a. Cohen SR. Yellow staining caused by 4, 4′-methylenedianiline exposure. Arch Dermatol 1985; 121:1022

30. Baran R, Dawber RPR. Diseases of the nails and their management. Oxford, Blackwell Scientific, 1984

31. Klock JC. Nails may reveal first sign of many internal disorders. Dermatol Pract 1976; 9:1

32. Baran R. Pigmentations of the nails (chromonychia). J Dermatol Surg Oncol 1978; 4:250

33. Caravata CM, Richardson DR, Wood BT, et al. Cutaneous manifestations of hyperthyroidism. South Med J 1969; 62:1127

34. Thomas HM Jr. Pigment in the nails during hyperthyroidism. Bull Johns Hopkins Hosp 1933; 52:315

35. Muehrcke RC. The fingernails in chronic hypoalbuminemia. Br Med J 1956; 1:1327

36. Samman PD, Strickland B. Abnormalities of the fingernails associated with impaired peripheral blood supply. Br J Dermatol 1962; 74:165

37. Hudson JB, Dennis AJ Jr. Transverse white lines in the fingernails after acute and chronic renal failure. Arch Intern Med 1966; 117:276

38. Zaias N. The nail in lichen planus. Arch Dermatol 1970; 101:264

39. Kint A, Herpe LV. Ungual anomalies in lupus erythematosus discoides. Dermatologica 1976; 153:298

40. Bisht DB, Singh SS. Pigmented bands on nails: A new sign in malnutrition. Lancet 1962; i:507

41. Samman PD. The nails. In: Rook AH, Wilkinson DS, Ebling FJG, eds. Textbook of dermatology. 2nd edn. Blackwell Scientific, London, 1968

42. Baran R. The nail. In: Pierre M, ed. The nail. Edinburgh, Churchill Livingstone, 1981

43. Moschella SL, Pillsbury DM, Hurley HJ, eds. Dermatology. Philadelphia, WB Saunders, 1975

44. Fryer JM, Werth VP. Pregnancy-associated hyperpigmentation: longitudinal melanonychia. J Am Acad Dermatol 199226:493

45. Baran MF, Gioanni T. Half and half nail. Fitiale L'ouest Sud-Ouest-Séance 1968; 16:399

46. Daniel CR III, Bower JD, Daniel CR Jr. The half-and-half fingernail: a clue to chronic renal failure. Proc Clin Dial Transplant Forum 1975; 5:1

47. Daniel CR III, Bower JD, Daniel CR Jr. The half-and-half fingernail: The most significant onychopathological indicator of chronic renal failure. J Miss State Med Assoc 19756; 16:376

48. Leyden JJ, Wood MG. The half-and-half nail. Arch Dermatol 1972; 105:591

49. Lindsay PG. The half-and-half nail. Arch Intern Med 1967; 119:583

49a. Giustina TA, Woo TX, Campbell JP, Ellis CN. Association of pili torti and leukonychia. Cutis 1985; 35:533

50. Barrow MV. The nails in multicentric reticulohistiocytosis. Arch Dermatol 1967; 95:200

51. Baran R. Nail changes in general pathology. In: Pierre M, ed. The nail. Edinburgh, Churchill Livingstone, 1981:5–101

52. Castello V, Pardo OA. Diseases of the nails, 3rd edn. Springfield, IL, Charles C Thomas, 1968

53. Marks R, Ellis HP. Yellow nails. Arch Dermatol 1970; 120:619

54. Petrozzi JW, Shore RN. Keratosis lichenoides chronica, possible variant of lichen planus. Arch Dermatol 1976: 112:709

55. Zaias N. Psoriasis of the nail. Arch Dermatol 1969; 99:567

56. Orentreich N, Harber LC, Tromovitch TA. Photosensitivity and photo-onycholysis due to demethyl-chlortetracycline. Arch Dermatol 1961; 83:730

57. Carmel R. Hair and fingernail changes in acquired and congenital pernicious anemia. Arch Intern Med 1985; 145:484

58. Chernovsky ME, Finley VK. Yellow nail syndrome in patients with acquired immunodeficiency disease. J Am Acad Dermatol 1985; 13:731

59. Daniel CR III. Yellow nail syndrome and acquired immunodeficiency disease. J Am Acad Dermatol 1986; 14:844

60. Norton L. Nail disorders. Lecture presented at the annual meeting of the American Academy of Dermatology, Las Vegas, 11 December 1985

61. Ronchyese F. The nail in Darier's disease. Arch Dermatol 1965; 91:617

62. Zaias N, Ackerman AB. The nail in Darier–White disease. Arch Dermatol 1973; 107:193

63. Redeker AC, Levan NE, Beake M. Erythropoietic protoporphyria with eczema solare. Arch Dermatol 1962; 86:569

64. Sulis E, Floris C. Nail pigmentation following cancer chemotherapy: a new genetic entity? Eur J Cancer 1980; 15:1517

64a. Koch SE, LeBoit PE, Odon RB. Laugier–Hunziker syndrome. J Am Acad Dermatol 1987; 16:431

65. Cram DL, Resneck JS, Jackson G. A congenital ichthyosiform syndrome with deafness and keratitis. Arch Dermatol 1979; 115:467

66. Sulzburger MB. Incontinentia pigmenti. Arch Dermatol 1938; 38:65

67. Bart RS, Pumphrey RE. Knuckle pads, leukonychia and deafness: a dominantly inherited syndrome. New Engl J Med 1967; 276:202

68. Samman PD. The nails in disease. 2nd edn. Springfield, IL, Charles C Thomas, 1972

68a. Lazar P. Reactions to nail hardeners. Arch Dermatol 1973; 94:446

69. Caron GA. Familial congenital pigmented nevi of the nails. Lancet 1962; i:508

70. Degowin EL, Degowin RL. Bedside diagnostic examination, 20th edn. New York, Macmillan, 1969

71. Achord JL, Proctor HD. Malignant degeneration and metastasis in Peutz–Jeghers syndrome. Arch Intern Med 1963; 111:498

72. Valero A, Sherf K. Pigmented nails in Peutz–Jeghers syndrome. Am J Gastroenterol 1965; 43:56

73. Johnson RB, Goldsmith IA. Dilantin digital defects. Am Acad Dermatol 1981; 5:191

74. Prandi G, Caccialanza M. An unusual congenital nail dystrophy (soft nail disease). Clin Exp Dermatol 1977; 2:265

75. Millns JL, Dicken HC. Hereditary acrolabial telangiectasia. Arch Dermatol 1979; 115:474

76. Braverman IM. Skin signs of systemic disease. Philadelphia, WB Saunders, 1970

77. Price VH, Odon, RB, Ward WH, et al. Trichothiodystrophy. Arch Dermatol 1980; 116:1375

78. Bearn AG, McKusick VA. Azure lunulae. JAMA 1958; 166:904

79. Nixon DW, Pirozzi D, York RM, et al. Dermatologic changes after systemic cancer therapy. Cutis 1981; 27:181

80. Modny C, Barondess JA. Nail pigmentation secondary to quinacrine. Cutis 1973; 11:789

81. Madorsky DD. Arsenic in dermatology. J Assoc Milit Dermatol 1977; 3:19

82. Furth PA, Lazakis AM. Nail pigmentation changes associated with azidothymidine (zidovudine). Ann Intern Med 1987; 107:350

83. Fisher CA, McPoland PR. Azidothymidine-induced nail pigmentation. Cutis 1989; 43:552

84. Naik RPC, Gurmohan S. Nail pigmentation due to oral 8-methoxypsoralen. Br J Dermatol 1979; 100:229

85. Scher R. The nail. Lecture presented at Columbia University Nail and Hair Symposium, September 1989

86. Zhu WY, Xia MY, Huang SD, Du D. Hyperpigmentation of the nail from lead deposition. Int J Dermatol 1989; 28:273

87. Hooper JF. Lithium carbonate and toenails. Am J Psychiatry 1981; 138:1519

88. Granstein RD, Sober JA. Drug- and heavy-metal-induced hyper-pigmentation. J Am Acad Dermatol 1981; 5:1

89. Morgan DB. Blue nails from minocycline. Schoch Letter 1979; 29:2

90. Krebs A. Drug-induced nail disorders. Praxis 1981; 70:1951

91. Bjellerup M. Nail changes induced by penicillamine. Acta Derm Venereol (Stockh) 1989; 69:339
92. Ross JB. Side effect of phenindione. Br Med J 1963; 1:886
93. Seckler SG. A handful of pearls. Hosp Physician 1976; 12:4
94. Koplon BS. Azure lunulae due to argyria. Arch Dermatol 1966; 94:333
94a. Noppakum N, Swasdikul D. Reversible hyperpigmentation of skin and nails with white hair due to vitamin B$_{12}$ deficiency. Arch Dermatol 1986; 122:896
95. Loveman AB, Fliegelman MT. Discoloration of the nails. Arch Dermatol 1955; 72:153
96. Sanders CV, Saenz RE, Lopez M. Splinter hemorrhages and onycholysis: Unusual reactions associated with tetracycline hydrochloride therapy. South Med J 1976; 69:1090
97. Fieler-Ofry V, Godel V, Lagan M. Nail pigmentation following timolol maleate therapy. Ophthalmologica 1981; 182:153
98. Feder W, Auerbach R. 'Purple toes': an uncommon sequela of oral coumarin drug therapy. Ann Intern Med 1961; 55:911
99. Lebsack CS, Weibert RT. 'Purple toes' syndrome. Postgrad Med 1982; 71:81
100. Shah PC, Rao KRP, Patel AR. Cyclophosphamide-induced nail pigmentation. Br J Dermatol 1978; 98:675
101. Shetty MR. Case of pigmented banding of the nail caused by bleomycin. Cancer Treat Rep 1977; 61:501
102. Morris D, Aisner J. Horizontal pigmented banding of the nails in association with adriamycin chemotherapy. Cancer Treat Rep 1977; 61:499
103. Kennedy BJ, Smith LR, Goltz RW. Skin changes secondary to hydroxyurea therapy. Arch Dermatol 1975; 111:183
104. Nixon DW. Alterations in nail pigment with cancer chemotherapy. Arch Intern Med 1976; 36:1117
105. Pratt CV, Shanks EC. Hyperpigmentation of the nails from doxorubicin (letter). JAMA 1974; 228:460
106. Fisher AA. Contact dermatitis, 3rd edn. Lea and Febiger, Philadelphia, 1973
107. Schwartz L, Tulipan L, Birmingham DJ. Occupational diseases of the skin. 3rd edn. Philadelphia, Lea & Febiger, 1957
108. Baran R. Nail damage caused by weed killers and insecticides (letter). Arch Dermatol 1974; 110:467
109. Samman PD, Johnston EN. Nail damage associated with handling of paraquat and diquat. Br Med J 1969; 1:818
110. Suringa DW. Treatment of superficial onychomycosis with topically applied glutaraldehyde. Arch Dermatol 1970; 102:153
111. Olsen TG, Jatlav P. Contact exposure to elemental iron causing chromonychia. Arch Dermatol 1984; 120:102
111a. Rudophy RI. Subungual basal cell carcinoma presenting as longitudinal melanonychia. J Am Acad Dermatol 1987; 16:229
112. Harris AO, Rosen T. Nail discoloration due to mahogany. Cutis 1989; 43:55
113. Bedi TR. Intradermal triamcinolone treatment of psoriatic onychodystrophy. Dermatologica 1977; 155:24
114. Restrepo A, Arango M, Vedlez H, et al. The isolation of *Botryodiplodia theobromae* from a nail lesion. Sabouraudia 1976; 14:1
115. Zaias N. Onychomycosis. Arch Dermatol 1972; 105:263
116. Jorizzo JL, Gonzalez EB, Daniels JC. Red lunulae in a patient with rheumatoid arthritis. J Am Acad Dermatol 1983; 8:711
117. Campbell CK, Kurwa A, Abdel-Aziz AHM, et al. Fungal infection of the skin and nails by *Hendersonula toruloides*. Br J Dermatol 1973; 89:45
118. Reiss F. Leukonychia trichophytica caused by *Trichophyton rubrum*. Cutis 20:223, 1977
119. Higashi N. Melanocytes and nail matrix and nail pigmentation. Arch Dermatol 1968; 97:570
120. Higashi N, Saito T. Horizontal distribution of the DOPA-positive melanocytes in the nail matrix. J Invest Dermatol 1969; 53:163
121. Yung CW, Estes SA. Subungual epidermal cyst. J Am Acad Dermatol 1980; 3:599
122. Lewin K. Subungual epidermoid inclusions. Br J Dermatol 1969; 81:671
123. Shelley WB, Rawnsley HM, Pillsbury DM. Postirradiation melanonychia. Arch Dermatol 1964; 90:174
124. Ronchese F, Kern AB. Longitudinal pigmentation of the nails (letter). JAMA 1971; 216:1352
125. Daniel CR III, Sams WM, Scher RK. Nails in systemic disease. Dermatol Clin 1985; 3:465
126. Rook A. Textbook of dermatology. 33rd edn. Blackwell Scientific, Oxford, 1979
127. Grossman M, Scher RK. Leukonychia, review and classification. Int J Dermatol 1990; 29:535
127a. Stewart WK, Raffle EJ. Brown nail-bed arcs and chronic renal disease. Br Med J 1972; 1:784
128. Fitzpatrick TB. Dermatology in general medicine. 2nd edn. McGraw-Hill, New York, 1979
129. Jawny L, Spada F. Contact dermatitis to a new nail hardener. Arch Dermatol 1981; 5:191
130. March CH. Allergic contact dermatitis to a new formula to strengthen nails. Arch Dermatol 1966; 93:720
131. Held JL, Chew S, Grossman ME, Kohn SR. Transverse striate leukonychia associated with acute rejection of renal allograft. J Am Acad Dermatol 1989; 20:513
132. Feldman SR, Gammon WR. Unilateral Muehrcke's lines following trauma. Arch Dermatol 1989; 125:133
133. Arnold HL. Sympathetic symmetric punctate leukonychia. Arch Dermatol 1979; 115:495
133a. Terry R. Red half-moons in cardiac failure. Lancet 1954; ii:842
134. Leyden JJ. Chromonychia. Cutis 1972; 10:161
135. Pappert AS, Scher RK, Cohen JL. Longitudinal pigmented nail bands. Dermatol Clin 1991; 9:703
136. Markenson AL, Chandra M, Miller DR. Hyperpigmentation after cancer chemotherapy. Lancet 1975; ii:128
137. Fisher BK, Warner LC. Cutaneous manifestations by the AIDS. Update 1987. Int J Dermatol 1987; 26:615
138. Haneke E. Fungal infections of the nail. Semin Dermatol 1991; 10:41–53
139. Saijos KT. Pigmented nail streaks associated with Bowen's disease of the nail matrix. Dermatologica 1990; 181:156
140. VomVouras S, Pakula AS, Shaw JM. Multiple pigmented bands during hydroxyurea therapy. An uncommon finding. J Am Acad Dermatol 1991; 24:1016
141. Leyden JJ, Spott DA, Goldschmidt H. Diffuse and banded melanin pigmentation in nails. Arch Dermatol 1972; 105:548
142. Klein ME. Linear lateral black nail discoloration after months on Lopid. Schoch Letter 1990; 40:29
143. Litt JZ. A dark streak in the nail. Diagnosis 1982; 4:23
144. Baran R. Nail biting and picking as a possible cause of longitudinal melanonychia: a study of 6 cases. Dermatologica 1990; 181:126
145. Canizares O. Chronic porphyria. Arch Dermatol Syphilol 1951; 63:269
146. Lewin K. Subungual epidermal inclusions simulating melanoma. Br J Dermatol 196981:671
147. Tosti A, Gaddoni G, Fanti PA, et al. Longitudinal melanonychia induced by 3'azidodeoxythymidine. Dermatologica 1990; 180:217
147a. Scheithauer W, Ludwig H, Kotz R, Depisch D. Mitoxantrone-induced discoloration of the nails. Eur J Cancer Clin Oncol 1989; 25:763
148. Baran R. Frictional longitudinal melanonychia: A new entity. Dermatologica 1987; 174:280
149. Baran R. Frictional longitudinal melanonychia: A new entity. Dermatologica 1987; 174:280
150. Blum M, Avinam AL. Splinter hemorrhages in patients receiving regular hemodialysis. JAMA 1978; 1239:44
151. Kilpatrick ZM, Greenberg PA, Sanford JP. Splinter hemorrhages-Their clinical significance. Arch Intern Med 1965; 115:730
152. Zala L. Photo-onycholysis induced by 8-methoxy-psoralen. Dermatologica 1977; 154:203
153. Gross NJ, Tall R. Clinical significance of splinter hemorrhages. Br Med J 1963; 12:1496
154. Robertson JC, Braune ML. Splinter hemorrhages, pitting, and other findings in fingernails of healthy adults. Br Med J 1974; 4:279

155. Guin JD, Elleman JH. Yellow-nail syndrome: possible association with malignancy. Arch Dermatol 1979; 115:734

156. Mattingly PC, Bossingham DH. Yellow-nail syndrome in rheumatoid arthritis: report of three cases. Ann Rheum Dis 1979; 38:475

157. Edwards EA. Nail changes in functional and organic arterial disease. New Engl J Med 1948; 239:362

158. Fromer JL. Multiple myeloma. In: Moschella SL, Pillsbury DM, Hurley HJ, eds. Dermatology. Philadelphia, WB Saunders, 1975: 1420–1422

159. Patterson JW. Pterygium-inversum-unguis-like changes in scleroderma. Arch Dermatol 1977; 113:1429

160. Baran R, Stroud JD. Congenital onychodysplasia of the index fingers. Arch Dermatol 1984; 120:243

161. Baran R. Nails. Lecture presented at the meeting of the American Academy of Dermatology, San Francisco, December 1981

162. Ringrose EJ. Alopecia symptomatica with nail base changes (society transactions). Arch Dermatol 1957; 76:263

163. Wilkerson MG, Wilkin JK. Red lunulae revisited: A clinical and histopathologic examination. J Am Acad Dermatol 1989; 20:453

164. Misch KJ. Red nails associated with alopecia areata. Clin Exp Dermatol 1981; 6:561

165. Rigrose EJ, Bahcall CR. Alopecia symptomatica with nail base changes. Arch Dermatol 1957; 76:263

166. Daniel CR III, Osment LS, Noojin RO. Triangular lunulae. Arch Dermatol 1980; 116:448

167. Beaver DW, Brooks SE. Color atlas of the nail in clinical diagnosis. Chicago, Year Book, 1984:39

168. McGeorge BCL. Lunula change induced by psoralen plus ultraviolet A radiation. Photodermatol Photoimmunol 1992; 9:15

169. Kose O, Baloglu H. Knuckle pads, leukonychia, and deafness. Int J Dermatol 1996; 35:728

170. Baran R, Kechijian P. Hutchinson's sign: A reappraisal. J Am Acad Dermatol 1996; 34:87

171. Cohen PR. The lunula. J Am Acad Dermatol 1996; 34:943

172. Hoffman MD, Fleming MG, Pearson PW. Acantholytic epidermolysis bullosa. Arch Dermatol 1995; 131:566–589

# 8

# Brittle Nails

## Philip Fleckman and Richard K Scher

## Key Features

1. Brittle nails display accentuated onychorrhexis and onychoschizia
2. Nail hardness is determined by several factors, including the physical properties, constituents, and hydration of the nail plate
3. Endogenous causes of brittle nails include systemic and cutaneous disease
4. Exogenous causes of brittle nails include trauma and environmental insult

Why is the nail plate hard? What makes nails brittle? Technically this topic could be included in Chapter 3 (as it was in previous editions), and many of the biophysical and biochemical aspects thought to be associated with brittle nails are discussed there. Nevertheless, the subject is of sufficient importance to merit a place of its own.

To discuss brittle nails one must first define hard and brittle. Most definitions of brittleness include onychorrhexis, longitudinal ridging (Fig. 8.1) and onychoschizia, horizontal (lamellar) cracking or splitting of the free end of the nail plate into laminae (Fig. 8.2).[1-3] Additional terms such as 'soft' nails, 'fragile' nails, 'thin' nails, koilonychia, and nails that break 'easily' are sometimes added. Hard nails have been defined as '"normal nails", where this does not happen.'[2] Others have attempted to define hardness and brittleness by more easily evaluated clinical parameters, such as photographs,[3] scanning electron microscopy,[4] or by more easily

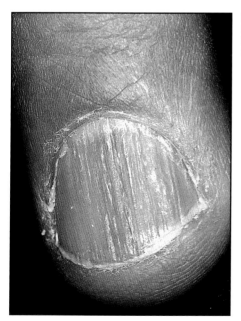

FIGURE 8-1. Onychorrhexis caused by lichen planus of the nail unit.

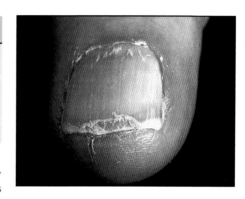

FIGURE 8-2. Onychoschizia caused by frequent hand washing.

quantified physical parameters, such as Knoop hardness number, which measures indentation under a fixed weight,[5-7] flexural characteristics,[8-10] modulus of elasticity, which quantifies the relationship between force/area and deformation produced,[11-13] and tensile strength, tearing resistance, and impact absorption.[9] A grading system for brittle nails has been suggested,[14] emphasizing that brittle nails reflect a spectrum of changes that result in nails that are less durable and more susceptible to injury.

## PATHOPHYSIOLOGY

Forslind attributed nail plate hardness to physical properties, including the double curvature (longitudinal and transverse) of the nail plate, the very flat adhesive pattern of cells in the plate, the orientation of the fibers in the plane of the plate perpendicular to the direction of growth, and the junctions between cells in the nail plate.[15] Baden suggested that the mechanical properties of the nail plate might be due in part to cell wall attachments.[11]

Cystine is decreased in brittle nails.[16,17] The high cystine content of nail matrix proteins is discussed in Chapter 3. In sheep, as the consumption of sulfur is reduced, the amount of matrix protein in wool decreases; however, once the intake of sulfur is reduced below a critical level, the growth of wool decreases progressively, suggesting that the high-sulfur matrix proteins are necessary for the synthesis of the appendageal product.[18] The solubility of matrix proteins is such that they would be extracted by alkaline solutions that increase lamellar splitting.[2,19,20] This suggests that extraction of matrix proteins may be responsible for splitting in brittle nails, although exogenous factors are more likely to effect onychoschizia through extracellular, rather than intracellular components.[21]

No association of calcium with brittle nails has been documented.[2] Calcium is increased in the nails of individuals with kwashiorkor.[22] Such nails have a higher Knoop hardness number than normal nails.[7] The increase in hardness has been attributed to the increase in calcium, but the arguments are not supported by analytic electron microscopic studies.[23] X-ray diffraction studies contain no suggestion of a separate phase (e.g. a calcium mineral, such as in bone) in the nail plate.[15] Heterotopic calcification of the nail plate can occur after injury.[24] The preoccupation with calcium in relationship to nail hardness 'probably stems from the hardness of bones and teeth, where large quantities of calcium are present. Thus the idea may have evolved that the more calcium in the system, the harder the nails.'[2]

The importance of water in nail hardness, brittleness, and flexibility has been emphasized repeatedly.[2,15,25] In housewives, brittle nails are an occupational hazard.[26] Solvents probably exert adverse effects on nail plates, not through lipid extraction[11] but through dehydration,[26] and may be overrated in causing adverse effects. The modulus of elasticity,[11,13] flexibility,[8] and the number of times a nail plate can be flexed before breaking[10] all increase when the nail plate is hydrated. Changes seen by scanning electron microscopy similar to those seen in onychoschizia have been produced by repeated wetting and drying and by exposure of nail clippings to detergent and water.[25]

Thus, the hardness of nails is determined by several factors: the physical properties of the nail plate, the matrix proteins that may glue the fibrous proteins together, intercellular components, and the hydration of the nail plate. The function of the cornified cellular envelope and whether an intercellular cement substance[27] has a role in nail hardness remain to be determined.

The prevalence of brittle nails in the general population is about 20%; women are affected more commonly than men. Most of those surveyed who had brittle nails found them 'a nuisance' because the split ends catch and tear and because the nails are unsightly.[28]

Silver and Chiego reviewed the association of brittle nails with systemic and cutaneous disease.[26] Their investigations included many exogenous factors, including occupation, trauma, avitaminosis, iron metabolism, the coefficient of nail plate expansion, unsaturated fats, the pH of the skin, and solvents. Their classification of the causes of brittle nails stands today and forms the basis for an approach to understanding the causes of and treating the disorder (Box 8.1). Others have listed disorders and exposures

with which brittle nails have been associated.[20,21,29] Rather than parrot their work, we will focus on questions and conditions that merit further investigation and suggest an approach to evaluate and treat the patient who complains of brittle nails.

Many systemic diseases have been associated with brittle nails.[20,26,30,31] Any systemic disease can clearly affect nail growth through general effects on the organism. One can easily extrapolate such changes to effects on nail plate formation; in addition, a nail that grows more slowly is subject to prolonged environmental insult and more 'wear and tear'. Chronic diseases are therefore more likely to result in brittle nails. Systemic disorders that bear particular attention include circulatory dysfunction, iron deficiency, and thyroid disease. Samman described nail changes resulting from circulatory dysfunction;[32] although such changes are often more profound, brittle nails should be included. Nail changes associated with iron deficiency are described[20,26,33] but poorly documented. The authors have seen patients with nail dystrophy associated with low ferritin (Fig. 8.3), but well designed studies demonstrating the association of low iron stores with nail dystrophy or improvement with iron replacement are lacking. The association of brittle nails with thyroid disease is better documented[34–37] (Fig. 8.4); improvement with treatment is less well substantiated.

Any skin disease can result in nail dystrophy, including brittle nails. One of the hazards of the close approximation of the nail matrix and the proximal nail fold is that inflammation of the

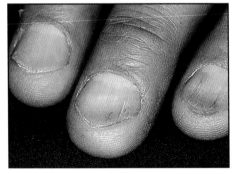

FIGURE 8–3. Koilonychia, onychoschizia, and longitudinal fissuring caused by low iron stores.

Box 8–1: Causes of brittle nails (modified from[26])

**Endogenous**
- Systemic disease:
  · Circulatory
  · Iron deficiency
  · Thyroid disease
  · Other
- Cutaneous disease (including diseases of the nail unit):
  · Inflammation of the proximal nail fold
  · Lichen planus
  · Psoriasis
  · Other

**Exogenous**
- Trauma
- Environmental insult:
  · Infection
  · Repeated wetting and drying

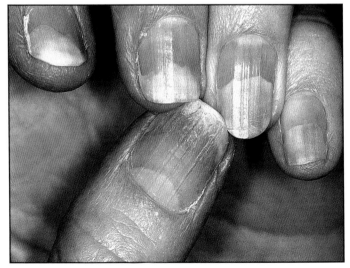

FIGURE 8–4. Onycholysis, onychorrhexis, and thinned nails caused by hyperthyroidism.

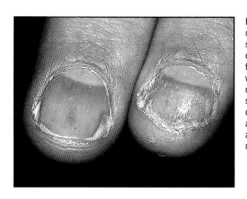

FIGURE 8–5. Irregular onychorrhexis, distal splitting, and onychoschizia in the index finger nail of a person with psoriasis. Distal onycholysis and oil drop sign, findings more characteristic of psoriasis, are present in the adjacent middle finger nail.

proximal nail fold is often reflected in brittle nails. Lichen planus and psoriasis stand out as the cutaneous disorders most commonly underlying brittle nails (see Figs 8.1 and 8.5). One can speculate that nail dystrophy associated with psoriasis reflects distal interphalangeal joint arthritis, but this begs the question of why psoriasis has a predilection for nails, and the affinity of lichen planus for nail (and hair) is totally unexplained.

Exogenous insult is the more common cause of brittle nails. Repetitive trauma of any type to the nail plate may produce the changes. Kechijian makes the point that longer nails are more susceptible.[21] This is intuitive, because not only does cumulative exposure to the environment increase with the length of the nail, but also the additional surface that is exposed once the nail plate lifts off the nail bed increases risk. Mechanical trauma, such as typing, knitting, and even telephone dialing may exacerbate the problem. Fungal infection is a less common cause of brittle nails, but should not be overlooked because of the opportunity to treat effectively.

Exposure to harsh solvents and detergents is thought to be associated with brittle nails,[20,21,26] particularly onychoschizia. The assumption is that solvents extract intercellular material that 'glues' the keratinocytes of the nail plate together. The nature of such glue is not defined. Extraction of intracellular keratin-associated proteins (discussed in Chapter 3) is less likely, because the destruction of the cells would be required in order to reach the material. Nail cosmetics are considered causes of brittle nails; the dorsal nail plate changes seen after removal of artificial nails are easily understood. However, Silver and Chiego[26] may be correct in suggesting that the true culprit in nail cosmetics is repeated hydration and desiccation of the nail plate; their conclusions are supported by others. Finlay et al[10] showed that cadaver nails could be repeatedly bent for longer periods when they were hydrated, and Shelley and Shelley showed that changes seen in onychoschizia could be reproduced by repeated hydration and desiccation of nail plates.[4]

## CLINICAL EVALUATION AND TREATMENT

The approach to and treatment of brittle nails follows the causes (Box 8.2). Underlying causes should be determined and addressed. Brittle nails are not a specific finding and may reflect multiple underlying systemic or cutaneous disorders. A general medical history and physical examination should identify underlying medical disorders. Attention should be focused on those disorders more commonly associated with brittle nails, including thyroid disease, low iron stores, distal digital arthritis, and circulatory dysfunction, including Raynaud's phenomenon and peripheral vascular disease. Laboratory studies should include measures of thyroid function and iron stores, and should exclude underlying onychomycosis. Treatment of underlying conditions should parallel general treatment measures. Ferritin reflects iron stores more accurately than any assessment other than bone marrow staining.[38,39] As with telogen effluvium, we treat a ferritin value below 50 μg/L in the absence of anemia. Low iron stores in a male or a postmenopausal woman should be evaluated.

### Rx TREATMENT

- Underlying causes should be determined and addressed
- A complete skin exam is suggested to exclude underlying skin disease
- Laboratory studies should assess thyroid function and iron stores, when appropriate
- General nail care is a critical component of treatment
- Patients should be cautioned that improvement may require at least several months and will begin proximally

Because underlying causes of brittle nails are often not identified, general nail care is a critical aspect of treatment. Such care reflects common sense more than science; few studies

### Box 8–2: Approach and treatment of brittle nails

1. Identify underlying causes
- History:
  · general
  · thyroid disease
  · anemia, iron deficiency
  · arthritis
  · Raynaud's phenomenon, peripheral vascular disease
  · trauma
  · occupational exposure
  · family, personal history of skin, hair, nail disease.
- Physical exam.
- Laboratory studies:
  · TSH
  · ferritin
  · KOH, culture if indicated.
2. Treat underlying cause
3. General nail care
- Keep nails short.
- File weekly.
- Moisturize at least four times a day and after each exposure to water.
- Avoid artificial nails and nail wraps: Occasionally nail wraps may be necessary to prevent severe and painful splitting.
- Avoid nail polish or hardeners: We prefer to avoid nail polish because it negates the effects of moisturization and requires periodic exposure to nail polish remover. If nail polish is necessary, it should be removed infrequently. After removal of nail polish, the fingertips should be soaked in tap water for 10 to 15 minutes and moisturized overnight before polish is reapplied.
- Biotin – 2.5 to 5 mg daily.

document the efficacy of these suggestions. Care is directed at minimizing trauma and optimizing nail plate integrity and growth. The nail plate incurs injury once it is exposed; once the attachment to the undersurface of the free edge of the nail is released additional surface is exposed. Thus, keeping the nails short is important. Because flexibility increases with hydration, nails should be trimmed after they have been hydrated. Filing the edges after trimming should reduce sharp edges that might catch and tear.[21] Buffing nails to reduce ridging and minimize irregularities is reasonable, provided the buffing is limited and does not thin the nail plate excessively or result in pain.[21,40]

Moisturizing the nail plate increases flexibility and decreases the signs of brittle nails, and is critical.[47] We suggest the use of a good hand lubricant, because palmar/plantar skin differs sufficiently from other skin to merit specific topical therapy; preference and tolerance to moisturizers vary.[41] Patients should moisturize their nails at least four times a day and after each exposure to water. Repeated hydration and dehydration makes brittle nails worse. We do not encourage routine use of gloves but suggest thin cotton gloves as liners beneath fabric-lined rubber gloves to avoid exposure to harsh solvents or chemicals. Moisturizing after washing is preferred to the use of gloves for simple hand washing.

Avoiding trauma includes avoidance of harsh chemicals and solvents. This includes nail cosmetics, including acrylic or other synthetic nails. This area is controversial. Those who favor nail polish argue that the polish seals the nail plate against repeated hydration and dehydration, and argue the culprit is not the polish but the polish remover.[26] Regardless of the nature of the polish remover, it acts as a solvent to remove polish and effectively dehydrates the nail. We encourage patients to avoid nail polish. If they insist on its use, nail polish should be '... "repaired" by frequent use of another "top coat" of polish every few days to prevent chipping or peeling ...'[40] Nail polish remover should be used infrequently. After its use, the nails should be hydrated in tap water for 10–15 minutes and then moisturized overnight before reapplication of polish. Anyone who has seen a nail plate before and after an artificial nail has been removed recognizes the damage the surface of the nail plate incurs. These devices cannot be bound to the nail plate without disturbing the surface of the nail. However, in some cases permanently dystrophic nail plates can be camouflaged by artificial nails. The same goes for nail wraps, where thin strips of fabric or paper are glued to the nail tips and polish applied; this can be an effective treatment for permanently split nails, but additional damage will be incurred by the user.[42] We encourage patients to avoid all artificial nail products until conservative treatments have been exhausted.

Biotin has been touted as a useful treatment for brittle nails.[43,44] Its use remains to be proven conclusively, but the B vitamin is relatively harmless and inexpensive. Biotin can be obtained from most health food stores or pharmacies. The recommended dose is 2.5 to 5 mg per day, approximately 100 to 200 times the recommended daily allowance.[45] Adverse effects of gastrointestinal complaints are rarely seen. The use of gelatin is reviewed in Chapter 3 and cannot be recommended.

It is essential to remind your patient that nails grow very slowly. Changes from these measures are likely to take several months, and should begin proximally. We recommend marking the dorsal surface of one affected nail at the proximal nail fold with a superficial notch[46] and following patients with photographs of marked nail. This allows the patient to see how slowly the nail grows and offers a more objective assessment of change. We endorse the recommendation that patients with brittle nails in whom no specific cause is identified be followed periodically to assure detectable underlying causes do not arise and with the hope that new, improved treatments will be identified.[21]

# REFERENCES

1. Tyson TL. Preliminary and short reports: the effect of gelatin on fragile finger nails. J Invest Dermatol 1950; 14:323–325
2. Kile RL. Some mineral constituents of fingernails. AMA Arch Dermatol Syphil 1954; 70:75–83
3. Rosenberg SW, Oster K. Gelatin in the treatment of brittle nails. Conn St Med J 1955; 19:171–179
4. Shelley WB, Shelley ED. Onychoschizia: scanning electron microscopy. J Am Acad Dermatol 1984; 10:623–627
5. Michaelson JB, Huntsman DJ. New aspects of the effects of gelatin on fingernails. J Soc Cosmetic Chemists 1963; 14:443–454
6. Robson JRK, El-Tahawi HD. Hardness of human nail as an index of nutritional status: a preliminary communication. Br J Nutr 1971; 26:233–236
7. Robson JRK. Hardness of finger nails in well-nourished and malnourished populations. Br J Nutr 1974; 32:389–394
8. Young RW, Newman SB, Capott RJ. Strength of fingernails. J Invest Dermatol 1965; 44:358–360
9. Maloney MJ, Paquette EG, Shansky A. The physical properties of fingernails: 1. Apparatus for physical measurements. J Soc Cosmet Chem 1977; 28:415–425
10. Finlay AY, Frost P, Keith AD, et al. An assessment of factors influencing flexibility of human fingernails. Br J Dermatol 1980; 103:357–365
11. Baden HP. The physical properties of nail. J Invest Dermatol 1970; 55:115–122
12. Baden HP, Goldsmith LA, Fleming B. A comparative study of the physiocochemical properties of human keratinized tissues. Biochem Biophys Acta 1973; 322:269–278
13. Forslind B, Nordstrom G, Toijer D, et al. The rigidity of human fingernails: a biophysical investigation on influencing physical parameters. Acta Dermatovener 1980; 60:217–222
14. van de Kerkhof PCM, Pasch MC, Scher RK, et al. Brittle Nail Syndrome: a pathogenesis based approach with a proposed grading system. J Am Acad Dermatol. In press.
15. Forslind B. Biophysical studies of the normal nail. Acta Dermatovener 1970; 50:161–168
16. Hess WC. Variations in amino acid content of finger nails of normal and arthritic individuals. J Biol Chem 1935; 109:xiii
17. Klauder JV, Brown H. Sulphur content of hair and of nails in abnormal states. II. Nails. Arch Dermatol Syphil 1935; 31:26–34
18. Fraser RDB. Keratins. Sci Amer 1969; 221:86–96
19. Dixon S. Nail-splitting: A survey. Nursing Times 1967; 63:1760–1761
20. Samman PD, Fenton DA. Samman's the nails in disease. 5th edn. London: Butterworth-Heinemann, 1995
21. Kechijian P. Brittle fingernails. Dermatol Clin 1985; 3:421–429
22. Robson JRK, Brooks GJ. The distribution of calcium in fingernails from healthy and malnourished children. Clin Chim Acta 1974; 55:255–257
23. Forslind B, Wroblewski R, Afzelius BA. Calcium and sulfur location in human nail. J Invest Dermatol 1976; 67:273–275
24. Blakey PR, Earland C, Stell JGP, et al. Heterotopic calcification of human nail and hair. Nature 1965; 207:190–191
25. Wallis MS, Bowen WR, Guin JD. Pathogenesis of onychoschizia (lamellar dystrophy). J Am Acad Dermatol 1991; 24:44–48
26. Silver H, Chiego B. Nails and nail changes: III. Brittleness of nails (fragilitas unguium). J Invest Dermatol 1940; 3:357–374
27. Rosenberg S, Oster KA, Kallos A, et al. Further studies in the use of gelatin in the treatment of brittle nails. AMA Arch Dermatol 1957; 76:330–335
28. Lubach D, Cohrs W, Wurzinger R. Incidence of brittle nails. Dermatologica 1986; 172:144–147

29. Scher RK, Bodian AB. Brittle nails. Semin Dermatol 1991; 10:21–25

30. Pardo-Castello V, Pardo OA. Diseases of the nails. 3rd edn. Springfield, IL: Charles C. Thomas, 1960

31. De Nicola P, Morisiani M, Zavagli G. Nail diseases in internal medicine. Springfield, IL: Charles C. Thomas, 1974

32. Samman PD, Strickland B. Abnormalities of the finger nails associated with impaired peripheral blood supply. Br J Derm 1962; 74:165–175

33. Hogan GR, Jones B. The relationship of koilonychia and iron deficiency in infants. J Pediatr 1970; 77:1054–1057

34. Luria MN, Asper SP. Onycholysis in hyperthyroidism. Ann Intern Med 1958; 49:102–108

35. Caravati CM, Jr., Richardson DR, Wood BT, et al. Cutaneous manifestations of hyperthyroidism. South Med J 1969; 62:1127–1130

36. Keipert JA, Kelly R. Acquired juvenile hypothyroidism presenting with nail changes. Australas J Dermatol 1978; 19:89–90

37. Orteu CH, Rustin MHA. 20 thickened, fragile nails. Lancet 1996; 347:662

38. Lipschitz DA, Cook JD, Finch CA. A clinical evaluation of serum ferritin as an index of iron stores. N Engl J Med 1974; 290: 1213–1216

39. Bezwoda WR, Bothwell TH, Torrance JD, et al. The relationship between marrow iron stores, plasma ferritin concentrations and iron absorption. Scand J Haematol 1979; 22:113–120

40. Terezakis N. Brittle nail care, Westwood Western Conference on Clinical Dermatology; 1981

41. Fleckman P. Management of the ichthyoses. Skin Therapy Lett 2003; 8:3–7.

42. Anonymous. Troubleshooter: strengthen weak nails with wraps. Nails Magazine 1-1-2002, 116–122

43. Colombo VE, Gerber F, Bronhofer M, et al. Treatment of brittle fingernails and onychoschizia with biotin: Scanning electron microscopy. J Am Acad Dermatol 1990; 23:1127–1132

44. Scher RK, Fleckman P, Tulumbas B, et al. Brittle nail syndrome: treatment options and the role of the nurse. Dermatol Nurs 2003; 15:15–23

45. Institute of Medicine. Dietary Reference Intakes for Thiamin, Riboflavin, Niacin, Vitamin B6, Folate, Vitamin B12, pantothenic acid, biotin, and choline. National Academy Press 2000:374–389. Online. Available: http://www.nap.edu/catalog/6015.html

46. Zaias N, Drachman D. A method for the determination of drug effectiveness in onychomycosis. Trials with ketoconazole and griseofulvin ultramicrosize. J Am Acad Dermatol 1983; 9:912–919

47. Daniel CR, Elewski BE. Simple brittle fingernails. Cosmetic dermatology 2001; 14:53–54

# 9

# Simple Onycholysis

C Ralph Daniel III

## Key Features

1. Find and eliminate or minimize the cause
2. Very strict contact irritant moisture avoidance regimen (see below)
3. Keep the nails short. A dual-action nail nipper is indispensable
4. Avoid trauma to the nail unit
5. Chronicity may cause the 'disappearing nail bed'
6. The role of *Candida* is controversial
7. Culture, X-ray, and/or biopsy unusual on recalcitrant cases, especially when only one nail is involved

Onycholysis is defined as distal or distal lateral separation of the nail plate from the underlying and/or lateral supporting structures (nail bed, hyponychium, lateral nail folds). When the separation begins proximally near the matrix, the process is called onychomadesis. This is a common disorder.[1] It is therefore important that the clinician is able to approach onycholysis systemically to find a cause and treat it.[1,2]

For onycholysis to occur, there must be a disruption of the poorly defined cement substance/adherence mechanism of the nail plate.[1] The pathogenesis in a number of cases may be unclear. We know that the normal nail bed does not have a granular layer. We know that any process that disturbs the normal formation of the nail bed, such as psoriasis, which can form a nail bed granular layer, or lichen planus, can cause onycholysis. We also know that trauma, whether it be physical, irritant, or allergic, can cause onycholysis. The Koebner phenomenon appears to be instrumental in the diathesis of onycholysis.

This chapter focuses on simple onycholysis, i.e., that which is not congenital, due to systemic disease,[3,4] systemic drugs,[5,6] neoplasm, dermatophyte infection, or primary dermatological disease such as psoriasis and lichen planus. See the corresponding chapters to the above disorders to learn numerous specific onycholysis associations and recognition factors.

We have done several studies of patients with simple onycholysis. The first[7] looked at 93 patients. The ages ranged from 1 to 85. The mean age was 47, 91% were females, 93% gave a strong contact irritant history, and 7% gave a history of trauma or trauma and contact irritants. A total of 98% of the onycholysis cases were in the fingernails, 85% of the fungal cultures showed yeast, 50% showed a luxuriant growth of yeast on Mycosel agar (suggesting *Candida albicans*) and 3% grew a dermatophyte. Potassium hydroxide (KOH) tests were not as helpful and did not correlate with cultures. Although no specific tabulation was made, it was found (through trial and error) that these patients did not improve without a strict irritant avoidance regimen, keeping the nails short, and broad-spectrum, usually topical, antifungal therapy.

We also did another small study[8,9] looking at 31 cases of simple onycholysis. Of these, 97% were female and the age range was 23 to 85. All the cases of onycholysis (100%) were in the fingernails, 81% gave a strong history of contact irritants, 6% gave a history of trauma, 90% grew yeast, with 64% growing luxuriant yeast on Mycosel agar. The KOHs were not particularly helpful, as was the case in the previously mentioned study. The nails were initially cut back to the point of attachment. Ciclopirox 0.77% lotion was applied twice a day for 6–12 weeks (treatment was stopped in less than 12 weeks if the condition cleared earlier). In total, 81.5% of the onycholysis patients cleared and another 6% improved. All patients were also on a strict irritant avoidance regimen. Optimal therapeutic outcomes were dependent both on primary causes (probably contact irritants and/or trauma) and secondary factors, such as yeast, being recognized and treated.[7,8] It is imperative that onycholysis is treated. The longer it lasts, the more likely that the nail bed will cornify (develop a granular layer). Once this occurs, it is much less likely that the nail will ever reattach.[1,8–12] We have termed this the 'disappearing nail bed'.[9]

The role of Candida as a nail pathogen in healthy patients and as a primary or secondary pathogen is controversial.[13,14] This author feels that Candida (especially albicans) does not cause onycholysis in most cases in a healthy individual. But it is possible that it may exacerbate or prolong the disorder. It seems that contact irritants and/or trauma in most cases initiate the disorder by breaking the seal between the nail plate and its surrounding structures.

If one does not eliminate the cause(s) and treat any secondary yeast, then it is less likely that the onycholysis will resolve.

## TREATMENT[1,7,8,9,12,15–19]

### Rx TREATMENT

- Find and eliminate or minimize the cause
- A very strict irritant avoidance must be maintained
- The nails must be kept short
- Avoid trauma to the nails
- The use of topical broad-spectrum antifungal therapy and gels, lacquer, solution, or lotion is controversial
- Patients usually expect therapy other than an irritant avoidance regimen

1. One must first try to find and eliminate or minimize the cause.
2. Contact irritants and moisture must be avoided during treatment and for at least 1–2 months after onycholysis resolution:
   a. Wear light cotton gloves underneath vinyl gloves for wet work. Non-powder lightweight disposable vinyl gloves are available

from pharmacies. Heavy-duty vinyl gloves by Allerderm are available at pharmacies and generic brands at paint stores.

b. Wear the above gloves when handling raw foods and fruit (especially citrus).

c. Avoid contact with hydrocarbons such as paint thinner, petroleum products, paints, metal polish, etc.

d. Avoid nail cosmetics of all kinds while the onycholysis is resolving and for at least 2 months after the onycholysis has resolved. Then use only non-formaldehyde-containing nail products such as those made by Clinique. Nail polish remover is drying and may be harmful. Acetate polish removers are less irritating than those containing acetone. Use no nail hardeners or acrylic products.

e. Wear heavy-duty cotton gloves for dry work.

f. Use lukewarm water and very little mild soap when washing hands. Be sure to wash the soap off and dry the hands gently.

g. Protect the hands from chapping and drying in windy or cold weather by wearing unlined leather gloves.

3. Avoid trauma to the nails. Keep the nails short. Cut toenails straight across and don't round at the edges. A dual-action nail clipper is indispensable for a dermatologist to have to cut back the nails as painlessly as possible. Shoes should fit properly to decrease the chance of toenail onycholysis. No higher heels or narrow-toed shoes should be used. A 'boxy' or wider toebox is preferable.

4. Antifungal therapy:

a. Topical: This author uses a topical antifungal in conjunction with a strict irritant/trauma avoidance program. Ciclopirox topical suspension and lacquer, and/or sulconazole solution are primarily used. Older treatments less frequently utilized are 4% thymol in 95% alcohol or chloroform, and sulfacetamide 15% in 50% alcohol. All are used twice a day except for ciclopirox lacquer, which is used once daily. Tioconazole and amoralfine are available outside the US.

b. Oral: In resistant cases, try fluconazole 150 mg once a week. Ketoconazole and itraconazole may also be utilized but less frequently. Usage of the above is not presently FDA approved for onycholysis.

# REFERENCES

1. Daniel CR. Onycholysis: an overview. Seminars in Derm 1991; 10:34–40
2. Kechijian P. Onycholysis of the fingernails: evaluation and management. J Am Acad Dermatol 1985; 12: 552–560
3. Daniel CR, Sams WM, Scher RK. Nails in systemic disease. Dermatol Clin 19853:465–483
4. Daniel CR, Sams WM, Scher RK. The nails in systemic disease. In: Scher R, Daniel CR, eds. Nails: therapy diagnosis and surgery. 2nd edn. Philadelphia, WB Saunders, 1997:219–250
5. Daniel CR, Scher RK: Nail changes secondary to systemic drugs and ingestants. J Am Acad Dermatol 1984; 10:250–258
6. Daniel CR, Scher RK. Nail changes caused by systemic drugs and ingestants. In: Scher R, Daniel CR, eds. Nails: therapy, diagnosis, and surgery. 2nd edn. Philadelphia, WB Saunders, 1997:251–261
7. Daniel CR, Daniel MP, Daniel CM, et al. Chronic paronychia and onycholysis: a 13-year experience. Cutis 1996: 58:397–401
8. Daniel CR, Daniel MP, Daniel JG, Sullivan S. Managing simple chronic paronychia and onycholysis with ciclopirox 0.77% and an irritant avoidance regimen. Cutis 2004; 73:81–85
9. Daniel CR, Tosti A, Piraccini MB. The disappearing nail bed: a possible outcome of onycholysis. Cutis (in press)
10. Daniel CR. Nail disorders: Conn's current therapy. Philadelphia, WB Saunders, 1983:653–661
11. Daniel CR. The nail. Dermatology clinics 3. Philadelphia WB Saunders, 1985
12. Daniel CR, Scher RK. The nail. In: Sams WM, Lynch P, eds. Principles and practice of dermatology. 2nd edn. New York, Churchill Livingtone, 1996:763–777
13. Daniel CR. Onycholysis. Dialogues in Dermatol 1992; 30(1)
14. Daniel CR, Gupta AK, Daniel MP, Sullivan S. Candida infections of the nails: role as primary or secondary pathogen. Internat J Dermatol 1998; 7: 904–907
15. Daniel CR, Elewski BE. Candida as a nail pathogen in healthy patients. J MS State Med Assoc 1995; 6: 379–381
16. Daniel CR. Pigmentation abnormalities. In: Daniel CR, Scher R, eds. Nails: therapy, diagnosis, and surgery. 2nd edn. Philadelphia, WB Saunders, 1997:219–250
17. Daniel CR. Onycholysis. In: Proceedings of the Nail and Hair Symposium, 'Autumn in New York', Columbia University, 15–16 September 1989:121–123
18. Daniel CR, Daniel MP, Daniel CM, et al. Treatment of simple chronic paronychia and simple onycholysis. Derm Therapy 1977; 3:73–74
19. Daniel CR, Daniel MP, Sullivan S. Chronic paronychia and onycholysis: management considerations for optimal therapeutic results. Summer AAD Meeting, Nashville, TN, August, 2000

# 10

# Simple Chronic Paronychia

## C Ralph Daniel III

Chronic paronychia may be defined as inflammation lasting over 6 weeks of one or more of the three nail folds (one proximal and two lateral). It is a common disorder that may have a number of associations (Table 10.1; this is reproduced with permission from the second edition of this title).

In the past, chronic paronychia was often associated with psoriasis. Ganor[1] found that 38% of his adult female dermatology patients with chronic paronychia had psoriasis. He explained this as follows:[1]

1. Psoriasis injures nails and allows candida to proliferate.
2. In patients with psoriasis, increased rate of turnover of the skin enhances the growth of candida.
3. Impairment of peripheral blood flow contributes to chronic paronychia (disturbance of microcirculation of skin in psoriasis).

Eczema commonly affects the distal digit, and therefore the nail apparatus. Inflammation of the nail folds may cause secondary nail plate changes such as discoloration, uneven nail plate, occasional pitting, and occasional onycholysis.

For the purposes of this chapter, 'simple' chronic paronychia is that which is not secondary to any other entity such as psoriasis, eczema, systemic disease, drugs, etc.

In simple chronic paronychia, the initial insult to the nail fold(s) (usually the cuticle) seems to be either physical or contactant. The former may occur from trauma as with aggressive manicuring or filing folders, etc., and the latter from water and contact irritants. Once the seal between the nail plate and the nail fold(s) has been broken, moisture and irritants that might not adversely affect an intact nail unit, may worsen a compromised nail and perpetuate the problem.

Bakers, barbers, bartenders, domestic workers, women looking after small children, waitresses and food handlers are some occupations commonly associated with chronic paronychia.

# POSSIBLE CONFOUNDING OR EXACERBATING INFECTIOUS FACTORS

Ganor is quoted above,[1] and the older literature is replete with theories and statements that microorganisms cause and/or worsen chronic paronychia. Also in that literature, it is often stated that, in adults, 'infectious' paronychia is usually caused by a combination of Candida and low-grade bacterial infection. In adults, Gram-negative organisms such as Escherichia coli, Proteus,[2] and Klebsiella[2] may be involved. In studies of adult Israeli women,[3] infected fingers are usually on the dominant hand, and the same holds true in our practice. Ganor and Pumpiansky further found that the number of fingers affected is associated with chronicity.[3] In their study of patients and their families, the mouth and bowel, but not the vagina, were sources of Candida albicans in chronic paronychia. A 'pathognomic sign' of severe infection by Candida may sometimes be seen: Fine transverse splits that are only a few millimeters wide and never involve the whole width of the nail.[4] This is seen primarily in mucocutaneous candidiasis, in severe candidal paronychia with onycholysis, and in acrodermatitis enteropathica.[4] Maceration of the posterior nail folds allows passage of foreign material from organisms into the dermis and nail folds, inciting a chronic inflammatory reaction.[4]

The chief predisposing factor in children is probably finger sucking.[5,6] Splinting of the finger in children has been suggested as a treatment. Poor skin hygiene also plays an important role.[7] Bacteria involved are usually mixed aerobic and anaerobic, with 18% of cultures growing Candida.[7] The aerobic bacteria are usually group A streptococcus, Staphylococcus aureus, or Eikenella corrodens.[7] Anaerobic bacteria are usually Bacteroides, Gram-positive anaerobic cocci, and Fusobacterium nucleatum.[6,7,8] Brook[8] found that anaerobic infections are more common than aerobic infections, in a ratio of 3 : 2, because of organisms residing in the mouth. He furthermore stated that E. corrodens is susceptible to ampicillin and penicillin but often resistant to methicillin, nafcillin, and clindamycin.

## Candida

We did two studies. In the first we looked at 44 patients with chronic paronychia.[9] The age range was 1–85 years, with a mean age of 47; 91% were female. Cultures and potassium hydroxide (KOH) tests were done; KOHs were negative in 96%. Fungal cultures showed yeast 81% of the time and C. albicans 55% of the

**TABLE 10–1.** Diseases, factors, occupations, and conditions associated with paronychia

| ENTITY | COMMENT |
|---|---|
| **Diseases** | |
| Subungual epidermoid inclusions | |
| Psoriasis (also sometimes sterile paronychia-like lesions) | |
| Reiter's syndrome | |
| Histiocytosis X | Sometimes granulating |
| Rubinstein–Taybi syndrome | Chronic, fingernails and toenails |
| Enchondroma | May first present as paronychia |
| Verrucous nevus and nevus unius lateris | Recurrent inflammatory changes possible |
| Multicentric reticulohistiocytosis | Paronychial nodules 'like coral beads' |
| Pemphigus | May herald exacerbation |
| Stevens–Johnson syndrome | |
| Systemic lupus erythematosus | |
| Progressive systemic sclerosis | Periungual vesiculation, chronic paronychia |
| Leiner's disease | |
| Darier's disease | |
| Pachyonychia congenita | |
| Pemphigoid | |
| Job syndrome | |
| Wiscott–Aldridge syndrome | |
| **Factors** | |
| Sarcoid | Painful paronychia |
| *Tunga penetrans* | |
| Bazex's paraneoplastic syndrome | |
| Chilblain (and a distinctive variant of chilblain) | |
| Vasculitis | |
| Traumatic injury | |
| Ionizing radiation | Chronic relapsing paronychia |
| Leukemia cutis (chronic lympocytic leukemia) | |
| Vascular thrombosis, thrombophlebitis | |
| Frostbite | |
| Leprosy | |
| Zinc deficiency, pustular paronychia | |
| Erysipeloid | |
| Tulip bulbs | Periungual eruption |
| Hypoparathyroidism | Chronic paronychia |
| Acrodermatitis enteropathica | |
| Celiac disease | |
| Cold hands | |
| Varicose veins | |
| Diabetes mellitus | |
| Dyskeratosis congenita | |
| Cosmetics around nails | |
| Parakeratosis pustulosa | |
| Glucogona syndrome | |

**TABLE 10–1.** (*Cont'd*) Diseases, factors, occupations, and conditions associated with paronychia

| ENTITY | COMMENT |
| --- | --- |
| **Occupations** (See Chapter 18) | |
| Bartenders | |
| Janitorial and domestic workers | |
| Oil rig workers | |
| Barbers and hairdressers | |
| Waitresses and waiters | |
| Homemakers | |
| Gardeners | |
| Grounds keepers | |
| Secretarial/clerical | When filing |
| Florists | |
| Dentists | |
| Dental hygienists | |
| Cosmetologists | |
| Cooks | |
| Carpenters, builders | |
| Fishermen | |
| Photographic and X-ray developers | |
| Meat (and other raw food) handlers | |
| Mechanics | |
| Engravers | |
| Etchers | |
| Glaziers | |
| Painters | |
| Radio workers | |
| Shoemakers | |
| Pianists | |
| Legume shellers | |
| Poultry line workers | |
| **Conditions** | |
| Hydrocarbon exposure | |
| Transplants (renal) | |
| Granulomatous disease (chronic) | |
| Yellow nail syndrome | |
| Bandages around the nail | |
| **Drugs** (See Chapter 16) | |
| Retinoids (sometimes painful paronychia) | |
| 5-Fluorouracil | Usually from direct contact |
| Cephalexin | |
| Cyclosporin | |
| Indinovil | |
| Lanivudine | |
| Methotrexate | |
| Zidovudine | |
| Protease inhibitors in general | |

time. One patient grew a dermatophyte. In a more recent study, we looked at 17 patients.[10] The age range was 17–85 with the mean age of 54; 88% were female. Cultures and KOHs were done; KOHs were negative in about 80% and cultures showed yeast similarly to the first study. Tosti's culture results were similar.[11] This information definitely supports the presence of yeast. The question is what role it plays in the diathesis of chronic paronychia. The answer is unclear.[12]

## Contact Irritants/Trauma

In the first study mentioned above, we found that 93% of the patients gave a strong contact irritant history, with 5% giving a history of both contact irritants and trauma and 2% with a history of trauma only. In the second study, we found that 85% of the patients gave a strong contact irritant history.[10] The history of contact irritants preceded and continued during the active chronic paronychia. Tosti's studies also found strong evidence of contact irritants being the instigating and perpetuating factors.[11] Although we made no specific tabulation, through trial and error it was found that our patients did not improve without first and foremost a strict irritant avoidance regimen combined with broad-spectrum, usually topical antifungal therapy.[9,13] In the more recent study of 17 patients, we found 100% clearing using ciclopirox 0.77% lotion and a strict irritant avoidance regimen.[10,13] Dr Tosti did not find that antifungal therapy was regularly useful.[11] It is unusual for us to treat with fluconazole or itraconazole.

## TREATMENT[9,13–22]

### Rx ⊙ TREATMENT

- Find and eliminate, or minimize, the cause
- A strict moisture/contact irritant avoidance regimen is essential
- Physical trauma to the cuticles must be avoided indefinitely
- Treatment of secondary yeast and bacteria may be needed
- Mid- or higher-potency topical steroids may be used for several weeks

1. Avoid or treat the previously mentioned predisposing conditions. Avoid moisture and contact irritants for at least 1–2 months after the condition has resolved.
2. The patient should be instructed to do the following:
   a. Wear light cotton gloves under heavy-duty vinyl gloves for wet work. Heavy-duty vinyl gloves are available at paint stores and pharmacies.
   b. Wear the cotton and vinyl gloves when peeling or squeezing citrus fruits, handling tomatoes, and peeling tomatoes or other raw food.
   c. Avoid direct contact with paints, metal polish, paint thinner, turpentine, other solvents, and polish, and wear the cotton and vinyl gloves when using them.
   d. Use lukewarm water and very little mild soap when washing hands; be sure to rinse the soap off and dry gently.
   e. Protect hands from chapping and drying in windy or cold weather by wearing unlined leather gloves.
   f. Push cuticles back as little as possible and do not use fingernails, a metal file, or orange stick to do this. Cuticle removers are not good for people with paronychia and those predisposed to acquiring paronychia.
   g. If necessary, cuticles can be pushed back gently at the end of a shower or bath using a wet washcloth on the end of a finger.
   h. Avoid nail cosmetics of all kinds while the disorder is healing. Frequent application and removal of nail cosmetics are harmful. Commercial cuticle treatments are often harmful.
3. Treatment of any mild bacterial component is usually not necessary. Short courses of cephalosporin or ciprofloxacin may be used, especially for an acute exacerbation of chronic paronychia. Cultures may be needed.
4. Topical broad-spectrum antifungal solutions are helpful as drying and antiyeast agents. Clotrimazole and sulconazole solutions are available and should be applied two or three times daily. Ciclopirox topical suspension may be applied twice daily. It is a broad-spectrum antifungal agent that may also have some antibacterial and anti-inflammatory effects.
5. Itraconazole or fluconazole may be used as antiyeast agents in more resistant cases. Pulse dosing with itraconazole has some success. Once-a-week fluconazole may be tried. At the time of this printing, however, these have not been approved by the Food and Drug Administration for this indication. Terbinafine is also being studied in these patients. Mid-potency or higher-potency topical steroids are useful for 1–2 weeks. Pulse therapy with systemic steroids should be reserved for particularly recalcitrant cases. Intralesional steroids are used less commonly: triamcinolone acetonide 3 mg/ml.
6. Marsupialization or excision of the proximal nail fold has been advocated by Baran for resistant cases.
7. Some older therapies used in the past include the following:
   a. Tetracycline with amphotericin V (Mysteclin-F) and nystatin with tetracycline (Achrostatin V).
   b. 4% thymol in 95% ethanol or in chloroform.
   c. Sulfacetamide, 15%, in 50% alcohol topically three to four times a day.
8. Paronychia occurring among children who suck their fingers may be considered as bite wounds with respect to their microbiology, because the normal oral flora often are involved. The finger may be splinted to stop sucking.
9. In unusual or recalcitrant cases one must consider fungal and bacterial cultures. Unusual mycobacteria, etc. can occasionally be found. One must consider the beauty salon as a possible source. Especially if a single digit is involved, consider X-rays and biopsies to rule out an osseous cause or skin cancer as squamous cell carcinoma.

## REFERENCES

1. Ganor S. Chronic paronychia and psoriasis. Br J Dermatol 1975; 92:685
2. Cohen PR, Scher RK. Geriatric nail disorders: diagnosis and treatment. J Am Acad Dermatol 1992; 26:521
3. Ganor S, Pumpianski R. Chronic *Candida albicans* in adult Israeli women. Br J Dermatol 1974; 90:77
4. Runne U, Offanos CE. The human nail. Curr Probl Dermatol 1981; 9:102
5. Daniel CR. Nonfungal infections. In: Scher RK, Daniel CR, eds. Nails: therapy, diagnosis, surgery. Philadelphia, WB Saunders, 1990:120–126
6. Stone OJ, Mullins JF. Chronic paronychia in children. Clin Pediatr 1968; 7:104
7. Stone OJ, Mullins JF. Experimental studies in chronic paronychia. Arch Dermatol 1964; 89:455

8. Brook K. Bacteriologic study of paronychia in children. Am J Surg 1981; 141:703

9. Daniel CR, Daniel MP, Daniel CM, et al. Chronic paronychia and onycholysis: a 13-year experience. Cutis 1996; 58:397–401

10. Daniel CR, Daniel MP, Daniel JG, Sullivan S. Managing simple chronic paronychia and onycholysis with ciclopirox 0.77% and an irritant avoidance regimen. Cutis 2004; 73:81–85

11. Tosti A, Piraccini BM, Ghetti E, Colombo MD. Topical steroids versus systemic antifungals in the treatment of chronic paronychia: an open, randomized double-blind and double dummy study. J Am Ac Dermatol 2002; 47:73–76

12. Daniel CR, Gupta AK, Daniel MP, Sullivan S. Candida infection of the nail: role of Candida as a primary or secondary pathogen. Int J Dermatol 1998; 37:904–907

13. Daniel CR, Daniel MP, Daniel J, Sullivan S. Management of simple chronic paronychia and onycholysis utilizing ciclopirox 0.77% lotion. (Poster) American Academy Dermatology, Washington, DC, March 2001

14. Daniel CR. Nail disorders. In: Conn's current therapy. Philadelphia, WB Saunders, 1983:653–661

15. Daniel CR. Paronychia. The nail. In: Dermatologic clinics. Vol. 3, Philadephia, WB Saunders, 1985:461–464

16. Daniel CR. Paronychia. In: KE Greer, ed. Common problems in dermatology. Chicago, Year Book, 1988:249–255

17. Daniel CR. Non-fungal infections. In: Scher RK, Daniel CR, eds. Nails: therapy, diagnosis and surgery. Philadelphia, WB Saunders, 1990:153–166

18. Daniel CR, Daniel MP, Gupta AK. Non-fungal infections and paronychia. In: Scher RK, Daniel CR, eds. Nails: therapy, diagnosis and surgery. 2nd edn. Philadelphia, WB Saunders, 1997:163–71

19. Daniel CR. Paronychia. In: Proceedings of the nail and hair symposium. New York, Columbia University, 15–16 September 1989:125–129

20. Daniel CR, Daniel MP, Daniel CM, Ellis G. Treatment of simple chronic paronychia and simple onycholysis. Derm Therapy 1997; 3:73–74

21. Daniel CR, Daniel MP, Bell FE. Controversy: the role of yeasts in chronic paronychia: contra. Dermatology online journal, 2002

22. Daniel CR, Daniel MP, Sullivan S. Chronic paronychia and onycholysis: management considerations for optimal therapeutic. Results (Poster) Summer American Academy Dermatology, Nashville, TN, August 2000

# 11 Dermatological Diseases

Antonella Tosti and Bianca M Piraccini

## Key Features

1. The examination of the nail apparatus is an essential part of any dermatological examination
2. Recognizing the different nail signs is important in diagnosing nail dystrophies

## Rx ◐ TREATMENT

- Avoid trauma
- Keep the nails short
- The diagnosis must be certain before starting treatment

A large number of dermatological diseases involve and may be limited to the nails; the examination of the nail apparatus is therefore an essential part of any dermatological examination. This chapter describes the nail signs observed in dermatological diseases and underlines clinical clues for diagnosing skin disorders by nail evaluation (Box 11.1 and Table 11.1).

## PSORIASIS

### Key Features

* Several nails affected
* Diagnostic signs (fingernails only): Irregular pitting, salmon patches, onycholysis with erythematous border, subungual hyperkeratosis
* Toenail psoriasis clinically indistinguishable from onychomycosis
* Often associated with psoriatic arthropathy

Nail abnormalities are evident in up to 50% of patients with skin psoriasis and possibly represent a marker for severe psoriasis. Nail changes are more severe in patients with early onset (0–30 years of age) and familiar psoriasis.[1,2] The nail changes may be the first manifestation of the disease, or might be associated with mild scalp involvement and therefore be a clue for early diagnosis of psoriasis.

Psoriatic arthropathy, particularly the distal interphalangeal type, is significantly associated with nail psoriasis and it is important to refer patients with nail psoriasis to a rheumatologist to evaluate possible joint involvement.[3]

Psoriatic onycho-pachydermo-periostitis is a rare manifestation of psoriatic arthritis. It is characterized by psoriatic nail changes, tender soft tissues thickening, and osteoperiostitis of the distal phalanges in the absence of distal interphalangeal arthritis.[4] Radiological examination shows bone erosions and periosteal reaction of

### Box 11–1: Dermatological diseases involving the nails

- Psoriasis
- Pustular psoriasis
- Pityriasis rubra pilaris
- Keratoderma
- Lichen planus
- Lichen striatus
- Alopecia areata
- Eczema
- Darier's disease
- Hailey–Hailey disease
- Pemphigus vulgaris
- Bullous pemphigoid
- Cicatricial pemphigoid
- Erythema multiforme (Stevens–Johnson syndrome)
- Toxic epidermal necrolysis
- Discoid lupus erythematosus

the terminal phalanges. Nail psoriasis usually involves several nails and both fingernails and toenails may be affected.

Signs that are diagnostic for nail psoriasis include extensive irregular pitting, salmon patches of the nail bed and onycholysis with erythematous borders.[5] All these signs are almost exclusively limited to the fingernails, where several signs are often associated.

*Pitting* describes small depressions of the nail plate surface (Figs 11.1 to 11.4). Pits are the most common sign of nail psoriasis[6] and are due to psoriatic involvement of the proximal nail matrix that result in clusters of parakeratotic cells in the dorsal nail plate. These clusters are easily detached, leaving the pits that migrate distally with nail growth. Psoriatic pits are typically large, deep, irregular in size and randomly distributed within the nail plate. In the proximal part of the nail, pits may be covered by whitish, easy detachable scales.

*Salmon (oily) patches* appear as yellow or salmon-pink areas of discoloration visible through the transparent nail plate (Fig. 11.5). They are irregular in size and shape and represent a sign of psoriatic involvement of the nail bed. Salmon patches may be localized in the central portion of the nail or surround an area of distal onycholysis.

*Onycholysis* describes the distal or lateral detachment of the nail plate from the nail bed and appears white due to the presence of air in the subungual space. In psoriasis it is a consequence of psoriatic involvement of the distal nail bed and is characteristically surrounded by an erythematous margin that marks its proximal border (Figs 11.6 and 11.7).

**TABLE 11-1.** Nail signs of dermatological diseases

| SIGN | DESCRIPTION | CONDITION |
|---|---|---|
| Pitting | Irregular deep | Psoriasis |
| | Irregular deep, often other superficial abnormalities | Eczema |
| | Geometric superficial | Alopecia areata |
| Onycholysis | Erythematous border | Psoriasis |
| | Often with thinning and longitudinal fissuring | Lichen planus |
| | Hemorrhagic | Bullous diseases |
| Subungual hyperkeratosis | Associated with onycholysis | Psoriasis |
| | | Eczema |
| Acute paronychia | Relapsing inflammation with pustulae | Pustular psoriasis |
| | Hemorrhagic | Bullous diseases |
| | Vesicles and itching | Eczema |
| Longitudinal striae | Ridging and fissuring | Lichen planus |
| | Erythronychia and leukonychia | Darier's disease |
| | Roughness | Twenty-nail dystrophy |

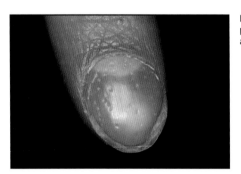

FIGURE 11-1. Psoriasis: pits are irregular in size and distribution.

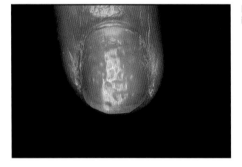

FIGURE 11-2. Psoriasis: irregular pitting.

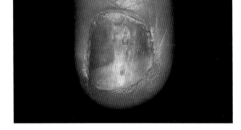

FIGURE 11-3. Psoriasis: pits are irregular in size and depth. Onycholysis and salmon patches are also evident.

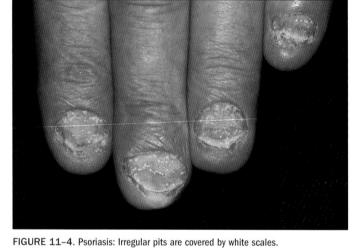

FIGURE 11-4. Psoriasis: Irregular pits are covered by white scales.

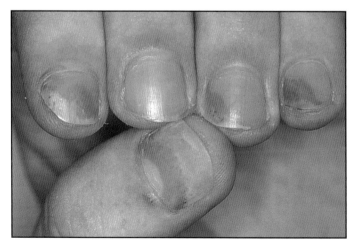

FIGURE 11-5. Psoriasis: Salmon patches of the nail bed and onycholysis.

Nail psoriasis often produces other nail abnormalities, including splinter hemorrhages, nail bed hyperkeratosis, nail thickening and crumbling, paronychia, and rarely leukonychia and erythema of the lunula and trachyonychia. None of these signs is diagnostic for nail psoriasis, because they are commonly observed in other inflammatory, traumatic, or infective nail conditions.

*Splinter hemorrhages* appear as thin red or black longitudinal lines localized in the distal portion of the nail. They result from psoriatic involvement of the nail bed capillaries, which are longitudinally oriented. They are usually seen in the fingernails (Fig. 11.8).

*Nail bed hyperkeratosis* (Figs 11.9 and 11.10) is characterized by a thickened nail plate due to the presence of subungual scales, which may either be silver–white in color and difficult to scrape, or yellow and greasy due to accumulation of scales and exudate. This sign indicates involvement of the distal nail bed and hyponychium and can be observed both in fingernails and in toenails where it often represents the only sign of nail psoriasis.

*Crumbling of the nail plate* (Fig. 11.11) results from diffuse psoriatic involvement of the nail apparatus and is typical of severe nail psoriasis. The nail is thickened, opaque, and grossly deformed. It presents a very irregular and scaly surface.

*Paronychia* results from involvement of the periungual skin and the proximal nail fold with retention of scales between the ventral fold and nail plate (Fig. 11.12). The digit may be inflamed and painful. The nail presents superficial abnormalities due to nail

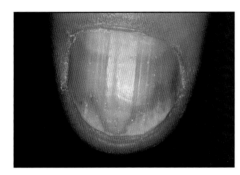

FIGURE 11–6. Psoriasis: Onycholysis surrounded by erythematous border.

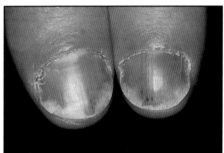

FIGURE 11–8. Psoriasis: Splinter hemorrhages and typical onycholysis.

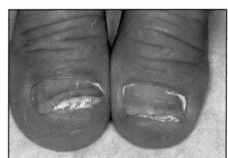

FIGURE 11–9. Psoriasis: Severe nail bed hyperkeratosis.

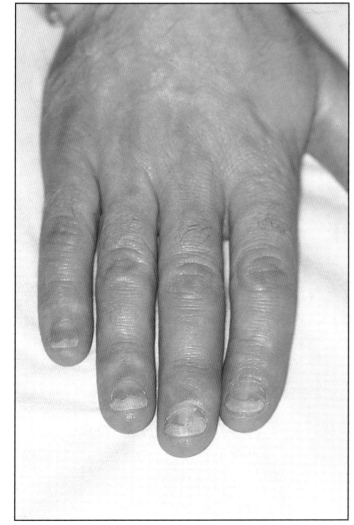

FIGURE 11–7. Psoriasis: Onycholysis with proximal erythematous margin.

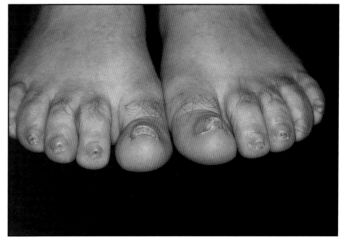

FIGURE 11–10. Psoriasis: Greasy subungual hyperkeratosis.

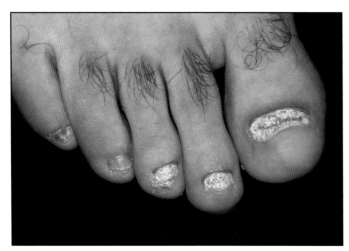

FIGURE 11-11. Psoriasis: Nail crumbling.

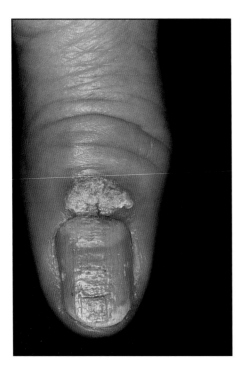

FIGURE 11-12. Psoriasis: Paronychia and superficial nail plate abnormalities.

The nail is divided with imaginary horizontal and longitudinal lines into quadrants. Each nail is given a score for nail bed psoriasis (0–4) and nail matrix psoriasis (0–4) depending on the presence of *any* of the features of nail psoriasis in that quadrant:

1. Evaluation 1: Nail matrix. In each quadrant of the nail, nail matrix psoriasis is evaluated by presence of *any* of the nail matrix features (pitting, leukonychia, red spots in the lunula, crumbling): 0 for none, 1 if present in one quadrant of the nail, 2 if present in two quadrants of the nail, 3 if present in three quadrants of the nail, and 4 if present in all four quadrants of the nail.
2. Evaluation 2: Nail bed. Nail bed psoriasis is evaluated by the presence of *any* of the nail bed features (onycholysis, splinter hemorrhages, subungual hyperkeratosis, 'oil drop' (salmon patch dyschromia): 0 for none, 1 for one quadrant only, 2 for two quadrants, 3 for three quadrants, and 4 for all four quadrants.
3. Each nail gets a matrix score and a nail bed score, the total of which is the score for that nail (0–8).
4. Each nail is evaluated, and the sum of all the nails is the total NAPSI score. The sum of the scores from all nails is 0–80; or 0–160 if toenails are included. At any time, the matrix or nail bed score can be assessed independently if desired. If a target nail scale is desired, the same technique can be used to evaluate all eight parameters (pitting, leukonychia, red spots in lunula, crumbling, oil drop, onycholysis, hyperkeratosis, and splinter hemorrhages) in each quadrant of the nail, giving that one nail a score of 0–32.

### Diagnostic signs

- Irregular pitting (proximal nail matrix)
- Salmon patches (nail bed)
- Onycholysis with erythematous border (nail bed)

### Nondiagnostic signs

- Subungual hyperkeratosis (hyponychium and nail bed)
- Splinter hemorrhages (nail bed)
- Nail crumbling (nail matrix and nail bed)
- Paronychia (proximal nail fold)
- Nail plate surface abnormalities (proximal nail matrix)
- Trachyonychia

matrix damage. Psoriatic paronychia is often precipitated by treatment with systemic retinoids.[7]

*Leukonychia* due to psoriasis is uncommon. The nail may present a few white opaque irregular spots or be diffusely whitish. Leukonychia results from parakeratosis of the ventral nail plate due to psoriatic inflammation of the distal matrix.

*Erythema of the lunula* is characterized by a mottled erythema on the lunula. This is a sign of matrix inflammation and may be observed in other inflammatory diseases of the matrix, such as lichen planus and alopecia areata.

*Trachyonychia* due to psoriasis is clinically indistinguishable from trachyonychia due to alopecia areata or lichen planus. The nail is rough due to excessive longitudinal ridging.

Severity of nail psoriasis can be evaluated using the recently proposed NAPSI (NAil Psoriasis Severity Index) scale, which considers extent of involvement and location of psoriasis in the nail unit[8] (Box 11.2).

Nail psoriasis is often precipitated and worsened by microtraumas due to Koebner phenomenon. This is especially evident for fingernail psoriasis, which is often more severe in the dominant hand (Fig. 11.13). Onycholysis and subungual hyperkeratosis are often prominent symptoms in manual workers and in subjects with occupations requiring continuous use of the nails or the digital pulp.

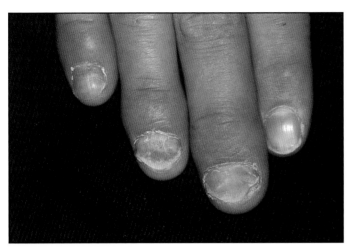

FIGURE 11-13. Psoriasis: Nail abnormalities and psoriatic arthropathy in a manual worker.

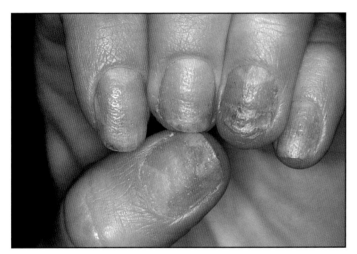

FIGURE 11-14. Psoriasis: Pitting and onycholysis with secondary *Pseudomonas* colonization.

Psoriatic onycholysis may be complicated by penetration and secondary colonization of the subungual space by microrganisms, especially bacteria and yeasts. Colonization by *Pseudomonas* produces a typical dark-green discoloration (Fig. 11.14).

# Differential Diagnosis

Diagnosis of fingernail psoriasis is easier than that of toenail psoriasis, where the disease usually produces nonspecific symptoms.

## Onychomycosis

Differential diagnosis between psoriasis and onychomycosis may be very difficult, especially when the disease is limited to the toenails. Mycology is mandatory in all cases. It is important to keep in mind that a positive mycology does not rule out psoriasis, because psoriatic nails are more susceptible to fungal infections than normal nails.[9] Pathology of nail clipping or nail bed biopsies may be mandatory in some cases.[10]

Distal subungual onychomycosis (DSO) causes subungual hyperkeratosis and onycholysis, as does nail bed psoriasis. The only clinical clue for a diagnosis of onychomycosis is the presence of yellow–white longitudinal streaks, which indicate proximal progression of the disease. The presence of plantar scaling is not helpful because it may be due to psoriasis or tinea pedis, which is frequently associated to onychomycosis.

### PSORIASIS VERSUS ONYCHOMYCOSIS
- Look for typical symptoms (pitting, salmon patches) in the fingernails.
- Look at the scalp or intergluteal clefts for psoriasis.
- History of spontaneous improvement and relapses suggests psoriasis.
- Presence of longitudinal streaks suggest onychomycosis.
- Potassium hydroxide (KOH) tests and culture are mandatory.
- Remember that both may be present in the same nail, especially toenails.

## Idiopathic onycholysis

This is restricted to the fingernails and often associated with chronic paronychia. The onycholytic area is not surrounded by the erythematous border. Nail discoloration due to secondary bacteria and yeast colonization is common.

## Traumatic onycholysis

This is common in the toenails, especially in the allux, where it is usually symmetric. Onycholysis may be associated with splinter hemorrhages and subungual hematoma. A diagnosis of traumatic onycholysis is suggested by the absence of subungual hyperkeratosis. In the fingernails, traumatic onycholysis is most frequently induced by over-zealous manicuring.

## Alopecia areata

Nail pitting in alopecia areata is characterized by superficial and small depressions, which are geometrically distributed on the nail plate surface. A diagnosis of alopecia areata is suggested by the regular distribution and morphology of the pits.

## Eczema

In eczema, nail abnormalities are usually associated with involvement of the proximal nail fold and digital pulp. The nail plate may be deformed by Beau's lines and irregular depressions. When eczema involves the distal pulp, the nail shows distal onycholysis and subungual hyperkeratosis. Differential diagnosis with psoriasis may be difficult. Minor nail pitting may be seen.

## Bazex paraneoplastic acrokeratosis

Nail lesions may be indistinguishable from psoriasis, but the acral distribution with involvement of the nose and ears is typical.

## Inflammatory linear verrucous epidermolytic nevus (ILVEN)

Nail lesions are identical to those of psoriasis but limited to one or a few adjacent digits. The linear distribution of the cutaneous eruption is typical.

### Keratotic scabies

Subungual hyperkeratosis is marked and onycholysis is usually absent or mild.

### Nail bed lichen planus

This produces onycholysis and mild subungual hyperkeratosis. The presence of nail plate thinning, ridging, and fissuring suggests lichen planus but a biopsy may be necessary for differential diagnosis.

### Parakeratosis pustolosa

This diagnosis should be considered in children with psoriasiform nail changes limited to one digit.

### Pytiriasis rubra pilaris

Subungual hyperkeratosis and splinter hemorrhages are prominent signs.

### Psoriasiform acral dermatitis

This rare condition is characterized by chronic dermatitis of the terminal phalanges associated with marked shortening of the nail bed of the affected fingers.[11] Some consider this condition a possible manifestation of psoriasis in children.[12]

## Course

Spontaneous improvement may occur and patients often see improvement of some nails together with spreading of the disease to other nails. Fingernail psoriasis often worsens in the summer months and is not positively influenced by UV exposure. Traumas precipitate or worsen nail symptoms. Most patients with nail psoriasis complain of disabilities in their daily activities and profession.[13]

## Treatment[14]

**Rx ◑ TREATMENT**

- Nail matrix psoriasis does not benefit from topicals
- Topical steroids are scarcely effective, even in nail bed psoriasis
- Treatment should be prolonged for several months
- Look for scalp scaling
- Rheumatological evaluation recommended
- Avoid microtraumas (Koebner phenomenon)

### Topical treatments

These include steroids, vitamin D derivatives and tazarotene.

Nail matrix psoriasis does not benefit from topicals, which cannot penetrate the proximal nail fold and nail plate. Topical steroids are rarely effective, even in nail bed psoriasis, and long-term application may cause skin and even bone atrophy, especially with the super potent steroids.

Topical calcipotriol or topical tazarotene improve nail bed hyperkeratosis and can be prescribed in patients with prevalent nail bed involvement.[15,16] Treatment should be prolonged for several months.

### Intralesional steroids

These can be injected in the proximal nail fold for the treatment of nail matrix psoriasis or into the nail bed for the treatment of nail bed psoriasis. Triamcinolone acetonide should be diluted 2.5–10 mg/mL in saline solution and injected to a maximum of 0.1 mL per digit, using a fine-gauge needle and a syringe with Luer lock. It is advisable to cool the skin before injection to reduce pain. Injections can be repeated monthly. Subungual hyperkeratosis and nail thickening respond better than onycholysis and pitting.[17] Most common side effects include hemorrhages and pigmentary changes.

### Systemic retinoids

Low dosages of acitretin (0.2–0.3 mg/kg/day) are a good treatment for severe nail matrix and nail bed psoriasis in males or post-menopausal women. It is important to avoid dosages exceeding 0.3 mg/kg/day because they may cause side effects in the nails, including brittleness and paronychia with/without pyogenic granulomas.[7]

### Systemic methotrexate and systemic CyA

These are effective but not recommended except in patients with diffuse cutaneous involvement.

### PUVA

This is not effective and may even worsen the nail signs.

### New biologic agents

New selective immunomodulatory drugs have been recently approved for use in psoriasis. These include alefacept, etanercept, infliximab, efalizumab and adalimumab. Infliximab seems to be very effective in nail psoriasis, whereas alefacept and etanercept are moderately effective. No data are available on the efficacy of adalimumab and efalizumab on nail psoriasis.

Data on nail psoriasis are currently available especially from abstracts and posters presented at dermatology meetings.

## PUSTULAR PSORIASIS

Pustular psoriasis (PP) of the nail is not rare and is often limited to one or a few digits (Hallopeau's acrodermatitis). It is restricted to the nail and the distal pulp in most cases.[18,19] About 30% of patients with palmoplantar pustolosis have nail involvement.[20]

Diagnosis of PP of the nail is suggested by a history of relapsing painful inflammation of the nail. Pain may be severe and impairs digital use.

The disease is frequently localized in the nail bed, producing onycholysis, periungual erythema and pain. Pustules may be visible through the nail plate (Figs 11.15 and 11.16). In severe cases the nail plate is discoloured and detached by accumulation of purulent-appearing material and scales that form thick yellow exudating

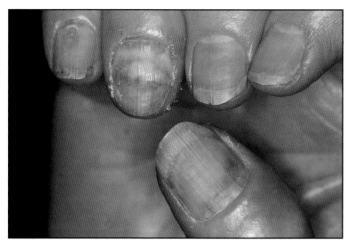

FIGURE 11-15. Pustular psoriasis: Pustules are visible through the transparent nail plate.

masses (Fig. 11.17). Involvement of the nail matrix produces acute paronychia and onychomadesis (Fig. 11.18).

However, in most cases, the patient is not seen during the acute flare-up and presents with subacute signs. The nail plate is onycholytic, shortened, and yellow–brown in color, and the exposed nail bed presents mild erythema and scaling. The periungual skin may show erythema, pustulae, and hyperkeratosis or mild scaling (Fig. 11.19).

### Diagnostic signs

- Periungual/subungual pustules
- Painful onycholysis
- Chronic onycholysis with nail bed scaling and exudation
- History of rapidly recurrent painful flares is typical

FIGURE 11-16. Pustular psoriasis: Nail bed pustules and periungual inflammation.

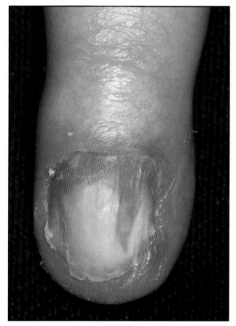

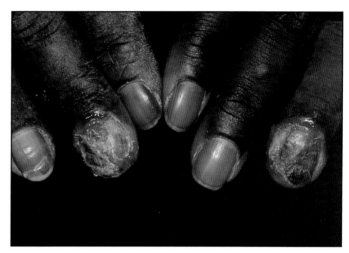

FIGURE 11-18. Pustular psoriasis: Acute paronychia and onychomadesis.

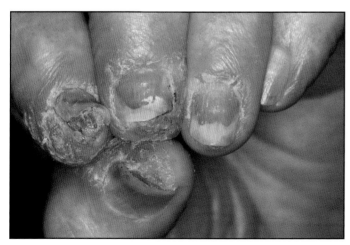

FIGURE 11-17. Pustular psoriasis: Nail bed pustules and periungual exudation and crusts.

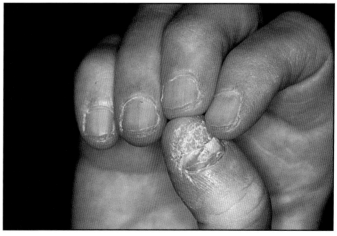

FIGURE 11-19. Pustular psoriasis: Onycholysis and nail bed scaling between acute flares.

## Differential diagnosis

### Key Features

* Bacterial infections: No history of recurrences
* Herpetic whitlow: Normal nail between recurrences
* Acute contact dermatitis: Absence of pustules and presence of itching
* Onychomycosis due to nondermatophytic molds: onycholysis, nail discoloration and periungual inflammation – toenails involvement

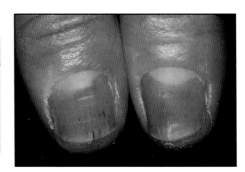

FIGURE 11–20. Pityriasis rubra pilaris: Splinter hemorrhages and orange-yellow discoloration of the distal nail plate.

### Bacterial or viral paronychia

Bacterial paronychia is not recurrent. Herpes simplex infection is usually less severe and the nail recovers completely between relapses. Cultures may clarify diagnosis in doubtful cases.

### Acute contact dermatitis

The affected digit shows acute paronychia with exudation and scaling. The patient complains of itching but not pain.

### Onychomycosis

When present, nondermatophytic molds often cause periungual inflammation and pain.[21] The affected nail is onycholytic and discolored and removal of the detached nail plate may sometimes reveal pus discharge. The disease is limited to the toenails in most cases and there is no history of periodic flare-ups. Cultures confirm the diagnosis.

## Course

The course of the disease is characterized by repetitive episodes of acute pustulation and pain. Pustular psoriasis of the nail may induce atrophy of the nail matrix and nail bed. Bone resorption may also occur.

## Treatment[19]

Acitretin 0.5 mg/kg/day is effective in preventing relapses and can produce complete cure in most cases; duration of treatment is 4–6 months. Recurrences are frequent after interruption.

Topical calcipotriol 0.005% can be utilized as maintenance treatment to prevent recurrences. It may be utilized as the sole treatment when the disease is limited to one nail or when systemic retinoids are contraindicated.

## PITYRIASIS RUBRA PILARIS

Nail changes are common, especially in the classic adult type 1.[22] The nail abnormalities are similar to those of nail bed psoriasis with subungual hyperkeratosis, splinter hemorrhages and distal yellow–brown discoloration (Fig. 11.20). Nail signs diagnostic for psoriasis (irregular pitting, salmon patches), however, are typically absent.

## Treatment

Treatment with retinoids and re-PUVA improves the skin and nail lesions.

## KERATODERMA

Psoriasiform nail changes, particularly subungual hyperkeratosis and splinter hemorrhages are common in all types of palmoplantar keratoderma, including epidermolytic palmoplantar keratoderma (Fig. 11.21).[23,24]

## LICHEN PLANUS

### Key Features

* Nail thinning and fissuring
* Possible cicatricial outcome (dorsal pterygium)
* Several nails usually affected
* Biopsy required for diagnosis

Nail abnormalities are evident in about 10% of patients with skin or mucosal lichen planus.[25] Nail lichen planus, however, most commonly occurs in the absence of skin or mucosal involvement.

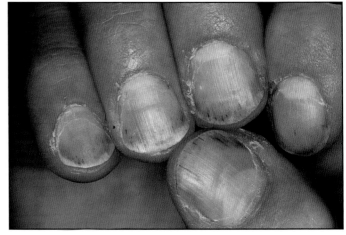

FIGURE 11–21. Palmoplantar keratoderma: Splinter hemorrhages and mild subungual hyperkeratosis and distal onycholysis.

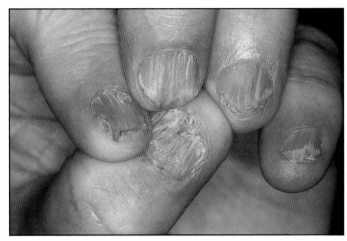

FIGURE 11–22. Lichen planus: Thinning, longitudinal ridging and fissuring.

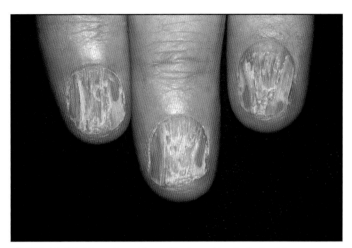

FIGURE 11–23. Lichen planus: Severe thinning and longitudinal splitting.

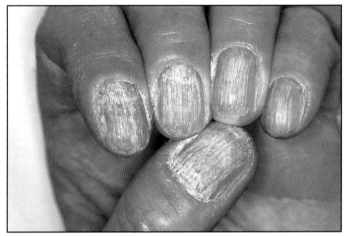

FIGURE 11–24. Lichen planus: Longitudinal ridging and fissuring.

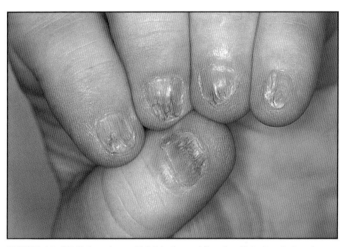

FIGURE 11–25. Lichen planus: Nail thinning and fissuring. Note dorsal pterygium on the fifth fingernail.

In our experience, oral lesions are present in 25% of patients. Skin or scalp involvement is very rare.[26]

The disease is more common in adults and usually affects several or most nails. Nail lichen planus may cause permanent nail destruction if not properly diagnosed and treated.

Diagnosis of lichen planus of the nails is suggested by thinning, longitudinal ridging, and fissuring of the nail plate. Pterygium formation is a possible outcome and indicates nail matrix scarring.[27,28]

In most patients the disease starts abruptly and the nails become markedly thinned and longitudinally fissured (Figs 11.22 to 11.24). The nail plate surface is longitudinally ridged, opaque, and extremely brittle. The distal margin is irregular and short. This presentation, *especially when associated with pain*, indicates nail matrix involvement and requires prompt treatment to avoid pterygium formation and nail atrophy.

Dorsal nail pterygium (Figs 11.25 and 11.26) describes distal extension of the proximal nail fold, which adheres to the nail bed. The extension has a V-shaped appearance and often splits the nail plate in two portions. Pterygium occurs where the nail plate is absent due to nail matrix destruction and widens with progressive scarring of the matrix.

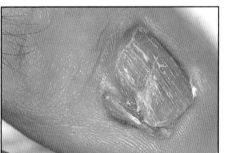

FIGURE 11–26. Lichen planus: Dorsal pterygium.

In addition to these very typical symptoms, nail lichen planus may produce other nail abnormalities including:

- onycholysis with/without subungual hyperkeratosis
- yellow nail syndrome-like changes
- idiopathic atrophy of the nails
- twenty-nail dystrophy
- pigmentary changes
- erythema of the lunula.

*Onycholysis with/without Subungual Hyperkeratosis*
Nail bed lichen planus is often associated with nail matrix lichen planus. The nails show onycholysis with or without subungual hyperkeratosis (Figs 11.27 and 11.28). In some cases, the hyperkeratosis is severe with a markedly uplifted nail plate.

*Yellow Nail Changes*
In the toenails, the disease may cause a diffuse yellow discoloration mimicking the yellow nail syndrome[29] (Fig. 11.29).

*Idiopathic Atrophy of the Nails[30–32]*
This variety of lichen planus is rare and almost exclusively observed in Asian populations. The disease is characterized by a rapid progressive atrophy of the nail with or without pterygium (Figs 11.30 and 11.31). The condition usually develops in childhood and the patient comes to see the doctor when nail atrophy is already established.

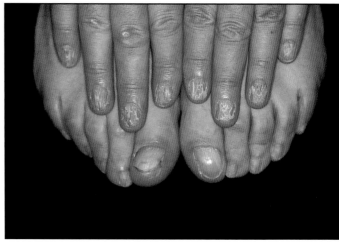

FIGURE 11–29. Lichen planus: Yellow nail syndrome-like changes in the toenails are associated with typical symptoms in the fingernails.

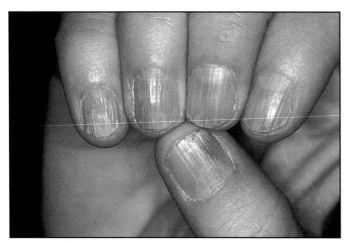

FIGURE 11–27. Lichen planus: Onycholysis due to nail bed involvement. Also note mild longitudinal ridging and fissuring and erythema of the lunulae.

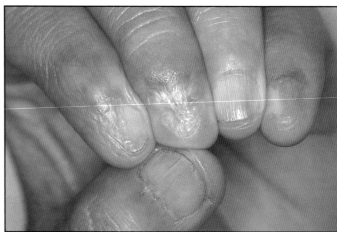

FIGURE 11–30. Lichen planus: Idiopathic atrophy of the nails. Note postinflammatory pigmentation of the proximal nail fold.

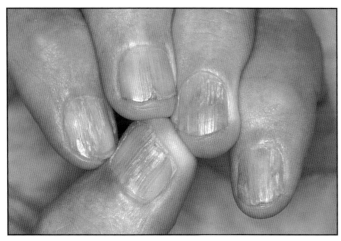

FIGURE 11–28. Lichen planus: Onycholysis due to nail bed lichen planus associated with nail thinning and longitudinal fissuring due to matrix involvement.

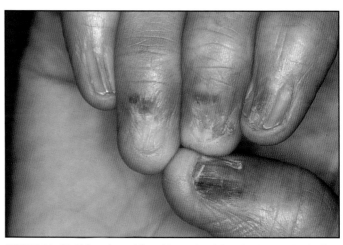

FIGURE 11–31. Lichen planus: Idiopathic atrophy of the nails. Note proximal nail fold teleangectasia and postinflammatory melanonychia.

Most digits are affected, with complete or partial absence of the nail plates. The proximal nail fold shows atrophy and teleangectasia.

### Trachyonychia (Twenty-Nail Dystrophy)

Idiopathic trachyonychia may be caused by lichen planus of the nail matrix. The condition is benign and does not produce pterygium. The nails are rough due to excessive longitudinal striations.

### Pigmentary Changes (Figs 11.30 and 11.31)

Postinflammatory hyperpigmentation of the proximal nail fold is common in dark-skinned individuals. Longitudinal melanonychia can also occur.[33]

### Erythema of the Lunula

The lunula shows mottled erythema due to distal matrix inflammation.

---

**Diagnostic signs**

- Nail thinning with longitudinal fissuring (nail matrix inflammation)
- Dorsal pterygium (nail matrix scarring)
- Nail atrophy with and without pterygium (nail matrix scarring)

**Nondiagnostic signs**

- Onycholysis with/without subungual hyperkeratosis (nail bed inflammation)
- Pigmentary changes (post-inflammatory melanocyte activation)

---

## Differential Diagnosis

**Key Features**

- \* Systemic amyloidosis: Thinning and splitting are associated with hemorrhagic lesions
- \* Lichen striatus: Thinning and splitting involving just one side of one to two nails
- \* Bullous diseases: Pterygium but not nail plate abnormalities
- \* Raynaud's disease: Proximal nail fold capillaries abnormalities

Nail lichen planus may be observed in graft versus host disease and in drug-induced lichenoid reactions.[34]

### Systemic amyloidosis

Nail changes may precede the development of skin and mucosal lesions. Systemic amyloidosis produces nail thinning and fissuring that resemble very closely typical nail matrix lichen planus. Splinter hemorrhages are often associated. The diagnosis is confirmed by pathology that reveals amyloid deposits in the nail matrix and nail bed dermis.[35]

### Lichen striatus

The nail changes are limited to one digit and usually to one side of the nail plate. Typical skin lesions are often associated.

### Bullous diseases

Cicatricial pemphigoid, erythema multiforme, and Lyell syndrome may affect the nail and cause pterygium. The clinical history and the presence of skin and/or mucosal lesions permits the diagnosis.

### Raynaud's disease

This causes nail plate thinning and occasionally dorsal pterygium. The history is typical and examination of the proximal nail fold reveals capillary changes.

### Psoriasis

Nail bed lichen planus may closely simulate nail psoriasis. When the nail bed lesions are not associated with thinning and fissuring, the differential diagnosis may require a biopsy.

## Diagnosis

Typical lichen planus is usually easy to diagnose from clinical examination. A 3-mm punch biopsy from the nail matrix should be taken to confirm the diagnosis in doubtful cases. A nail bed biopsy may be necessary to discriminate nail bed lichen planus from nail psoriasis.

## Course

Typical lichen planus is slowly progressive and pterygium formation usually takes at least several months. Permanent atrophy of the nail bed and hyponychium may be a long-term sequela of untreated nail bed lichen planus.

Trachyonychia due to lichen planus has a benign course and never produces nail scarring.[36]

## Treatment

Lichen planus responds very well to treatment with intralesional or systemic steroids. The latter should be preferred when the disease involves more than three digits.

### Intralesional steroids

These can be injected in the proximal nail fold for the treatment of nail matrix psoriasis or in the nail bed for the treatment of nail bed psoriasis. Triamcinolone acetonide should be diluted 2.5–5 mg/mL in saline solution and injected to a maximum of 0.5 mL for each digit, using a fine-gauge needle and a syringe with Luer lock. It is advisable to cool the proximal nail fold before injection to reduce pain. Injections can be repeated monthly. The most common side effects include hemorrhages and pigmentary changes.

### Systemic steroids

We routinely utilize triamcinolone acetonide 0.5 mg/kg IM once a month for 4–6 months. Almost all patients respond to treatment and recurrences are uncommon. Pterygium is irreversible and should not be treated.

## LICHEN STRIATUS[37]

Nail involvement is uncommon and usually associated with typical skin lesions. The disease usually involves only one finger and produces nail abnormalities that resemble typical nail matrix lichen planus. A diagnosis of lichen striatus is suggested by nail thinning associated with longitudinal ridging and splitting restricted to a lateral or medial portion of a single nail. Dorsal pterygium is not a feature. Skin lesions typical of lichen striatus are often associated and may precede or follow the development of the nail changes (Fig. 11.32).

## Course

Spontaneous regression is the rule, usually within 1–2 years from diagnosis. No treatment is required.

## LICHEN NITIDUS

Nail involvement is rare. A large number of nail plate surface abnormalities have been reported, including pitting, deep ridging, brittleness and longitudinal striations, but none is typical for the disease.

## LICHEN SCLEROSUS

Nail involvement is rare.

## ALOPECIA AREATA

### Key Features

* Geometric pitting
* Twenty-nail dystrophy
* Children most commonly affected

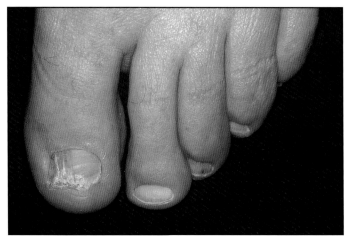

FIGURE 11–32. Lichen striatus: Lichenoid nail changes restricted to the medial site of the left great toenail. Note typical skin lesions.

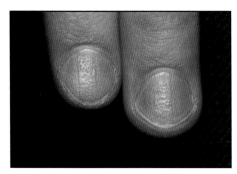

FIGURE 11–33. Alopecia areata: Geometric pitting.

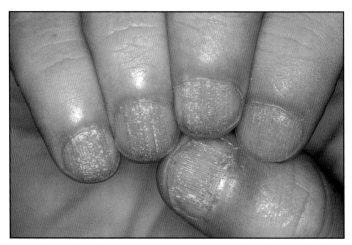

FIGURE 11–34. Alopecia areata: Geometric punctate leukonychia.

Nail abnormalities occur in about 20% of adults and 50% of children with alopecia areata. They are more common in males and in patients with severe alopecia areata.[38-40] The nail abnormalities may precede or follow the onset of hair loss and are a consequence of nail matrix involvement by the disease. Signs that are typical for alopecia areata are geometric pitting and geometric leukonychia.

Trachyonychia (twenty-nail dystrophy) is due to alopecia areata in most cases (see p. 109).

Nail abnormalities may be limited to one nail or involve most of the nails:

* *Geometric pitting* (Fig. 11.33): The nail plate shows multiple, small, superficial pits which are regularly distributed in a geometric pattern along longitudinal and transverse lines.

* *Geometric punctate leukonychia*: This is rare but very typical (Fig. 11.34). The nail plate presents multiple, small white spots, which are geometrically oriented in a grill pattern.[41]
* *Trachyonychia*: The nails are rough due to excessive longitudinal ridging (Fig. 11.35).

Alopecia areata also produces nail signs that are not diagnostic, including: Beau's lines, onychomadesis and erythema of the lunulae:

* *Onychomadesis and Beau's lines*: These rarely develop in coincidence of an acute attack of alopecia areata. The nail abnormalities involve all or most nails.

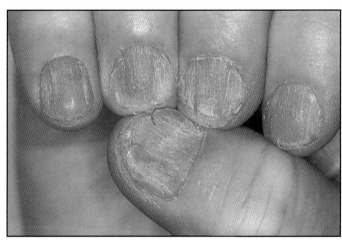

FIGURE 11-35. Alopecia areata. Trachyonychia: nail roughness due to excessive longitudinal ridging.

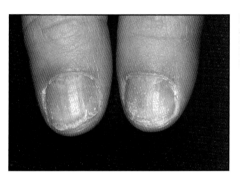

FIGURE 11-36. Alopecia areata: Geometric pitting, leukonychia and mottled lunula.

- *Erythema of the lunulae:*[42] The lunula shows mottled erythema (Fig. 11.36). This sign is most frequently observed in association with trachyonychia.

### Diagnostic signs

- Geometric pitting
- Geometric punctate leukonychia
- Trachyonychia

### Nondiagnostic signs

- Onychomadesis
- Beau's lines
- Erythema of the lunulae

## Differential Diagnosis

### Trachyonychia

There are no clinical clues to differentiate trachyonychia due to alopecia areata from trachyonychia due to lichen planus or psoriasis.

### Nail psoriasis

Pitting is usually associated with other signs and it is not regular as it is in alopecia areata.

## Course

The nail abnormalities are usually stable and gradually improve over the years. The course of nail abnormalities does not necessarily correlate with the course of hair loss.

## Treatment

The nail abnormalities improve when alopecia areata is treated with systemic steroids. They are not affected by other effective treatment of alopecia areata, such as topical immunotherapy or PUVA.

## ECZEMA

Nail changes are common in patients with hand dermatitis:
- *Acute eczema* produces erythema, edema, and vesiculation of the periungual tissues (Fig. 11.37). Involvement of the proximal nail fold produces acute paronychia that may be followed by development of onychomadesis. Beau's lines and irregular depressions usually appear a few weeks after the episode, as a sign of nail matrix damage.
- *Chronic eczema* usually affects the proximal nail fold and/or the hyponychium. Chronic paronychia is the most common presentation with swelling of the proximal nail fold and loss of the cuticle. The nail plate frequently shows irregular superficial abnormalities, such as pitting and Beau's lines resulting from nail matrix damage (Fig. 11.38). Yellow or green discoloration of the lateral margins of the nail is common and due to secondary bacterial colonization. Chronic eczema of the hyponychium presents with subungual hyperkeratosis and distal onycholysis, usually associated with fingertip scaling. Koilonychia is often associated.

Patients with atopic dermatitis of the hands frequently present irregular nail plate surface abnormalities due to eczematous

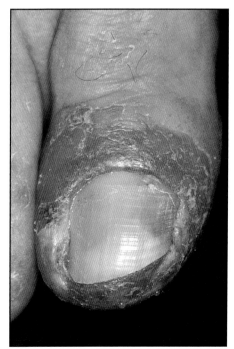

FIGURE 11-37. Eczema: Acute contact dermatitis due to topical tioconazole.

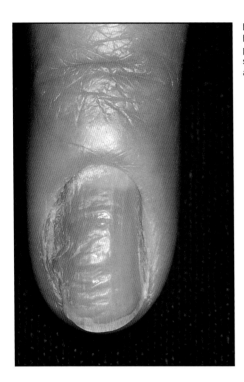

FIGURE 11–38. Eczema: Chronic paronychia and irregular superficial nail plate abnormalities.

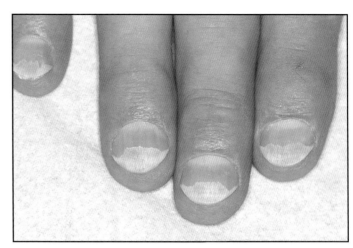

FIGURE 11–39. Hyperhidrosis: Distal onycholysis.

involvement of the nails. Atopics also have often shiny nails due to scratching. Colonization of the subungual space by *Staphylococcus* is frequent and may rarely cause osteomyelitis of the distal phalanges.[43]

| Diagnostic signs of Hand Eczema |
| --- |
| • Paronychia (acute or chronic). <br> • Irregular nail plate surface abnormalities. <br> • Onycholysis and hyperkeratosis. |

## Causes

Acute eczema of the digits may or may not be occupational. Cosmetics and topical drugs are the most common causes of nonoccupational eczema. Acrylates utilized in sculptured nails may cause both irritant and allergic contact dermatitis.

Chronic paronychia may be caused and exacerbated by contact with foods and can be an occupational disease in food handlers.[44]

## Treatment

Avoidance of allergens/irritants and protective measures (cotton gloves under vinyl gloves); topical steroids, emollients, and barrier creams can all help.

## HYPERHIDROSIS

Distal onycholysis of fingernails may occur in patients with hyperhidrosis during the summer months. Onycholysis is not associated with subungual hyperkeratosis and affects – symmetrically – most or all fingernails (Fig. 11.39). The onset is sudden and the proximal border of the onycholysis is very regular. The nail lesions improve spontaneously during the winter and often recur every summer.

## DARIER'S DISEASE

Darier's disease often involves the nails, which can be a clue for the diagnosis. The disease more frequently affects fingernails than toenails. Typical signs are longitudinal red and white streaks with fissuring of the distal margin (Figs 11.40 and 11.41). All these signs often coexist in the same nail, but are not necessarily present in all the affected nails, which may show other nonspecific signs:[45]

• *Red streaks, longitudinal erytronychia:* These may be single or multiple and represent an early lesion which, with time, transforms into a white streak.

• *White streaks, longitudinal leukonychia:* These extend from the proximal nail fold to the distal margin, which may show a small incision and mild onycholysis due to a subungual hyperkeratotic papule. The width of the longitudinal white streak varies from 0.1 to a few millimeters.

Other signs of Darier's disease are not diagnostic and include: splinter hemorrhages, nail fissuring and fragility, severe nail bed hyperkeratosis, and keratotic papules of the proximal nail fold.

In some patients, the nails may be grossly thickened and deformed. Secondary bacterial infection of more severe cases is not unusual.

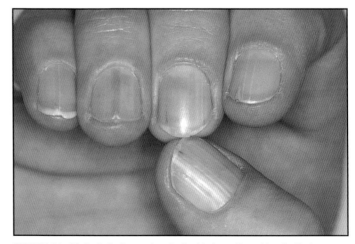

FIGURE 11–40. Darier's disease: Longitudinal leukonychia and longitudinal erytronychia.

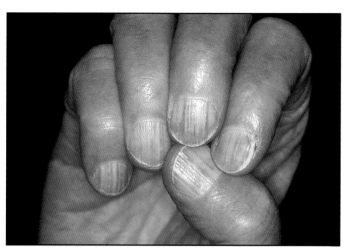

FIGURE 11-41. Darier's disease: Longitudinal red and white streaks with fissuring of the distal margin.

### Diagnostic signs

- Red longitudinal streaks (vasodilatation and nail bed epithelial hyperplasia)
- White longitudinal streaks (nail bed hyperplasia with multinucleated epithelial cells)
- Distal nail plate incision with subungual papules

### Nondiagnostic signs

- Splinter hemorrhages
- Nail fissuring and fragility
- Massive subungual hyperkeratosis
- Nail fold keratotic papules

## Differential Diagnosis

### Hailey–Hailey disease

Nail changes are similar to those of Darier's disease but the red streaks are not present.

### Nail bed fibrokeratoma

This produces a single red or white longitudinal streak with linear subungual hyperkeratosis.

### Subungual warts

These may spread to the nail bed from the hyponychium.

## Course

Nail lesions of Darier's disease can be worsened by traumas (Koebner phenomenon) and tend to become bacterially infected.

## Treatment

There is no effective treatment for nail lesions, which do not improve with systemic retinoids.

# HAILEY–HAILEY DISEASE

Asymptomatic longitudinal white bands are present in the fingernails of most patients and represent a helpful physical sign for the diagnosis.[45]

# PEMPHIGUS VULGARIS[46-48]

### Key Features

* Fingernails most commonly affected
* Erosive acute paronychia
* Pseudopyogenic granuloma of the nail folds may be the first symptom of a relapse

Nail involvement in pemphigus vulgaris occurs in up to 22% of patients and is almost always localized to the fingernails, especially the thumb and the index finger.

Erosive acute paronychia results from acantholysis of the proximal nail fold. It is often associated with hemorrhagic discoloration of the proximal nail fold with blood and serum fluid discharge. Pseudopyogenic granuloma of the proximal or lateral nail fold may be observed (Figs 11.42 and 11.43). It may be the first symptom of a relapse of the disease. Beau's lines and onychomadesis may follow acute paronychia.[49]

Other nonspecific nail abnormalities that have been reported in pemphigus include subungual hemorrhages and onycholysis, trachyonychia, subungual hyperkeratosis, nail plate yellow or brown discoloration, nail destruction.

Onychomycosis due to dermatophytes appears to be common in patients with pemphigus, probably as a consequence of therapeutic immunosuppression.

## Differential Diagnosis

*Paronychia with pyogenic granuloma of the proximal nail fold*

It follows cast immobilization after hand fractures and is usually limited to one finger. Patients complain of pain.[50]

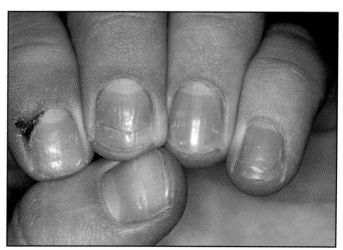

FIGURE 11-42. Pemphigus vulgaris: Erosive hemorrhagic paronychia and onychomadesis.

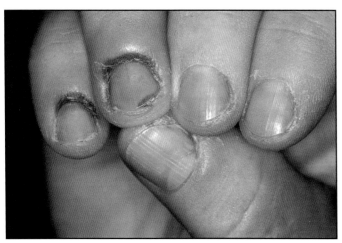

FIGURE 11-43. Pemphigus vulgaris: Hemorrhagic bullae of the nail fold and hyponychium.

Involvement of several nails may be a consequence of treatment with systemic retinoids, indinavir and epidermal growth factor receptor inhibitors.

Nail abnormalities improve with systemic treatment of the disease with no residual nail damage.

## BULLOUS PEMPHIGOID

Nail involvement is uncommon. Paronychia with pyogenic granulomas and hemorrhagic onycholysis results from blistering of the nail fold or the nail bed. Onychomadesis and nail destruction may occur with chronic nail bed erosions.[51]

## CICATRICIAL PEMPHIGOID

This may rarely cause scarring of the nail bed and nail matrix with pterygium formation and nail deformity (Fig. 11.44).

## ERYTHEMA MULTIFORME (STEVENS–JOHNSON SYNDROME)

Nail involvement results from localization of bullae in the nail matrix or nail bed. Nail matrix damage results in development of onychomadesis, Beau's lines and leukonychia striata. Several nails are usually affected at the same level.

Permanent anonychia of several nails may be a permanent sequela of Stevens–Johnson syndrome.

## TOXIC EPIDERMAL NECROLYSIS[52-54]

Onychomadesis and onycholysis are frequently observed during the acute phase of toxic epidermal necrolysis. Nail distrophies are a frequent dermatological sequela, occurring in 37.5% of patients. These include pterygium, anonychia and nail bed scarring.

Fingernail deformities are a common sequela (up to 30% of cases) of toxic epidermal necrolysis in children.

## PITYRIASIS LICHENOIDES CHRONICA

Nail involvement occurs in about one-third of patients. Periungual warty papules and patches are typically associated with severe hyperkeratosis of the cuticle.

## DISCOID LUPUS ERYTHEMATOSUS

Discoid lupus erythematosus may involve the periungual tissues with erythema, scaling, atrophy, and hypopigmentation. Nail fold capillary abnormalities similar to those observed in systemic lupus erythematosus may be observed. The cuticle frequently shows severe warty-like hyperkeratosis (Fig. 11.45). Nail matrix involvement is rare, and nail pterygium or scarring are exceptional.

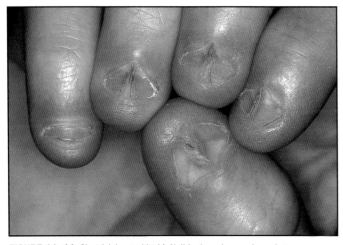

FIGURE 11-44. Cicatricial pemphigoid: Nail bed erosions and scarring.

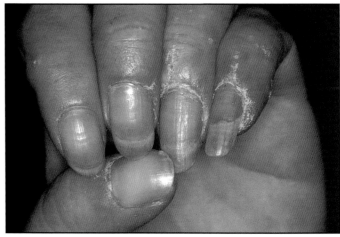

FIGURE 11-45. Discoid lupus erythematosus: Severe cuticle hyperkeratosis.

# REFERENCES

1. Ferràndiz C, Pujol RM, Garcia-Patos V et al. Psoriasis of early and late onset: a clinical and epidemiological study from Spain. J Am Acad Dermatol 2002; 46:867–873

2. Stuart P, Malick F, Nair RP et al. Analysis of phenotypical variation in psoriasis as a function of age at onset and family history. Arch Dermatol Res 2002; 294:207–213

3. Ruzicka T. Psoriatic arthritis. New types, new treatments. Arch Dermatol 1996; 132:215–219

4. Boiseau-Garsand AM, Beylot-Barry M, Doutr MS et al. Psoriatic onycho-pachydermo-periostitis. A variant of psoriatic distal interphalangeal arthritis. Arch Dermatol 1996; 132:176–180

5. Zaias N. Psoriasis of the nail. Arch Dermatol 1969; 99:567–579

6. Kaur I, Saraswatt A, Kumar B. Nail changes in psoriasis, a study of 167 patients. Int J Dermatol 2001; 40:601–603

7. Baran R. Retinoids and the nails. J Dermatol Treat 1990; 1:151–154

8. Rich P, Scher RK. Nail psoriasis severity index: a useful tool for evaluation of nail psoriasis. J Am Acad Dermatol 2003; 49:206–212

9. Gupta AK, Lynde CW, Sain HC et al. A higher prevalence of onychomycosis in psoriatics compared with non psoriatics: a multicentre study. Br J Dermatol 1997; 236:786–789

10. Grammer-West NY, Corvette DM, Giandoni MB et al. Nail plate biopsy for the diagnosis of psoriatic nails. J Am Acad Dermatol 1998; 38:260–262

11. Tosti A, Fanti PA, Morelli R et al. Psoriasiform acral dermatitis: report of 3 cases. Acta Derm Venereol 1992; 72:206–207

12. Patrizi A, Bardazzi F, Neri I et al. Psoriasiform acral dermatitis: a peculiar clinical presentation of psoriasis in children. Pediatr Dermatol 1999; 16:439–443

13. De Jong EM, Seegers BA, Gulnick MK et al. Psoriasis of the nails associated with disability in a large number of patients: results of a recent interview with 1728 patients. Dermatology 1996; 193:300–303

14. de Berker DAR. Management of nail psoriasis. Clin Exp Dermatol 2000; 25:357–362

15. Scher RK, Stiller M, Zhu YI. Tazarotene 0.1% gel in the treatment of fingernail psoriasis: a double-blind, randomized, vehicle-controlled study. Cutis. 2001; 68: 355–358

16. Tosti A, Piraccini BM, Cameli N et al. Calcipotriol ointment in nail psoriasis: a controlled double-blind comparison with betamethasone dipropionate and salicylic acid. Br J Dermatol. 1998; 139: 655–659

17. deBerker DAR, Lawrence CM. A simplified protocol of steroid injections for psoriatic nail dystrophy. Br J Dermatol 1998; 138:90–95

18. Piraccini BM, Fanti PA, Morelli R et al. Hallopeau's acrodermatitis continua of the nail apparatus: a clinical and pathological study of 20 patients. Acta Derm Venereol 1994; 74:65–66

19. Piraccini BM, Tosti A, Iorizzo M et al. Pustular psoriasis of the nails: treatment and follow-up of 46 patients. Br J Dermatol 2001; 144:1000–1005

20. Burden AD, Kemmet D. The spectrum of nail involvement in palmoplantar pustolosis. Br J Dermatol 1966; 134:1079–1082

21. Tosti A, Piraccini BM, Lorenzi S. Onychomycosis caused by non dermatophytic molds: clinical features and response to treatment of 59 cases. J Am Acad Dermatol 2000; 42:217–224

22. Sonnex TS, Dawber RP, Zachary CD et al. The nails in adult type I pityriasis rubra pilaris. A comparison with Sézary syndrome and psoriasis. J Am Acad Dermatol 1986; 15: 956–960

23. Tosti A, Misciali C, Piraccini BM et al. Woolly hair, palmo-plantar keratoderma and cardiac abnormalities: report of a family. Arch Dermatol 1994; 130:522–524

24. Tosti A, Morelli R, Fanti PA et al. Nail changes of punctate keratoderma: a clinical and pathological study of two patients. Acta Derm Venereol 1993; 73:66–68

25. Scher RK. Lichen planus of the nail. Dermatol Clin 1985; 3:395–399

26. Tosti A, Peluso AM, Fanti PA, Piraccini BM. Nail lichen planus: clinical and pathologic study of 24 patients. J Am Acad Dermatol 1993; 28: 724–730

27. Zaias N. The nail in lichen planus. Arch Dermatol 1970; 101:264–271

28. Ronchese F. Nail in lichen planus. Arch Dermatol 1965; 91:347–350

29. Tosti A, Piraccini BM, Cameli N. Nail changes in lichen planus may resemble those of yellow nail syndrome. Br J Dermatol 2000; 142:848–849

30. Tosti A, Piraccini BM, Fanti PA et al. Idiopathic atrophy of the nails: clinical and pathological study of 2 cases. Dermatology 1995; 190:116–118

31. Barth JH, Millard PR, Dawber RP. Idiopathic atrophy of the nails: a clinico-pathological study. Am J Dermatopathol 1988; 10:514–517

32. Suarez SM, Scher RK. Idiopathic atrophy of the nails: a possible hereditary association. Pediatr Dermatol 1990; 7:39–41

33. Juhlin L, Baran R. On longitudinal melanonychia after healing of lichen planus. Acta Derm Venereol (Stockh) 1990; 70:183

34. Palencia SI, Rodriguez-Peralto JL, Castano E et al. Lichenoid nail changes as sole external manifestation of graft versus host disease. Int J Dermatol 2002; 41:44–45

35. Fanti PA, Tosti A, Morelli R et al. Nail changes as the first sign of systemic amyloidosis. Dermatologica 1991; 183:44–46

36. Tosti A, Piraccini BM. Trachyonychia or twenty nail dystrophy. Curr Opin Dermatol 1996; 3:83–86

37. Tosti A, Peluso AM, Misciali C, Cameli N. Nail lichen striatus: clinical features and long-term follow up of 5 patients. J Am Acad Dermatol 1997; 36:908–913

38. Tosti A, Morelli R, Bardazzi F et al. Prevalence of nail abnormalities in children with alopecia areata. Pediatr Dermatol 1994; 11: 112–115

39. Tosti A, Fanti PA, Morelli R et al. Trachyonychia associated with alopecia areata: a clinical and pathologic study. J Am Acad Dermatol 1991; 25:266–270

40. Sharma WK, Dawn G, Muralidhar S et al. Nail changes in 1000 Indian patients with alopecia areata. J Eur Acad Dermatol Venereol 1998; 10:189–191

41. Dotz WI, Lieber CD, Wogt PJ. Leukonychia punctata and pitted nails in alopecia areata. Arch Dermatol 1985; 121:1452–1454

42. Bregner T, Donhauser G, Ruzicka T. Red lunulae in severe alopecia areata. Acta Derm Venereol 1992; 72: 203–205

43. Boico S, Kaufman RA, Luky AW. Osteomyelitis of the distal phalanges in 3 children with severe atopic dermatitis. Arch Dermatol 1988; 124:418–423

44. Tosti A, Guerra L, Morelli R et al. Role of foods in the pathogenesis of chronic paronychia. J Am Acad Dermatol 1992; 27:706–710

45. Zaias N, Ackerman AB. The nail in Darier–White disease. Arch Dermatol 1973; 107:193–199

46. Burge SM. Hailey-Hailey disease: the clinical features, response to treatment and prognosis. Br J Dermatol 1992; 126:275–282

47. Engineer L, Norton LA, Ahmed R. Nail involvement in pemphigus vulgaris. J Am Acad Dermatol 2000; 43:529–535

48. Kolivras A, Gheeraert P, Andre J. Nail destruction in pemphigus vulgaris. Dermatology 2003; 206:351–352

49. Schlesinger N, Katz M, Ingber A. Nail involvement in pemphigus vulgaris. Br J Dermatol 2002; 146:836

50. Zaias N (Editor). The nail in health and disease, 2nd edition. Norwalk: Appleton & Lounge, 1990:189–199

51. Tosti A, Piraccini BM, Camacho-Martinez F. Onychomadesis and pyogenic granuloma following cast immobilization. Arch Dermatol 2001; 137:231–232

52. Namba Y, Koizumi H, Kumakiri M et al. Bullous pemphigoid with permanent loss of the nails. Acta Derm Venereol 1999; 79:480–481

53. Magina S, Lisboa C, Leal V et al. Dermatological and ophtalmological sequels in toxic epidermal necrolysis. Dermatology 2003; 207:33–36

54. Sheridan RL, Weber JM, Schulz JT et al. Management of severe toxic epidermal necrolysis in children. J Burn Care Rehabil 1999; 20:497–500

# 12

# Onychomycosis

## Jenny O Sobera and Boni E Elewski

## Key Features

1. Onychomycosis is most commonly caused by dermatophytes, although *Candida* species and nondermatophyte molds may also cause disease
2. There are four patterns of fungal infection of the nail, each with distinct clinical manifestations
3. Diagnosis may be made by potassium hydroxide preparation, culture, and/or histologic examination
4. Systemic therapy is typically required to eradicate disease; however topical therapies may be useful in certain circumstances. Nondermatophyte molds are difficult to eradicate with any current therapies

The term 'onychomycosis' refers to fungal infection of one or more of the components of the nail unit and can be caused by dermatophytes, yeasts, or nondermatophyte molds. The term 'tinea unguium' is generally applied to dermatophytosis of the nail unit. There are four patterns of fungal invasion into the nail unit: distal lateral subungual onychomycosis (DLSO), white superficial onychomycosis (WSO), proximal subungual onychomycosis (PSO), and *Candida* onychomycosis. Each of these varieties has distinct clinical manifestations and may be caused by a different group of fungal organisms.

Onychomycosis is a challenging disease for patients and physicians, despite recent advances. Diagnosis remains difficult and often cumbersome, and treatment is still costly. While many have considered this disease a cosmetic problem, patients often complain of pain and discomfort and are often limited in their activities.

The exact prevalence of onychomycosis is unknown, but in one study it occurred in 13.8% of the population.[1] The prevalence is higher in patients with HIV, in whom it has been reported to be approximately 25%.[2] Studies in the UK,[3] Spain,[4] and Finland[5] found an overall prevalence of 3%, 1.7%, and 8.4%, respectively. It is probably the most common nail disorder, accounting for up to 50% of all nail diseases.

The incidence of onychomycosis has been rising sharply in the US and in other developed countries. Predisposing factors include increasing age, male gender, diabetes mellitus, immunosuppression, hyperhidrosis, poor peripheral circulation, trauma, and nail dystrophy.

Dermatophytes cause the majority of nail infections. In a large study by Summerbell and others[6] of 2662 nail-invading infective agents, dermatophytes were isolated in 91% of cases, *Candida albicans* in 5.5%, and various nondermatophyte molds in 3%. In a more recent study of 217 cases of onychomycosis, dermatophytes, nondermatophytes, and yeasts were cultured in approximately 60%, 20%, and 20% of cases, respectively.[1] Because the clinical manifestations may be identical, a fungal culture is essential in determining the infective agent. Not all patients with dystrophic nails have onychomycosis and a thorough understanding of the disease process is needed to establish the proper diagnosis and make informed decisions regarding therapy.

## TINEA UNGUIUM

It is not surprising that dermatophyte fungi are the most common cause of onychomycosis because they are keratinolytic pathogens and invade normal keratin of the skin, hair, and nail. Few other fungi have the ability to decompose native keratin. The most common dermatophyte nail pathogens are *Trichophyton rubrum* and *T. mentagrophytes*, which are also the most common causes of tinea pedis. *Epidermophyton floccosum*, *T. violaceum*, and miscellaneous *Microsporum* species account for a small percentage of cases. The various causative agents of tinea unguium are listed below:

- Dermatophyte fungi:
  - *Trichophyton rubrum*
  - *Trichophyton mentagrophytes*
  - *Epidermophyton floccosum*
- Nondermatophyte fungi:
  - *Acremonium*
  - *Aspergillus* species
  - *Cladosporium carrionii*
  - *Fusarium* species
  - *Onycochola canadensis*
  - *Scopulariopsis brevicaulis*
  - *Scytalidium dimidiatum*
  - *Scytalidium hyalinum*
- Yeasts:
  - *Candida albicans*

The one hand, two feet syndrome of onychomycosis is not uncommon. A retrospective study of 80 patients with this disorder revealed that the age at which symptoms first developed on the feet was 37.1 ± 2.4 years and 45.7 ± 2.2 years for the hands.[7] A traumatic event often preceded the appearance of the fungus in the nails. The hand involved was usually the one used to scratch the feet or pick the toenails. *T. rubrum* was the usual causative organism.

Toenails are about 25 times more likely than fingernails to be infected, and dermatophyte fingernail involvement rarely occurs without toenail involvement. Fingernails are more likely than toenails, however, to be infected with *Candida*.[8] The longest toe, either the first or the second, which bears the brunt of pressure and trauma from footwear, is particularly susceptible to invasion, although multiple nails are typically infected. Some authors believe that eliminating the instigating factor may often result in spontaneous resolution.[9] Approximately 30% of patients who have dermatophyte infections elsewhere on their bodies also acquire tinea unguium. Premenopausal females with no predisposing factors are less frequently affected than men of the same age group,[10] suggesting that estrogen may offer a protective effect. Although prepubertal children are rarely affected with this disease, possibly because of the protective element of faster nail growth in this age group, the prevalence is increasing.[11,12] Children with Down syndrome are particularly susceptible to infection. Numerous patients associate onset of disease with military service, especially those stationed for prolonged periods in hot, humid areas wearing heavy, occlusive footwear. Years of repeated trauma and impaired peripheral vascular supply are believed to account for an increased prevalence in the elderly.

## Distal Subungual Infection

The most common variety of onychomycosis, distal lateral subungual onychomycosis (DLSO), starts as an infection of the cornified layer of the hyponychium and distal or lateral nail bed (Fig. 12.1). It is best described as 'nail bed dermatophytosis', and is most commonly caused by *T. rubrum* and *T. mentagrophytes*. Proximal invasion of the nail bed and ventral invasion of the nail plate then occur. The first clinical signs of infection include the following: discrete, distal (or lateral) focus of onycholysis, yellow–brown discoloration, and hyperkeratosis of the nail bed. A mild inflammatory reaction occurs in the hyponychium and nail bed, resulting in further hyperkeratosis with accumulation of subungual debris, discoloration, and onycholysis. The nail bed becomes cornified and normal nail contour is lost. According to Zaias,[13] most cases begin with tinea pedis with subsequent invasion of the nail unit. Some authors speculate that this disorder may be autosomal dominant with incomplete penetration[14,15] but, because it is an infectious organism, it also might occur in families as a result of exposure to the pathogen rather than as a 'syndrome'. However, a 'hole' in the immune system might predispose certain individuals to infection, yet others develop disease due to environmental factors.

DLSO may progress to total dystrophic onychomycosis in which the entire nail plate and bed are involved. The dystrophic nail plate is retained as a residual stump at the proximal nail fold or is traumatically lost.

## White Superficial Onychomycosis (WSO; Leukonychia Trichophytica)

WSO (Fig. 12.2), a less common variety, is a distinctive pattern in which the nail plate is the primary site of invasion. The infection then proceeds to include the nail bed and hyponychium. It is most frequently seen in toenails and is primarily caused by *T. mentagrophytes*, which possesses enzymes that allow it to digest and invade the nail plate directly. *Microsporum persicolor* is an occasional etiologic agent, as is *C. albicans* in infants. WSO may also be caused by nondermatophyte molds, including *Aspergillus terreus*, *Fusarium oxysporum*, and *Acremonium* species. *T. rubrum* has been reported to present in this manner in children.[16]

The infection manifests as speckled or punctate porcelain-white lesions randomly distributed along the surface of the nail plate, gradually coalescing to involve the whole surface.[17] The nail plate becomes white and crumbly, with the consistency of plaster. The crumbled appearance can be used as a differentiating point from

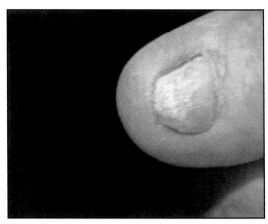

FIGURE 12–1. Distal subungual onychomycosis, *Trichophyton rubrum*, chronic; note keratinization of distal nail bed.

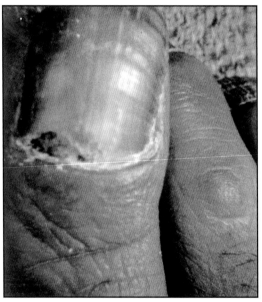

FIGURE 12–2. Proximal subungual onychomycosis, *Trichophyton rubrum*.

leukonychia. Older lesions may acquire a yellow hue. The morphology of the fungus in WSO is typically that of a saprophyte with modified hyphal elements (eroding fronds) as opposed to the usual parasitic hyphal forms seen in stratum corneum invasion.[13]

## Proximal Subungual Onychomycosis (PSO)

PSO (Fig. 12.3), a rarely seen pattern that affects fingernails and toenails equally, is primarily caused by *T. rubrum*; *T. mentagrophytes*, *T. schoenleinii*, *T. tonsurans*, and *T. megninii* have also been reported to cause the condition.[18] The fungus initially invades the stratum corneum of the proximal nail fold and subsequently penetrates the newly formed nail plate. The clinical result is a white discoloration under the proximal nail plate in the area of the lunula; the distal nail unit remains normal. As opposed to WSO, the nail plate is intact. Subungual hyperkeratosis, onychomadesis, and eventual destruction and shedding of the entire nail plate may occur in advanced disease. Because it is infrequent, some authors believe that a preceding episode of trauma is a prerequisite for it to occur in immunocompetent patients.[9]

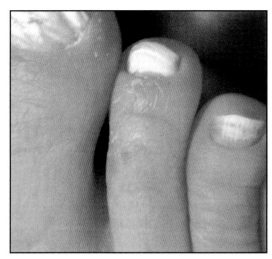

FIGURE 12–3. White superficial onychomycosis, *Trichophyton mentagrophytes*.

Proximal white subungual onychomycosis (PWSO) has been described with increasing frequency in patients with acquired immunodeficiency syndrome (AIDS). In fact, this rare form of onychomycosis was seldom encountered before AIDS became prevalent.[18] Toenail, rather than fingernail, involvement is more common and, unlike other instances of onychomycosis, concurrent tinea pedis is rare. In one study of 61 individuals with onychomycosis who were also infected with human immunodeficiency virus (HIV), 54 (87.1%) had PWSO.[18] *T. rubrum* is the most common pathogen. The explanation for the increased prevalence in this patient population remains unclear. PWSO may be the presenting sign of HIV infection and should prompt healthcare providers to obtain serologic tests for HIV infection in individuals at risk.

## *CANDIDA* INFECTIONS

*Candida albicans* is the etiologic agent in 70% of cases of onychomycosis caused by yeast (Fig. 12.4); *C. parapsilosis*, *C. tropicalis*, and *C. krusei* account for the remainder of cases.[19,20] *Candida* onychomycosis refers to a rare syndrome limited to patients afflicted with chronic mucocutaneous candidiasis. In this type of onychomycosis, the organism invades the nail plate directly. Both toenails and fingernails may be involved, and the full thickness of the nail can be affected. Nail bed thickening and yellow–brown

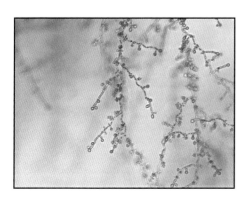

FIGURE 12-4. Cornmeal agar cut of *Candida albicans*. Courtesy of Judy Warner, UAB Fungal Reference Laboratory.

discoloration occur, as does swelling of the proximal and lateral nail folds, resulting in the characteristic 'drumstick' appearance of the digits.

*Candida* can also be a secondary pathogen in nails previously damaged by dermatophytes, trauma, or other skin diseases or in a setting of chronic paronychia. *Candida* infection is two to three times more common in women.[21] Seventy per cent of cases affect the hands, especially the middle finger, which may be infected from an intestinal or vaginal reservoir.[19] Recurrent infection of the nail matrix may result in transverse striations (Beau's lines) and nail plate dystrophy. Onycholysis and subungual hyperkeratosis may also occur, resulting in a clinical picture similar to that of distal subungual onychomycosis.

A third type of *Candida* infection – primary *Candida* onycholysis – may also occur. Whether this represents a distinct entity is open to debate. Some argue that *Candida* merely colonizes onycholytic nails, whereas others believe that *Candida* infection is the primary process.

Factors that predispose to *Candida* infection include immunosuppression, diabetes mellitus, hypoparathyroidism, thyroid disease, Addison's disease, malabsorption, malnutrition, malignancies, and intake of steroids, antibiotics, and antimitotic medications. Peripheral vascular disease, particularly Raynaud's disease, may also predispose an individual to *Candida* onycholysis.[22] Local factors include chemical or mechanical damage to the cuticle, frequent exposure to water, frequent contact with sugar-containing food items, hyperhidrosis, chilblains, and psoriatic onycholysis.

## OTHER FUNGAL INFECTIONS

Non-dermatophyte molds cause 1.5–6% of onychomycosis.[19,23] In the study by Summerbell and colleagues, non-dermatophyte molds constituted up to 3.3% of the organisms cultured from nail infections.[6] Only *Scytalidium dimidiatum*[24] and *S. hyalinum* have demonstrated the ability of keratinolysis, and there is presumptive evidence that *Scopulariopsis brevicaulis* also has an ability to invade keratin directly. Other nondermatophyte molds only invade nails that have altered keratin, secondary either to trauma or disease. An exception is the molds that cause WSO. *Onychocola canadensis* has also been reported to be associated with onychomycosis.[25] Onychomycosis secondary to nondermatophyte molds is seen most frequently in the elderly, in patients with skin diseases that affect the nails, and in immunocompromised patients. It is more frequent in toes than in fingers. Only one nail may be affected. Confinement in tight shoes, trauma from repeated pressure, and close contact between digits are believed to account for this.

Although several nondermatophyte molds have been reported to cause onychomycosis, *Scopulariopsis brevicaulis* is the most common.[6] Other pathogens include *Alternaria*, *Aspergillus*, *Acremonium*, *Fusarium*, *Scytalidium dimidiatum*, *Scytalidium hyalinum*, and *Cladosporium carrionii*.[6] *Fusarium oxysporon*, *Aspergillus terreus*, and *Acremonium roseogriseum* cause WSO, which may progress to total dystrophic onychomycosis. *S. dimidiatum*, a dematiaceous mold that occurs commonly in West Africa, the West Indies, and Southeast Asia, is distinctive in its ability to cause paronychia as well as infections that resemble classic tinea manuum and tinea pedis.[26] *S. hyalinum* may also cause a classic 'one hand, two feet' pattern of skin infection (Figs 12.5 and 12.6).

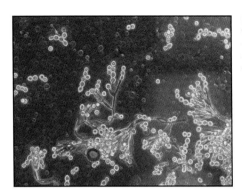

Figure 12-5. A Scotch tape preparation of *Scopulariopsis brevicaulis*. Courtesy of Judy Warner, UAB Fungal Reference Laboratory.

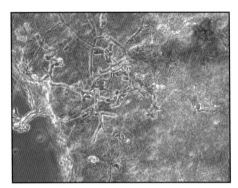

FIGURE 12-6. A preparation of *Scytalidium* species in nail material. Courtesy of Judy Warner, UAB Fungal Reference Laboratory.

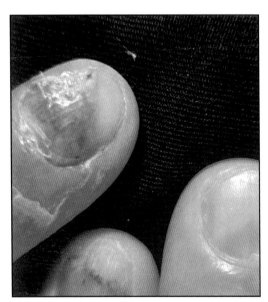

FIGURE 12-7. *Aspergillus niger.*

and a history of nonresponsiveness to systemic antimycotics (fluconazole, itraconazole, and terbinafine). Also, nondermatophyte molds are frequently associated with periungual inflammation.[27]

## LABORATORY DIAGNOSIS

### Collection of Specimens[20]

A stepwise approach to diagnosis is outlined in Fig. 12.8. The first step in diagnosis is obtaining an adequate specimen. In patients with distal subungual onychomycosis, the specimen should be obtained from the nail bed, which is the primary site of infection, ideally with a 1–2-mm serrated curette and as proximal as possible. Care must be taken to avoid penetration of the nail bed and

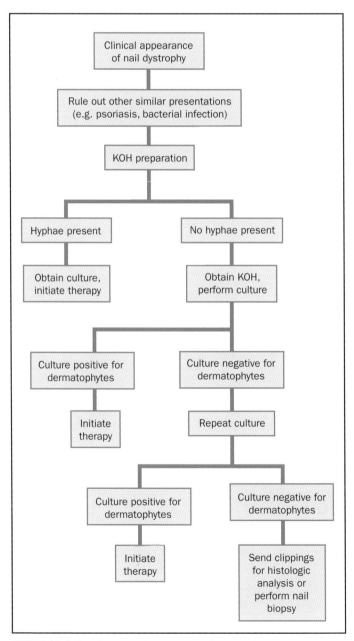

FIGURE 12-8. Stepwise approach to diagnosis. KOH, potassium hydroxide.

*Aspergillus* (Fig 12.7) is frequently cultured from the nails. In most instances, it is a saprophytic inhabitant rather than a pathogen and may impart a bluish-green tint to the involved nail structure, reminiscent of the discoloration caused by *Pseudomonas*.

Many of these fungi are highly sensitive to cycloheximide and may be missed if the specimen is not also inoculated on a cycloheximide-free medium, such as Sabouraud's glucose, Littman's Oxgall agar or potato dextrose agar. Clinical clues that a non-dermatophyte mold is the causative pathogen include the absence of tinea pedis (except in *S. brevicaulis* and *Scytalidium*[27]), only one or two infected toenails, a history of trauma before nail dystrophy,

bleeding. Scrapings from the undersurface of the nail should also be collected. It is important to obtain nail material from the advancing infected edge closest to the cuticle, where the likelihood of viable hyphae is the greatest. If nail bed debris is unavailable or insufficient, the affected nail plate can be sampled with special nail clippers. Nail clippings and portions of nails that have been avulsed are the least desirable specimens because they have a very low yield of viable hyphae and require special processing.[28,29]

In WSO, the fungi directly invade the nail plate surface. This infected nail debris can be removed with a no. 15 blade or sharp curette.

In PSO, the fungus invades under the cuticle and then settles in the proximal nail bed; the overlying nail plate is intact. To obtain culture material, the overlying healthy nail plate should be gently pared away with a no. 15 blade scalpel, and material from the proximal nail bed should be collected with a sharp curette.

The sampled material can be divided in two portions: one for direct microscopy and the remainder for culture. If nail material is to be used, fine shavings or minute clippings are preferred to large pieces. The old technique of pulverizing thick nail clippings in a nail micronizer is seldom used now and the authors do not recommend this procedure because of CLIA regulations and health concerns. The specimen should be obtained when the patient has been off both topical and systemic antifungal drugs for 2 to 4 weeks.[30] If the specimen is shipped to an outside laboratory, a sterile container (i.e. urine cup), a pill packet, a clean sheet of white paper folded and sealed with tape,[10] or a specially designed mailer such as a Dermapak™ can be used. Specimens should not be placed in broth, saline, or other moist media. Bacteria and fungal spores that may be contaminants can multiply quickly under such conditions, making it difficult to recover any pathogenic fungus. Ideally, nail specimens should be processed within a week, but infective fungal elements can remain viable for months after specimen collection.

## Direct Microscopy

Direct microscopy of potassium hydroxide (KOH) preparations is only a screening test for the presence or absence of fungi; it cannot identify pathogens. KOH dissolves keratin in nail material, leaving fungal elements intact. However, because large pieces of debris are often obtained in nail specimens, this procedure can be time consuming. The use of 15 to 20% KOH in dimethyl sulfoxide will hasten the process. The counterstain, chlorazol black E, which is highly specific for chitin, will selectively accentuate hyphae and is, therefore, particularly useful for nail specimens because fungal elements are typically scarce. Furthermore, it will not stain potential contaminants such as cotton or elastic fibers, which eliminates many false-positive findings.[31] Another counterstain is Parker's blue–black ink, but this is not chitin specific. Calcofluor white, a fluorescent dye that stains chitin in the fungal cell wall, can be used to enhance a standard KOH preparation (Figs 12.9 and 12.10). However, the use of this stain is not always practical in a clinical setting because a fluorescent microscope is required.[32,33] For best results, the microscope should be set on medium power (using the ×20 objective), and the light should be reduced. If direct microscopy is negative, and the KOH reagent used contains glycerol, the preparation may be left standing on the workbench overnight and re-examined the next day.[10] A Scotch tape preparation directly from a representative colony on the culture plate may also be utilized (Figs 12.11 to 12.14).

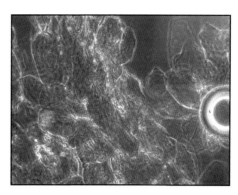

FIGURE 12–9. KOH preparation under white light. Courtesy of Judy Warner, UAB Fungal Reference Laboratory.

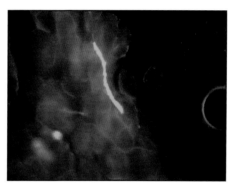

FIGURE 12–10. Same field as Fig. 12–9 but enhanced with Calcofluor white. Courtesy of Judy Warner, UAB Fungal Reference Laboratory.

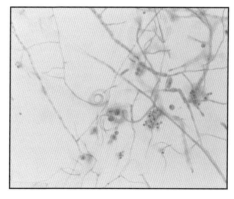

FIGURE 12–11. A Scotch tape preparation of *Trichophyton mentagrophytes*. Courtesy of Judy Warner, UAB Fungal Reference Laboratory.

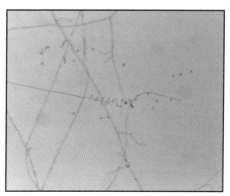

FIGURE 12–12. A Scotch tape preparation of *Trichophyton rubrum*. Courtesy of Judy Warner, UAB Fungal Reference Laboratory.

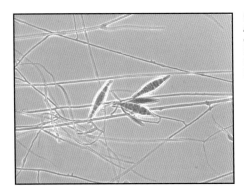

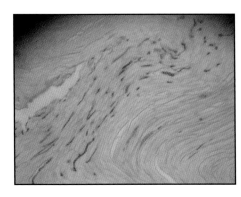

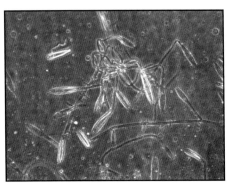

## Culture Techniques

Fungal culture is the only method that can identify the genus and species of the causative pathogen. Although most cases of onychomycosis are caused by dermatophytes, the occasional nondermatophyte fungus that requires treatment with a broader-spectrum antifungal needs to be ruled out before selecting appropriate treatment. Two types of media are needed for culturing nail specimens. One should contain cycloheximide, an antifungal agent that is added to agar to selectively isolate dermatophytes while inhibiting many saprophytic molds. Examples of media containing cycloheximide are dermatophyte test media (DTM), Mycosel (BBL), and Mycobiotic (DIFCO).[30] Sabouraud's glucose agar and potato dextrose agar are examples of agars that have no added cycloheximide and serve as the other type of media to ensure isolation of nondermatophyte nail pathogens that are sensitive to cycloheximide, such as *S. brevicaulis*, *S. dimidiatum*, and *S. hyalinum*[26], as well as the *Candida sp.* other than *Candida albicans*. The addition of antibiotics such as chloramphenicol and gentamicin to Sabouraud's glucose agar or potato dextrose agar is an additional precaution to eliminate bacterial contamination from nonsterile sites.[30] Ideally, the specimen should be cultured at 25–30°.

Although some molds may be recognized by their characteristic colonies, microscopic examination of isolates is usually required for precise identification. Microscopic morphology is studied by obtaining teased or Scotch tape preparations in lactophenol cotton blue.[10] Biochemical tests, which include *Trichophyton* agars, urea testing, and hair perforation tests, can also be useful in differentiating among various species of Trichophyton.

## Histopathology

If KOH preparation and fungal culture fail to yield a diagnosis, a large nail plate fragment can be sent in a 10% buffered formalin container for histologic analysis. Because special techniques may be required in processing specimens, it is helpful to inform the pathologist that nail material is enclosed and to request fungal stains, such as periodic acid-Schiff (PAS). PAS stains glycogen and mucoproteins in the fungal cell wall (Fig. 12.15). In one recent study, histologic analysis with PAS was found to be more sensitive than KOH preparation or culture alone (92% versus 80% or 59%, respectively), and PAS staining plus culture had the best sensitivity overall.[32,33] Another advantage of histopathologic evaluation with PAS is the short amount of time required to render a diagnosis compared to culture. The finding of hyphae and arthroconidia in a nail plate may permit differentiation from psoriasis, lichen planus, and other causes of nail dystrophy, but, like KOH, this preparation does not identify the particular pathogen. Nail biopsy is the last resort.

## STRATEGIES OF THERAPY

### Rx ❯ TREATMENT

- Treatment with systemic antifungals (typically of the azole and allylamine families) is required for eradication of disease.
- Topical therapy is not typically curative, but may provide palliative benefits or prophylaxis after systemic therapy.
- Systemic agents may be administered in continuous or pulsed doses.
- *Candida* onychomycosis requires treatment with an azole antifungal.
- Nondermatophyte molds do not generally respond well to systemic therapy and may require surgical therapy or debridement, followed by treatment with a topical agent.

Onychomycosis is a medical, not a surgical, problem; however, for decades, because there was no effective therapy, nail avulsion was commonly used for palliative purposes. Now, there are several antifungal agents available to treat this condition. In most instances, initial therapy consists of a systemic agent because topical antimycotics are generally ineffective as sole therapy due to their inability to penetrate the hyperkeratotic nail plate. Factors to consider when choosing therapy are:
- causative pathogen
- potential adverse events
- potential drug interactions (see Table 12.1)
- dosage schedule
- compliance of patient

**TABLE 12–1. Potential adverse events**

| DRUG | ADVERSE EVENT |
|------|---------------|
| Terbinafine | Nausea, gastrointestinal disturbance, taste disturbance (reversible on discontinuation of therapy), hepatic toxicity, leukopenia, rash |
| Itraconazole | Nausea, gastrointestinal disturbance, rash, pruritus, hypokalemia, reversible telogen effluvium, hepatotoxicity, congestive heart failure, drug–drug interactions (i.e. quinidine, pimozide, cisapride, statins, benzodiazapines, and others)[34] |
| Fluconazole | Nausea, gastrointestinal disturbance, rash, pruritus, thrombocytopenia, hepatotoxicity, reversible telogen effluvium, drug–drug interactions (i.e. cisapride, terfenadine, cimetidine, rifampin, HCTZ, and others) |

- cost of treatment regimen
- age and health of patient
- whether onychomycosis is present.

Determining the minimum inhibitory concentration of the cultured pathogen may also help narrow the choice, although that test is not routinely performed. Should patients not improve, consider incorrect dosage, poor patient compliance, drug interaction, and wrong diagnosis.

Remember to review the patient's needs and prospective compliance. The dosage schedule would be relatively important to a patient taking multiple medications, for example, who might prefer the convenience of a once-a-week dose of fluconazole, although this is not an FDA-approved therapy. Others might prefer to select the one-week-a-month regimen of itraconazole or a fixed 3-month course of either terbinafine or itraconazole. Also important to consider are the potential serious drug interactions that may occur with itraconazole (see Table 12.1). There are no significant drug interactions with terbinafine, and with once weekly dosing of fluconazole, the chance of an interaction is minimal.

Treating children with onychomycosis requires special consideration. Children should be carefully examined for tinea capitis and tinea pedis, and other causes of nail abnormalities should be ruled out (e.g. warts, psoriasis, chronic finger sucking, subungual hematoma). While there are no approved systemic therapies for onychomycosis in children, terbinafine, itraconazole, and fluconazole may be effective. Fluconazole is approved for use in children for other indications, and a liquid formulation is available, but it is not indicated for onychomycosis in the US. Itraconazole has been associated with abnormalities of tooth pulp in rats.[34] Terbinafine may be an excellent option, although tablets may need to be cut for younger children. Specific dosing regimens will be discussed below.[12]

# Dermatophyte Onychomycosis

## Systemic antifungals

Possible drug interactions should be kept in mind with all oral antifungals.

**TERBINAFINE** This is a member of the allylamine family of antifungals and is currently the only fungicidal oral antimycotic. It is broad spectrum and is effective against dermatophyte fungi, some nondermatophytes, and some species of *Candida*. It is the most potent antifungal agent in vitro against dermatophytes. Terbinafine is lipophilic and persists in the nail plate for several months after discontinuation. It is detected in the nail plate in 1 week, apparently delivered via the nail bed and matrix.

On the basis of pharmacokinetics, a 12-week course of 250 mg every day is generally effective in toenail disease; a 6-week course of the same dose is effective in fingernail disease. The US study had clinical success rates of 71% at 12 weeks and 77% at 24 weeks, and an overall clinical success rate of 74%.[35] Most patients require 3 months of therapy but patients with severe disease may need 4 or more months to cure the infection. In children, the treatment duration is the same, and the dose may be calculated as follows: Children less than 20 kg, 62.5 mg/day ($\frac{1}{4}$ tablet); children 20 to 40 kg, 125 mg/day ($\frac{1}{2}$ tablet); and children over 40 kg, 250 mg/day (1 tablet).[12] As anticipated, the nail is not clinically normal when the drug is discontinued. Although hepatotoxic reactions are rare, baseline assessment of hepatic parameters is reasonable (see Table 12.1). This drug has no significant drug interactions, and can be co-administered with statins, digoxin, coumadin and most other commonly used drugs. However, because terbinafine is known to be a potent inhibitor of CYP2D6, clinicians should be aware of potential drug–drug interactions.[36]

**ITRACONAZOLE** This is a member of the azole family of antifungal agents. Effective against dermatophytes, *Candida*, and some nondermatophyte molds, itraconazole has a broad spectrum of activity. Additionally, the pharmacokinetics in the nail show that itraconazole is detected in the nail plate within 7 days of administration, penetrating the nail bed and matrix and persisting in the nail plate for 6 to 9 months after therapy is discontinued.[37] This is probably related to its lipophilic property, causing the drug to adhere to the lipophilic cytoplasm of the keratinocytes in the nail plate.

Two schedules have been investigated: the fixed (continuous)[38] and the pulse or intermittent. The fixed dosage is 200 mg daily for 12 weeks in pedal onychomycosis or for 6 weeks in fingernail disease. The US study's results for toenail onychomycosis showed a mycologic cure rate of 54%, a clinical success rate of 65%, and an overall success rate of 35% (clinical success and mycologic cure). In children, the dosage is 5 mg/kg/day for 1 week/month (as pulse treatment). The treatment duration is the same as the adult regimen.[12] It is important to emphasize to the patient that, as is true with terbinafine, when therapy is discontinued the nail is not normal. Because of the persistence of itraconazole in the nail plate, however, the nail grows out fungus free. The pulse or intermittent regimen is based on the rationale that the drug reaches the nail within 7 days of therapy and persists in the nail for 6 to 9 months, whereas serum levels are not detectable 1 week after discontinuation. Two pulse doses have been FDA approved for fingernail onychomycosis.[39] Intermittent cycles of 400 mg daily for 1 week per month can be continued for 2 months when treating fingernails and for 3 months for toenail infection. Like the fixed dosage, the nail is not normal when therapy is discontinued. Itraconazole should be given with food. Baseline and periodic monitoring of hepatic parameters is not unreasonable, especially in patients with a history of liver function abnormality or in those expected to use the drug for longer than one month of daily usage.

Rare postmarketing reports have implicated itraconazole in either contributing to or causing congestive heart failure[40] (see Table 12.1).

**FLUCONAZOLE** This is a biz-triazole and has activity against dermatophytes, *Candida*, and some nondermatophyte fungi. Fluconazole has an oral bioavailability of about 90% and a half-life of 20–50 hours.[41] The drug reaches the nail plate via the nail bed, and there is evidence it persists in the nail for several months.[42] A 'pulse' or intermittent regimen reported to be effective is 150 mg administered once a week until the nail has grown out. In those patients not responding, the dose can be increased to 300 or 450 mg once per week. Patients on multiple medications may enjoy the freedom of the 1-day-per-week dosage. Assaf and Elewski[43] evaluated 11 patients with onychomycosis of the fingernail or toenail, with a total of 43 infected nails. *Trichophyton rubrum* was the predominant organism cultured, although two patients with fingernail infections had *C. albicans*. Eight patients received fluconazole 300 mg once weekly, 1 patient received 200 mg once weekly (a child), and two patients received an alternate-day dosage of 100 to 200 mg. Eight of the patients also used an adjunctive topical antimycotic preparation. All six patients, with 32 toenails involved, were clinically cured after a mean duration of 6 months, and five patients, with 11 fingernails involved, were cured after 3.7 months. No clinical or laboratory adverse events were recorded. One of these patients had previously experienced a morbilliform eruption while on itraconazole but was successfully treated with fluconazole without a similar problem.

In a large study by Scher and coworkers, treatment of toenail onychomycosis with fluconazole yielded greater than 86% clinical success with a low relapse rate at dose schedules of 150 mg, 300 mg, and 400 mg once weekly for a mean period of 6 to 7 months.[44] In a similar study by Drake and others evaluating fingernail onychomycosis, 100% of patients receiving 450 mg once weekly for 6 months achieved clinical success (91% and 97% achieved clinical success at doses of 150 mg and 300 mg once weekly, respectively).[45] All three doses were well tolerated by patients in both studies. Based on limited data, children should receive 6 mg/kg once weekly.[12]

Fluconazole can be administered with or without food and without regard to gastric acidity. The drug is well tolerated, and instances of hepatotoxicity are rare. Laboratory monitoring is controversial, but baseline testing of hepatic and hematopoietic functions may be indicated for those planning to be on long-term therapy. Several drugs may cause interactions and are contraindicated with use of fluconazole (see Table 12.1).

**GRISEOFULVIN** Of the available oral antimycotics, griseofulvin is the least effective in onychomycosis. Its spectrum of action includes only dermatophyte fungi, with no activity on *Candida* or other nondermatophyte fungi. Griseofulvin must be administered daily until the infected nail plate grows out, which is generally 6 to 9 months for fingernails and 12 to 18 months for toenails. Griseofulvin is delivered to the nail plate via the matrix, but the pharmacokinetics of the drug have not been well studied. This fungistatic medication does not persist in the nail plate more than 1 to 2 weeks, which explains the long duration of therapy.[37] The ultra-micro-size form is best suited for onychomycosis, and most patients require 1000–2000 mg daily in divided doses to eradicate the infection. Both underdosing and patient compliance are common reasons for failure.

Laboratory monitoring during griseofulvin therapy is controversial but periodic monitoring of hematopoietic and hepatic functions is reasonable, especially when long-term therapy is planned. Griseofulvin is contraindicated in pregnancy, lupus erythematosus, hepatocellular failure, and acute intermittent porphyria. Additionally, the drug may interfere with oral contraceptives and cause fetal abnormalities (particularly conjoint twins). Appropriate precautions are, therefore, necessary in women of childbearing potential. Long-term regimens are frequently accompanied by minor annoyances such as gastrointestinal disturbances and headaches, causing patients to discontinue therapy prematurely and resulting in treatment failure. Patients on warfarin-type anticoagulants and barbiturates will require dose adjustments.[41] Cure rates are low and recurrence rates are high.

**KETOCONAZOLE** The first broad-spectrum oral antifungal and first oral azole, ketoconazole has activity not only against dermatophyte fungi but also *Candida* and some nondermatophytes. The potential risk of hepatotoxicity has limited the use of ketoconazole in onychomycosis.

**TOPICAL THERAPIES** Topical therapy has the greatest potential as primary therapy in mild infections, as palliative therapy in those unable to take oral therapy, and as a prophylactic agent. Eight per cent ciclopirox lacquer has been approved for use in onychomycosis. In the US studies, treatment cure (clinically clear and negative mycology) was achieved in 5.5 to 8.5%, whereas mycologic cure alone was achieved in 29 to 36%.[46] Although not approved for this indication, another promising topical agent is 40% urea gel, used alone or in combination with another topical antifungal. A recent study has shown increased mycological cure rates in patients treated with 8% ciclopirox lacquer plus 40% urea gel compared to treatment with the antifungal lacquer alone. This is likely due to the ability of the urea to chemically debride the hyperkeratotic nail plate, allowing better penetration of the antifungal. Avulsion of the nail combined with a topical antifungal agent under occlusion may be effective in select patients. However, because of the inherent problems of nail avulsion, this is best limited to those with only one or two dystrophic nails and those intolerant of oral antifungals.

## Nondermatophyte Mold Onychomycosis

Nondermatophyte molds seldom cause onychomycosis (see Table 12.1). In general, when a nondermatophyte mold is determined to be the pathogen, successful treatment is difficult and technically impossible to acheive. Surgical treatment or debridement followed by application of a topical antifungal may benefit some select patients. *S. dimidiatum* and *S. hyalinum* have not responded to systemic treatment, topical therapy or nail avulsion. In one report, however, amorolfine lacquer (not available in the US) was successful.[27] When *Scopulariopsis* species are cultured, they are frequently contaminants. However, they also can function as a pathogen, and some infections have responded to itraconazole and terbenafine. Addition of an antifungal lacquer has increased cure rates by 25%.[27]

Onychomycosis caused by *Fusarium* is very difficult to treat. Systemic antifungals are effective in only about one-third of cases, and nail avulsion is typically unsuccessful.[27]

*Aspergillus terreus* can cause WSO. The treatment of WSO is curettage or debridement of the dystrophic superficial nail plate followed by application of a topical antifungal. Terbinafine and itraconazole have been used with very good results.[27] However, when the infection has progressed to total dystrophic onychomycosis, treatment is difficult. In these instances, surgical debridement or avulsion may be beneficial in select patients.

## Candida 'Onychomycosis'

*Candida albicans* is the most common species of *Candida* that can secondarily cause or exacerbate nail disease. When other species of *Candida* are isolated, they are generally saprophytes and not pathogenic. If *C. albicans* is determined to be the pathogen,[47] an oral azole such as fluconazole would be appropriate, at a dosage of 150–200 mg once per week until resolved. Antifungal lacquers have been shown to increase the efficacy of systemic therapies.[27] Griseofulvin and terbinafine are ineffective. *Candida* has also been implicated in onycholysis and paronychia infections.[20] Many believe *Candida* paronychia represents an environmental condition exacerbated by irritants and allergens and should be treated as such with barrier creams and topical steroids.[27]

## REFERENCES

1. Ghannoum MA, et al. A large-scale North American study of fungal isolates from nails: The frequency of onychomycosis, fungal distribution, and antifungal susceptibility patterns. J Am Acad Dermatol 2000; 43(4):641–648
2. Tosti A, Piraccini BM. Nail disorders. In: Bolognia JL, Jorizzo JL, Rapini RP, et al, eds. Dermatology. London: Mosby; 2003:1061–1078
3. Roberts DT. Prevalence of dermatophyte onychomycosis in the United Kingdom: results of an omnibus survey. Br J Dermatol 1992; 126(Suppl 39):23
4. Sais G, Juggla A, Peyri J. Prevalence of dermatophyte onychomycosis in Spain: a cross-sectional study. Br J Dermatol 1995; 132:758
5. Heikkila H, Stubb S. The prevalence of onychomycosis in Finland. Br J Dermatol 1995; 133:699
6. Summerbell RC, Kane J, Kradjden S. Onychomycosis, tinea pedis and tinea mannum caused by non-dermatophyte filamentous fungi. Mycoses 1989; 32:609
7. Daniel CR, et al. Two feet-one hand syndrome – a retrospective multicentre serving. Int J Dermatol 1997; 36 (9):658–660
8. Gupta AK, et al. Prevalence and epidemiology of onychomycosis in patients visiting physicians' offices: A multicenter Canadian survey of 15,000 patients. J Am Acad Dermatol 2000; 43 (2):244–248
9. Cohen JL, Scher RK, Pappert AS. The nail and fungus infections. In: Elewski BE, ed. Cutaneous fungal infections. New York: Igaku-Shoin; 1992:106–123
10. Haley L, Daniel RC III. Fungal infections. In: Scher RK, Daniel CR III, eds. Nails: therapy, diagnosis, surgery. Philadelphia: WB Saunders; 1990:106–119
11. Martin AG, Kobayashi GS. Fungal diseases with cutaneous involvement. In: Fitzpatrick TB, Eisen AZ, Wolff K, et al, eds. Dermatology in general medicine, vol 2. New York: McGraw-Hill; 1993:2421–2451
12. Tosti A, Piraccini BM, Iorizzo M. Management of onychomycosis in children. Dermatol Clin 2003; 21 (3):507–509
13. Zaias N. Onychomycosis. Dermatol Clin 1985; 3:445
14. Zias N, Tosti A, Rebell G, et al. Autosomal dominant pattern of distal subungual onychomycosis caused by *Trichophyton rubrum*. J Am Acad Dermatol 1996; 34:302
15. Daniel CM, Daniel MP, Daniel CR. Onychomycosis update. J Miss State Med Assoc 1995; 36:37
16. Ploysangam T, Lucky AW. Childhood white superficial onychomycosis caused by *Trichphyton rubrum*: Report of seven cases and review of the literature. J Am Acad Dermatol 1997; 36 (1):29–32
17. Norton LA. Disorders of the nail. In: Moschella SL, Hurley HJ, eds. Dermatology. Philadelphia: WB Saunders; 1992:1563–1585
18. Elewski BE. Clinical pearl: proximal white subungual onychomycosis in AIDS. J Am Acad Dermatol 1993; 29:631
19. Andre J, Achten G. Onychomycosis. Int J Dermatol 1987; 26:481
20. Daniel CR III. The diagnosis of nail fungal infection. Arch Dermatol 1991; 127:1566
21. Achten G, Wanet-Rouard J. Onychomycosis in the laboratory. Mykosen 1978; 14 (suppl):125
22. Hay RJ, et al. Candida onychomycosis – an evaluation of the role of *Candida* species in nail disease. Br J Dermatol 1988; 118 (1):47–58
23. Greer DL. Evolving role of nondermatophytes in onychomycosis. Int J Dermatol 1995; 34:521
24. Elewski BE. Onchomycosis caused by *Scytalidium dimidiatum*. J Am Acad Dermatol 1996; 35:336
25. Gupta AK, Horgen-Bell J, Summerbell R. Onychocola canadensis: Two cases with toenail onchomycosis and a review of the literature. Poster presentation, International summit on cutaneous antifungal therapy. Vancouver, British Columbia. 26–28 May 1996
26. Elewski BE, Greer DL. *Hendersonulea toruloidea* and *Scytalidium hyalinum*. Arch Dermatol 1991; 127:1041
27. Tosti A, et al. Treatment of nondermatophyte mold and *Candida* onychomycosis. Dermatol Clin 2003; 21 (3):491–497
28. Daniel CR. Nail micronizer. Cutis 1985; 36:118
29. Daniel CR, Elewski BE, Gupta AK. Surgical pearl: nail micronizer. J Am Acad Dermatol 1996; 34:278
30. Elewski BE. Clinical pearl: diagnosis of onychomycosis. J Am Acad Dermatol 1995; 32:500
31. Burke WA, Jones BE. A simple stain for rapid office diagnosis of fungal infections of the skin. Arch Dermatol 1984; 120:1519
32. Mahoney JM, Bennett J, Olsen B. The diagnosis of onychomycosis. Dermatol Clin 2003; 21 (3):463–467
33. Weinberg, et al. Comparison of diagnostic methods in the evaluation of onychomycosis. J Am Acad Dermatol 2003; 49 (2):193–197.
34. Physicians' Desk Reference, 2003
35. Gupta AK, Sauder DN, Shear NH. Antifungal agents: An overview. Part II. J Am Acad Dermatol 1994; 30:911
36. Shapiro LE, Shear NH. Drug interactions: proteins, pumps, and P-450s. J Am Acad Dermatol 2002; 47 (4):467–484
37. Elewski BE. Mechanism of action of systemic antifungal agents. J Am Acad Dermatol 1993; 28S:28
38. Odom R, Daniel CR, Aly R. A double-blind, randomized comparison of itraconazole capsules and placebo in the treatment of onchomycosis of the toenail. J Am Acad Dermatol 1996; 35:110
39. Odom RB, Devillez R, Daniel CR, et al. A multicentre placebo-controlled double blind study of intermittent therapy with itraconazole capsules for the treatment of onychomycosis of the fingernail. J Am Acad Dermatol 1996; 35:110
40. Ahmad SR, Singer SJ, Leissa BG. Congestive heart failure associated with itraconazole. Lancet 2001; 357 (9270):1766–1767
41. Gupta AK, Ryder JE. The use of oral antifungal agents to treat onychomycosis. Dermatol Clin 2003; 21 (3):469–479
42. Montero-Gei F, Robles-Soto M, Schlager H. Fluconazole in the treatment of severe onchomycosis. Int J Dermatol 1996; 35:587
43. Assaf RR, Elewski BE. Intermittent fluconazole dosing in patients with onychomycosis: results of a pilot study. J Am Acad Dermatol 1996; 35:216
44. Scher RK, et al. Once-weekly fluconazole (150, 300, or 450 mg) in the treatment of distal subungual onychomycosis of the toenail. J Am Acad Dermatol 1998; 38(6 Pt 2):S77–S86
45. Drake L, et al. Once-weekly fluconazole (150, 300, or 450 mg) in the treatment of distal subungual onychomycosis of the fingernail. J Am Acad Dermatol 1998; 38(6 Pt 2): S87–S94
46. Gupta AK, Fleckman P, Baran R. Ciclopirox nail lacquer: the first prescription topical therapy for onychomycosis. J Am Acad Dermatol 2000; 43:[4]S70–S80
47. Daniel CR, Elewski BE. *Candida* as a nail pathogen in healthy patients. J Miss State Med Assoc 1995; 36:379

# 13

# Podiatric Approach to Onychomycosis

## Warren S Joseph and John D Mozena

Since the beginnings of the profession of podiatric medicine, toenail pathology has been of primary importance. In 1970 Krausz, reporting on nearly 30 years experience and almost 11,000 patients, found that 61% of patients' presenting complaints was for nail pathology.[1] Early podiatrists, then known as chiropodists, were fairly limited in their scope of practice. Emphasis was placed on the treatment of hyperkeratotic lesions and dystrophic or ingrown nails. Treatment of these conditions was primarily local, including debridement and accommodative padding. Surgical therapy, including the use of local anesthetics, and systemic medical therapy were outside the scope of practice of these early pioneers. As the profession evolved and became more sophisticated, so did many of the approaches to different lower extremity pathologies. Surgical therapies were more commonly used. The pharmacopoeia for podiatric physicians increased dramatically. However, although the scientific training and knowledge is now on a par with the rest of the medical community, old traditions still die hard. The roots of the profession continue to be taught to this day. Local, hands-on mechanical therapy is still a mainstay for the treatment of nails and keratotic lesions. However, with the development and release of safer, more effective oral antifungal agents and, more recently, a Food and Drug Administration (FDA) approved topical antifungal medication, there is renewed interest and excitement in the exploration of new therapies for onychomycosis.

The causes and pathophysiology of onychomycosis are covered elsewhere in this book. The purpose of this chapter is to illustrate the way in which podiatric physicians approach the diagnosis and therapy of onychomycosis. It will cover:

- patient demographics
- historic issues
- debridement therapies
- surgical therapies
- medical therapies.

## PODIATRY VERSUS DERMATOLOGY

The two specialty groups most interested in the treatment of onychomycosis are podiatry and dermatology. Although the condition is seen by many general family practitioners, there seems to be only minimal interest in the importance of this condition to the vast majority in other specialties. Much of the literature published on the topic of systemic therapy for onychomycosis has appeared in the dermatologic and mycologic literature. However, most of the work on the local, surgical, and cosmetic aspects of treatment has been performed by podiatrists.

Podiatry may, in fact, see more patients presenting with onychomycosis than does the dermatology community. Sheer numbers alone could account for this dichotomy. The American Podiatric Medical Association quotes 13,000 actively practicing podiatrists in the USA. This compares to the worldwide figure of 14,000 fellows and members of the American Academy of Dermatology (as of 2004). According to the National Center for Health Statistics' National Health Interview Survey, the prevalence of toenail problems in the United States was 46 per 1000 people. It is estimated that 35 million Americans suffer from onychomycosis yet only 6.3 million have actually been diagnosed. Of those patients complaining of toenail problems who sought professional care, 70% presented to a podiatrist. In fact, onychomycosis is the number one diagnosed and treated disease in podiatry.[2,3]

## PATIENT DEMOGRAPHICS AND CONCERNS

The greatest difference between the two specialties and their respective approaches to onychomycosis can be traced to patient populations. Podiatrists have traditionally concentrated their efforts toward nail complaints in the older population. These patients generally complain of pain as a sequela of their thickened, dystrophic toenails. They are not as concerned about the cosmetic nature of the problem or some of the psychosocial stigmas that have been applied to this disease in younger patients. Furthermore, these patients may have significant underlying conditions and risk factors that make this frequently benign condition life- and limb-threatening:

- diabetes
- vascular disease
- degenerative arthritis
- loss of visual acuity
- immune deficiencies
- polypharmacy
- chronic disease.

For this reason, the Health Care Financing Association has recognized toenail onychomycosis as a condition that may require professional care among the Medicare population. To be covered under Medicare, patients with onychomycosis must meet strict evidential criteria to prove the significance of the disease. Although regulations may differ somewhat among States, the criteria established by Pennsylvania Blue Shield, the Medicare carrier for a number of Eastern States, are paraphrased in Table 13.1.

Fungal nail infections represent 23.9% of the conditions podiatrists see. Despite having to satisfy these strict criteria for coverage of onychomycosis, podiatrists provided more than 8.3 million qualified services by 15,500 podiatrists to Medicare patients in 2000. Past statistics showed 70% of patients were

TABLE 13-1. Medicare guidelines and the systemic conditions for which onychomycosis care is covered

| MEDICARE GUIDELINES TO COVER ONYCHOMYCOSIS | SYSTEMIC CONDITIONS FOR WHICH ONYCHOMYCOSIS CARE IS COVERED |
|---|---|
| Clinical evidence of mycosis<br>Marked limitation of ambulation<br>Pain or secondary infection caused by the thickening<br>Debridement of mycotic nails is covered if there is a systemic condition that would pose a hazard if treatment was administered by a nonprofessional | Arteriosclerosis obliterans<br>Buerger's disease<br>Thrombophlebitis<br>Peripheral neuropathy secondary to:<br>• malnutrition<br>• cancer<br>• diabetes<br>• multiple sclerosis |

75 years of age or older, and a full 29% were 85 years of age or older. These numbers indicate the potential for serious sequelae of this condition in this population.[4]

# DIABETES MELLITUS AND ONYCHOMYCOSIS

By far the most significant risk factor for severe complications in patients with onychomycosis is diabetes mellitus. The skin of the diabetic patient is similar to geriatric skin. Loss of pliability secondary to increased collagen cross-linking may predispose the tissue to ulceration. Patients with diabetes frequently present with the triad of neuropathy, angiopathy, and immunopathy. Of these, the former is the most significant. Neuropathy may present as sensory, motor, or autonomic. Because of the sensory neuropathy, the patient may be unaware of the thickness or length of the toenail until the nail has damaged adjacent skin, potentiating a deep infection (Fig. 13.1). Furthermore, the patient with diabetic neuropathy tends to wear shoes that are too tight. Because the patient has lost the ability to feel the presence of the shoe on the foot, he or she will try on shoes until they are tight enough to give the expected sensation. Combining a thickened, dystrophic, mycotic nail with a neuropathic nail bed placed into a shoe a few sizes too small potentially leads to subungual ulcerations of the nail bed (Fig. 13.2). Statistics show that one-third of ulcers occur on the hallux and that 12% are caused by nail trauma.[5] Given the minimal amount of tissue present between the nail bed and the distal phalanx, osteomyelitis is a frequent result. In fact, it has been shown that there is an increased incidence of ulcers, gangrene, and infections in patients with onychomycosis and diabetes versus those patients with diabetes and no onychomycosis.[6]

Even plantar ulcerations of the hallux may be traced to the combination of a neuropathic foot, a thickened nail, and a tight shoe. Excessive pressure from the shoe onto the top of the toe may cause increased plantar pressure, leading to ulceration (Fig. 13.3).

Another risk factor found in patients with and without diabetes is peripheral vascular disease. With poor perfusion to the digits, ulcerations and wounds heal with difficulty. Thirty per cent of diabetics have onychomycosis and 15% develop ulcers. Of these,

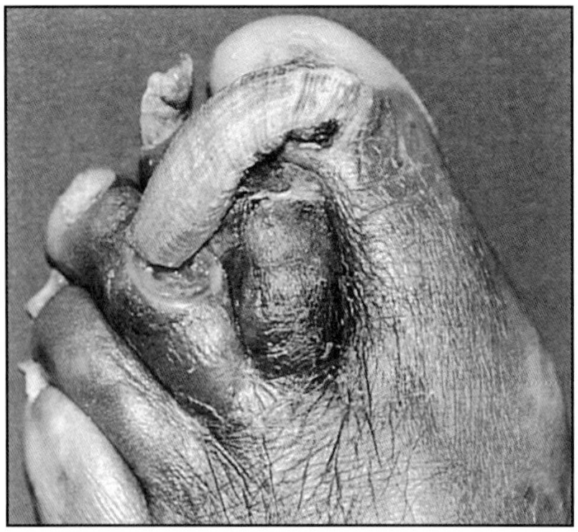

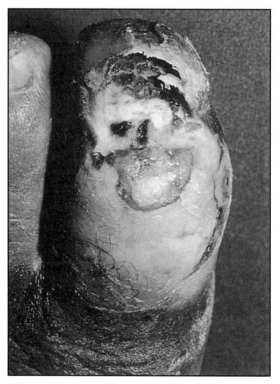

FIGURE 13-1. Ulceration of the third toe caused by an elongated mycotic toenail in a patient with diabetic peripheral neuropathy.

FIGURE 13-2. Neuropathic ulceration of the hallux toenail bed caused by pressure from the thickened mycotic toenail.

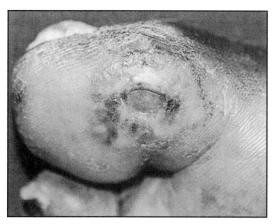

FIGURE 13-3. Plantar malperforans ulceration in a patient with diabetic neuropathy. Excessive dorsal shoe pressure on the thickened toenail may increase pressure on the plantar aspect of the toe, predisposing the patient to this type of ulcer.

20% go on to amputations and 35% of those demonstrate a 5-year mortality rate. If the patient attempts self-care and accidentally causes a laceration, this may progress to secondary infection, frank ischemia, and gangrene.[7]

## HISTORIC ISSUES

As mentioned, podiatric medicine has focused on diseases of the toenail since the beginnings of the profession. Although this history lends a rich tradition to the local and surgical approaches that the specialty brings to the therapy of nail conditions, in the area of systemic therapy for onychomycosis the profession has only really become involved since the release of the newer oral anti-fungals and the aggressive marketing campaigns that accompanied them. Reasons for this may include the following:

1. The importance of the disease. Although known to be a major potential problem in the patients with the risk factors described previously, is the disease important for otherwise healthy patients? The toenails look unsightly, but is this only a cosmetic situation? Through the quality-of-life work originally performed by Lubeck and colleagues,[8] and more recently by Drake, Scher,[9] and others, it is now documented that a great number of these patients suffered with pain, missed days of work, and were subject to social castigation. In their article, Lubeck and coworkers concluded that 'persons with onychomycosis also had significantly poorer ratings for mental health, social functioning, health concerns, physical appearance and functional limitations associated with activities involving standing on one's feet'. Before these studies, this was mostly anecdotal knowledge.

2. Impossibility of a cure. Even if this disease was thought to be a true issue for the patient, there was little effective therapy. Although it could perhaps be controlled with local nail care and topical medication, results were less than spectacular. Patient dissatisfaction was high, as was physician frustration. All podiatrists have either heard a patient say or have muttered to themselves, 'If only you (I) could find a cure for this, you'd (I'd) make a fortune!'

3. Distrust of griseofulvin. Even if systemic therapy was contemplated, what choices were there? Closely related to point 2 is the concern instilled in podiatrists that griseofulvin is a dangerous, ineffective drug. Before the introduction of the newer antifungals, only griseofulvin was approved by the FDA. There is a pervasive feeling throughout much of the podiatric profession that the hepatic and leukocyte toxicities of this agent, combined with a less than stellar success rate, render the only previously available choice as moot.

For these reasons, podiatric medicine has relied on its roots of local mechanical, chemical, and surgical therapy for the treatment of onychomycosis. Only recently, with the introduction of terbinafine, itraconazole, and topical ciclopirox 8%, is effective, safe systemic and topical therapy being used and the old paradigm has changed somewhat.

## DEBRIDEMENT THERAPY

The mainstay of the podiatric approach to onychomycosis is the physical debridement of the dystrophic nail through manual, electric, and chemical means. The goal of this debridement therapy is to reduce the length and thickness of the nail significantly. Although not a cure for the condition, an aggressive debridement can render the patient pain free, reduce the risk for pressure-related sequelae, debulk the nail thereby reducing fungal load, and make the nail more aesthetically pleasing. Removing the hypertrophied nail plate also facilitates the penetration of topical antifungals on the nail bed. Furthermore, the treatment is noninvasive and, therefore, safe for all patients, including those with advanced peripheral vascular disease and diabetes.

Manual debridement is performed using a hand-held nail nipper specifically designed for this task (Fig. 13.4). Any loose nail should be removed and the nail is reduced from distal to proximal with angulation added to thin the nail as it is being shortened (Fig. 13.5).

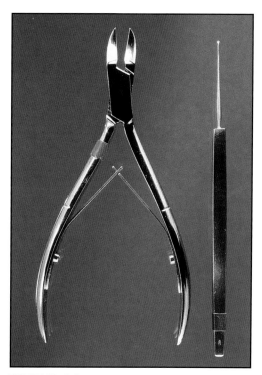

FIGURE 13-4. Curved jaw nail nipper designed for debridement of thickened mycotic toenails.

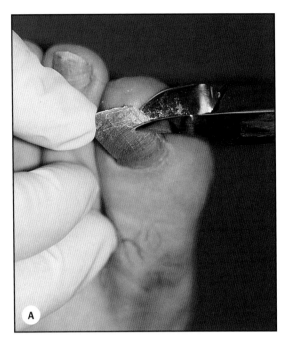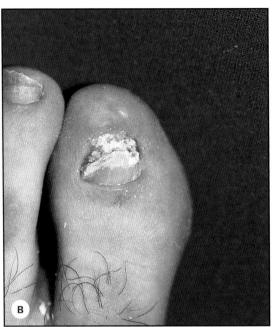

FIGURE 13–5. A, Proper use of the nipper to reduce the length and thickness of the mycotic nail. B, End result of a proper debridement. Note both the marked shortening and thinning of the nail plate.

In many cases, after manual debridement, an electric drill with a rotary burr is used to reduce the thickened toenail further (Fig. 13.6). This allows for closer reduction than would have been possible with the hand instrument alone. It also has the secondary benefit of smoothing any rough edges. This prevents the potential for irritation to an adjacent toe (Fig. 13.7).

The greatest drawback to the use of the electric burr is the production of nail dust. To solve this problem, many different types of dust extraction devices have been marketed to the profession. These units range from small, inexpensive, easily installed canister vacuums to central externally ducted vacuums and the newer water or alcohol spray systems. According to a 1993 study by Harvey,[10] the efficacy of these different types of units ranges from 24.6 to 91.6%. The water spray units were found to be the most effective at capturing debris; however, these units have the disadvantage of creating a 'sludge'. According to detractors, this becomes a neatness problem in the office. For this reason, along with the relatively high cost of these units, they have not gained a significant foothold in the office setting. The conclusion drawn by Harvey was that the most important factors in the overall efficacy of the various units were: (1) the distance of the vacuum nozzle to the nail, (2) the age of the collection bag, and (3) the power of the system.

Chemical debridement using 40% urea is practiced to some extent in podiatric medicine. Overall, the technique is considered by many to be too time and labor intensive. However, the recent introduction of 40% urea 'nail gels' has reignited interest in the use of this compound. In many cases, aggressive manual debridement obviates the need for the chemical therapy and can be performed in one visit. Some of the topical preparations frequently used in the profession, such as Fungoid tincture and Gordochom, contain agents to help soften the nail to facilitate regular debridement. They have been used by some as actual therapy for onychomycosis; however, by themselves they show very low mycological cure rates of 11–18%.[11] Independent of the type of debridement performed, once the nail plate is removed topical antifungal therapy may be applied to the nail bed. Theoretically, this will provide activity against the organisms residing in the nail bed stratum corneum, allowing the new portion of nail to grow in more normally.

## SURGICAL THERAPIES

In patients unresponsive to regular debridement therapy, or in those requesting a permanent cure, surgical removal of the nail and nail matrix is a standard podiatric treatment. Contrary to the often-heard dermatologic axiom that 'onychomycosis is a medical,

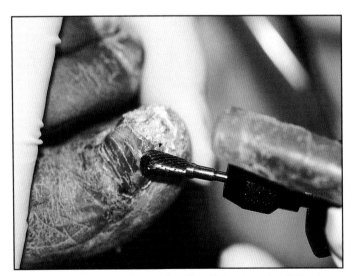

FIGURE 13-6. Electric rotary burr used to thin a thickened mycotic nail. The clear plastic hose attached to the hand piece is part of a dust extraction vacuum system.

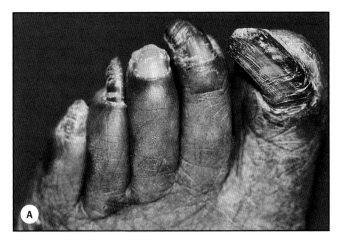

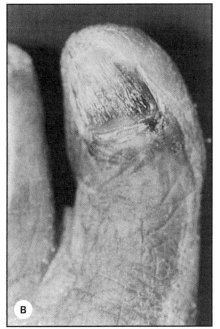

FIGURE 13–7. A, Markedly thickened and elongated mycotic hallux toenail. B, Marked shortening and thinning of the nail, which was possible with proper mechanical and electrical debridement technique.

| TABLE 13–2. Advantages and disadvantages of the two commonly used matricectomy procedures | |
|---|---|
| **ADVANTAGES** | **DISADVANTAGES** |
| **Chemical** | |
| Technically easy | Prolonged drainage |
| Relatively painless | Recurrences may be more frequent |
| Low infection rate | |
| **Surgical** | |
| Lower recurrence | More painful |
| Faster healing | More technically demanding |

Entire chapters of textbooks have been written on the podiatric surgical approach to the toenail. There are multiple variations of similar approaches, all with advocates claiming superiority. Basically, partial or total nail excisions can be broken down into two general classes: those performed with chemical matricectomy or those performed with surgical 'cold steel' matricectomy. Both, again, have advocates and detractors. Advantages and disadvantages for each procedure are listed in Table 13.2. Other techniques, such as carbon dioxide laser, radiotherapy, and electrocoagulation, have been used to varying degrees and with varying success by some segments of the profession. The purpose of this section is not to present a primer on surgical procedures but rather to discuss briefly some of the techniques commonly practiced in podiatric surgery.

## Anesthesia

Most podiatrists favor a digital block for local anesthesia. This may differ from the common dermatology technique of local, periungual infiltration of the anesthetic agent, which can be extremely painful due to the lack of potential space. The digital block is performed near the base of the toe using a two-stick (medial and lateral) or a three-stick 'H' technique (medial, lateral, plantar) (Fig. 13.8). This technique is advantageous in that the greater volume of soft tissue in the area allows for greater expansion as the agent is injected and, therefore, minimal discomfort. It also addresses the neuroanatomy better as the innervation is likened to the four corners of a box. Adequate anesthesia can usually be accomplished with 2 to 3 mL of lidocaine in the hallux. For lesser toes, a single stick 'V' block can be used, initiated at the dorsal aspect of the base of the toe using less lidocaine.

## Chemical Matricectomy

After digital block, a tourniquet is placed around the base of the hallux. Once the toenail is avulsed (Fig. 13.9), the proximal and lateral folds are inspected for any remaining nail spicule. Phenol, 89%, is applied to the matrix and proximal nail bed (Fig. 13.10). The timing and number of applications vary with different surgeons, but generally three applications of 30 seconds each is sufficient. This is followed with a copious flush of either an alcohol solution (thus the common name phenol and alcohol, or P & A, technique) or normal saline. A sterile, nonadherent dressing is applied, and the patient is discharged. The first postoperative visit usually occurs at 1 week, and the patient may then be monitored

not a surgical, disease', excellent results yielding patient satisfaction have been reported by podiatric surgeons. Concerns about loss of function after removal, which may be relevant for fingernails, seldom apply to toenails. The nail plate acts as a buttress that opposes the opposite force, placing pressure on the finger or toe. This increases the discrimination ability of the acral pulp and skin wherever the object is felt. This is much more important in the finger than the toe. With the advent of a fungal infection the intermediate layer hypertrophies and distorts the nail. Toenail removal can therefore be performed with very few consequences.[12,13] In most cases, even the aesthetic result is quite acceptable. The remaining nail bed actually takes on the appearance of a more normal nail. It is not uncommon to see female patients apply nail polish to the bed and treat it as though a nail was present. Indications for surgical intervention include, but are not limited to, the following:

- severely deformed nails
- painful nails unresponsive to conservative therapy
- failures with systemic oral antifungals
- a desire for a reliable, permanent cure.

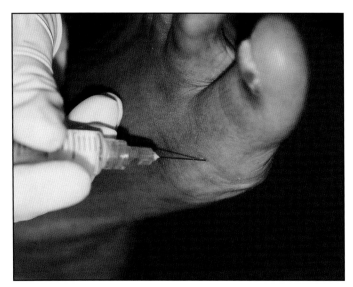

FIGURE 13–8. 'Two-stick' technique performed at the base of the toe for proper preoperative anesthesia.

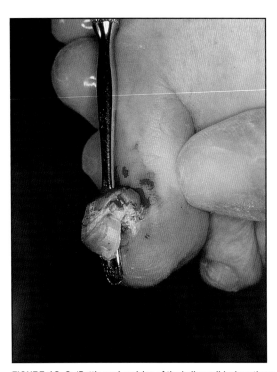

FIGURE 13–9. 'Bottle cap' avulsion of the hallux nail by inserting a Freer periosteal elevator into the proximal nail fold and rotating to lift the thickened nail plate from the nail bed. From Bolognia et al. *Dermatology* © 2003 Elsevier Ltd.

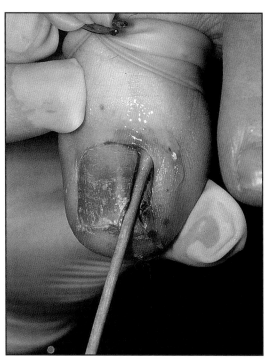

FIGURE 13–10. The use of a cotton-tipped applicator to apply the 89% phenolic acid in a phenol and alcohol (P & A) procedure. From Bolognia et al *Dermatology* © 2003 Elsevier Ltd.

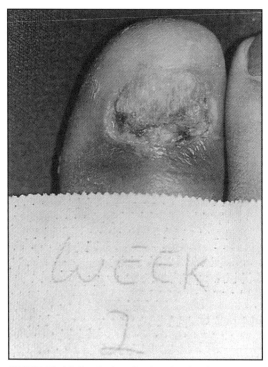

FIGURE 13–11. Results 2 weeks after phenol and alcohol procedure. Note the minimal amount of normal drainage still present at the proximal nail fold.

weekly (Fig. 13.11). Because the phenol causes a chemical burn, there is usually some inflammation and drainage. Both gradually subside, with the drainage lasting anywhere from 2 to 6 weeks or more. The patient should be made aware of the possibility for prolonged drainage to avoid untoward apprehension about infection. The end result is generally excellent (Fig. 13.12).

Although the phenol and alcohol procedure is by far the most common chemical matricectomy performed by podiatrists,

variations do exist. The use of 10% sodium hydroxide followed by a 5% acetic acid flush was popularized in the early 1980s.[14] Proponents emphasized the lower recurrence rate with fewer postoperative complications, but the procedure has not achieved wide acceptance.[15]

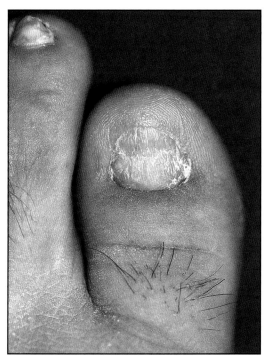

**FIGURE 13–12.** End result of a properly performed phenol and alcohol procedure. The result is usually aesthetically pleasing to the patient, and there is no possibility of pain from a thickened mycotic nail.

## Surgical Matricectomy

As mentioned, there are numerous variations on the approach to a surgical matricectomy. Whether the surgeon performs a proximal flap, performs an 'acisional', or removes varying amounts of the nail bed is dependent on individual preference. Whichever method is chosen, the technique is performed under sterile conditions after avulsion of the nail plate. The matrix is identified in the pocket of the eponychial fold and excised via sharp dissection. The eponychium may then be sutured to the remaining nail bed. The wound is dressed with a sterile, nonadherent dressing. Frequently, a longer acting anesthetic agent may be instilled into the base of the toe at the completion of the procedure. This is helpful in maintaining the patient's comfort through the immediate postoperative period. Laser removal of the matrix also has been proven to be an effective method tool, with the same basic technique employed as the cold steel method. However, closure is usually by secondary intention.[16,17]

## MEDICAL THERAPIES

Although most podiatrists' experience with griseofulvin was not overly encouraging, the drug was helpful in a great number of patients. When used at a high enough dose for a long enough period of time, nails would clear. However, because of the previously discussed issues surrounding the safety and efficacy of this drug, many podiatrists avoided the use of oral antifungal therapy. One limited survey of podiatric prescribing habits found that, before the introduction of the new drugs, the responding podiatrists averaged fewer than one prescription per week for oral antifungal medications.[18] Instead, there was reliance on the use of topical therapy with or without nail avulsion. The same survey showed that this group of podiatrists was prescribing almost ten topical antifungal prescriptions per week. Extrapolated out to the number of actively practicing podiatrists, this amounts to almost 130,000 antifungal prescriptions per week. Unfortunately, there is no way to determine from the survey how much of this topical usage was for onychomycosis versus tinea pedis.

Over the past decade immense interest has been generated in the profession regarding the newer oral antifungal drugs. Currently, the most prescribed oral anti fungal medication is terbinafine (Lamisil), which represents the lion's share of the oral market. Itraconazole (Sporanox) has dropped out of favor with most podiatrists because of concerns over drug–drug interactions and FDA-issued 'black box warnings'. Fluconazole (Diflucan), although shown to be safe and effective, never received an FDA indication for onychomycosis and therefore has never been marketed to the profession. Although some podiatrists still use the drug, debate still rages on the internet about the proper dosing regimen.

## Topical Therapies

In the early 1990s, the FDA proclaimed that no topical medication could claim efficacy against onychomycosis. However, for years the medical profession has continued to use many 'potions' in hopes of finding a safe topical agent with proven efficacy. It was not until late 1999 that the first FDA-approved topical agent, ciclopirox 8% nail lacquer (Penlac) hit the market. Ciclopirox lacquer 8% is indicated for mild to moderate fungal infections of the nail. It should be applied daily, much like a toenail polish, and should be removed once a week to promote better penetration of the nail. The lacquer should be used for 48 weeks or until the nail fungus is clinically cured. Ciclopirox lacquer is a hydroxypyridone that works by chelating the polyvalent cations $Fe^{3+}$ or $Al^{3+}$, resulting in the inhibition of the metal-dependent enzymes that degrade the toxic peroxides within the fungal cell. It is effective against dermatophytes, molds, and yeasts. Although its proven efficacy does not approach that of oral medications, it has certainly found a place due to its excellent safety profile and ease of use.

For those who cannot, or who choose not to take oral antifungals, topical medications can be a viable choice. They are also much more cost effective for those showing only partial involvement of one or a couple of nails. In the past, the nail itself has proven to be the largest impediment in the usage of any topical medication because the active agent could not reach the nail bed where the fungus infection perpetuates itself. Ciclopirox lacquer 8% has proven itself to be the only topical medication with the ability to penetrate the nail, proven by carbon labeling of the medication that was able to pass through the nail itself. Recent pending studies show that combination therapy of a topical and oral medication used in parallel may have synergistic effects. Reoccurrence rates of 22% have led some to believe that topical ciclopirox 8% may be a good prophylactic medication used biweekly.[19]

With each clinical exposure to the new drugs, podiatrists will become more and more comfortable with their safety profile, successes, and failures. Proper patient selection criteria will be determined. Mechanical, surgical therapy will continue to play an important role and may be useful in augmenting the new oral and topical therapies. Only with time, clinical usage, and well-designed, large-scale postmarketing studies will any clearly superior treatment or combination of treatments be delineated.

# REFERENCES

1. Krausz CE. Nail survey, 1942–1970. Br J Surg 1970; 35:117
2. Greenberg L, Davis H: Foot problems in the US: the 1990 National Health Interview Survey. J Am Podiatr Med Assoc 1993; 83:475
3. PDA, Scott Levin. March 2000. Data on file
4. BMAD Report. Data on file
5. Boffelli TJ, Bean JK, Natwick GAR. Biomechanical abnormalities in ulcers of the great toe in patients with diabetes. J Foot Ankle Surg 2002; 41 (6):359–364
6. Doyle JJ et al. Onychomycosis among diabetes patients: prevalence and impact of nonfungal foot infections. Presented at the American Diabetes Association's 60th scientific seminar; 9–13 June 2000; San Antonio, TX
7. Reiber Boyko Smith. Lower exremity ulcerations and amputations in diabetes. Bethesda, MD, National Institutes for Health, 1995
8. Lubeck DP, Patrick DL, McNulty P, et al. Quality of life of persons with onychomycosis. Quality Life Res 1993; 2:341
9. Drake LA Scher RK Smith EB et al. Effects of onychomycosis on the quality of life. J Am Acad Dermatol 1998; 38:702–704
10. Harvey CK. Comparison of the effectiveness of nail dust extractors. J Am Podiatr Med Assoc 1993; 83:669
11. Bodman M, Fender L, Nance A. Topical treatments for onychomycosis. JAPMA 2003; 93 (2):136–141
12. Fishman HC. Practical therapy for ingrown toenails. Cutis 1983; 32:159.
13. Scher RK, Daniel CR. Nails: therapy, diagnosis, surgery, pg 13 WB Sanders, Philadelphia 1990
14. Travers GR, Ammon RG. The sodium hydroxide chemical matricectomy procedure. J Am Podiatr Assoc 1980; 70:476
15. Greenwald L, Robbins HM. The chemical matricectomy. J Am Podiatr Assoc 1981; 71:388
16. Siegle RJ, Stewart R. Recalcitrant ingrowing nails: surgical approaches. J Dermatolog Surg Oncology 1992; 18:744.
17. Goldberg DJ. Laser surgery of the skin. Am Family Physician 1989; 40:109
18. Donoghue SK. Keeping pace in the face of managed care. Podiatr Management 1996; 14:44
19. Olafsson JH. Combination therapy for onychomycosis. Br J Dermatol 2003; 1:49. Hays RJ. The future of onychomycosis therapy may involve a combination of approaches. Br J Dermatol 2001; 145 (Suppl 60):3–8

# 14 Nonfungal Infections and Acute Paronychia

Monica Lawry and C Ralph Daniel III

## INFECTIONS RESULTING FROM HIGHER ORGANISMS

Some parasitic organisms must be included in the differential diagnosis of ungual diseases. For the most part, the disorders discussed next are rare.

## Scabies

*Sarcoptes scabiei* is the most common higher organism to cause nail disease. Significant nail damage most often occurs in individuals with Norwegian (or crusted) scabies. Crusted scabies is most common in immunocompromised, homeless or institutionalized patients. Patients with Down syndrome are also predisposed. The nail plate is usually dystrophic and brittle, with subungual hyperkeratosis.[1] With this disorder, keratotic areas may be present in the scalp, the face (rare in regular scabies), the palms, and the soles.[2] It is well known that large numbers of organisms may be involved. Nail changes similar to those in nail scabies may be seen in chronic granulomatous disease of childhood[2] or in other disorders producing dystrophic, crumbling nails with subungual hyperkeratosis.

The nail may also be instrumental in perpetuating recurrent scabies by harboring the organism and protecting it from topical scabicides.[3,4]

### Diagnosis and treatment

Simple microscopic examination after placing the specimen in mineral oil is all that is usually needed to diagnose the organism. A biopsy also readily shows the organism.

Chemical or surgical avulsion of the involved nail plates may sometimes be necessary to allow scabicides to reach the diseased tissue. Urea may be used to avulse the nail.[5] Removing patients from a predisposing environment or improving their immunologic status, if possible, may also be necessary.

Various treatment regimens have been used in the past, including lindane 1%, permethrin 5%, precipitated sulfa, and so on. Gamma benzene hexachloride (GBH) has been used according to the following procedure:[6]

1. Isolate the patient.
2. Provide weekly total body treatment with daily trimming of nails and scrubbing the nails with GBH, and daily application of GBH to hyperkeratotic crusts. Consider debridement of extremely hyperkeratotic nails.[7]
3. Treat fomites with acaricide.

A 10-month-old infant was treated with a 10% water–soap suspension of benzyl benzoate, which cleared the skin and nail plates.[8]

Ivermectin has emerged as a new therapeutic option. Oral ivermectin (200 µg/kg) alone or in combination with topical therapy can be used as treatment for crusted scabies.[9] Although not approved by the US Food and Drug Administration (FDA) for scabies in any age group, there is also growing experience with ivermectin for scabies in children.[10]

## Trichinosis

The organism *Trichinella spiralis* is hematogenously spread before it becomes encysted in muscle. It may find its way into the small vessels of the nail bed. Splinter hemorrhages may result and, if they undergo biopsy, the organism can be found.[11] Transverse splinter hemorrhages have also been seen.[12] Because the nail bed vessels are oriented longitudinally, the mechanism for this is at best unclear. Splinter hemorrhages caused by systemic disorders as well as trichinosis tend to occur simultaneously in multiple nails and begin proximally.

## Tungiasis (Jigger Flea)

*Tunga penetrans* (also known as sand flea, jigger, nigua, or chico) is found in warm, sandy soil close to farms. It is endemic in Central and South America, the Caribbean, sub-Saharan Africa, Pakistan, and the west coast of India. Tungiasis occurs when the female flea, which requires a warm-blooded host to continue its life cycle, burrows into the epidermis. When the flea enlarges to produce eggs, painful and pruritic skin lesions appear. The nodule may have slight or intense erythema and often displays a central black pit, which is the posterior portion of the organism. The periungual central black pit is typical.[13] Secondary bacterial infection or tetanus are concerns, but other complications are uncommon.[14]

### Treatment

Curettage of the nodule to remove the flea and egg deposits is recommended. Culture of purulent material and appropriate treatment for secondary bacterial infection, as well as tetanus immunization, is important.

## Subungual Myiasis

Myiasis is an infestation of *Dermatobia hominis*, the human botfly, which is found in areas ranging from Argentina to southern Mexico. It is prevalent in warm, humid, lowland forests and depends on warm-blooded hosts to complete larval stages of its life cycle. The female fly attaches eggs to a biting insect such as a mosquito. The larvae burrow through the site of the arthropod bite and develop into a third-stage larva, measuring 2 cm in length with a barbed end. An erythematous papule forms within 24 hours of an insect bite; this grows over 4 to 14 weeks to a 3-cm nodule often with a 2-mm breathing hole.[14]

Myiasis is rarely caused by larvae of *Musca domestica*, the common housefly, and is uncommon in the United States. However, subungual hematoma associated with trauma was found to be teeming with these larvae.[15]

### Treatment

Surgical excision of the nodule and appropriate therapy of secondary bacterial infection, if present, is recommended.[14]

## Cutaneous Larva Migrans

The larvae of the nematode *Ancylostoma braziliense* are most often the cause of cutaneous larva migrans.[16] Secondary nail dystrophy, probably caused by the migration of the organism near the matrix, occurred on the thumbnail of one individual.[16]

### Treatment

Topical or systemic thiabendazole is administered.

## Pediculosis[17,18]

Diemer reported pediculosis involving the toenails.[17] Debridement of a great toenail manifested 10 to 12 body lice.

## Post-Kala-Azar Dermal Leishmaniasis[19]

A verrucous eruption has been reported at the base of the nails. Chronic ulcerations leading to destruction of the nail plate and distal phalanx may be caused by cutaneous leishmaniasis.[20]

## VIRAL INFECTIONS

## Herpes Simplex

### Key Features

* Healthcare personnel
* Pain out of proportion to physical findings
* Oral antiviral therapy
* Consider possible bacterial superinfection

Herpes simplex type 1 or type 2[21] may affect the nail apparatus. The condition is usually described as herpetic whitlow or herpetic paronychia. Medical and dental personnel are most commonly affected because of their direct contact with patients harboring the infection. Infection follows minor local trauma, although patients often deny this.[21] Individuals with oral infection may inoculate themselves if they are nail biters or finger suckers.[22,23] One finger is usually involved; usually the forefinger or thumb.[21] Involvement of the toes has been reported but is rare.[22] Any cut or compromise in the periungual tissue allows the infection to penetrate more easily.

As with other herpetic infections, after inoculation there is a latency period of about 3 to 10 days. Local tenderness appears first, followed by erythema, vesicle formation, and pain.[21] Burning pain, out of proportion to physical findings helps distinguish herpetic whitlow from acute bacterial paronychia.[24] The vesicles may coalesce and a yellowish, honeycomb appearance may be evident.[21] Sometimes, vesicles are less apparent and ulcerations are seen. Gradual healing takes place over 2 to 3 weeks. Superinfection with *Staphylococcus aureus* and streptococci, as well as other bacteria, may occur. Periodic recurrences occur in a small minority of persons.[25] Diagnosis is based on the clinical picture plus Tzanck smear, culture, or rapid immunofluorescence. A fourfold rise in viral antibody titer is diagnostic, but is usually used as a confirmatory measure after treatment is initiated because of the time lag. Herpes simplex may secondarily affect the nails by triggering erythema multiforme.

### Treatment

The infection may be highly contagious. Medical and dental personnel, as well as others, should be aware of this fact. Contact with infants and immunosuppressed individuals should especially be avoided. The wearing of exam gloves may decrease transmission but the safest option is avoidance of direct contact while the infection is active. We tell patients that they may still be contagious up to 7 days or longer after the vesicles completely heal. This is erring on the side of safety. Appropriate patient education, treatment of secondary bacterial infection, and close follow-up are often all that is indicated in minor cases.[23] Elevation, analgesics, immobilization of the involved extremity, and hospitalization may be necessary in more severe infections.[23] Treatment options include acyclovir or valacyclovir for uncomplicated cases. Famciclovir orally or foscarnet intravenously may be used in severe, recurrent cases, which are more likely in immunosuppressed patients.

As a general rule, surgical drainage should be avoided because it does not usually provide added comfort, and it exposes the patient to the risk of superinfection.[25] Large or tense vesicles may be carefully opened to ease discomfort. This is especially true in the area of the nail matrix because permanent nail deformity may occur if this structure is damaged. Upon incising and draining a lesion, we use prophylactic penicillinase-resistant antibiotics for about 7 days. Idoxuridine has been given by cathodic iontophoresis. Rapid relief of symptoms and rapid healing were reported in two patients.[26]

## Herpes Zoster

Shingles may coincidentally affect the nail apparatus if that particular dermatome is involved; this is rare. Treatment is the same as for herpes zoster elsewhere on the body. Oral acyclovir, valacylovir or famciclovir may be instituted.

## Human Papilloma Virus

Human Papilloma Virus (HPV) is the etiologic agent for verruca vulgaris, or the common wart. More recent information has been published on intralesional bleomycin,[27,28] infrared coagulation,[29] and the carbon dioxide laser.[30]

## Human Immunodeficiency Virus

See the discussion of the nails in patients with human immunodeficiency virus in Chapter 15.

## Miscellaneous Infections

Orf virus can affect the nail unit, often the dorsum of the right index finger.[31] Milker's nodules, caused by paravaccinia virus, affect mainly agricultural workers and veterinarians.[31] Leprosy may affect the nails by a number of mechanisms, including neuropathy, vascular deficit, and infection.[32] Some of the clinical manifestations include Beau's lines,[33] pterygium inversum unguis,[33] pseudomacrolunula,[34] leukonychia,[34] macronychia,[34] melanonychia,[32] subungual bleeding,[28] and hapalonychia.[30]

## BACTERIAL INFECTION

Bacteria are ubiquitous. Our hands provide much of our physical contact with our environment; therefore, we are constantly coming in contact with bacteria. Nails are known to harbor bacteria.[35] Artificial nails may provide an additional home for these organisms.[36] Bacterial infections may manifest themselves in a number of ways in the vicinity of the nail apparatus, including bacterial felon, which requires aggressive systemic antibiotic therapy, blistering distal dactylitis,[37] and acute paronychia.

## Pathogens Associated with Artificial Nails

It is well known that artificial nails are more likely to harbor pathogens than native nails.[38–41] This is especially pertinent to healthcare workers and those handling food. The highest number of organisms is located in the subungual area of both artificial and native nails, although more organisms are found on the surface of artificial nails. The longer the artificial nails are worn, the higher the likelihood of isolating a pathogen.[38] Artificial nails seem to impair hand washing and are associated with more tears in gloves. A study examining hand-washing techniques in subjects with natural and artificial nails demonstrated that the greatest reduction of bacteria was possible when short natural nails were washed with liquid soap and a nail brush.[39]

There have also been reports of patients who develop acute paronychia, subungual abscess, and felon in association with artificial nails. Diabetics and immunocompromised patients are especially at risk.[42]

## Anthrax Infection of the Hands and Fingers

*Bacillus anthracis* rarely causes cutaneous anthrax in humans but most frequently presents on exposed areas such as hands and face in persons in contact with infected animals. Cases are rare in Europe and the US but should be considered when patients present with a painless ulcer with black eschar and have a history of handling animals, especially cattle.[43] Anthrax can be fatal in humans and has become an important consideration with bioterrorism. However, the cutaneous form (usually not fatal) is responsible for 95% of infections and may lead to extensive local tissue destruction requiring plastic surgery.[44] Areas endemic for anthrax include the Middle East, especially Turkey. Treatment is penicillin and possibly surgical debridement.[45]

## PARONYCHIA

The word 'paronychia' means inflammation of the nail folds. Acute paronychia is often infectious and chronic paronychia (see Chapter 10) is generally noninfectious. Acute paronychia usually involves only one nail. When several nails are involved, subacute or chronic paronychia secondary to either chronic dermatitis or psoriasis vulgaris should be suspected.[46]

## Acute Paronychia

### Key Features

1. Most common infection of the hand
2. *Staphylococcus aureus*, streptococci and *Pseudomonas* are the most common organisms
3. Trauma from nail biting or over-manicuring often involved
4. Culture if possible, drain if necessary, oral antibiotic therapy and soaks

Allergic contact, contact irritant, fixed drug eruption,[47] and dyshidrotic eczema are among the entities that may cause acute periungual inflammation not associated with infections (Fig. 14.1A). High-dose methotrexate and other antineoplastic drugs, such as

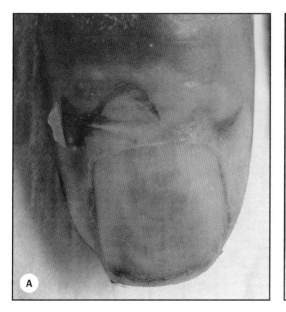 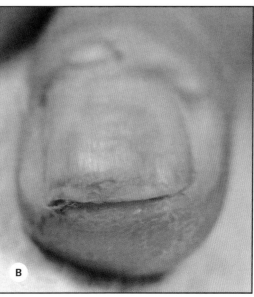

FIGURE 14.1 (A) Docetaxel induced acute paronychia; (B) docetaxel induced acute paronychia.

the taxoids, are reported to rarely cause acute paronychia[48] and subungual abscess. Cultures reveal a mixture of organisms and mechanism may be due to immunosuppression or due to direct drug toxicity on the nail unit.[49,50] Retinoids, certain antiretroviral drugs, and monoclonal antibodies (cetuximab, gefitinib) have been associated with acute paronychia and periungual granulation.[51–55] This section focuses on bacterial causes.

Acute bacterial paronychia is the most common infection in the hand.[56] Trauma to the nail folds, as may occur with overaggressive manicuring or pulling a hangnail, can allow pathologic bacteria to invade the nail apparatus. Young children may be predisposed to acute paronychia by sucking on digits.[24] Once a primary, active infection has occurred in a nail fold, the seal between the fold and nail is broken, which often predisposes to chronic paronychia (see Fig. 14.2B). This is true for several reasons. The alignment and integrity of the nail folds may be chronically or permanently disrupted. Irritants such as detergents, bath soaps, or nail cosmetics may disrupt the healing structure. The patient's increased personal attempts to heal the area may cause further damage.

*S. aureus*, streptococci, and *Pseudomonas* are the most common offenders. Anaerobic paronychia, usually caused by oropharyngeal commensals, is generally less acute than aerobic paronychia and usually responds to penicillin.[56] Some cases of acute paronychia, such as those caused by *Prevotella bivia*, may progress rapidly to osteomyelitis, therefore accurate bacteriological diagnosis is crucial.[57] Acute paronychia has been reported to be caused by *Candida albicans*[58] and *Trichosporon cutaneum*.[59]

## Treatment

Obtain bacterial culture if possible. One must try to eliminate predisposing factors. For mild cases, the following regimen should be implemented:

1. Warm saline or aluminum acetate (1 : 80 Domeboro) for 10 to 15 minutes two to four times a day, continued for 1 to 2 days after the infection has clinically disappeared.[56]
2. 2% mupirocin ointment or polymyxin B-bacitracin ointment should be applied after each soak.
3. An oral antistaphylococcal antibiotic should be prescribed and continued for several days after the infection has clinically resolved. Cephalosporin (bacteriocidal), 250 to 500 mg by mouth four times a day, is the initial drug of choice until Gram's stain results or culture and sensitivity studies have returned. Methicillin resistant staphylococcus is being seen more and more frequently in the physician's office. Continue antibiotics for at least 5 to 7 days after the infection has resolved clinically.

In some cases incision and drainage should be carried out: Painful bulging nail folds should be carefully drained, especially if the nail matrix area is involved, because permanent damage to the nail matrix may occur. An 18-gauge needle or a no. 11 scalpel blade may be used to gently 'tease' an opening to release purulent material. Soaking is begun as previously discussed. The hand should be elevated if much swelling is apparent.[47] Nonadherent gauze[48] or Telfa pads may help drainage.

For unresponsive cases consider imaging studies to rule out osteomyelitis and biopsy to rule out malignancy, such as squamous cell carcinoma.[60]

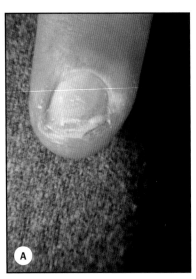

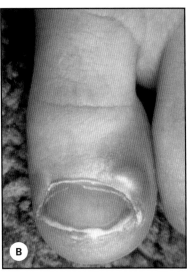

FIGURE 14.2 (A) Acute paronychia, fingernail; (B) acute paronychia, toenail.

# REFERENCES

1. Runne U, Offanos CE. The human nail. Curr Probl Dermatol 1981; 9:102
2. Zais N. The nail in health and disease. New York: SP Medical and Scientific Books; 1980
3. Scher RK. Subungual scabies. Am J Dermatopathol 1983; 5:87
4. Koesard E. The dystrophic nail of keratotic scabies. Am J Dermatopathol 1984; 6:308
5. De Paoli RT, Marks VJ: Crusted (Norwegian) scabies: treatment of nail involvement. J Am Acad Dermatol 1987; 17:136
6. O'Donnell BF, O'Loughlin S, Powell FC. Management of crusted scabies. Int J Dermatol 1990; 29:258
7. Ohtaki N, Taniguchi H, Ohtomo H. Oral ivermectin treatment in two cases of scabies: effective in crusted scabies induced by corticosteroid but ineffective in nail scabies. J Dermatol 2003; 30:411–416
8. Sokolova TV, Sizov IE: Involvement of fingernails in scabies in an infant. Vestn Dermatol Venerol 1989; 2:68
9. Chouela E, Abeldano A, Pellerano G, Hernandez MI. Diagnosis and treatment of scabies: a practical guide. Am J Clin Dermatol 2003; 3:9–18
10. Cestari SC, Petri V, Rotta O, Alchorne MM. Oral treatment of crusted scabies with ivermectin: a report of two cases. Pediatr Dermatol 2000; 17:410–414

11. Farah FS. Protozoan and helminth infections. In: Fitzpatrick TB, Eisen AZ, Wolf K, et al. eds. Dermatology in general medicine. 2nd edn. New York: McGraw-Hill; 1979

12. Samman PD. The nails in disease. 3rd edn. London: William Heinemann; 1978

13. Wentzell JM, Schwartz BK. *Tunga penegrans*. J Am Acad Dermatol 1986; 15:117

14. Wolf R, Orion E, Matz H. Stowaways with wings: two case reports on high-flying insects. Dermatology Online Journal 2004; 9 (3):10

15. Munyon TG, Urbanc AN. Subungual myiasis: a case report and literature. J Assoc Military Dermatol 1978; 4:60

16. Edelglass JW, Douglass MC, Steifler R, et al. Cutaneous larva migrants in northern climates. J Am Acad Dermatol 1982; 7:353

17. Diemer JT. Isolated pediculosis. J Am Podiatr Med Assoc 1985; 75:99

18. Hay RJ, Baran R, Haneke E. Fungal and other infections involving the nail apparatus. In: Baran R, Dawber RPR, eds. Diseases of the nails and their management. 2nd edn. Oxford: Blackwell Scientific; 1994:97–134

19. Moschella SL. Benign reticuloendothelial diseases. In: Moschella SL, Pillsbury DM, Hurly HJ, eds. Dermatology, vol 1. Philadelphia: WB Saunders; 1975:751–836

20. Ogawa MM, Macedo FS, Alchorne MM, Tomimori-Yamashita J. Unusual location of cutaneous leishmaniasis on the hallux in a Brazilian patient. Int J Dermatol 2002; 41:439–440

21. Giacobetti R. Herpetic whitlow. Int J Dermatol 1979; 18:55

22. Muller SA, Hermann EC Jr. Association of stomatitis and paronychias due to herpes simplex. Arch Dermatol 1970; 101:396

23. Daniel CR III. Diseases of the nail. In: Conn HF, ed. Current therapy. Philadelphia: WB Saunders; 1983:656

24. Hedrick J. Acute bacterial skin infections in pediatric medicine: current issues in presentation and treatment. Paediatr Drugs 2003; 5 Suppl 1:35–46

25. Andiaman WA. Questions and answers, herpetic whitlow in a nursing student. JAMA 1981; 245:2531

26. Gangarosa LP, Payne LJ, Hayakawa K, et al. Iontophoretic treatment of herpetic whitlow. Arch Phys Med Rehabil 1989; 70:336

27. Epstein E. Intralesional bleomycin and Raynaud's phenomenon. J Am Acad Dermatol 1991; 24:785

28. Shelley WB, Shelley D. Intralesional bleomycin sulfate therapy for warts: a novel bifurcated needle puncture technique. Arch Dermatol 1991; 127:234

29. Halasz CLG. Treatment of common warts using the infrared coagulator. J Derm Surg Oncol 1994; 20:252

30. Street ML, Roenigk RK. Recalcitrant periungual verrucae: the role of carbon dioxide laser vaporization. J Am Acad Dermatol 1990; 23:115

31. Baran RJ, Dawber RPR. Diseases of the nails and their management. Oxford: Blackwell Scientific; 1984

32. Kikuchi I. Some observations on the nail changes in patients with leprosy. In: Burgdorf WHC, Katz SI, eds. Dermatology progress and perspectives. The Proceedings of the 18th World Congress of Dermatology. Parthenon, New York, 1993

33. Patki AH. Pterygium inversum unguius in a patient with leprosy. Arch Dermatol 1990; 126:1110

34. Patki AH, Baran R. Significance of nail changes in leprosy: a clinical review of 357 cases. Semin Dermatol 1991; 10:77

35. Leyden JJ, McGinley KJ, Kates SG, Myung KB. Subungual bacteria of the hand: contribution to the glove juice test; efficacy of anti-microbial detergents. Infect Control Hosp Epidemiol 1989; 10:451

36. Senay H. Acrylic nails and transmission of infection. Can J Infect Control 1991; 6:52

37. Telfer NR, Barth JH, Dawber RP. Recurrent blistering distal dactylitis of the great toe associated with an ingrowing toenail. Clin Exp Dermatol 1989; 14:380

38. Hedderwick SA, McNeil SA, Lyons MJ, Kauffman CA. Pathogenic organisms associated with artificial fingernails worn by healthcare workers. Infect Control Hosp Epidemiol 2000; 21:505–509

39. Lin CM, Wu FM, Kim HK, et al. A comparison of hand washing techniques to remove *Escherichia coli* and calciviruses under natural or artificial fingernails. J Food Prot 2003; 66:2296–2301

40. Toles A. Artificial nails: are they putting patients at risk? Review of the research. J Pediatr Oncol Nurs 2002; 19:164–171

41. Porteous J. Artificial nails … very real risks. Can Oper Room Nurs J 2002; 20:16–17, 20–21

42. Roberge RJ, Weinstein D, Thimons MM. Perionychial infections associated with sculptured nails. Am J Emerg Med 1999; 17 (6):581–582

43. Aslan G, Terzioglu A. Surgical management of cutaneous anthrax. Ann Plast Surg 1998; 41:468–470

44. Coban YK, Balik O, Boran C. Cutaneous anthrax of the hand and its reconstruction with a reverse-flow radial forearm flap. Ann Plast Surg 2002; 49:109–111

45. Caksen H, Arabaci F, Abuhandan M, et al. Cutaneous anthrax in eastern Turkey. Cutis 2001; 67:488–492

46. Cohen PR, Scher RK. Geriatric nail disorders: diagnosis and treatment. J Am Acad Dermatol 1992; 26:521

47. Baran R, Perrin C. Fixed drug eruption presenting as acute paronychia. Br J Dermatol 1991; 125:592

48. Wantzig GL, Thomsen K. Acute paronychia after high dose methotrexate therapy. Arch Dermatol 1983; 119:623

49. Albares MP, Belinchon I, Pascual JC, et al. Subungal abcessess secondary to paclitaxel. Dermatology Online Journal 2004; 9 (3):16

50. Nicolopoulos J, Howard A. Docetaxel-induced nail dystrophy. Australas J Dermatol 2002; 43:293–296

51. Sass JO, Jakob-Solder B, Heitger A, et al. Paronychia with pyogenic granuloma in a child treated with indinavir: the retinoid-mediated side effect theory revisited. Dermatology 2000; 200:40–42

52. Garcia-Silva J, Almargo M, Pena-Penabad C, Fonseca E. Indinavir-induced retinoid-like effects: incidence of clinical features and management. Drug Safety 2002; 25:993–1003

53. Boucher KW, Davidson K Mirakhur B, et al. Paronychia induced by cetuximab, an antiepidermal growth factor receptor antibody. J Am Acad Dermatol 2002; 47:632

54. Nakano J, Nakamura M. Paronychia induced by gefitinib, an epidermal growth factor receptor tyrosine kinase inhibitor. J Dermatol 2003; 30:261–262

55. Dainichi T, Tanaka M, Tsuruta N, et al. Development of multiple paronychia and periungual granulation in patients treated with gefitinib, an inhibitor of epidermal growth factor receptor. Dermatology 2003; 207:324–325

56. Whitehead SM, Eykyn SJ, Phillips I. Anaerobic paronychia. Br J Surg 1981; 68:420–422

57. Riesbeck K. Paronychia due to Prevotella bivia that resulted in amputation: fast and correct bacteriological diagnosis is crucial. J Clin Microbiol 2003; 41:4901–4903

58. Fisher BK, Warner LC. Cutaneous manifestations of the acquired immunodeficiency syndrome. Int J Dermatol 1987; 26:615

59. Zaias N. Paronychia. In: The nail in health and disease. 2nd edn. Norwalk, CT: Appleton & Lange; 1990:131–135

60. Jebson PJ. Infections of the fingertip. Hand Clinics 1998; 14:547–555

# 15

# Nails in Systemic Disease

## Monica Lawry and C Ralph Daniel III

## Key Features

1. Examine all 20 nails
2. Do a full skin exam
3. Obtain a detailed history with attention to chronology of events
4. Obtain laboratory studies indicated by history and physical exam

Nail abnormalities secondary to systemic disease are important to dermatologists because they are readily examined and may be the initial signal that systemic disease is present.

Jemec et al. suggest that while nail abnormalities are not common in nondermatologic patients, some nail changes do occur more frequently in certain disease states.[1] Nail abnormalities associated with systemic disease can be organized into groups such as nonspecific findings (reaction patterns), nail abnormalities that show specific associations, and findings that are considered part of a specific syndrome.[2] An understanding of the nature of the clinical nail abnormality will allow appropriate work-up or help avoid incorrect and costly diagnostic and treatment plans. There are no hard and fast rules concerning nails in systemic disease, but several points are worthy of mention:

1. Always examine all 20 nails because multiple nails are usually involved.
2. In general, fingernails provide more subtle information than toenails because trauma is more likely to mask or change certain manifestations in toenails.
3. Examine the rest of the skin and mucous membranes for additional abnormalities, and perform a complete physical examination if indicated.
4. A detailed history is important, including close attention to the chronologic sequence of events.
5. Obtain appropriate laboratory tests as indicated by the history and physical examination.

Nail pigmentation changes associated with systemic disease often arise in the area of the matrix. In this case, the leading edge of the abnormal pigmentation is often shaped similarly to the distal matrix (lunula or half-moon).[3] If this color change is transmitted to the nail plate, it will grow out with that structure. By measuring the distance from the proximal nail fold (cuticle) to the leading edge of the pigmentation change and calculating from the rate of nail growth (0.1–0.15 mm per day), one can estimate the time at which the initial insult occurred.

## CHAPTER OVERVIEW

Nail Abnormalities Less Specifically Associated with Systemic Disease
- Splinter hemorrhages

- Beau's lines/onychomadesis
- onycholysis
- pitting
- koilonychia
- pigmented bands

Nail Abnormalities More Specifically Associated with Systemic Disease
- True leukonychia – Mee's lines: arsenic toxicity
- Apparent leukonychia – Muehrcke's lines (hypoalbuminemia), Half & Half/Lindsay's Nails (renal disease), Terry's nails (hepatic cirrhosis)
- Clubbing – cardiopulmonary disease

Nail Abnormalities Associated with Disease of a Specific Organ System (organized by system)
- Cardiovascular/Hematologic
- Gastrointestinal
- Pulmonary Disease – Yellow Nail Syndrome
- Renal Disease – Half & Half/Lindsay's Nails
- Autoimmune Disease-periungual telangectasia, pterygium inversus ungium
- Endocrine
- Infectious Disease
- HIV Disease – proximal white subungual onychomycosis, pyogenic granulomas with antiretroviral therapy
- Central and Peripheral Nervous System Disease
- Psychological Disease – Onychotillomania
- Miscellaneous Diseases

Nail Abnormalities Associated with Specific Syndromes or Genodermatoses
- Darier's Disease – longitudinal streaks & distal V-shaped notch
- Dyskeratosis Congenita – koilonychias, onychorrhexis, onychoschizia
- Pachyonychia Congenita – extreme nailbed hyperkeratosis
- Nail Patella Syndrome – triangular lunulae
- Incontinentia Pigmenti – periungual/subungual tumors

# NAIL ABNORMALITIES LESS SPECIFICALLY ASSOCIATED WITH SYSTEMIC DISEASE (REACTION PATTERNS)

## Splinter Hemorrhages and Subungual Purpura

Splinter hemorrhages are formed by the extravasation of blood from the longitudinally oriented vessels of the nail bed (Fig. 15.1). The blood attaches itself to the underlying nail plate and moves distally.

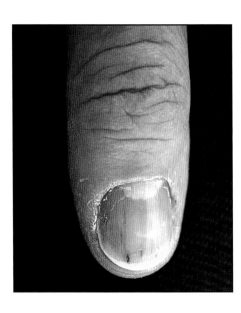

FIGURE 15–1. Splinter hemorrhages (courtesy of Dr Jeffrey Callen).

The splinter hemorrhages occasionally appear to remain stationary, probably because of attachment to the nail bed rather than to the plate.

Splinter hemorrhages can be caused by physical factors, including trauma, drugs, dermatologic diseases, systemic diseases, and idiopathic conditions, among others. Trauma is by far the most common cause.[4,5] At times, certain presentations of splinter hemorrhages should make one consider a systemic cause, particularly bacterial endocarditis.[6] Their simultaneous appearance in multiple nails is more frequently associated with systemic disease. Also, their occurrence closer to the lunula as opposed to the distal nail plate seems to be more directly correlated with systemic disease.[4,5]

Miscellaneous information about splinter hemorrhages:

1. Splinter hemorrhages are more common in the elderly, are more common in Black people, and are located distally.[13,14] When found in women, splinter hemorrhages are more likely to indicate systemic disease.[14]

2. In one study, the left hand was involved greater than three times more frequently than the right hand in patients with single hemorrhages; the left thumb was the digit most frequently involved.[7]

3. In patients with multiple hemorrhages, more occurred on the left hand than the right hand. The thumb was the most frequently involved digit, followed by the left index finger and the left thumb.[7]

4. In one study, peritoneal dialysis was the single most frequently encountered factor in patients with splinter hemorrhages.[8]

5. Splinter hemorrhages were found to occur in 10.3% of patients admitted to a general medicine ward of a large city-county hospital in one study, and 19.5% and 19.1%, respectively, in two other studies.[7]

6. Biopsy of splinter hemorrhages that are associated with trichinosis may reveal the organism.[9]

7. In trichinosis, splinter hemorrhages may be oriented transversely instead of longitudinally.[10]

8. Splinter hemorrhages have been described histologically.[11]

9. Splinter hemorrhages do not blanch upon pressure to the nail plate in the way that some other disorders, e.g., ataxia-telangiectasia, do.[12]

10. Splinter hemorrhages and pain have been associated with subacute bacterial endocarditis,[15] trichinosis,[15] an indwelling arterial catheter,[15] and leukocytoclastic vasculitis.[16] (C.R. Daniel, personal observation)

Table 15.1 lists various diseases that have been associated with splinter hemorrhages, subungual purpura, and their many causes. Most commonly, systemic disease is not the cause but, when keeping the points just listed in mind, one may more rationally evaluate their true significance.

## Beau's Lines/Onychomadesis

Beau's lines are probably one of the most common but least specific nail changes associated with systemic disease. The exact cause is unclear.[17] Temporary cessation of nail growth or decreased nail plate deposition results in a transverse depression across the nail plate (Fig. 15.2). There is probably an approximate direct correlation with the degree of general body trauma sustained and the likelihood of manifesting Beau's lines. Local injury or trauma to the proximal nail fold region may also cause a similar lesion. It seems that the most useful information that this finding gives is found by measuring the distance from the proximal nail fold distally to the leading edge of the Beau's line. Then one may approximate the time the insult occurred because the fingernail grows about 0.1 mm to 0.15 mm a day.

The width of the furrow is an indicator of the duration of the disease that has affected the matrix.[18] If there is complete inhibition of nail growth for at least 1–2 weeks, the Beau's line will reach its maximum depth and may result in onychomadesis (nail shedding). This form of onychomadesis is referred to as latent, because the split created by prolonged interruption of nail growth emerges gradually from beneath the proximal nail fold.[18] Beau's lines are the most common ischemic deformity of the nail seen by the hand surgeon after the use of the upper extremity tourniquet.[19] Onychomadesis may also occur abruptly as a spontaneous separation of the nail from the matrix. Associated factors are similar to Beau's lines: Serious systemic illness, drug reactions, bullous dermatoses, severe psychological stress, inherited form or idiopathic.[18] Beau's lines and onychomadesis have been reported in children recovering from hand-foot-mouth disease.[20,21] Figure 15.3 illustrates onychomadesis that occurred in a 3-year-old child after streptococcal infection and high fever. Onychomadesis and periungual pyogenic granuloma may also be associated with patients who have cast immobilization, especially when there is paresthesia and pain of the immobilized hand.[22]

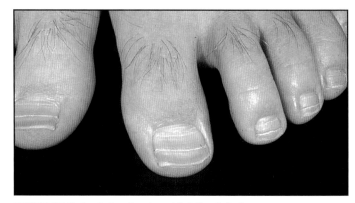

FIGURE 15–2. Beau's lines (courtesy of Dr Jeffrey Callen).

**TABLE 15-1.** Conditions associated with splinter hemorrhages and subungual purpura

Alopecia mucinosa[233]
Altitude (high)[1]
Amyloid[10]
Anemia[233]
Antigen-antibody complex disease
Antiphospholipid coagulopathy[234]
Antiphospholipid syndrome[304]
Behçet's syndrome[1]
Blood diseases[1]
Buerger's disease[76]
Cirrhosis[235]
Cryoglobulinemia[76]
Cystic fibrosis[1]
Darier's disease[236]
Diabetes mellitus
   (in about 10% of patients)[16]
Dialysis[5,235]
Drug reactions (in general),[237]
   especially phototoxic
Arterial emboli[76]
Endocarditis[238,239]
Eczema[76]
Exfoliative dermatitis[16]
Fungal[7]

General illness[5,235]
Glomerulonephritis[12]
Heart disease[233]
Hemochromatosis[1]
Hepatitis[6]
Histiocytosis X[205]
Human immunodeficiency virus[12a]
Hypertension[7]
Hypoparathyroidism[76]
Irradiation[16,240]
Keratosis lichenoides chronica[241]
Letterer-Siwe disease[205]
Leukemia[16]
Malignant neoplasms[7]
Mitral stenosis[235,237]
Multiple sclerosis[14]
Mycosis fungoides[55]
Normals[18,235]
Onychomycosis
Osler-Weber-Rendu disease[16]
Pemphigoid[10]
Pemphigus[47]
Pen-push purpura[242]
Peptic ulcer disease[7]

Periarteritis nodosa[243]
Pityriasis rubra pilaris[163b]
Porphyria[12]
Psittacosis[12]
Psoriasis[26,75,237,244]
Pterygium[12]
Pulmonary disease[233]
Purpura[8]
Radial artery puncture[12]
Raynaud's disease[76]
Rheumatic fever[12]
Rheumatoid arthritis[7]
Sarcoid[47]
Scurvy[237]
Septicemia[12]
Systemic lupus erythematosus[6,75]
Tetracycline[245]
Thrombocytopenia[16]
Thyrotoxicosis[235,237,238]
Transplant patients[c]
Trauma[2,3,5,26,235,238,244]
Trichinosis[6,75]
Vasculitis[237a]
Wegener's granulomatosis[246]

[a]C.R. Daniel, personal observation.
[b]H.W. Randle, personal communication, 1982.
[c]J.M. Mascaro, personal communication, December 8, 1992.

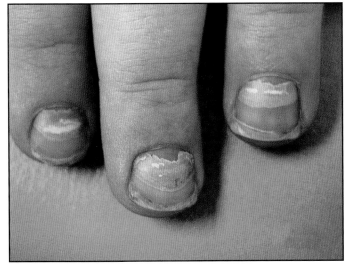

FIGURE 15-3. Onychomadesis in a 3-year-old after a streptococcal infection with high fever.

Histologic studies have shown an inflammatory infiltrate consisting of lymphocytes, plasma cells, and a moderate number of polymorphonuclear leukocytes. The epidermis shows abnormal keratinization; many of the cells retain their cellular outline and granularity.[23]

DeNicola and colleagues described Rosenau's depression, which seems to be similar if not identical to Beau's lines.[24]

## Onycholysis

Onycholysis has been discussed elsewhere (see Chapters 9, 11, and 18). Its correlation with systemic disease is overrated, especially because it is associated much more frequently with such diverse conditions as trauma, drug reactions, psoriasis, fungus, local allergy, and irritant reactions.[25]

Onycholysis is believed by some to be correlated with thyroid disease. It has been said that separation often occurs in thyrotoxicosis,[26,27] in which the earliest stage is conversion of the curved adhesion to a straight line. This adhesion line later dips proximally into the nail bed as a jagged projection.[26] This description is that of Plummer's nails, which usually starts at the fourth and then the fifth fingers.[24] X-ray examination has been used to help differentiate between onycholysis associated with thyroid disease and that resulting from other causes.[24] Most cases of thyroid disease do not manifest onycholysis.

Table 15.2 lists several systemic diseases that have been associated with onycholysis.

## Pitting

Pitting has been described earlier (see Chapter 11). Its diagnostic relationship to systemic disease is doubtful because numerous dermatitides in the vicinity of the proximal nail fold may cause parakeratotic foci in the proximal matrix and thus pitting. Once the pits are visible in the more distal nail, sufficient time has passed so that the etiologic lesion may have disappeared or the patient may not remember whether there ever was an abnormality in that area.

| TABLE 15–2. Systemic diseases associated with onycholysis | |
| --- | --- |
| Amyloid and multiple myeloma[203] | Pellagra[1] |
| Anemia[16] | Pemphigus vulgaris[55] |
| Bantu porphyria[17] | Pleural effusion[a] |
| Bronchiectasis (see yellow nail syndrome)[a] | Porphyria cutanea tarda[55] |
| Carcinoma (lung)[247] | Pregnancy[17] |
| Circulatory disorders | Pseudoporphyria of hemodialysis[249] (possible photo-induced) |
| Cronkhite-Canada syndrome[248] | Psoriatic arthritis |
| Cutaneous T cell lymphoma (mycosis fungoides)[17] | Pustular eruption of pregnancy[250] (impetigo herpetiformis) |
| Diabetes mellitus[17] | Raynaud's phenomenon[14] |
| Drug reaction (see Chapter 16) | Reiter's syndrome |
| Erythropoietic porphyria[55] | Scleroderma[124] |
| Erythropoietic protoporphyria[17] | Sézary syndrome[251] |
| Histiocytosis X[206] | Syphilis[16] (secondary and tertiary) |
| Ischemia (peripheral) | Thyroid disease[18] |
| Leprosy[16] | Vitamin C deficiency[63] |
| Lupus erythematosus[22] | Yellow nail syndrome[125,126] |
| Neuritis[16] | |

[a]See discussion of yellow nail syndrome in text.

We find pitting occasionally helpful in building a clinical case for psoriatic arthritis in the absence of other definitive markers, especially when it is the only cutaneous manifestation of psoriasis. Lovoy[28] and Pajarre[29] and their colleagues associated pitting with human leukocyte antigen (HLA) inheritance, psoriatic arthritis, and Reiter's syndrome. Urowitz and others reported pitting in association with systemic lupus erythematosus.[30] We have seen, and Dupre and associates[31] have noted, pitting in patients with dermatomyositis. The pitting may exhibit tight longitudinal rows in HLA-B27 inheritance.[29] We have only seen the latter orientation of pits in alopecia areata. Large pitting (elkonyxis) confined to the lunula has been described in syphilis.[24] Sarcoid[32] and pemphigus vulgaris[33] have been reported to cause nail pitting.

## Koilonychia (Spoon Nails)

Spoon-shaped nails are not uncommon. Their relationship to systemic disease is at times relatively clear, but most frequently nebulous. Classically, when koilonychia is mentioned, one's thoughts turn to iron deficiency anemia or Plummer–Vinson syndrome. This is not, however, one of the more common causes. In our experience, the most most common presentation occurs in babies as a traumatic response to rigid shoes that are perhaps too tight. A drop of water placed on a spoon nail will not roll off.[34] The spooning is best viewed from the side.

The exact cause of koilonychia is at best elusive, but several hypotheses have been given. Stone suggested that angulation of the nail matrix secondary to connective tissue changes is the cause: 'Spooning of the nail occurs when the distal matrix is relatively low compared to the proximal matrix and vice-versa for clubbing.'[35] Jalili and Al-Kassaf[36] found that the cystine content was somewhat low in the nails of patients with anemia and very low when koilonychia was present. They thus concluded that a deficiency of sulfur-containing amino acids played a role in the pathogenesis of koilonychia.[36] This association might be more superficial than real and could possibly reflect malnutrition. Samman believed that the cause is thinning and softening of the nail plate.[10] Most publications categorize spoon nails into three major groups: idiopathic, hereditary, and acquired. We believe that acquired is the largest group. Trauma, dermatologic diseases such as psoriasis and fungal infection, and distal ischemia as in Raynaud's phenomenon seem to be the most common offenders. Occupational koilonychia has been reported in numerous instances and unusually in the toenails of boys who pull rickshaws.[37] The authors of this article state that spoon nails caused by systemic diseases exhibit a concavity from side to side, with the edges everted and the nail plates themselves thinned. Rickshaw boys tended to have the concavity from end to end, with eversion of the free margin of the nail plate associated with thickening.[37] The inertia of stopping and starting the rickshaw was the probable cause. Koilonychia has also been associated with an upper gastrointestinal tract carcinoma.[3]

The petaloid nail is an early stage of koilonychia and is characterized by flattening of the nail.[38]

The idiopathic group is probably the second largest and may be the most common if the investigator does not rigorously pursue a cause. We most frequently find that children fit into this group more often than adults. One should rule out trauma from shoes and finger sucking before categorizing children as such. Serrated koilonychia syndrome has been described as a combination of koilonychia and deep longitudinal grooving of all nails.[39]

Koilonychia can be inherited in a dominant manner with a high degree of penetration.[40] Inherited koilonychia may be seen in association with total leukonychia.[41] This group is probably the least commonly encountered.

Stone compiled an extensive list of possible diseases associated with koilonychia (Table 15.3).[34,35] Some additions include alopecia areata,[42] carpal tunnel syndrome,[19] and scurvy.[43]

## Longitudinal Pigmented Bands

The vast majority of cases of longitudinal pigmented bands have no clear association with systemic disease. It seems that the more heavily pigmented the individual's skin, the more likely it is that longitudinal pigmented bands will form in the nails. Trauma, dermatologic conditions (especially lichen planus), nevi, drugs, fungi, and other factors may cause these bands.[24,44,45]

Melanoma is certainly a possible cause and must be considered in any patient with these bands (see Chapters 7 and 17). Melanocyte-

**TABLE 15–3. Classification of spoon nails**

I. Idiopathic
II. Hereditary, congenital, and associated with other ectodermal defects
   A. Spoon nails only, as a dominant
   B. Monilethrix
   C. Palmar hyperkeratoses
   D. Steatocystoma multiplex
   E. Spoon-fissured nail
   F. LEOPARD syndrome (leukokoilonychia)[47]
   G. Nail-patella syndrome[47,166]
   H. Nezelof syndrome[47]
   I. Incontinentia pigmenti[47]
   J. Gottron's syndrome (acrogeria)[47]
   K. Ectodermal dysplasia with anhydrosis[47]
   L. Chondroectodermal dysplasia (Ellis-van Creveld syndrome)[47]
   M. Palmoplantar keratoderma, maleda type[47]
   N. Focal dermal hypoplasia (Goltz's syndrome)[47]
III. Acquired
   A. Cardiovascular
     1. Anemia
       a. Hypochromic anemia (Plummer-Vinson syndrome)
       b. Epithelial iron deficiency (in our opinion a secondary phenomenon)
       c. Cystine deficiency (in our opinion a secondary phenomenon)
       d. Hemoglobinopathy SG[47]
     2. Polycythemia vera
     3. Coronary disease
   B. Infections: syphilis, fungus

C. Metabolic
   1. Acromegaly
   2. Hypothyroidism
   3. Thyrotoxicosis
   4. Porphyria cutanea tarda[47]
   5. Malnutrition[52]
   6. Pellagra[16]
D. Traumatic and occupational
   1. Petroleum products
   2. Alkalis and acids
   3. Homemakers, chimney sweeps
   4. Thioglycolate (hairdressers)[47]
   5. Frostbite[16]
   6. Thermal burns[16]
E. Miscellaneous
   1. Psoriasis
   2. Lichen planus
   3. Acanthosis nigricans
   4. Banti's syndrome: nails cured with splenectomy
   5. Postgastrectomy
   6. Raynaud's disease
   7. Cachexia
   8. Scleroderma
   9. Toenails of some normal children (our experience)
   10. Hypovitaminoses ($B_2$ and especially C)[47]
   11. Darier's disease[47]
   12. Alopecia areata[7,47]
   13. Renal transplant[47]
   14. Polyglobulias (erythropoietin-producing tumors)[16]
   15. Primary amyloid (slight spooning)[47]
   16. Alopecia areata

From Stone OJ: Spoon nails and clubbing. Cutis 16:235, 1975; Stone OJ, Maberry JD: Spoon nails and clubbing. Tex State J Med 61:620, 1965. Used with permission.

stimulating hormone often plays a role in the pathogenesis of longitudinal pigmented bands associated with systemic diseases. The more lightly pigmented an individual, the more likely it is that longitudinal pigmented bands are associated with melanoma or systemic disease (Table 15.4). Longitudinal pigmented bands associated with systemic changes are usually in multiple nails, although they occur idiopathically in darkly pigmented patients (see Chapters 7 and 17).

# NAIL ABNORMALITIES MORE SPECIFICALLY ASSOCIATED WITH SYSTEMIC DISEASE

## Key Features

* True leukonychia: White coloration in the nail plate due to pathology that arose in the nail matrix; doesn't change with pressure
* Apparent leukonychia: Pathology in the nail bed is seen through the nail plate giving a white appearance
* Pseudoleukonychia: Exogenous effect (such as fungal infection) on the nail plate

## Leukonychia (White Nails)

There are several subtypes of leukonychia (white nails): true leukonychia (pathology originates in the matrix and emerges in the nail plate), apparent leukonychia (pathology is in the nail bed), and pseudoleukonychia (nail plate pathology is exogenous, e.g. onychomycosis).[18] Leukonychia associated with systemic disease is usually true leukonychia or apparent leukonychia.

## True Leukonychia

True leukonychia can be total, subtotal, or partial (transverse, punctuate, longitudinal most commonly). Total or subtotal leukonychia can be inherited, sporadic or associated with systemic illness.[18,46] Partial leukonychia is especially common in the transverse and punctate forms and is most commonly caused by trauma to the matrix from overly aggressive manicuring of the proximal nail fold area. There are however, numerous associations with drugs or systemic illness (Table 15.5).[47]

Histologically, parakeratosis and large, immature keratohyaline granules have been described in the areas of leukonychia.[46] However, electron microscopic findings suggest that clear lipid vacuoles may actually be the cause of leukonychia.[48]

| TABLE 15-4. Longitudinal pigmented bands and systemic disorders* |
| --- |
| Acrodermatitis enteropathica[257] |
| Addison's disease[72] |
| Acquired immunodeficiency syndrome[92] |
| Amyloid (primary)[47] |
| Arsenic intoxication[16] |
| Carcinoma of the breast[258] |
| Carpal tunnel syndrome[259] |
| Cushing's syndrome (postadrenalectomy)[260] |
| Fluorosis[26,120] |
| Gastrointestinal diseases[16] |
| Hemosiderosis[257] |
| Hyperbilirubinemia[92] |
| Hyperthyroidism[92] |
| Hypopituitarism[257] |
| Irradiation[257] |
| Malnutrition[120] |
| Melanoma (metastatic)[257] |
| Ochronosis[257] |
| Peutz-Jeghers syndrome[26,261] |
| Porphyria[26] |
| Pregnancy[76] |
| Syphilis (secondary)[257] |
| *See also Chapter 7. |

## TABLE 15-5. Disorders associated with true leukonychia (Mees' lines)

### Poisoning/drug induced

| | |
| --- | --- |
| Antimony poisoning[252] | Fluorosis[14] |
| Arsenic poisoning[27,253,254] | Lead poisoning[252] |
| Carbon monoxide poisoning[204] | Thallium poisoning[27] |
| Chemotherapeutic drugs | |

### Metabolic/endocrine

| | |
| --- | --- |
| Cachectic state[14] | Parathyroid insufficiency[14] |
| Gout[14] | Pellagra[27] |
| Hyperalbuminemia[14] | Protein deficiency[14] |
| Hypocalcemia[5] | Vitamin $B_{12}$ deficiency[14] |
| Menstrual cycle[14,b] | Zinc deficiency[14] |

### Malignancy/hematologic disorders

| | |
| --- | --- |
| Carcinoid[255] | Warm-reacting antibody |
| Hodgkin's disease[27] | immunohemolytic |
| Sickle cell anemia[27] | anemia[256] |

### Infectious disease

| | |
| --- | --- |
| Endemic typhus[252] | Syphilis[14] |
| Herpes zoster[14] | Tuberculosis[14] |
| Leprosy[27] | Parasitic Infection[17] |
| Malaria[27] | (Mee's lines) |
| Measles[14] | |

### Dermatologic disease

Erythema multiforme[14]
Psoriasis[27]

### Cardiopulmonary disease

| | |
| --- | --- |
| Cardiac failure[27] | Shock[14] |
| Myocardial infarction[27] | Empyema[13] |
| Pneumonia[27] | |

### Renal disease

| | |
| --- | --- |
| Renal failure[26,27,33,34] | Glomerulonephritis[33] |
| Acute rejection of | Renal transplant[252] |
| renal allograft[252] | |

### Miscellaneous

| | |
| --- | --- |
| Childbirth[a] | Fracture[14] |
| Crush injury[b] | Peripheral neuropathy[14] |
| Cryotherapy (local)[14] | Ulcerative proctitis[b] |

[a]C.R. Daniel, unpublished observation.
[b]C.R. Daniel, personal observation.
the abnormal nail

Mees' lines are transverse types of true leukonychia associated with systemic disease.[18] Arsenic intoxication was classically believed to be the major cause of Mees' lines. It is now well known that numerous severe systemic insults may be the stimuli to initiate the abnormality (see Table 15.5).[44,49] It has been said that Mees' lines that occur as a result of arsenic poisoning are due to actual deposition of arsenic in the nail plate (Fig. 15.4).[50] One may approximate the time of onset of systemic illness by measuring the distance from the Mees' line to the proximal nail fold, as one can do with Beau's lines.

Mees' lines tend to be single but may be multiple transverse white lines that occur in the nail plate and move distally as the nail grows. If one squeezes the distal digit, the line does not disappear because it is a permanent alteration of that particular focus of nail plate. Biopsy of a probable Mees' line has shown the nail plate to appear 'fragmented', with the underlying nail bed and nail matrix showing nothing of note.[23] This fragmentation probably represents a focus of abnormally formed cells exhibiting parakeratosis imparted to the nail plate by the compromised matrix.

Several important points help differentiate local trauma-induced lesions from those associated with systemic disease:

1. Mees' and Muehrcke's lines tend to occur on several nails at once (traumatically induced lines may too, but less frequently).
2. These systemic-disease-associated lines usually spread across the entire breadth of the nail bed or plate and tend to be more homogeneous and have smoother borders.[44]
3. In our experience, as well as that of Zaias,[3] these lines tend to have a similar contour to the distal lunula, with a rounded distal edge. Trauma-induced lines tend to be more linear and resemble the contour of the proximal nail fold[3] and often do not span the entire breadth of the nail plate.

4. One usually finds no specific history of sufficient physical trauma to the cuticle area in patients with Mees' or Muehrcke's lines (Fig. 15.5).
5. A systemic insult usually may be correlated with the onset of the lines.

In our experience, only one consistent mimic of a Mees' line exists: The situation in which only the distal aspect of the lunula is

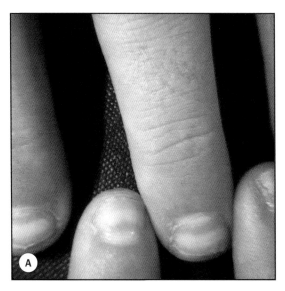

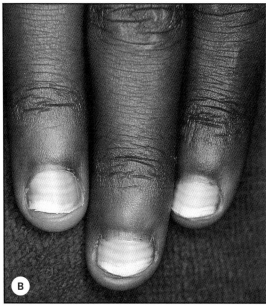

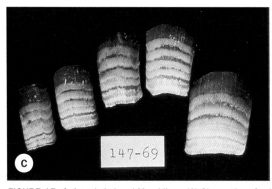

147-69

FIGURE 15–4. Arsenic-induced Mees' lines. (A) Observation of nails led to discovery of criminal case of arsenic poisoning; (B) Mees' lines caused by chemotherapy; (C) Nails taken at autopsy of patient with arsenic poisoning (courtesy of Dr N. Grannemann).

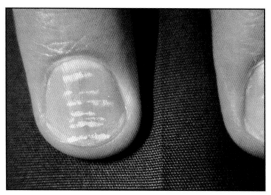

FIGURE 15–5. Trauma to cuticle producing transverse leukonychia, not Mees' lines.

apparent. This may sometimes be caused by an erythematosus masking of the more proximal lunula. The tip-off is that this line (or lines) does not move out with the growing nail plate.

## Apparent Leukonychia

Apparent leukonychia is caused by changes in the nail bed that are seen through the nail plate.[18] Several patterns of apparent leukoncychia have been classically described: Muehrke's lines, half-and-half (Lindsay's) nails, Terry's nails and others.

## Muehrcke's Lines

Muehrcke's lines are double white transverse lines that represent an abnormality of the nail vascular bed. Squeezing the distal digit will cause the lines to disappear temporarily.[44] They are not palpable and do not indent the nail, and it has been noted that they are usually found on the second, third, and fourth fingernails.[51] They sometimes occur when chronic hypoalbuminemia persists and tend to disappear when the serum albumin is above 2.2 g/100 mL.[52] Their exact pathogenesis has not been adequately explained, but possibly a localized edematous state in the nail bed exerts pressure on the underlying vasculature, thus decreasing the normal erythema seen through the nail plate[23] (Fig. 15.6).

A number of disease states causing hypoalbuminemia may be associated with Muehrcke's lines, such as the nephrotic syndrome and glomerulonephritis. Liver disease[52] and malnutrition[51] are among those that have been mentioned. A case has been reported attempting to correlate Muehrcke's lines with normal serum albumin, but this patient may have had Mees' lines.[53] A case of Muehrcke's lines has been reported after trauma.[54]

Muehrcke's lines have been reported in association with heart transplantation in patients who had transient hypoalbuminemia.[55,56] Blanchable transverse white bands have been reported in association with wintertime acrocyanosis in an otherwise healthy young patient.[57]

## Half-and-Half (Lindsay's Nails)

Lindsay's nails (half-and-half nails) are associated with chronic renal insufficiency (see p. 164). They are a form of apparent leukonychia exhibiting either a whitish or normal proximal half and a distinctly abnormal brownish distal portion. This distal portion begins proximally where the normal or whitish nail ends

153

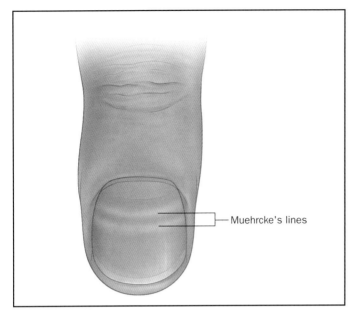

FIGURE 15–6. Muehrcke's lines.

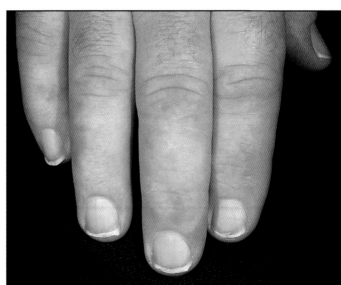

FIGURE 15–8. Terry's nails (courtesy of Dr Jeffrey Callen).

and terminates distally where the free end of the nail loses its attachment to the hyponychium[44,58,59] (Fig. 15.7). It has been our experience that this description most aptly describes the half-and-half nail and leaves less room for imitations. Lindsay's description, as well as crescents, are seen frequently in renal failure but not infrequently otherwise.[58–60] Psoriasis is the most common cause of a pseudo half-and-half nail appearance.

## Terry's Nails

In 1954, Terry described apparent leukonychia over the entire nail bed with narrow distal pink band in 82 of 100 cirrhotic patients.[61] In a large prospective study, Holzberg and Walker revised the description to include a pink or brown band 0.5–3.0 mm wide, which histologically demonstrated telangectasias in the dermis (Fig. 15.8).[62] Their study showed association with cirrhosis, congestive heart failure, diabetes mellitus, and age. When seen in younger individuals, Terry's nails should prompt consideration of an investigation for systemic disease.

Holzberg and Walker's description is very close to Daniel's description of the the erythematous crescent.[44,58,59] Thyrotoxicosis, 'pulmonary eosinophilia', malnutrition, or 'keratoses' were found in other patients who had Terry's nails but who did not exhibit cirrhosis.[63] We have noticed numerous patients who had a similar nail appearance (but who never had liver disease), and we concluded that this disorder is a reaction pattern and is not pathognomonic for cirrhosis (also see the following discussion of erythematous crescents). The white color has been said to be caused by overgrowth

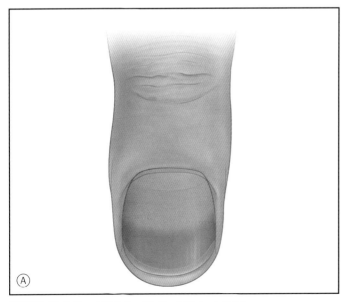

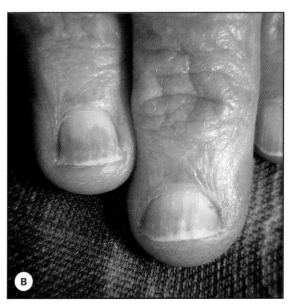

FIGURE 15–7. (A and B) Half-and-half nail (Lindsay's Nails).

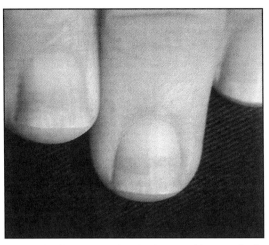

FIGURE 15-9. Terry's nail. Note the close resemblance to what has been labeled by some as half-and-half nail.

| TABLE 15-6. Other names for clubbed fingers |
| --- |
| Acropachy |
| Digital hippocratism[16] |
| Drumstick fingers[18] |
| Dysacromelia[38] |
| Hippocratic nails (or fingers)[18] |
| Parrot-beak nails[18] |
| Serpent-head nails[18] |
| Trommelschlagelfinger[56] |
| Watch-glass nails[18] |

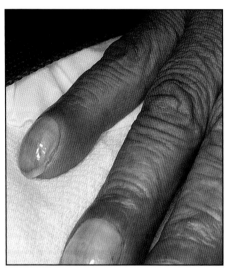

FIGURE 15-10. Clubbing (courtesy of Dr Jeffrey Callen)

of connective tissue between the nail and bone, reducing the amount of blood in the subcapillary plexus[9] (Fig. 15.9).

## Erythematous Crescent

The erythematous crescent represents a nail disorder that has received little attention.[44,58,59] It is defined as an abnormally prominent erythematous band that is seen at the distal portion of the nail vascular bed and is an anomaly of that structure. The proximal nail is normal. It may be thought of as a prominent onychodermal band. This band, described by Terry[63] in combination with a proximal whitish portion of the nail, illustrates Terry's nail associated with cirrhosis.

In our experience, the erythematous crescent may or may not be associated with an abnormally white proximal nail portion. Holzberg and Walker describe pink to white color of the nail bed proximal to the band in Terry's nails.[62] Crescents were seen more frequently in patients with chronic medical illnesses such as renal failure[58-60] but may appear in healthy persons as well. Thus, the crescent is more of academic interest and not of particular diagnostic importance.[44,58,59] It may mimic the half-and-half nail.[64]

## Clubbing

Clubbing is an important physical finding that seems unique to humans.[51] Although this abnormality may be familial or idiopathic, its relationship to systemic disease is at times unquestionable. Much has been written on the subject from antiquity to the present. It has been called by many names (Table 15.6). Stone and

Maberry studied clubbing extensively and rationally classified it into three major categories: idiopathic, hereditary–congenital, and acquired.[34,35] Each of these three categories is addressed later.

In our opinion, two major findings are important to classify nail changes as clubbing. First, and most important, the ungual–phalangeal angle (Lovibond's angle) must be increased in true clubbing. The normal nail proceeds from the finger at an obtuse angle of about 160°[65] (Fig. 15.10). This can be visualized by placing the base of a 'V' at the proximal nail fold and pointing one of its arms toward the distal end of the nail and the other proximally toward the wrist. With gross clubbing, the angle at the base of the nail becomes greater than or equal to 180°[65] (Fig. 15.11). Two common conditions may seem to mimic the increasing of the angle. Curved nails usually manifest their abnormal appearance by the distal part of the nail curving downward.[65] Paronychia exhibiting

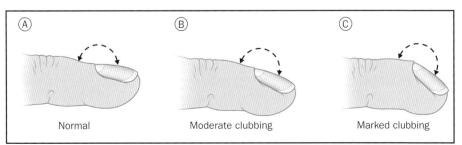

| (A) | (B) | (C) |
| --- | --- | --- |
| Normal | Moderate clubbing | Marked clubbing |

FIGURE 15-11. Clubbing. (A) Normal; (B) moderate clubbing; (C) marked clubbing (from ref 39, used with permission).

inflamed proximal nail fold tissue may cause an apparent pseudo-clubbing by the bulging of the cuticular area. Pseudoclubbing may have hypercurvature of both transverse and longitudinal axes (which is seen in true clubbing), however, the unguo–phalangeal angle is preserved.[66] Pseudoclubbing may be seen in osteitis fibrosa cystica[67] as well as in other conditions causing resorption of the distal phalanx. **Another important physical finding is the development of a spongy feel as one pushes downward on the tissue just proximal to the cuticle. This finding is probably due to fibrovascular hyperplasia of the underlying soft tissue.**

Numerous hypotheses have been presented to explain clubbing. Stone and Maberry theorized that clubbing is caused by angulation of the nail matrix secondary to connective tissue changes. They believed that the distal nail matrix is relatively high compared with the proximal matrix.[34,35]

Mendlowitz[68] found, in all the cases of simple clubbing he studied, except hereditary clubbing, that the blood flow per unit surface or per volume of fingertip was abnormally high. These excessive flow rates were at least partially caused by elevated digital arterial pressure. He also concluded that abnormally high blood flow and digital arterial pressure, after release of sympathetic tone, are peculiar to ordinary clubbing and are integral forces in its development. Blood flow and pressure values were normal in hereditary clubbing. In addition, he noted that the blood flow per unit of tissue and the digital arterial pressure were within normal limits in hypertrophic osteoarthropathy.[68] Hall believed that the capillary blood flow is less than in normal fingers even though overall flow is increased through dilated arteriovenous anastomoses.[69] He indicated that this abnormal circulation was due to the presence of reduced ferritin. Hall also suggested that many intrathoracic diseases that induce clubbing manifest pulmonary arteriovenous shunts or their equivalents, which allow reduced ferritin to pass into the peripheral circulation instead of being rendered inert by oxidation in normal lung tissue. Bashour had a similar opinion and stated that reduced tissue oxygen tension secondary to blood shunting caused by a peripheral vasodilator, rather than an increased oxygen supply over tissue demand was the cause of clubbing.[70] Ginsburg and Brown found increased urinary estrogen excretion in a group of 11 men with hypertrophic pulmonary osteoarthropathy.[71]

**Acquired, simple, bilateral clubbing is most often associated with cardiopulmonary disease.** Approximately 80% of simple clubbing is associated with respiratory ailments, and 10 to 15% is associated with cardiovascular and extrathoracic diseases.[34,35] In our experience, this clubbing is most frequently bilateral. It often begins in the thumb and index finger.[71] 'In chronic bronchial infections, the appearance of clubbing depends on three criteria: long duration, often more than 10 years, hypoxia, and hyperglobulinemia. If one is missing, there is little likelihood of clubbing developing.'[38]

Acquired unilateral or single-digit clubbing is usually related to vascular lesions in that extremity, such as a peripheral shunt, aneurysm, or arteriovenous fistula, but Pancoast tumors, erythromelalgia, or lymphadenitis may cause unilateral clubbing.[34,35] When a single nail is involved, the cause is usually traumatic but may be congenital.[34,35]

Acquired hypertrophic osteoarthropathy has six characteristics, according to Stone and Maberry:[34,35]

1. Simple clubbing, including the toes.
2. Hypertrophy of the upper and lower extremities, with soft tissue proliferation and, at times, edema simulating elephantiasis.

3. Peripheral neurovascular diseases such as local cyanosis, hyperhidrosis, paresthesia, and erythema.
4. **Bone pain** aggravated by lowering the extremity, proliferative periostitis radiographically manifesting a laminated sheath along the shaft or a compact layer like wax dripping along a candle.
5. Joint pain and swelling.
6. Muscle weakness.

They also emphasized that when the syndrome is complete a malignant thoracic tumor, especially bronchogenic carcinoma, is seen in at least 90% of the cases.[34,35]

Several miscellaneous diseases associated with acquired clubbing and not mentioned in Stone's extensive compilation of causes of clubbing (Table 15.7) include systemic lupus erythematosus,[68,72] poisoning[22] with phosphorus, vinyl chloride, alcohol, mercury or beryllium, hyperparathyroidism,[73] Down syndrome,[74] Ayerza's syndrome (asthma in infancy),[22] amebiasis,[22] familial polyposis,[22] Gardner's syndrome,[22] chronic active hepatitis,[22] POEMS syndrome,[22] Graves' disease,[22] causalgia,[22] sarcoidosis and painful clubbing with discomfort relieved by colchicine therapy,[75] alpha heavy-chain disease (diffuse intestinal lymphoma),[76] Osler–Weber–Rendu disease,[76] laxative abuse,[77] chronic obstructive jaundice,[26] Crohn's disease,[78] and vinyl chloride disease.[39] Burgdorf stated that clubbing found in Crohn's disease may help differentiate it from ulcerative colitis,[78] but we have not found this useful. Idiopathic and hereditary clubbing may be transmitted as a simple Mendelian-dominant or autosomal-dominant sex-limited trait with variable penetrance. It has an insidious onset, usually starting after puberty, and may affect both fingernails and toenails.[79] Pachydermoperiostosis is rare and is generally considered idiopathic. It is familial in more than half of the cases and consists of clubbing, pawlike or spade-like enlargement of the hands, thickening of the legs and forearms involving the bones as well as the soft tissue, thickening of the forehead and scalp (cutis verticis gyrata), and symmetric periosteal bone ossification.[34,35] It is more likely to initially affect adolescent males and be self-limited. The sella turcica is normal, distinguishing pachydermoperiostosis from classic acromegaly.[34,35] Chronic lymphedema and endocrine abnormalities have been associated with pachydermoperiostosis.[80]

Generally, there is no specific treatment for clubbing other than eliminating the predisposing cause. As mentioned, colchicine has been used for the subsequent pain. Remission of clubbing has been observed after cutting the vagus nerve in the thorax, even when the associated pulmonary malignancy was not removed.[81]

The histologic picture of the tissue involved illustrates three histologic patterns corresponding to the severity of clubbing:[23]

1. Early clubbing is associated with an increase in dermal fibroblasts and connective tissue.
2. Moderate clubbing is accompanied by mucoid degeneration of the ground substances.
3. Severe clubbing is accompanied by marked interstitial edema and a mild infiltrate of plasma cells, lymphocytes, and primitive fibroblasts.

It is not clear from Lewin's article, but the prior description probably relates to simple, acquired clubbing. Interestingly, bulbous rete pegs (or keratin cysts) were noted in all cases.[23]

DeNicola and colleagues mentioned that the nail plate is thickened.[24] 'It has rightly been said that clubbing is one of those phenomena with which we appear to know more about it than we really do.'[65]

**TABLE 15–7. Classification of clubbing**

I. Idiopathic
II. Hereditary, congenital[262]
   A. Citrullinemia[263]
   B. Other[76]
III. Acquired
   A. Pulmonary
     1. Neoplasms of lung
     2. Bronchitis, bronchiectasis, emphysema, lung abscess, cyst, tuberculosis, pulmonary fibrosis, blastomycosis, acute pneumonia, pulmonary endarteritis, chronic passive congestion
     3. Mediastinal: fibrosarcoma, mesoendothelioma, Hodgkin's disease, lymphoma, pseudotumor (dilation of esophagus)
     4. Metastatic neoplasm (fibrosarcoma, giant cell tumor)
   B. Cardiovascular
     1. Congenital heart disease (cyanotic)
     2. Subacute bacterial endocarditis
     3. Congestive heart failure
     4. Chronic myelogenous leukemia
     5. Myxoid tumor
     6. Acyanotic congenital heart diseases (rare)
   C. Hepatic
     1. Cirrhosis (cholangiolitic, malarial, hemochromatotic)
     2. Portal cirrhosis, secondary amyloidosis
   D. Gastrointestinal
     1. Chronic diarrhea, sprue
     2. Ulcerative colitis
     3. Neoplasms
     4. *Ascaris*
   E. Renal: chronic pyelonephritis (rare)
   F. Toxic: phosphorus, arsenic, alcohol, mercury, beryllium, reduced ferritin
   G. Miscellaneous (rare): syphilis, syringomyelia, Maffucci's syndrome, congenital dysplasia, angiectasis, chronic familial neutropenia, post-thyroidectomy, myxedema, cretinism, primary polycythemia, leprosy, rheumatic fever, Raynaud's disease, scleroderma, acrocyanosis, chilblains, Kaposi's sarcoma, transitory physiology in newborn resulting from reversal of circulation at birth,[47] Gottron's syndrome (acrogeria)[47]
   H. Unilateral or unidigital
     1. Arterial aneurysm (aortic auxillary)
     2. Brachial arteriovenous fistula
     3. Subluxation of shoulder
     4. Pancoast's tumors
     5. Erythromelalgia
     6. Lymphangitis
     7. Median nerve injury
     8. Local trauma
     9. Felon
     10. Tophaceous gout
     11. Sarcoidosis

From Stone OJ: Spoon nails and clubbing. Cutis 16:235, 1975; Stone OJ, Maberry JD: Spoon nails and clubbing. Tex State J Med 61:620, 1965. Used with permission.

# NAIL ABNORMALITIES ASSOCIATED WITH DISEASE OF A SPECIFIC ORGAN SYSTEM

The following is a brief system-by-system or category approach to nail changes associated with particular disorders. Emphasis is placed on major findings, and tables include a partial listing of associated disorders. For additional information, see the remainder of this chapter and Chapter 7 on nail pigmentation.

## Cardiovascular, Hematologic, and Ischemic Disorders

Reddish lunulae have been associated with heart failure,[82] even though other causes of this color change have been noted (see Chapter 7). Raynaud's phenomenon and other causes of peripheral ischemia, including koilonychia, may cause nail dystrophy. The yellow nail syndrome has been reported in association with ECG abnormalities.[83]

Kawasaki disease, seen predominantly in children, is characterized by vasculitis with predilection for the coronary arteries. Early diagnosis and initiation of immunoglobulin therapy may prevent serious coronary artery damage. The most sensitive early sign is nonpurulent conjunctivitis, the most specific signs are perianal eruption and edema, erythema and desquamation that usually begins on the periungual skin. Nail shedding has also been reported in Kawasaki syndrome.[84]

Blood groups may be demonstrated from nail clippings and may be important if only hands and feet are obtainable for study or if mummification or putrefaction has set in.[39,86] Also, a victim's blood-tinged material under an assailant's nails may be important in legal cases. Generally, few if any nail changes are pathognomonic in this group. Table 15.8 lists changes associated with cardiovascular, hematologic, and ischemic conditions (see also Tables 15.1, 15.3, and 15.7).

Samman treated his patients who have cold hands or Raynaud's phenomenon with isonicotinic acid hydrazide, thymoxamine hydrochloride, warm gloves, and ultraviolet B exposure of the terminal phalanges. He stated that the latter treatment may provide relief for several months.[87]

## Gastrointestinal Disorders

It is our opinion that there are rarely specific nail findings in gastrointestinal disorders.

Several onychopathies are worthy of mention, however, because they have in the past been thought to be relatively specific (Table 15.9).

Azure lunulae are associated with hepatolenticular degeneration (Wilson's disease). This discoloration is localized to the lunulae as opposed to a similar azure color in other parts of the nail bed in argyria, with antimalarials, and *Pseudomonas* infections.[49,88] A patient taking a phenolphthalein-containing laxative exhibited a similar color change localized to the lunulae; the change was especially marked in the thumbnails and was unaffected by pressure on the nail.[88] Terry's nails, supposedly indicative of cirrhosis, are described as an abnormal white appearance of the nail except for the distal portion that is just proximal to the free end of the nail. This portion, the distal pink zone, is exaggerated

TABLE 15–8. Nail changes associated with cardiovascular, hematologic, and ischemic conditions

| DISEASE | NAIL ABNORMALITY |
|---|---|
| Aortic insufficiency | Quincke's pulse |
| Anemia (general)[6] | Nail dystrophy |
| Endocarditis (bacterial) | Splinter hemorrhages,[7] clubbing[264] |
| Fabry's disease[77] | Turtle-back nail configuration |
| Heart failure[64] | Reddish lunulae |
| Hypertension[7] | Splinter hemorrhages |
| Ischemia | Nonspecific dystrophy; pterygium, nail thickening[265] |
| Leukemia[16] | Splinter hemorrhages |
| Marfan syndrome (aneurysm)[18] | Long and narrow nails |
| Mitral stenosis[26] | Splinter hemorrhages |
| Myocardial infarction (see Chapter 7) | Mees' lines |
| Osler-Weber-Rendu disease | Telangiectasia[16] |
| Pernicious anemia[266] | Splinter hemorrhage[1] |
| Porphyria (erythropoietic)[52] | Blue fingernails |
| Periarteritis nodosa[243] | Splinter hemorrhages |
| Scurvy[26] | Splinter hemorrhages |
| Sickle-cell anemia (see Chapter 7) | Mees' lines |
| Thrombocytopenia[16] | Splinter hemorrhages |
| Thrombosis[16] | Onychomadesis |
| Vasculitis[26] | Splinter hemorrhages |
| Polyglobulias (erythropoietin-producing tumor)[16] | Koilonychia, reddish nail |
| Erythropoietic porphyria[55] | Onycholysis |
| Varicose lesions (trophic)[47] | Pachyonychogryphosis |
| Wegener's granulomatosis[267] | Periungual infarcts |

in this disorder and is named the onychodermal band. Its appearance does not diminish upon squeezing the digit.[63]

In Jemec's study of 569 hospital patients, statistical analysis showed an association between pincer nails (nails with abnormally increased transverse curvature) and gastrointestinal disease.[1]

There is an interesting report of hand and nail contact with methacrylate causing nausea and diarrhea.[89] Because nail cosmetics may contain methacrylate, the association is worth remembering. See the pulmonary section in this text for a discussion of Bazex's paraneoplastic syndrome.

## Metabolic-Hormonal-Endocrine Condition

Almost all onychopathies associated with the endocrine system are nonspecific (Table 15.10).[90,91] Bissell and colleagues described longitudinal pigmented bands that may occur in patients with Addison's disease.[92] These have more meaning when they occur in lightly pigmented individuals than in more heavily pigmented patients[44] (see the discussion above of longitudinal pigmented bands and, in Chapter 7, nail pigmentation). DeNicola and others suggested a radiologic method to distinguish onycholysis in thyroid disease from that caused by other diseases.[24] Nails in general are often brittle with hormonal disease.[93,94]

## Some Infectious Diseases

Findings associated with infectious diseases are basically nonspecific. Syphilis has been associated with numerous nail changes. Some of these include elkonyxis (loss of nail plate substance in the lunula only);[24] paronychia (sometimes ulcerative),[24] thought in the past to be a typical sign of congenital lues;[95] thinning and onychomadesis;[24] fragility with fissuring of the free margin;[24] racket nail;[24] and deep violet arch of Milan.[24] Several characteristics have been reported: reddish lunulae in lymphogranuloma venereum,[24] gray ardesia nail color during fever[24] or Mees' lines in malaria patients,[49] paronychia in tularemia,[9] nonspecific changes in typhoid fever,[9] atrophic nail changes in Job's syndrome,[96] and grayish discoloration in visceral leishmaniasis.[97] Leprosy may show numerous manifestations, including leukonychia and painful subungual abscess,[24] disappearing lunula,[24] lilac line of Milan,[24] and pterygium unguium.[98]

Toxoplasmosis has been associated with lichen planus verrucosus et reticularise of Kaposi and 'nail dystrophy'.[99] Beau's lines and nail shedding may occur with toxic shock.[100]

Accumulation of occult blood under the fingernails, especially the thumb and index finger in dentists, may be a mechanism for the spread of blood-borne infection such as hepatitis B.[101] It is recommended that dentists and others who have contact with blood and body fluids wear surgical gloves.[101] Scabies may take refuge under nails, leading to reinfection.[102,103]

Other associations are listed elsewhere (see Chapter 7).[104]

## The Nails in Patients with Human Immunodeficiency Virus

Because of the mobility of our society, human immunodeficiency virus (HIV) infection is becoming more prevalent worldwide. Whether one practices in a university setting, rural environment, or developing country, one can expect to encounter this disorder. Patients who are HIV positive (as well as those with other immunodeficiency disorders) often have numerous cutaneous manifestations.[105,106] Nail symptoms are much more frequent in HIV patients than healthy controls. Cribier et al found that the following were significantly more frequent in HIV patients: clubbing, transverse grooves, onychoschizia, leukonychia, and longitudinal melanonychia.[107] These authors found onychomycosis to be the most common nail abnormality and seemed to be linked to the level of immunosuppression. Usually these cutaneous manifestations follow their normal patterns. Sometimes, however, the presentation of these infections and neoplasms may be atypical.[105,106]

### Dermatophyte infections

**Key Features**

* Fingernails are more often involved than toenails
* Mycotic keratoderma and proximal white subungual onychomycosis are more common
* *Trichophyton rubrum* causes superficial white onychomycosis in fingernails and toenails

**TABLE 15–9. Nail changes associated with gastrointestinal diseases**

| DISEASE | NAIL FINDING |
|---|---|
| Acrodermatitis enteropathica | Paronychia |
| Bazex's syndrome[248,268] | Psoriasiform changes |
| Biliary cirrhosis[6] | Clubbing |
| Cirrhosis | Flat nails,[269] Terry's nails |
| Chylous ascites, intestinal lymphangiectasia[270] | Yellow nail syndrome |
| Crohn's disease[271] | Nail bed vasospasm |
| Cronkhite-Canada syndrome[6,272] | Ventral nail shaped like a triangle and nonspecific nail dystrophy, sometimes yellowish,[55] onychomadesis, onychoschizia,[273] and onycholysis[301] |
| Cystic fibrosis[1] | Periungual telangiectasia |
| Diabetes mellitus (pancreatic) | Paronychia more likely dysfunction) |
| Duodenal ulcer, gallstones[274] | Hereditary leukonychia |
| Hepatic disease (other nonspecific changes) | Erythema at base of nails,[6] Muehrcke's lines,[30] Beau's lines, melanonychia striata[16] |
| Hepatitis[6] (chronic active) | Clubbing, white nails, splinter hemorrhages |
| Hemochromatosis[275] | Koilonychia, leukonychia, longitudinal striation, brittleness |
| Intestinal leiomyosarcoma[276] | Brownish nail pigmentation |
| Jaundice (chronic obstructive)[18] | Clubbing, nail yellowing[277] |
| Malabsorption[52] | Abnormal growth |
| Plummer-Vinson syndrome (esophageal web) | Koilonychia |
| Porphyria cutanea tarda | Onycholysis,[55] dystrophy, clubbing, disappearance of lunula,[47] longitudinal band[26] |
| Progressive systemic sclerosis (gastrointestinal manifestation) | Ischemic changes and periungual telangiectasias |
| Peutz-Jeghers syndrome[278] | Brownish pigmentation |
| Regional enteritis[264] (Crohn's disease) | Clubbing |

See Table 15.7 for other gastrointestinal diseases not mentioned here.

Post-therapy relapses are common; topical therapy should be used for maintenance.

It is well known that dermatophyte infection is common in patients with HIV disease. The presence of onychomycosis generally correlates with helper T cell numbers less than 100 cells/mm$^3$.[108,109] Even though the causative organisms and clinical presentation in onychomycosis are usually similar to those in patients without HIV, there appear to be some notable differences:

1. The disorder may spread rapidly to all the fingernails and toenails.[108] In immunocompetent individuals, only the fingernails of one hand are usually involved (if at all).
2. Mycotic keratoderma of both palms may be found in HIV-positive individuals.[105,106] This would be quite rare in immunocompetent individuals.
3. A proximal white subungual onychomycosis often appears[105,106,108,110] (Fig. 15.12). This is unusual in the general population, especially in the fingernails. There has been a report of a patient with systemic lupus erythematosus with this presentation in the toenails.[111] Indeed, this presentation has prompted us[105] and others[112] upon seeing it to check for HIV and thus diagnose HIV in a previously unknown HIV-positive patient.
4. In immunocompetent individuals, chalky white involvement of the outer nail plate (superficial white onychomycosis) is rare in fingernails and is usually caused by *Trichophyton mentagrophytes*. In HIV-infected individuals, this presentation is not unheard of in fingernails or toenails and is usually caused by *Trichophyton rubrum*.[108]

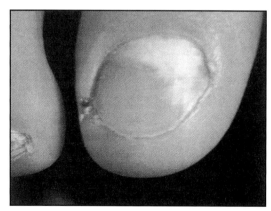

FIGURE 15–12. Proximal white subungual onychomycosis.

5. The periungual region may be involved with the dermatophyte infection.[109]
6. Fingernail involvement may occur without toenail involvement (T. Berger, personal communication, 6 February 1995).

Treatment is disappointing, and relapse is the rule. Consideration of therapy is important, however, because the nails act as a reservoir of infection. We have had poor results with griseofulvin. Itraconazole and, to a lesser extent, fluconazole have shown better efficacy than griseofulvin. We have not used terbinafine in these patients.

**TABLE 15–10. Hormonal-endocrine-metabolic associations**

| DISEASE | NAIL FINDINGS |
|---|---|
| Acromegaly | Thick nails[6]; short, wide, flat nails[16]; onychoschizia[16]; absent lunulae[16] |
| Addison's disease | Longitudinal pigmented bands[72] of deep yellow color with brown background[16] |
| Adiposogenital syndrome (Frölich's syndrome)[16] | Absent lunulae, onychauxis, longitudinal striations |
| Alkaptonuria[12] | Pigmented nail beds |
| Amyloid (bullous)[279] | Subungual hematoma |
| Amyloid (primary)[47] | Slight spooning, longitudinal melanotic band, subungual papillomatosis, striations, crumbling of the free margin, punctated erosions, fragility, anonychia: nail changes may be the first sign[280] |
| Cushing's disease[12] | Onycholysis, chronic paronychia |
| Diabetes mellitus | Yellowish toenails,[281] proximal nail bed telangiectasia, capillary dilation or blush,[281] splinter hemorrhages,[12] periungual erythema,[12,296] paronychia, tinea unguium, onycholysis, periungual skin-colored papules[299] |
| Fabray's disease[77] | Turtle-back configuration of the nails |
| Fucosidosis[12] | Purple nail bands, onychogryphosis |
| Glucagonoma syndrome[91] | Brittle nails |
| Gout[12] | Longitudinal streaks, brittleness, onychogryphosis |
| Hartnup disease[282] | Nail streaks |
| Histidinemia[12] | Pachyonychia, onychoschizia, Beau's lines |
| Homocystinuria[12] | Periungual telangiectasias and longitudinal ridging |
| Hypercalcemia[283] | Hypergranulation of nail bed |
| Hyperoxaluria[12] | Ungual oxalate granulomas |
| Hypogonadism[12] | Onychauxis |
| Lipoid proteinosis[6] | Poor nail growth |
| Menstruation (dysmenorrhea) | Striate leukonychia,[47] Beau's lines[284] |
| Metabolic acidosis[16] | Onychoschizia |
| Parathyroid disease | Beau's lines,[285] nail textural changes,[6] candidal paronychia[6] |
| 1. Hypoparathyroidism | Longitudinal striations,[16] opaque,[6] brittle,[6] splinter hemorrhages[12] |
| 2. Hyperparathyroidism (osteitis fibrosa cystica)[41] | Chronic paronychia,[47] pseudoclubbing |
| Pituitary disease (hypopituitarism) | Lunula may disappear[16]; brown spots[16]; long, thin nails[18]; *Candida* infection[12]; brittleness[12]; Beau's lines[12] |
| Pseudohypoparathyroidism[12] | Brachydactyly |
| Thyroid disease | |
| 1. Hypothyroidism | Nail plate wider than it is long,[16] hapalonychia,[16] slow growth,[16] longitudinal sulci,[16] transverse striations,[286] brittle,[16] onycholysis (dry, flat, thick, lackluster)[12] |
| 2. Hyperthyroidism | Plummer's nail: free edge is undulated and curves upward,[6] clubbing,[52] yellow nail syndrome,[126] splinter hemorrhage,[16] increased growth rate,[16] increased nail calcium,[287] soft, shiny, onycholysis,[286,288] koilonychia[12] |

For patients who decide against systemic therapy, the nails should be kept short and treated with topical[105] antifungal preparations such as ketoconazole, terbinafine, ciclopirox, oxiconazole, econazole, or sulconazole.

## Candida

It is uncommon for *Candida* to be a primary pathogen that directly invades the nail plate of a healthy individual.[113,114,115] *Candida* nail dystrophies are common in HIV-infected patients, especially when the helper T cell count is less than 100 cells/mm³.[108,109] Onycholysis and paronychia may occur. As with dermatophyte infection, numerous nails are often involved.[109] A hypertrophic nail bed *Candida* infection is more typical in HIV-infected patients,[113] as it is in chronic mucocutaneous candidiasis. We have not seen this in nonimmunocompromised individuals. Acute *Candida* paronychia

has been reported in one publication[116] in an HIV-positive patient. However, it has also been reported in a healthy individual.[117]

Some cases have responded to itraconazole, fluconazole, or ketoconazole, but relapse is the rule.[105]

*Candida albicans* is the major fungal agent in pediatric acquired immunodeficiency syndrome (AIDS).[118] In this age group, chronic *Candida* paronychia seems to occur most commonly between the ages of 2 and 6 years and is sometimes associated with severe nail dystrophy.[118]

## Other fungi

Undoubtedly, the entire spectrum of fungal infection in the general population (see Chapter 11) will appear in HIV-positive individuals.[113] *Pityrosporum ovale* was thought to cause onychomycosis in two patients with AIDS.[15,108] *Alternaria* nail infection has also been reported.[119,120] We certainly will find organisms affecting the nails that are most unusual in nonimmunosuppressed individuals. When performing fungal studies, one must do a potassium hydroxide (KOH) test and culture on Sabouraud's agar, one with cycloheximide and chloramphenicol and one without chlorheximide so as not to hinder the growth of some organisms that are not ordinarily pathogens.[112,113,121]

## Viral infection[105]

Herpetic whitlow has been reported in adults and in children with HIV.[122] Relapses are common, and recalcitrant, progressive disease may be ulcerative and scar the nail apparatus.[105] Acyclovir, famciclovir, or foscarnet may be instituted (see Chapter 14).

Papillomavirus may infect the nail unit. Biopsy should be performed on unusual or persistent lesions to rule out squamous cell carcinoma. We had a young adult patient who manifested a typical 'wart' on a finger. This later developed into an invasive squamous cell carcinoma of the nail bed. The patient was then tested for HIV and found to be positive. **The presence of a nail apparatus squamous cell carcinoma in persons younger than 30 years old should prompt one to consider immunosuppression, expecially HIV.**[105] Human papillomavirus type 16 deoxyribonucleic acid has been found in periungual squamous cell carcinoma.[123] Human papillomavirus type 35 and other strains have also been reported.[123]

## Scabies[105]

Crusted scabies[124,125] may occur in patients with HIV infection. The nail bed and plate may be hypertrophic and high numbers of organisms are present. Proper treatment of the nail, especially in refractory cases, is important.[126,127] This may consist of nail debridement and then multiple treatments with lindane or permethrin cream (see Chapter 14 on Non-fungal Nail Infections).

## Neoplastic disease[105]

Squamous cell carcinoma (see discussion of viral infections in Chapter 17), metastatic lesions, and Kaposi's sarcoma may appear in the region of the nail. The clinical presentation of squamous cell carcinoma may be subtle in HIV patients. The tumor can go undiagnosed for long periods as it may mimic chronic paronychia or verruca.[128] Almost 100% of AIDS patients with Kaposi's sarcoma have onychomycosis (T. Berger, personal communication, 6 February 1995). A nail unit lymphoma was the first manifestation in a patient with human T cell leukemia–lymphoma virus type I infection.

## Inflammatory disease[105]

Psoriasis or a psoriatic-like eruption may commonly affect patients with HIV. The typical nail manifestations of psoriasis may be present, but an eruption similar to pustular psoriasis may affect the nail. A proliferative, almost granulomatous process may permanently damage the nail. A psoriasis–Reiter's syndrome overlap process may occur.[106,108] Zidovudine may improve psoriasis in HIV-positive patients.[129] The antipsoriatic effect appears to be dose dependent and is associated with the development of erythrocyte macrocytosis, a side effect of zidovudine.[129] One psoriasis patient experienced improvement with high-dose co-trimoxazole,[130] and another did so with peptide T treatment.[131] Methotrexate should

not be used because it increases the chance of encephalopathy, leukopenia, infection, and death.[116] Systemic antimicrobial agents have been effective in some instances.[132] Etretinate has improved a Reiter's syndrome diathesis.[133]

Pityriasis rubra pilaris has been reported in two patients with HIV infection.[134] One had nail 'dystrophy' and one had normal nails. The disorder did not respond to etretinate.[134]

An atopic-like disease may occur with xerosis and brittle nails. Lichen spinulosus and 'nail dystrophy' in an HIV-positive person have been reported.[135]

In general, nail manifestations of inflammatory disease among HIV-infected persons and among the general population are similar.[105] However, as the helper T cell counts become lower, more secondary infection is seen, as is delayed healing.[105]

## Systemic disease[105,106]

Systemic disease in general can affect the nail apparatus.[136] There have been no specific nail changes associated with systemic disease (other than those mentioned previously) that suggest HIV infection (see Table 15.11 for some nonspecific findings.) We have noticed an apparent increase in erythematous crescents[58] in HIV-infected patients (unpublished observation). The condition has been reported to be more frequent in 'ill' patients.[58] We have not confirmed an increased frequency of yellow nail syndrome.[137-140] There may be a correlation between nail yellowing and *Pneumocystis carinii* pneumonia.[141] With wasting, slower nail growth and nail brittleness are observed.[105] Beau's lines may also occur with exacerbation and remission of the underlying disease.[105]

## Systemic drugs[106]

### Key Feature of Systemic Antiretroviral Therapy for HIV Disease

* Several antiretroviral drugs have retinoid-like effects causing nonbacterial acute paronychia and pyogenic granulomas around the nail unit

Systemic drugs can affect the nails in a number of ways (see Chapter 16).[142] The incidence of drug reactions is increased in patients with HIV infection, especially with trimethoprim–sulfamethoxazole. Cancer chemotherapeutic agents used to treat

---

**TABLE 15–11. Non-specific nail findings in HIV disease**

Slow growth
Beau's lines
Splinter hemorrhages
Slow healing
Clubbing, especially with pneumocystis pneumonia[12]
Brittle nails
Leukonychia[91]
Nail plate yellowing[96,114]
Psoriatic changes (Reiter's syndrome)[289]
Smooth nails (scratching)

developing malignancies are known to produce a wide array of pigmentary changes in patients without HIV infection, and similar patterns in patients with HIV are expected.[142] Zidovudine may produce dark brown, bluish, or blackish discoloration of the nail apparatus. However, blue nails may occur in HIV-positive disease and not be associated with zidovudine.[143] The pattern may vary and may be longitudinal, transverse, or diffuse. The color change is more commonly seen in Black people.

The protease inhibitor indinavir increases retinoic acid signaling, which may explain the paronychia, nailfold pyogenic granuloma-like lesions, and ingrown nails that are frequently seen. The combination of indinavir with ritonavir seems to increase the risk of ingrown toenails, which tend to present acutely and require surgical management.[144] In addition, zidovudine and lamivudine, nucleoside reverse transcriptase inhibitors, are associated with paronychia and pyogenic granuloma-like lesions.[145]

### Miscellaneous

The lunula may be smaller than usual in HIV-positive disease.[146] Blue nails have been reported as a sign of HIV infection.[147] Also, periungual erythema was found in 2.4% of one HIV study population.[148] Sometimes the erythema is painful and it can demonstrate nail fold telangiectasias that may be produced by angiogenic factors produced by HIV.[149,150]

## Nail Care in Patients with HIV Disease

Nails should be kept relatively short. Longer nails are more likely to abrade the skin when scratching. Longer nails are also more likely to harbor infectious agents. Toenails should be cut straight across and not rounded at the edges to help avoid in-grown nails. Onychophagia and onychotillomania are not uncommon,[15] and these should be discouraged. Hangnails should not be pinched or pulled off but gently clipped off. A dual-action nail nipper, when used correctly, may painlessly clip onycholytic nails with less chance of nail bed damage. Power-driven drills should not be used to pare down nails in patients with HIV infection because they scatter many small pieces of nail debris and may release a 'plume' of infectious material. Cotton gloves should be worn underneath vinyl gloves for wet work. Patients should notify their nail care professional if they are HIV positive so that appropriate precautions may be taken.[106] All cases of nail surgery should be done as though the patient had HIV.

### Summary

There are no known pathognomonic nail signs of HIV infection in nails. However, several presentations should increase the index of suspicion:

1. Proximal white subungual onychomycosis or *Trichophyton rubrum* appear most commonly in HIV-infected patients. Periungual dermatophyte involvement and involvement in all fingernails is unusual in non-HIV-infected individuals.
2. *Candida* as a primary pathogen of the nail bed and nail plate, especially if many nails are involved.
3. A destructive, almost granulomatous-like psoriatic diathesis of the nails.
4. Squamous cell carcinoma of the nail bed in a young adult.

## Malnutrition

Much has been written about nails in malnutrition, but these findings seem to be nonspecific. Slow growth and fissuring,[9] koilonychia,[24] pustular paronychia with zinc deficiency,[151] spear-like nails,[152] Muehrcke's lines,[51] pellagra and koilonychia,[24] vitamin A deficiency associated with eggshell nails,[26] and brittle nails[24] have been reported. Hypocalcemia is usually not a cause of brittle nails. Chronic, severe hypocalcemia as seen in severe malnutrition probably can contribute to abnormal nails.

## Central and Peripheral Nervous Systems

Probably no onychopathy is specific in this group, but one is of particular interest (Table 15.12). Several decades ago, Maricq noted that a significant correlation exists between a family history of schizophrenia and visibility of the subcapillary plexus in the nail fold.[153] The duration of illness was greater in these patients, and they did not perform well academically.[153] Several years later, she added that the abnormal capillary appearance is not a permanent characteristic.[154] In a later article, she noted that, when these patients had a more clearly visible subcapillary plexus, they more frequently had smooth, glossy skin and more capillary hemorrhages in the nail fold area and tended to have longer and straighter sweat ducts.[155]

A double-edged nail in psychoses, onycholysis with central and peripheral nervous system problems, destruction of the tips of the digits in Lesch–Nyhan syndrome, onychomadesis with peripheral neuritis and hemiplegia, splinter hemorrhages in central nervous system disease, long and convex nails with vertical ridging in the causalgic syndrome,[9] Beau's lines in epilepsy, striated leukonychia in manic-depressive illness, longitudinal striations in hemiplegia, multiple sclerosis, syringomyelia, pterygium inversus unguium-like change in a patient with neurofibromatosis,[156] and hard, thickened nails in Morgagni– Stewart–Morel syndrome[38] have been noted.[24] A well-defined, transverse, reddish band has been reported in all nails of a patient with multiple system atrophy (a primary degenerative disease of the central nervous system).[157]

## Nail Changes Associated with Psychological Disorders

Abnormalities of the nail unit may occur in association with a broad range of psychological or psychiatric illness. These are easily overlooked or misdiagnosed, leading to continued frustration and often despair for the patient. Conversely, if they are recognized and the patient's care is coordinated with the appropriate specialist, outcomes can be very positive for the patient and extremely rewarding for the dermatologist. This section is a brief introduction to aid in recognition of these conditions and does not address therapy, as this is often coordinated with a psychiatrist or clinical psychologist. The dermatologist monitors nail changes, treats secondary infection, aids wound healing and generally supports the patient's efforts.

Onychotillomania, an extreme form of self-mutilation of the nails, is thought to be a manifestion of obsessive-compulsive disorder (OCD). Figures 15.13 and 15.14 illustrate onychotillomania before therapy (Fig. 15.13) and after several months of therapy (Fig. 15.14).

**TABLE 15–12. Associations with central and peripheral nervous systems**

| DISORDER | NAIL FINDING |
|---|---|
| Carpal tunnel syndrome[290] | Beau's lines, yellow-brown discoloration and transverse furrows, koilonychia[12] |
| Causalgia[16] | Long convex nails with vertical ridging, unilateral clubbing[12] |
| Central nervous system disease[16] | Splinter hemorrhages |
| Central and peripheral nervous system disorders[16] | Onycholysis |
| Epidemic encephalitis[12] | Multiple paronychia |
| Epilepsy[16] | Beau's lines |
| Hemiplegia[16] | Longitudinal striations |
| Lesch-Nyhan syndrome | Self-destruction of the tips of the digit |
| Manic-depressive disease[16] | Striated leukonychia |
| Morgagni-Stewart-Morel syndrome[47] | Hard, thickened nails |
| Multiple sclerosis | Longitudinal striations[16] |
| Neurofibromatosis | Pterygium inversus unguium-like changes[124] |
| Peripheral neuritis and hemiplegia[16] | Onychomadesis |
| Psychosis[16] | Double-edged nail |
| Reflex sympathetic dystrophy[291] | Increased nail growth, excessive transverse curvature, brittleness and periungual whitlow-like changes |
| Spinal cord injuries[12] | Ingrown toenails |
| Syringomyelia | Longitudinal striations,[16] periungual crusting[12] |

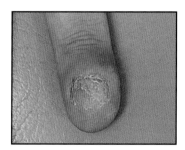

FIGURE 15–13. Onychotillomania before therapy.

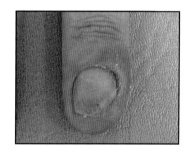

FIGURE 15–14. Onychotillomania after several months of therapy.

It often begins with nail biting or habit tic deformity of the nail, which are fairly common.[158] The term 'onychotillomania' should be reserved for those patients who demonstrate severe self-mutilation with complete or nearly complete removal of the nail plate. Lesch–Nehan syndrome should be considered in the differential diagnosis as well as apotemnophilia ('love of amputation').[159] Onychotillomania patients often complain of pain and may deny any manipulation of the nail vehemently. In our experience, patients should not be confronted with the question of self-induced injury or the need for psychiatric consultation until good rapport has been established. Patients are often angry that many prior physicians were unhelpful or even 'insulting'. They often experience embarrassment and anxiety, which can interfere with interpersonal relationships and business.[160] It is best to demonstrate empathy by addressing these issues, helping to manage pain (nonsteroidal anti-inflammatory drugs are better than narcotics in these patients), treating secondary infection, and encouraging close follow up. It is best to leave extra time in the schedule so that these needs can be addressed properly and the patient does not feel rushed. Once rapport is established, it is necessary to differentiate between OCD type behavior and the presence of delusions. Medications useful for OCD include clomipramine, fluoxetine, fluvoxamine, paroxetine, sertraline, venlafaxine, and citalopram. Pimozide and some of the newer antipsychotics may be especially useful if there are delusional thoughts. At this time, the patient may be comfortable going for psychological therapy but it is best to continue to follow the patient even if little dermatologic intervention is needed. Occlusive dressings may be helpful in some cases, but these will be unlikely to help if the pain is poorly controlled. Gabapentin in doses of 300–600 mg three times daily (similar to postherpetic neuralgia doses) can also be helpful. Long-acting digital blocks and topical anesthetics such as eutectic lidocaine cream may reduce pain. Consultation with a pain control specialist (often available in anesthesiology practices) can be extremely helpful, especially if there are concurrent issues of narcotic dependence.

There are also psychological disorders that encompass many nondermatological symptoms but happen to demonstrate skin and nail findings in some patients. For example, Hediger et al. studied cutaneous findings in patients with anorexia nervosa. In addition to xerosis, hypertrichosis, and alopecia, they found acrocyanosis, periungual erythema, and other nail changes in up to 48% of patients.[161] Alcoholic patients can manifest numerous nail changes related to liver disease. Terry's nails, red lunulae, koilonychias, and clubbing have been reported in association with alcoholic cirrhosis.[162]

## Pulmonary System

The nails in yellow nail syndrome exhibit a greatly slowed rate of growth, yellowish discoloration of the nail plate (which may be thickened and excessively curved from side to side), absent lunulae and cuticles, swelling of the periungual tissue, and a variable degree of onycholysis[163,164] (Fig. 15.15).

Yellow nail syndrome has been found in a wide array of pulmonary diseases,[165] including tuberculosis,[156] asthma,[163] pleural effusion,[163] bronchiectasis,[164] chronic sinusitis,[164] chronic bronchitis,[166] and chronic obstructive pulmonary disease.[167] The nail manifestations may be mimicked by bullous lichen planus.[90] Biopsy of an involved nail suggests primary stromal sclerosis, which may lead to lymphatic obstruction, thus possibly explaining the clinical manifestation.[168] Along with the nail and respiratory problems, lymphedema has been noted to be a third major component of the syndrome.[169,170]

Removal of a carcinoma of the larynx has been associated with a resolution of the yellow nails in one patient. Other associated malignancies are lymphoma, melanoma, adenocarcinoma of the endometrium, anaplastic undifferentiated tumor, and carcinoma of the gallbladder.[167,171]

Some other associations include breasts of unequal size,[90] thyroid disease,[164] chronic nasal obstruction and rock-hard cerumen,[172] empyema,[173] nephrotic syndrome,[15] use of penicillamine,[174,175] psoriasis,[176] intestinal lymphangiectasia,[177] and sleep apnea.[178]

Various therapeutic regimens have been cited in the literature but with no consistent results. Guin and Elleman mentioned that gold therapy and bed rest for rheumatoid arthritis had possibly improved one case.[167] Biotin,[179] intralesional triamcinolone,[180] diethylstilbestrol,[181] zinc,[176] and management of diabetes mellitus[182] have possibly caused improvement in various patients with the abnormality. Vitamin E[176,183] given in the dosage of 400 IU two[165] to three[184,185] times daily has been reported to improve the nails. There is also a report of topical vitamin E solution improving the nails.[186] Oral vitamin E and itraconazole have been used in one case.[187]

Shell nail syndrome was reported to be associated with bronchiectasis. Affected nails exhibited excessive longitudinal curvature of the nail plate, dystrophic fingertips resulting from atrophy of the distal nail bed, and onycholysis.[188] This description is certainly similar to that of yellow nail syndrome, except no mention is made of abnormal color or slow rate of growth.

Clubbing has been mentioned earlier and is associated with respiratory problems. Painful clubbing in a patient with sarcoidosis was documented, and the discomfort diminished after colchicine therapy.[75] The nail in sarcoidosis may also appear dystrophic and yellowish and may manifest painful paronychia and splinter hemorrhages.[38]

Bazex's paraneoplastic syndrome may present with psoriasis-like changes in the nails and other acral areas such as the nose and ears.[189–191] Other nail changes that may be found include horizontal and vertical ridging, yellow color, thickening, onycholysis, subungual debris, softness, thinning, slow growth, and increased glycine, lysine, and methionine.[15] These changes may occur months or years before an upper respiratory tract malignancy as well as upper gastrointestinal malignancies. Squamous cell carcinoma is most commonly found.[15] There have also been reports of associated carcinomas of the prostate or vulva.[15]

Some miscellaneous associations with pulmonary disease include interstitial pulmonary disease and dyskeratosis congenita.[192] Also

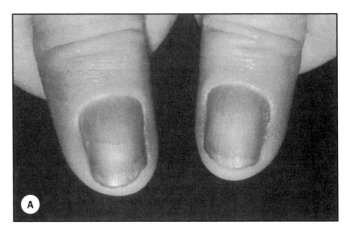

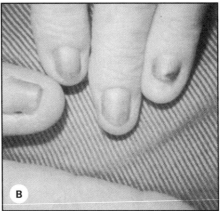

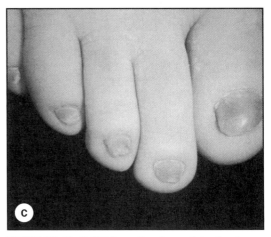

**FIGURE 15–15.** (A–C) Yellow nail syndrome of chronic pulmonary disease.

nail clippings in cystic fibrosis have an elevated sodium content,[39] and splinter hemorrhages and periungual telangiectasia have been noted.[15]

## Renal Disease

The half-and-half fingernail may be the most useful onychopathologic indicator of chronic renal failure.[58] The finding was originally popularized by Lindsay[193] but possibly first described by Bean.[194] Lindsay's working description reads as follows: 'a nail exhibiting a red, pink, or brown transverse distal band occupying

20 to 60% of the total nail length and with the remaining proximal portion exhibiting a dull, whitish ground-glass appearance.'[193] We did not find that the proximal portion necessarily needed to be whitish. Kint and colleagues came to the same conclusion.[195] If the distal band was less than 20% of the total nail length, the patient was considered to have Terry's nails.[193]

Numerous causes of nail discoloration could mimic the half-and-half nail, but understanding how to evaluate pigment changes can remove most from the differential diagnosis.[44] Probably the most frequently encountered causes that may mimic the half-and-half nail are topical agents[44] and psoriasis. A brownish discoloration (oil-spot change) often occurs just proximal to an area of onycholysis in a psoriatic nail, but the onycholysis as well as other nail and skin findings of psoriasis often make the diagnosis clear (Fig. 15.16). Systemic 5-fluorouracil and androgens may possibly cause a half-and-half-like nail.[196–198] Scher reported a patient with concomitant yellow nail syndrome and half-and-half nail.[199]

The exact cause of the half-and-half nail is unknown. Leyden and Wood[200] performed a biopsy on the distal brownish area and found the pigment to be melanin. They hypothesized that renal failure stimulates matrix melanocytes and causes melanin to be deposited in the nail plate.[200] Also, because the nail grows more slowly in renal failure, pigment is more likely to accumulate.[200] Stewart and Raffle found melanin granules in the basal layer of the nail bed epidermis.[201] Kint and colleagues found increased capillaries and a distinct thickening of the walls.[195] This could be due to increased blood flow through an artificial shunt. Capillary changes that are probably reversible have been suggested as the cause.[202] Plasma melanotropic hormone has been found to be greatly increased in patients treated by maintenance dialysis for chronic renal failure.[203] This and the fact that the nails are in a sun-exposed area could possibly be responsible for the melanin deposition.[203]

An intriguing question about the half-and-half nail is why the distal brownish color is not apparent throughout the more proximal nail, considering that the melanocytes responsible are probably in the matrix and the color does not seem to migrate. The pigment apparently is more visible distally than it is proximally

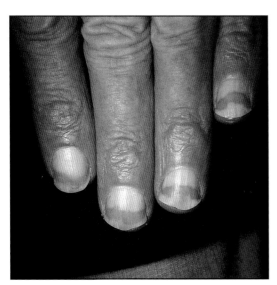

**FIGURE 15–16.** Pseudo-half-and-half nail caused by psoriasis.

because of a looser attachment of the nail plate or because of a variation of the Tyndall effect. It has been noted that after a chronic hemodialysis patient received a kidney transplant the brown pigment moved distally and his half-and-half nails slowly disappeared.[59] The half-and-half nail is not correlated with specific quantitative blood urea nitrogen or creatinine findings[193,200,201] (C.R. Daniel and J.D. Bower, unpublished data, 1975). It does seem apparent that renal disease per se is not the cause of this nail finding, but azotemia and renal failure do instigate the problem either by acting directly on the matrix melanocytes or by a melanocyte-stimulating substance released from another site. The half-and-half nail as more specifically described seems to occur in about 9[58,59] to 15%[202] of chronic renal failure patients sometime during the course of their disease. We described a condition called crescents that was found to occur more frequently in renal failure but also in other chronically ill patients as well as in some normal individuals. Lubach and colleagues lumped half-and-half nails, brown arcs, and possibly crescents under the term subungual erythema. Subungual erythema was found most commonly, but not exclusively, in renal failure patients.[60,204]

Levitt[205] analyzed the creatinine concentration of human fingernail and toenail clippings to determine the duration of renal failure. He concluded that patients with acute renal failure had normal nail creatinine concentration, whereas those with chronic renal failure had elevated levels that correlated with the serum creatinine concentration that had been present several months previously.[205]

Saray et al. studied nail changes in 127 patients on chronic renal dialysis and 116 renal transplant patients. They concluded that the most common changes seen in dialysis patients (which may actually be attributed to chronic renal failure) were absence of lunula, onychomycosis, splinter hemorrhages, leukonychia, longitudinal ridging, and half-and-half nails respectively. In the transplant group the most commonly seen nail pathology was: leukonychia, absence of lunula, onychomycosis, and longitudinal ridging.[206] Tercedor et al. also found absence of lunula the most common abnormality in dialysis patients and both studies concluded that nail disease is more common in patients on chronic hemodialysis than healthy patients.[207]

Kelly et al. suggest that significant micronutrient imbalance occurs in approximately one-third of hemodialysis patients and that nail changes may be markers for this. They note the following possible associated deficiencies: Beau's lines (zinc), koilonychia (iron, copper, zinc, protein), leukonychia (zinc), pale nail beds (iron), Muehrcke's lines (protein), splinter hemorrhages (vitamin C), onycholysis (iron, niacin), and chronic paronychia (zinc).[208]

Pincer nail deformity has been reported in association with pseudo-Kaposi's sarcoma as complications of arteriovenous fistula for hemodialysis.[209]

Probably the only other relatively specific nail findings associated with renal failure are those seen in the nail-patella syndrome. It is discussed in the section on nail changes associated with genodermatoses.

Mees' lines, Muehrcke's lines, splinter hemorrhages, and slow growth have been associated with renal failure, as mentioned earlier. Renal adenocarcinomas producing erythropoietin may impart a more reddish color to the nail bed.[24] Rheumatologic diseases that may produce secondary renal disease also have numerous associated nail abnormalities (see the following section). Angiokeratoma corporis diffusum (Fabry's disease) may have associated renal problems and a 'turtle-back' nail configuration.[97]

# Autoimmune and Arthritic Diseases

Numerous rheumatologic diseases[210] can either directly or indirectly affect the nail unit. The vast majority of these onychopathies represent nonspecific reaction patterns. A few are more specific, but, in our opinion, none is pathognomonic of that particular rheumatologic disorder. The proximal nail fold is often the most important site of alterations.[211] Capillary changes of the nail fold may be characteristic of scleroderma, as mentioned later. Ischemia often associated with Raynaud's phenomenon probably forms the basis of most changes.

## Periungual telangiectasia

This is a distinctive microvascular pattern of dilated and distorted capillary loops seen in patients with connective tissue vascular diseases. Maricq and colleagues[212] proposed a simple, inexpensive, reproducible technique to predict internal multisystem involvement in scleroderma, Raynaud's phenomenon, and dermatomyositis.[212] They have not found this specific change in systemic lupus erythematosus or rheumatoid arthritis. Their method is not easily applicable to darkly pigmented patients.[212] Periungual telangiectasia also may be seen in schizophrenia,[153–155] cystic fibrosis,[3] graft-versus-host reaction,[96] diabetes mellitus,[3] congenital heart disease,[3] homocystinuria,[96] and Down syndrome.[3] Minkin and Rabhan expounded on the periungual capillary changes seen in some arthritic disorders.[213] Implementing a method described by Herd[214] and using an ophthalmoscope, they examined 130 patients with various connective tissue diseases. They placed a drop of mineral oil on each nail fold to be examined. They believed that the capillaries were best visualized in the nail fold of the fourth finger. The ophthalmoscope was set at $+40$, resulting in a $\times 10$ magnification. They found the following:

1. Patients with systemic scleroderma exhibited enlarged and deformed capillaries with dilation of both limbs of the loop. This was associated with disorganization of the loop arrangement and many avascular areas. This pattern was seen in 74% of the patients studied. These capillary abnormalities seem to correlate with pulmonary arterial hypertension.[215]

2. The pattern in patients with systemic lupus erythematosus consisted of widened, tortuous, 'meandering' capillary loops at times resembling a renal glomerulus. There is usually some disorganization of the capillary pattern, but only rarely were avascular areas seen. These patients manifested this pattern 53% of the time.

3. Of patients with dermatomyositis, 82% illustrated the systemic scleroderma pattern.

4. No specific patterns were found for vasculitis, Raynaud's disease, morphea, or mixed connective tissue disease.

5. Capillary microscopy is most useful as a prognostic factor in Raynaud's disease or mixed connective tissue disease, to differentiate 'undifferentiated' connective tissue disease to distinguish cutaneous lupus from dermatomyositis, and to confirm the diagnoses of systemic scleroderma, dermatomyositis, and systemic lupus erythematosus.

6. Acrocyanosis, a reversible condition occurring in young women, shows specific nailfold capillary changes that may be distinguished from those seen in patients with scleroderma.[216]

7. Paraneoplastic acral vascular syndrome is an acral ischemic process presenting in older patients and is not associated with autoimmune disease. Patients develop painful lesions demonstrating acral necrosis, which often present prior to the diagnosis of underlying malignancy.[217]

8. Patients with primary biliary cirrhosis often show nail fold capillary patterns similar to those seen in scleroderma. These changes may be associated with the development of extrahepatic connective tissue disease.[218]

9. Dark-skinned people and traumatized fields may diminish capillary visibility.

Biopsy of proximal nail folds in these patients often shows deposits positive for periodic acid-Schiff that are not specific but may help identify those patients with idiopathic Raynaud's phenomenon who are at risk for the development of a connective tissue disease.[219] Direct immunofluorescence may be helpful diagnostically. Others have also confirmed the usefulness of capillary microscopy as a screening test for patients with apparent idiopathic Raynaud's phenomenon who are at risk for developing autoimmune disease.[220,221]

Maricq and Maize, pioneers in the study of nail fold capillary abnormalities, added that capillary hemorrhages are more frequent in patients with scleroderma than in controls. These hemorrhages may seem to 'grow out' with the cuticle.[222] Also, scleroderma nail fold capillary abnormalities may be quite characteristic in early disease. Ohtsuka reports that patients with abnormal nailfold capillaries tend to have increased nail fold bleeding.[223] Callen found that nail fold manifestations of dermatomyositis were diminished in a child he was treating with hydroxychloroquine sulfate (J. Callen, personal communication, 10 December 1985).

## Rheumatoid arthritis

This is often associated with nonspecific nail findings. Pronounced longitudinal ridges often having a beaded appearance, thickening, discoloration, splinter hemorrhages, and periungual vascular lesions (Bywaters' syndrome) associated with beading and longitudinal ridging have been noted.[224] Michel et al. studied nail findings in RA patients and found that longitudinal ridges were the most significant association:[225] 'A deep violet arch like a half moon, well delimited by the adjacent plate, 0.5 to 1 mm in size, at about 4 to 5 mm from the free nail margin, to which it is parallel, can occur.'[24] Milan believed that this was specific for syphilis, but it can also occur in rheumatoid arthritis, leprosy, and during the convalescence of debilitating, infectious diseases.[24]

Nail fold infarcts and yellow nail syndrome have also been associated with rheumatoid arthritis.[226] Periungual erythema is not uncommon. One case of a red lunula has been reported.[227] Nail abnormalities have been seen frequently in patients with lupus erythematosus. Erythema and fissuring of the proximal nail fold with dilated capillary loops may be seen in systemic lupus erythematosus,[9] as was a case of red lunulae.[227] Clubbing,[72] paronychia,[72] pitting,[30] white nails, leukonychia striata,[30] onycholysis that may cause nail shedding,[24] and 'coffin-lid' nail characterized by a flat laminar surface at the center descending steeply on both sides and penetrating the ungual sulci[24] have been noted. According to Kint and Herpe, the combination of a typical red-blue color of the crumbling nail plate and longitudinal striae should make one suspect discoid lupus erythematosus.[228] Periungual erythema and telangiectasia have been reported in coffee plantation workers without any association with lupus.[229] Their single patient's nail abnormality cleared with systemic chloroquine therapy. Also in discoid lupus a 'curious atrophic spindling of the fingers sometimes with hyperextension of the terminal phalanges and nail dystrophy' has been observed.[95]

## Lupus erythematosus

Erythema and telangiectasias of the proximal nail fold probably are the most frequently-found changes in systemic lupus erythematosus. Changes secondary to Raynaud's phenomenon and distal ischemia are also common in systemic lupus erythematosus. Sclerodactyly, seen in this disease group, may also be seen in toxic oil syndrome.[230] Hyperkeratosis of the cuticle in combination with erythema and telangiectasia is probably helpful, but hyperkeratosis alone seems to be too nonspecific because xerosis alone often causes this change (Fig. 15.17). Urowitz and coworkers found that patients with systemic lupus erythematosus who had nail changes tended to have a higher incidence of Raynaud's phenomenon and mucous membrane ulceration.[30] The oil-spot change so typical of psoriasis may be seen in the nail bed of a patient with systemic lupus erythematosus.[39] Painful, red lunulae which responded to systemic corticosteroid therapy have been reported in association with systemic lupus.[231] Diffuse nail hyperpigmentation has been found more commonly in darkly pigmented patients with systemic lupus erythematosus.[232] Baran et al. describe functional melanonychia due to involvement of the nail matrix in systemic lupus erythematosus as longitudinal bands.[233] Also, nail fold capillary density has been associated with pulmonary capillary loss.[234] Periungual erythema and onychodystrophy have been noted in chilblain lupus erythematosus.[235]

## Reiter's syndrome

This may cause nail changes that appear identical to psoriasis, but this occurs much less frequently in Reiter's syndrome. Onycholysis, yellowing, and subungual hyperkeratosis are the most frequent changes. Lovoy and colleagues reported a patient with nail pitting and incomplete Reiter's syndrome and suggested that this change may reflect a predisposition to the development of psoriasis or psoriasiform lesions conferred by HLA-A2 with B27 inheritance.[28]

Longitudinal tight superficial nail grooving, subungual hyperkeratosis, and onycholysis have been reported as the first manifestations of HLA-B27 inheritance.[29] Small yellow pustules may develop beneath the nail, often near the lunula; they may enlarge, and erosion through the nail plate may occur.[9] Paronychia-like changes have been noted.[28]

## Dermatomyositis

Patients with dermatomyositis frequently have nail changes similar to those seen in systemic lupus erythematosus, including erythema and dilated capillary loops in the proximal nail folds (Fig. 15.18), bluish-red plaques around the base of the nails, hyperkeratotic cuticles, and pitting.[9,31,95,236]

## Scleroderma

Patients with scleroderma (progressive systemic sclerosis) may exhibit nail abnormalities, including telangiectasia and erythema of the proximal nail fold, tightening of the skin of the digits, and distal digital infarcts resulting from ischemia and Raynaud's phenomenon. Pterygium inversus unguium-like changes may be seen and are characterized by adherence of the distal portion of the nail bed or hyponychium to the ventral surface of the nail plate, thereby obliterating the normal distal separation of these structures[156] (Fig. 15.19). **This often first becomes evident when the patient complains of pain when cutting the nails.** Progressive systemic sclerosis and systemic lupus erythematosus are the two most common associations.[237] Patterson noted that this finding may become symptomatic upon trauma or upon attempts to clip the nails.[156] Trauma may induce a similar disorder. A reaction to formaldehyde-containing nail cosmetics may also produce a pterygium inversus unguium-like picture.[238] Odom and colleagues described a similar finding in patients having the anomaly since birth, without apparent distal ischemia, and postulated that this change may represent an anomaly of the developing fetal nail primordia and is analogous to the claw of lower primates.[239] It has been reported that decreased manual skills and vibration exposure

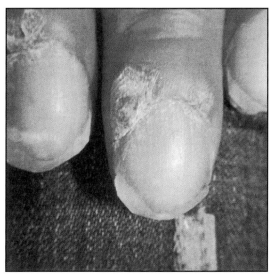

FIGURE 15–17. Hyperkeratosis of proximal nail fold in a patient with lupus erythematosus.

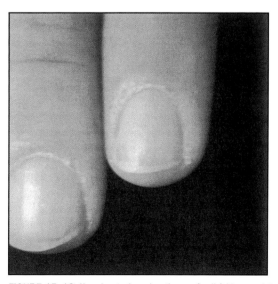

FIGURE 15–18. Hyperkeratosis and erythema of nail folds associated with dermatomyositis.

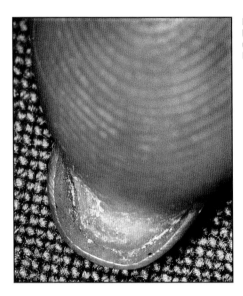

FIGURE 15-19.
Pterygium inversus
unguium (courtesy of
Dr R. Caputo).

may be associated with systemic scleroderma and nail fold abnormalities.[240]

Caputo and Prandi[241] found one patient who acquired the disorder without a definite predisposing cause, an observation confirmed by others.[242] Pterygium inversus unguium of the toenails has been reported only in families.[243] Ragged cuticles,[95] widened cuticles with the proximal skinfold thin,[9] clubbing (probably secondary to pulmonary manifestations),[244] onychorrhexis,[24] vesiculation of the periungual area, absence of the lunula, deep longitudinal sulci, hapalonychia, onycholysis, and onychogryphosis have been associated with progressive systemic sclerosis.[156] Distal pulp resorption tends to occur as in other diseases with Raynaud's phenomenon, and the subsequent ulcers may be painful. Nail fold bleeding is strongly associated with anticentromere antibodies, especially in scleroderma.[245] Abnormal periungual capillaries have also been noted in morphea.[246]

## Multicentric reticulohistiocytosis

With its often destructive polyarthritis, this may have associated atrophy, longitudinal ridging, brittleness, and hyperpigmentation[247] of the nails in addition to papules around the nail folds,[248] onycholysis, and racket-shaped (plates wider than long) nails.[247] Barrow attributed most of these changes to a synovial reaction affecting nail growth and to the giant cell nodules producing a pressure effect on the matrix.[247]

## Other rheumatologic nail associations

These include faster nail growth in Still's disease and acute rheumatic fever,[24] pitting with psoriatic arthritis, slow growth, and nails exhibiting decreased cystine content and absent lunulae in chronic polyarthritis.[24] In Behçet's syndrome, a half-and-half-like nail diathesis was reported.[249] A peculiar nail dystrophy composed of leukonychia,[96] longitudinal striations, brittleness, and crumbling of the nail plate may be seen in patients with gout.[95] Baran and Dawber, reporting the work of others, suggested that nails in psoriatic arthritis may be differentiated from those in rheumatoid arthritis by biochemical and statistical analysis of the amino acids of the fingernails.[96,250,251] Significant nail involvement

of psoriasis (e.g., advanced subungual hyperkeratosis) in children may suggest more severe psoriasis or an increased chance of the development of psoriatic arthritis.[252] Capillary changes of the proximal nail fold may also be found in psoriatic arthritis patients.[253] Splinter hemorrhages may be seen in patients with antiphospholipid syndrome.[254]

## Miscellaneous Systemic Disorders

Several more nail abnormalities that are nonspecifically associated with other systemic diseases include paronychia,[255] temporary,[255] and permanent[256] nail shedding and other changes after Stevens–Johnson syndrome, canalized and yellow nails (Vieira's sign) in fogo selvagem,[257] subungual pustules in impetigo herpetiformis,[97] disappearing lunula or onycholysis in multiple myeloma,[97,258] Mees' lines and leukonychia in carbon monoxide poisoning,[259] splinter hemorrhages, paronychia onycholysis, purpura, subungual hyperkeratosis in histiocytosis X[260,261] (biopsy of the involved nail unit in histiocytosis X showed the presence of atypical histiocytes[262]), subungual purpura in Letterer–Siwe disease,[263] nail shedding in toxic shock syndrome[264] and toxic epidermal necrolysis,[3] nail dystrophy (including horizontal ridging, hemorrhage, hyperkeratosis, and shedding in bullous pemphigoid), nail dystrophy in epidermolysis bullosa simplex,[265] and onychogryphosis[266] and other bullous diseases (Fig. 15.20). Lead poisoning may manifest leukonychia, onychalgia, and onychomadesis.[50] Periodic shedding of the nails may be associated with epidermolysis bullosa[267] and leukonychia seen in cryoglobulinemia.[9] Periungual erythema may be seen in histiocytosis X, graft-versus-host disease, and Wiskott–Aldridge syndrome.[148]

Graft-versus-host disease has also been associated with severe lichenoid lesions in the nails.[268]

**In our experience, sarcoid of the nail involves a crumbling nail plate sometimes associated with pain and paronychia. Painful paronychia and splinter hemorrhages may occur,[38] as may some nail pitting.[32] Sarcoidal granulomas of the nail bed may present as**

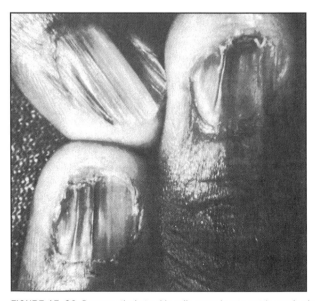

FIGURE 15-20. Permanently dystrophic nails secondary to matrix scarring in a patient with Stevens–Johnson syndrome.

subungual hyperkeratosis.[269] Treatment with prednisone and hydroxychloroquine cleared one patient of his nail abnormalities.[32] Pterygium formation may occur.[270] Sarcoid may cause nail dystrophy with or without underlying bony involvement.[271]

Myeloma-associated systemic amyloidosis has been reported to present with episodes of acute pustular paronychia. Ahmed et al. describe histologic changes consistent with cutaneous amyloidosis from a lateral nailfold biopsy.[272] Wong et al. report nail plate brittleness and onychodystrophy in association with systemic amyloidosis.[273]

Hodgkin's disease may manifest Mees' lines,[49] which may be associated with a poor prognosis.[38] Leukonychia may be seen in patients with hyperalbuminemia, zoster, and exfoliative dermatitis[96] and in Orthodox Jews who fast. Painful nails with subungual hyperkeratosis were reported in cutaneous T cell lymphoma.[274] In a child with mycosis fungoides, nail dystrophy resolved with photochemotherapy.[275] Paronychia and nail plate loss have been reported in a child with Langerhans cell histiocytosis.[276] Hypertrichosis lanuginosa may be associated with nail pitting and subungual epidermal hyperplasia.[277]

Pemphigus vulgaris has been noted to exhibit numerous nail findings, as have other bullous diseases. In our experience, pemphigus, in a majority of cases, causes nail changes by contiguous effects.[85] Onychomadesis,[278] discoloration, pitting, transverse lines, paronychia, onychoschizia,[217] and other dystrophic changes characterize the nail changes.[33] Beau's lines, pterygium, pigmentation changes, onycholysis, subungual hemorrhages, subungual hyperkeratoses, and fungal involvement may be seen.[33] Paronychia may be a sign heralding an exacerbation.[279]

An unsubstantiated report has raised the issue of whether a 'radium fingernail polish' has been associated with development of cancer.[280]

'Neopolitan nails,' the main features of which are loss of lunula and white appearance of the proximal half of the nail, a more normal pink band, and the opaque free edge of the nail, seems to be associated with old age, reduced bone mass, and thin skin.[281] This presentation has some of the features of the half-and-half nail,[58,193] Terry's nail,[63] and crescents,[58,59] described earlier.

Primary subungual calcification of fingers and toes may be an effect of advancing age in women. Secondary subungual calcification occurs occasionally after trauma and in psoriasis.[282] In pregnancy, nail changes occur as early as the sixth week and consist of grooving, increased brittleness and softening, distal onycholysis, and subungual keratosis;[283] longitudinal pigmented bands may occur.[96] Erythema elevatum diutinum has been reported in a periungual distribution.[284] Low nail nitrogen is found in ill neonates.[96] In graft-versus-host disease, lichen planus-like changes, including superficial ulceration of the lunula, fluting of the nails, onychatrophia,[96] onychomycosis,[285] longitudinal ridging (J.M. Mascaro, personal communication, 8 December 1992), and periungual erythema (J.M. Mascaro, personal communication, 8 December 1992) may occur.

Reversible hyperpigmentation of the nails has been reported in a patient with vitamin $B_{12}$ deficiency.[286] Nail dystrophy has been associated with vitiligo.[287] Onycholysis, thickening, and discoloration have been reported in the Sézary syndrome.[288,289]

Other miscellaneous reports have included nodules under the nails in chronic lymphocytic leukemia,[290] and nail necrosis in gamma heavy-chain disease.[291] In addition, severe psoriasis (usually with nail involvement) patients have an increased incidence of autoimmune disease in close relatives.[292]

# NAIL CHANGES ASSOCIATED WITH SPECIFIC SYNDROMES OR GENODERMATOSES

Although many genetic syndromes may demonstrate nail abnormalities, these are usually not the most prominent finding. The syndromes discussed below are those with fairly prominent and distinctive nail manifestations that are useful in diagnosis. Other syndromes that may demonstrate less specific nail changes are listed in Table 15.13. This table categorizes various genetic syndromes that may demonstrate nail abnormalities. It is not meant to be a complete list but to generally group the types of nail manifestations most frequently seen in association with particular syndromes to aid in diagnosis.

*Darier's disease* (keratosis follicularis) is an autosomal dominant or sporadic disorder of keratinization characterized by progressive appearance of 'greasy' keratotic papules in a seborrheic distribution. The characteristic nail changes are longitudinal streaks with distal V-shaped notches of the nail plate and subungual hyperkeratosis[293] (Fig. 15.21).

*Dyskeratosis congenita* (Zinsser–Cole–Engman syndrome) may be X-linked recessive, autosomal recessive, or autosomal dominant and involves a mutation in the DKC1 gene, which codes for dyskerin, a protein with important nucleolar functions. Premalignant leukoplakia of the oral mucosa, cutaneous reticulated hyperpigmentation and progressive (often fatal) pancytopenia are the most significant findings. Koilonychia, onychorrhexis, onychoschizia and rarely anonychia may be the presenting signs of this syndrome, which usually occurs in the mid first to second decade.[293,294]

*Pachyonychia congenita* (PC) is a group of disorders characterized by extreme nail bed hyperkeratosis, brown discoloration of the nail plate and increased transverse curvature of the nail plate. The various subtypes of PC demonstrate several associated features, such as palmoplantar keratoderma, leukoplakia of mucous membranes and follicular keratoses. Nail manifestations are the unifying feature and may begin as early as infancy but can be later. Most types of PC are inherited autosomal dominant but there are recessive forms. PC type I is characterized by oral leukoplakia and involves keratin K6a and K16 gene mutations. In contrast, PC type II presents with premature dentition and multiple pilosebaceous cysts and has a mutation in the keratin K6b and K17 genes.[295]

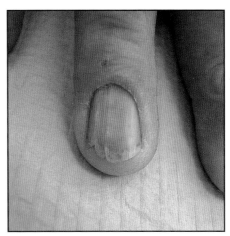

FIGURE 15–21. Darier's disease.

**TABLE 15–13. Less specific nail abnormalities associated with genetic syndromes**

## Ichthyosis/disorders of keratinization

Lamellar ichthyosis (autosomal recessive): rapid nail growth, subungual hyperkeratosis, onychorrhexis; hourglass-like pattern with lateral red triangular areas in the nail bed

Harlequin ichthyosis (autosomal recessive): hypoplastic or absent nails

Tay syndrome (AR, ichthyosis, brittle hair, impaired intelligence, decreased fertility, short stature): nail hypoplasia, onychorrhexis, koilonychias

Keratitis-ichthyosis-deafness (KID) syndrome (AD, AR): aplastic or hypoplastic nails at birth, nail dystrophy later

Ichthyosis with alopecia, eclabium, ectropion, and mental retardation: claw-like nails

Darier disease (AD, spontaneous mutations): longitudinal red, gray or white bands, distal notching of nail plate, subungual hyperkeratosis

Acrokeratosis verruciformis of Hopf (AD): white, thickened nail plates; ridging

Palmoplantar keratoderma syndromes (mal de meleda, papillion-lefevre): koilonychia, subungual hyperkeratosis, ridging

Punctate palmoplantar keratoderma (AD): nail dystrophy, onychomadesis, onychauxis

Porokeratosis of Mibelli (AD, sporadic): onychauxis, onychorrhexis, nail plate splitting

Keratosis palmoplantaris with periodontitis and onychogryphosis (AR): onychogryphosis, arachnodactyly, acro-osteolysis

Pachyoncychia congenita (AD): thickening, subungual hyperkeratosis, onychogryphosis (see section above)

## Mechanobullous disorders

Most types of epidermolysis bullosa may occasionally show nail dystrophy. The types with more specific findings are listed:

Epidermolysis bullosa simplex herpetiformis (AD): onychomadesis, nails regrow normally

Epidermolysis Bullosa Simplex, Ogna Variant (AD): onychogryphosis

Junctional epidermolysis bullosa (many subtypes, AR): nail dystrophy, anonychia (may be initial presenting sign), paronychia (hallmark of neonatal period)

Dystrophic epidermolysis bullosa (many subtypes, AD, AR): nails dystrophy, anonychia

## Other bullous disorders

Acrodermatitis enteropathica (AR): nail dystrophy and paronychia common, nail shedding may occur

## Poikilodermatous disorders

Many subtypes may demonstrate nail findings, however, only a few are specific:

Dyskeratosis congenita (XLR,AR,AD): nail dystrophy, rarely anonychia; nail changes may be presenting sign of the disease in mid-first to second decade (see above).

Hereditary sclerosing poikiloderma (AD): clubbing

## Premature aging syndromes

Progeria (sporadic, AR, AD): yellowish discoloration, thin, brittle nail plate

Werner syndrome (AR): nails brittle, atrophic or absent

Facial mandibuloacral dysplasia (AR): broad, brittle nails; acro-osteolysis and short club-shaped terminal phalanges

Acrogeria (sporadic, AR, AD): onychogryphosis, koilonychias, atrophy

Scleroatrophic and keratotic dermatosis of limbs (AD): nail hypoplasia and leukonychia, sclerodactyly

## Ectodermal Dysplasia Syndromes

Many subtypes show dystrophy, hypoplasia or anonychia. A few specific syndromes are listed:

AEC (ankyloblepharon, ectodermal dysplasia, and cleft palate; AD): dystrophy or anonychia

Coffin-Siris syndrome (AD): anonychia or hypoplasia of fifth fingernails and toenails

Ellis-van Creveld syndrome (AR): brittle, hypoplastic or absent nails

Goltz syndrome (XLD): koilonychia, hypoplasia, anonychia

Hydrotic ectodermal dysplasia (AD): onychauxis, paronychia, convex hypercurvature, anonychia

## Other dysplasia/malformation syndromes

Lacrimo-auriculo-dento-digital (LADD) syndrome (AD): ectopic nails, large thumb nail

Tooth and nail syndrome (AD): toenails more than fingernails hypoplastic and show koilonychias

Trichothiodystrophy (AR, XLR): onychauxis, subungual hyperkeratosis, onychoschizia, koilonychia

Triphalangeal thumbs-onychodystrophy-deafness (DOOR) syndrome (AR,AD): hypoplasia, anonychia

| TABLE 15-13. *(Cont'd)* Less specific nail abnormalities associated with genetic syndromes |
| --- |

## Syndromes with skeletal abnormalities

In general these frequently demonstrate short, broad or hypoplastic nails. Some specific syndromes are listed:
Apert syndrome (AD, sporadic): broad, short, fused nails, micronychia, anonychia
CHILD syndrome (XLD): onychogryphosis and brittleness on affected side
Marfan syndrome (AD): pseudo-clubbing
Oculodentodigital syndrome (AD, AR): anonychia
Pachydermoperiostosis (AD): clubbing, thin, yellow discoloration
Rubinstein-Taybi syndrome (AD): flat wide thumbnails and great toenails
Sclerosteosis (unknown inheritance): anonychia or dysplasia of second and third fingernails
Tricho-rhino-phalangeal syndrome (AD, AR): thin, short; koilonychia, leukonychia

## Miscellaneous syndromes and chromosomal abnormalities

Anonychia (AD): total or partial anonychia
Bart-Pumphrey syndrome (AD): total leukonychia
Familial koilonychia (AD): thin, concave nail plates
Hemochromatosis (AR): white, grey or brown nails; koiloncyhia
Hirschsprung disease (AR): hypoplastic nails
Leukonychia (AD): total, partial, striate, punctuate
Multiple lentigenes sydrome (AD): leukonychia, koiloncyhia
Peutz-Jeghers syndrome (AD): brown discoloration
Tuberous sclerosis (AD): subungual and periungual fibromas (Koenan tumors) usually appear around puberty
Cronkhite-Canada syndrome (sporadic): hypoplasia, soft, spongy nail plates and boggy nail beds
Down syndrome: clubbing, macronychia
Trisomies 18, 8,8p, 3q: hypoplastic, anonychia at birth
Turner syndrome: narrow, hyperconvex

*Nail–patella–elbow syndrome* (hereditary osteo-onychodysplasia; Fong's syndrome) is an autosomal dominant disorder characterized by dysplasia of the patella, decreased mobility of the elbow joints and nephropathy which may progress to renal failure. **The characteristic nail changes are hypoplasia or aplasia of the nails, and triangular lunulae most prominent in the thumbs and index fingers (Fig. 15.22).** The defect is a mutation in the homeodomain of the LMX 1B gene, an essential factor for limb development.

*The yellow nail syndrome*, characterized by slowly growing, yellow–green discolored nail plates in association with lymphedema and chronic respiratory tract disease is mostly sporadic but may be inherited in an autosomal dominant fashion. There are possible cases of recessive inheritance. This syndrome is discussed in detail in the pulmonary section above.[293]

*Incontinentia pigmenti* (IP) is an X-linked dominant disorder of ectodermal tissue. Infants present with a generalized vesicular eruption following the lines of Blaschko. This evolves into verrucous, hyperpigmented, and scarred stages over the first few years of life. Neurological and ocular abnormalities are seen in about 30% of patients; rarely, other musculoskeletal anomalies occur. The genetic defect is deletion of exons 4–10 of the NEMO gene, which encodes for a regulatory component of the IkB kinase pathway. The resulting cells are more susceptible to apoptosis in response to TNF-alpha. The presence of nail changes is variable but may be up to 40% of IP patients. Nonspecific findings like

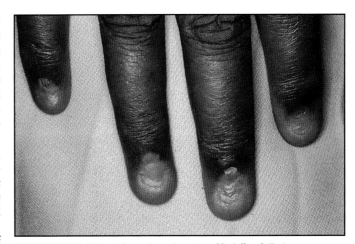

FIGURE 15-22. Nail-patella syndrome (courtesy of Dr Jeffrey Callen).

onychorrhexis, pitting or thinning of the nail plate may appear early and diminish with time. Subungual and periungual tumors may appear between puberty and the third decade and cause nail dystrophy, pain and even osteolysis of the terminal phalanx. There have been case reports of adult women with nail dystrophy and painful subungual tumors as the only sign of sign of incontinentia pigmenti.[293,297–299]

# REFERENCES

1. Jemec GB, Kollerup G, Jensen LB, Morgensen S. Nail abnormalities in nondermatologic patients: prevalence and possible role as diagnostic aids. J Am Acad Dermatol 1995; 32:977–981

2. Dupond AS, Magy N, Humbert P, Dupond JL. Manifestations ungueales des maladies generales. La Revue du Practicien 2000; 50: 2236–2240

3. Zaias N. The nail in health and disease. New York: Spectrum Publications; 1980

4. Daniel CR, Daniel MP. Nail signs of systemic disease. Consultant 1995; 35:392

5. Daniel CR. Nails in systemic disease. Audiotape presented at the meeting of the American Academy of Dermatology, New Orleans, 7 February 1995

6. Daniel CR, Scher RK. The nail. In: Sams WM, Lynch PJ, eds. Principles and practice of dermatology. 2nd edn. New York: Churchill-Livingstone; 1996:763–777

7. Kilpatrick ZM, Greenberg PA, Sanford JP. Splinter hemorrhages – their clinical significance. Arch Intern Med 1965; 115:730

8. Blum M, Avinam AL. Splinter hemorrhages in patients receiving regular hemodialysis. JAMA 1978; 239:44

9. Fitzpatrick TB. Dermatology in general medicine. 2nd edn. New York: McGraw-Hill; 1979

10. Samman PD. The nails in disease. 3rd edn. Chicago: Year Book; 1978

11. Zaias N. The nail in health and disease. New York: Spectrum Publications; 1980, citing Alkiewicz J. Zur Histopathologie der Hamatome des Menschlichen Nagels. Arch Dermatol Syphilol 1033; 168:411

12. Moschella SL, Hurley HJ, eds. Cutaneous manifestations of immuno-deficiency in dermatology. 2nd edn. Philadelphia: WB Saunders; 1985:218

13. Cohen PR, Scher RK. Geriatric nail disorders: diagnosis and treatment. J Am Acad Dermatol 1992; 26:521

14. Norton L. Determining if subungual bleeding signals systemic disease, trauma. Skin Allergy News 1991; 22:5

15. Tosti A, Baran R, Dawber RPR. The nail in systemic diseases and drug-induced changes. In: Baran R, Dawber RPR, eds. Diseases of the nails and their management. 2nd edn. Oxford: Blackwell Scientific 1994:175–261

16. Penas PF, Porras JI, Fraga J, et al. Microscopic polyangiitis. A systemic vasculitis with a positive P-ANCA. Br J Dermatol 1996; 134 (3):542–547

17. De Barber D. What do Beau's lines mean. Int J Dermatol 1994; 33:545

18. Baran R, Dawber RPR. Diseases of the nails and their management. 2nd edn. Oxford: Blackwell Science; 1994.

19. Baran R, Dawber RPR. Physical signs. In: Baran R, Dawber RPR eds. Diseases of the nails and their management. 2nd edn. Oxford: Blackwell Scientific; 1994:35–80

20. Bernier V, Labreze C, Bury F, Taieb A. Nail matrix arrest in the course of hand, foot and mouth disease. Eur J Pediatr 2001; 160:649–651

21. Clementz GC, Mancini AJ. Nail matrix arrest following hand-foot-mouth disease: a report of five children. Pediatr Dermatol 2000; 17:7–8

22. Tosti A, Piraccini BM. Onychomadesis and pyogenic granuloma following cast immobilization. Arch Dermatol 2001; 137:231–232

23. Lewin K. The fingernail in general disease. Br J Dermatol 1965; 77:431

24. DeNicola P, Morsiani M, Zavagli G. Nail diseases in internal medicine. Springfield, IL: Charles C Thomas; 1974

25. Daniel CR. Onycholysis: an overview. Semin Dermatol 1991; 10:34

26. Degowin EL, Degowin RL. The nails in bedside diagnostic examination. 2nd edn. New York: Macmillan; 1969

27. Luria MN, Asper SP. Onycholysis in hyperthyroidism. Ann Intern Med 1958; 49:102

28. Lovoy MR, Gluhm GB, Morales A. The occurrence of nail pitting in Reiter's syndrome. J Am Acad Dermatol 1980; 2:66

29. Pajarre R, Kemo M. Nail changes as the first manifestation of HLA-B27 inheritance. Dermatologica 1977; 154:350

30. Urowitz M, Gladman DD, Chalmers A, et al. Nail lesions in systemic lupus erythematosus. J Rheumatol 1978; 5:441

31. Dupre A, Viraben R, Bonafe JL, et al. Zebra-like dermatomyositis. Arch Dermatol 1981; 117:63

32. Patel KB, Sharma OP. Nail in sarcoidosis: response to treatment. Arch Dermatol 1983; 119:277

33. Baumal A, Robinson MJ. Nail bed involvement in pemphigus vulgaris. Arch Dermatol 1973; 107:751

34. Stone OJ. Spoon nails and clubbing. Cutis 1975; 16:235

35. Stone OJ, Maberry JD. Spoon nails and clubbing. Tex State J Med 1965; 61:620

36. Jalili MA, Al-Kassaf S. Koilonychia and cystine content of nails. Lancet 1959; i:108

37. Bentley-Phillips B, Bayles MA. Occupational koilonychia of the toenails. Br J Dermatol 1971; 85:140

38. Baran R. Nail changes in general pathology. In: Pierre M, ed. The nail. New York: Churchill Livingstone; 1981:5–105

39. Runne U, Orfanos CE. The human nail. In: Mali WH, Karger S, eds. Current problems in dermatology, vol 9. Basel: S Karger; 1981:102–149

40. Bergeron JR, Stone OJ. Koilonychia: a report of familial spooned nails. Arch Dermatol 1967; 95:351

41. Baran R, Achten G. Les associations congenitales de koilonychia et de leuconychie totale. Arch Belges Syphiligr 1969; 25:13

42. Hordinsky MK. Hair. In: Sams M, Lynch P, eds. Principles and practice of dermatology. New York: Churchill Livingstone; 1990:761–780

43. Cohen PR, Prystowsky JH. Metabolic and nutritional disorders. In: Sams W, Lynch P, eds. Principles and practice of dermatology. New York: Churchill-Livingstone; 1990:665–681

44. Daniel CR, Osment LS. Nail pigmentation abnormalities, their importance and proper examination. Cutis 1980; 25:595

45. Takeuchi Y, Iwase N, Suzuki M, Tsuyuki S. Lichen planus with involvement of all twenty nails and the oral mucous membrane. J Dermatol 2000; 27:94–98

46. Claudel CD, Zic JA, Boyd AS. Idiopathic leukonychia totalis and partialis in a 12-year-old patient. J Am Acad Dermatol 2001; 44:379–380

47. Foti C et al. Transverse leukonychia in severe hypocalcemia. Eur J Dermatol 2004; 14:67–68

48. Marcilly MC et al. [Sub-total hereditary leukonychia, histopathology and electron microscopy study of 'milky' nails]. Ann Dermatol Venereol 2003; 130:50–54

49. Hudson JB, Dennis AJ Jr. Transverse white lines in the fingernails after acute and chronic renal failure. Arch Intern Med 1976; 117:276

50. Pardo-Castello V. Diseases of the nails. 3rd edn. Springfield, IL: Charles C Thomas; 1960

51. Conn RD, Smith RH. Malnutrition, myoedema Muehrcke's lines. Arch Intern Med 1965; 116:875

52. Muehrcke RC. The fingernails in chronic hypoalbuminemia. Br Med J 1956; 1:327

53. Schwartz RA, Vickerman CE. Muehrcke's lines of the fingernails. Arch Intern Med 1979; 139:242

54. Feldman SR, Gummon WR. Unilateral Muehrcke's lines following trauma (letter). Arch Dermatol 1989; 125:133

55. Alam M, Scher RK, Bickers DR. Muehrcke's lines in a heart transplant recipient. J Am Acad Dermatol 2001; 44:316–317

56. Nabai H. Nail changes before and after heart transplantation: personal observation by a physician. Cutis 1998; 61:31–32

57. Ruggeri S, Viviano MT, Papi M, et al. Seasonal leukonychia: microvascular alteration? Eur Acad Dermatol Venereol 2000; 14 (Suppl 1):113

58. Daniel CR III, Bower JD, Daniel CR Jr. The half and half fingernail: the most significant onychopathological indicator of chronic renal failure. J Miss State Med Assoc 1975; 16:376

59. Daniel CR III, Bower JD, Daniel CR Jr. The half and half fingernail: a clue to chronic renal failure. Proc Clin Dial Transplant Forum 1975; 5:1

60. Lubach D, Strubbe I. The frequency of subungual erythema. Z Hautkr 1982; 57:1486

61. Terry R. White nails in hepatic cirrhosis. Lancet 1954; i:757–759

62. Holzberg M, Walker HK. Terry's nails: revised definition and new correlations. Lancet 1984; i:896–899

63. Terry RB. The onychodermal band in health and disease. Lancet 1955; i:179

64. Daniel CR. The nail. In: Sams M, Lynch P, eds. Principles and practice of dermatology. New York: Churchill Livingstone; 1990:743–760

65. Lovibond JL. Diagnosis of clubbed fingers. Lancet 1938; i:363

66. Goyal S, Griffiths AD, Omarouayache S, et al. An improved method of studying fingernail morphometry: application to the early detection of clubbing. J Am Acad Dermatol 1998; 39:640–642

67. Brickman AS. Grand rounds: progressive shortening of the fingertips. Drug Ther 1981; 49

68. Mendlowitz M. Measurements of blood flow and blood pressure in clubbed fingers. J Clin Invest 1941; 20:113

69. Hall GH. The cause of digital clubbing. Lancet 1959; i:750

70. Bashour FA. Clubbing of the digits: physiologic considerations. J Lab Clin Med 1961; 58:613

71. Ginsberg J, Brown JB. Increased estrogen exertion in hypertrophic pulmonary osteoarthropathy. Lancet 1961; ii:1274

72. Mackie RM. Lupus erythematosus in association with finger-clubbing. Br J Dermatol 1973; 89:533

73. Davis GM, Rubin J, Bauer JD. Digital clubbing due to secondary hyperparathyroidism. Arch Intern Med 1990; 150:452

74. Scherbenske JM, Benson PM, Rotchford JP, James WD. Cutaneous and ocular manifestations of Down syndrome. J Am Acad Dermatol 1990; 22:933

75. West SG, Gilbreath RE, Lawless, OJ. Painful clubbing and sarcoidosis. JAMA 1981; 246:1338

76. Braverman IM. Skin signs of systemic disease. 2nd edn. Philadelphia: WB Saunders; 1981

77. Pines A, Olchovsky D, Bregman J, et al. Finger clubbing associated with laxative abuse. South Med J 1983; 76:1071

78. Burgdorf W. Cutaneous manifestations of Crohn's disease. J Am Acad Dermatol 1981; 5:689

79. Demis DJ (ed). Clubbing of the fingers in clinical dermatology, vol 1. New York: Harper & Row; 1980

80. Brenner S, Srebrnik A, Kisch ES. Pachydermoperiostosis with new clinical and endocrinologic manifestation. Int J Dermatol 1992; 31:341

81. Just-Viera JO. Clubbed digits: an enigma. Arch Intern Med 1964: 113:122

82. Terry R. Red half-moons in cardiac failure. Lancet 1954; ii:842

83. Jeremias FJ, Sole MD, Conti M, Camarasa JG. Sindrome de las unas amarillas asociado a miocardiopatia. Med Cutan Iber Lat Am 1996; 24: 279–282

84. Barone SR et al. The differentiation of classic Kawasaki disease, atypical Kawasaki disease, and acute adenoviral infection. Arch Pediatr Adolesc Med 2000; 154:453–456

85. Dhawan SS, Zaias N, Pena J. The nail fold in pemphigus vulgaris. Arch Dermatol 1990; 126:1374

86. Garg RK. Determination of ABOCH blood group-specific substances from fingernails. Am J Forensic Med Pathol 1983; 4:143

87. Samman PD. Management of disorders of the nails. Clin Exp Dermatol 1982; 7:189

88. Bearn AG, McKusick VA. Azure lunulae. JAMA 1958; 166:904

89. Mathias CGT, Caldwell TM, Maibach HI. Contact dermatitis and gastrointestinal symptoms from hydroxyethylomethacrylate. Br J Dermatol 1979; 100:447

90. Greene RA, Scher RK. Nail changes associated with diabetes mellitus. J Am Acad Dermatol 1987; 16:1015

91. Feingold KR, Elias PM. Endocrine–skin interactions. J Am Acad Dermatol 1987; 17:921

92. Bissell GW, Sarakomoi K, Greenslit F. Longitudinal banded pigmentation of nails in primary adrenal insufficiency. JAMA 1971; 215:1656

93. Scher RK, Bodian AB. Brittle nails. Semin Dermatol 1991; 10:21

94. Scher RK. Brittle nails. Int J Dermatol 1989; 28:515

95. Rook A, Wilkinson DS, Eblins FJG, et al. Textbook of dermatology. 3rd edn. Oxford: Blackwell Scientific; 1979

96. Baran R, Dawber RPR. Diseases of the nails and their management. Oxford: Blackwell Scientific; 1984

97. Moschella SL, Pillsbury DM, Hurley HJ. Dermatology. Philadelphia: WB Saunders; 1975

98. Patki AH, Mehta JM. Pterygium unguium in a patient with recurrent type 2 lepra reaction. Cutis 1989; 44:311

99. Menter MA, Morrison JGL. Lichen verrucosus et reticularis of Kaposi: a manifestation of acquired adult toxoplasmosis. Br J Dermatol 1976; 94:645

100. Hirschmann JV. Cutaneous signs of systemic bacterial infection. In: Sams WM, Lynch PJ, eds. Principles and practice of dermatology. New York: Churchill-Livingstone; 1990:89–98

101. Allen LA. Occult blood accumulation under the fingernails: a mechanism for the spread of blood-borne infection. J Am Acad Dermatol 1982; 105:455

102. Scher RK. Subungual scabies. Am J Dermatopathol 1983; 5:187

103. Witkowski JA, Parish LC. Scabies, subungual areas harbor mites. JAMA 1984; 252:1318

104. Kosinski MA, Stewart D. Nail changes associated with systemic disease and vascular insufficiency. Clin Podiatr Med Surg 1989; 6:295

105. Daniel CR, Norton LA, Scher RK. The spectrum of nail disease in patients with human immunodeficiency virus infection. J Am Acad Dermatol 1992; 27:93

106. Daniel CR. Nail disease in patients with HIV infection. In: WHC Burgdorf, SI Katz, eds. Dermatology, progress and perspectives: the proceedings of the 18th World Congress of Dermatology. New York: Parthenon; 1993:382–385

107. Cribier B et al. Nail changes in patients infected with human immunodeficiency virus. Arch Dermatol 1998; 134:1216–1220

108. Dompmartin D, Dompmartin A, Deluol AM, et al. Onychomycosis and AIDS: clinical and laboratory findings in 62 patients. Int J Dermatol 1990; 29:337

109. Kaplan MH, Sadick N, McNutt NS, et al. Dermatologic findings and manifestations of acquired immunodeficiency syndrome (AIDS). J Am Acad Dermatol 1987; 16:485

110. Lizama E, Logemann H. Proximal white subungual onychomycosis in AIDS. Int J Dermatol 1996; 35:290

111. Rongioletti F, Persi A, Tripodi S, Rebora A. Proximal white subungual onychomycosis: a sign of immunodeficiency. J Am Acad Dermatol 1994; 30:129

112. Elewski BE. Clinical pearl: proximal white subungual onychomycosis in AIDS. J Am Acad Dermatol 1993; 29:631

113. Haley L, Daniel CR. Fungal infection of the nails. In: Scher RK, Daniel CR, eds. Nails: therapy, diagnosis, surgery. Philadelphia: WB Saunders; 1990:106–119

114. Daniel CR, Elewski BE. Candida as a nail pathogen in healthy patients. J MS State Med Assn 1995; 36:379–381

115. Scher RK. Nail signs of systemic diseases (audiotape). Dialogues in Dermatol 1991; 28

116. Fisher BK, Warner LC. Cutaneous manifestations of the AIDS: Update 1987. Int J Dermatol 1987; 26:615

117. Montemarano AD, Benson PM, James WD, Croup MA. Acute paronychia apparently caused by *Candida albicans* in a healthy female. Arch Dermatol 1993; 129:786

118. Prose NS. HIV infection in children. J Am Acad Dermatol 1990; 22:1223

119. Prose NS, Abson KG, Scher RK. Disorders of the nails and hair associated with HIV infection. Int J Dermatol 1992; 31:453

120. Valenzano L, Giacalone B, Grillo LR, Ferraris AM. Compromissione ungueale in corso di AIDS. G Ital Dermatol Venereol 1988; 123:527

121. Daniel CR. The diagnosis of nail fungal infection. Arch Dermatol 1991; 127:1566

122. Straka BP, Whitaker DL, Morrison SH, et al. Cutaneous manifestations of the acquired immunodeficiency syndrome in children. J Am Acad Dermatol 1988; 18:1089

123. Eliezri Y, Silverstein SJ, Nuoro GJ. Occurrence of human papillomavirus type 16 DNA in cutaneous squamous and basal cell carcinomas. J Am Acad Dermatol 1990; 23:836

124. Rau RC, Baird IM. Crusted scabies in a patient with acquired immuno-deficiency syndrome (letter). J Am Acad Dermatol 1986; 15:1058

125. Drabick JJ, Lupton GP, Tompkins K. Crusted scabies in human immunodeficiency virus infection (letter). J Am Acad Dermatol 1987; 17:142

126. Depaoli RT, Marks VJ. Crusted (Norwegian) scabies: treatment of nail involvement (letter). J Am Acad Dermatol 1987; 17:136

127. Scher RK. Subungual scabies (letter). Am J Dermatopathol 1983; 5:187

128. High WA, Tyring SK, Taylor RS. Rapidly enlarging growth of the proximal nail fold. Dermatol Surg 2003; 29:984–986

129. Kaplan MH, Sadick NS, Wieder J, et al. Antipsoriatic effects of zidovudine in human immunodeficiency virus-associated psoriasis. J Am Acad Dermatol 1989; 20:76

130. Rasokat H. Psoriasis in AIDS: remission with high dosage cotrimoxazole. A Hautkr 1986; 61:991

131. Marcusson JA, Wetterberg L. Peptide-T in the treatment of AIDS associated psoriasis and psoriatic arthritis. Acta Derm Venereal (Stockh) 1989; 69:86

132. Rosenberg EW, Noah D, Skinner RB. AIDS and psoriasis. Int J Dermatol 1991; 30:449

133. Belz J, Breneman DL, Nordlund JJ, Solinger A. Successful treatment of a patient with Reiter's syndrome and acquired immunodeficiency syndrome using etretinate. J Am Acad Dermatol 1989; 20:898

134. Bluvelt A, Nahass GT, Pardo RJ, et al. Pityriasis rubra pilaris and HIV infection. J Am Acad Dermatol 1991; 24:703

135. Cohen S, Dicken CH. Generalized lichen spinulosus in an HIV-positive man. J Am Acad Dermatol 1991; 25:116

136. Daniel CR, Sams WM, Scher RK. Nails in systemic disease. In: Scher RK, Daniel CR, eds. Nails: therapy, diagnosis, surgery. 2nd edn. Philadelphia: WB Saunders; 1990:167–191

137. Chernosky ME, Finley VK. Yellow nail syndrome in patients with acquired immunodeficiency disease. J Am Acad Dermatol 1985; 13:731

138. Daniel CR. Yellow nail syndrome and acquired immunodeficiency disease. J Am Acad Dermatol 1986; 14:844

139. Norton AL. Yellow nail syndrome controlled by vitamin E therapy (letter). J Am Acad Dermatol 1986; 15:715

140. Scher RK. Acquired immunodeficiency syndrome and yellow nails (letter). J Am Acad Dermatol 1988; 18:758

141. Goodman DS, Teplitz E, Wishner A, et al. Prevalence of cutaneous disease in patients with acquired immunodeficiency syndrome (AIDS) or AIDS-related complex. J Am Acad Dermatol 1987; 17:210

142. Daniel CR, Scher RK. Nail changes secondary to systemic drugs or ingestants. In: Scher RK, Daniel CR, eds. Nails: therapy, diagnosis, surgery. 2nd edn. Philadelphia: WB Saunders; 1990:192–201

143. Glaser DA, Remlinger K. Blue nails and acquired immunodeficiency syndrome: not always associated with azidothymidine use. Cutis 1996; 57:243

144. James CW, McNeils KC, Cohen DM, et al. Recurrent ingrown toenails secondary to indinavir/ritonavir combination therapy. Ann Pharmacother 2001; 35: 881–884

145. Ward HA, Russo GG, Shrum J. Cutaneous manifestations of anti-retroviral therapy. J Am Acad Dermatol 2002; 46:284–293

146. Cohen PR. The lunula. J Am Acad Dermatol 1996; 34:943

147. Leppard B. Blue nails are a sign of HIV infection. Int J STD AIDS 1999; 10: 479–482

148. Itin PH, Gilli L, Nuesch R, et al. Erythema of the proximal nailfold in HIV-infected patients. J Am Acad Dermatol 1996; 35:631

149. Ruiz-Avila P, Tercedor J, Rodenas JM. Periungual erythema in HIV-infected patients. J Am Acad Dermatol 1997; 37:1018

150. Ruiz-Avila P, Villen A, Rodenas JM. Painful periungual telangiectasia in a patient with acquired immunodeficiency syndrome. Int J Dermatol 1995; 34:199

151. Miller SJ. Nutritional deficiency and the skin. J Am Acad Dermatol 1989; 21:1

152. Gisht DB, Singh SS. Pigmented bands on nails: A new sign in malnutrition. Lancet 1962; i:507

153. Maricq HR. Familiar schizophrenia as defined by nail fold capillary pattern and selected psychiatric traits. J Nerv Ment Dis 1963; 136:216

154. Maricq HR. Capillary morphology and the course of illness in schizophrenic patients. J Nerv Ment Dis 1966; 142:63

155. Maricq HR. Association of a clearly visible subpapillary plexus with other peculiarities of the nail fold skin in some schizophrenic patients. Dermatologica 1969; 138:148

156. Patterson JW. Pterygium inversum unguius-like changes in scleroderma. Arch Dermatol 1977; 113:1429

157. Goihman-Yahr M. Peculiar dyschromic changes of finger nails in a patient with multiple system atrophy. Int J Dermatol 1998; 37:156–160

158. Inglesse M, Haley HR, Elewski BE. Onychotillomania: 2 case reports. Cutis 2004; 73:171–174

159. Bensler JM, Paauw DS. Apotemnophilia masquerading as medical morbiditiy. South Med J 2003; 96:674–676

160. Alam M, Moossavi M, Ginsburg I, Scher RK. A psychometric study of patients with nail dystrophies. J Am Acad Dermatol 2001; 45:851–856

161. Hediger C, Rost B, Itin P. Cutaneous manifestations in anorexia nervosa. Schweiz Med Wochenschr 2000; 130:565–575

162. Smith KE, Fenske NA. Cutaneous manifestations of alcohol abuse. J Am Acad Dermatol 2000; 43:1–16

163. Marks G, Ellis JP. Yellow nails. Arch Dermatol 1970; 102:619

164. Kandil E. Yellow nail syndrome. Int J Dermatol 1973; 12:236

165. Pavlidakey GP, Hashimoto K, Blum D. Yellow nail syndrome. J Am Acad Dermatol 1984; 11:509

166 Ayres S, Michan R. Yellow nail syndrome, response to vitamin E. Arch Dermatol 1973; 108:267

167. Guin JD, Elleman JH. Yellow nail syndrome possible association with malignancy. Arch Dermatol 1979; 115:734

168. Decosta SD, Imber MJ, Baden HP. Yellow nail syndrome. J Am Acad Dermatol 1990; 22:608

169. Bilen N et al. Lymphoscintigraphy in yellow nail syndrome. Int J Dermatol 1998; 37:433–453

170. Samman PD, White WF. The 'yellow nail' syndrome. Br J Dermatol 1964; 76:153

171. Burrows NP, Jones RR. Yellow nail syndrome in association with carcinoma of the gall bladder. Clin Exp Dermatol 1991; 16:471

172. Moran MF. Upper respiratory problems in the yellow nail syndrome. Clin Otolaryngol 1976; 1:333

173. Lodge JP, Hunter AM, Saunders NR. Yellow nail syndrome associated with empyema. Clin Exp Dermatol 1989; 14:328

174. Krebs A. Drug-induced nail disorders. Praxis 1981; 70:1951

175. Lubach D, Marghescu S. Yellow-nail syndrom durch D-enizillamin. Hautzt 1979; 30:547

176. Mautner G, Scher RK. Yellow nail syndrome. J Geriatr Dermatol 1993; 1:106

177. Ocana I, Bejarno E, Ruiz I, et al. Intestinal lymphangiectasia and the yellow nail syndrome (letter). Gastroenterology 1988; 94:858

178. Knuckles MLF, Hodge SJ, et al. Yellow nail syndrome in association with sleep apnea. Int J Dermatol 1986; 25:588

179. Meirs HG, Gruel H, Perschmann Y, et al. Yellow nail syndrome. Dtsch Med Wochenschr 1973; 98:1529

180. Abell E, Samman PD. Yellow nail syndrome treated by intralesional triamcinolone acetomide. Br J Dermatol 1973; 88:200

181. Lebioda J. Yellow nail syndrome. Przegl Dermatol 1972; 59:523

182. Nelson LM. Yellow nail syndrome. Arch Dermatol 1969; 100:499

183. Norton L. Further observations on the yellow nail syndrome with therapeutic effects of oral alphatocopherol. Cutis 1985; 36:457

184. Hazebrigg DE, McElroy RJ. The yellow nail syndrome. J Assoc Milit Dermatol 1980; 6:14

185. Cohen PR, Prystowsky. Metabolic and nutritional disorders. In: Sams WM, Lynch PJ, eds. Principles and practice of dermatology. New York: Churchill Livingstone; 1996:693–712

186. Williams HC, Buffham R, Vivier A. Successful use of topical vitamin E solution in the treatment of nail changes in yellow nail syndrome. Arch Dermatol 1991; 127:1023

187. Andre J, Walraevens C, DeDoncker P. Yellow nail syndrome infected by dermatophyte SPP: experience with itraconazole pulse treatment combined with vitamin E. Poster exhibit at the annual meeting of the American Academy of Dermatology, New Orleans, February 1995

188. Cornelius CE, Shelley WB. Shell nail syndrome associated with bronchiectasis. Arch Dermatol 1967; 96:694

189. Baran R. Paraneoplastic acrokeratosis of Bazex. Arch Dermatol 1977; 113:1613

190. Pecora AL, Landsman L, Imgrund SP, et al. Acrokeratoses paraneoplastics (Bazex' syndrome). Arch Dermatol 1983; 119:820

191. Bazex A, Salvador R, Dupre A. Syndrome paraneoplasique a type d'hyperkeratose des extremities: Guerison apres le traitement de Peoithelioma larynge. Bull Soc Fr Dermatol Syphiligr 1965; 72:182

192. Paul SR, Perez-Atayde A, Williams DA. Interstitial pulmonary disease associated with dyskeratosis congenita. Am J Pediatr Hematol Oncol 1992; 14:89

193. Lindsay PG. The half and half nail. Arch Intern Med 1967; 119:583

194. Bean WB. A discourse on nail growth and unusual fingernails. Trans Am Clin Climatol Assoc 1963; 74:152

195. Kint A, Bussels L, Fernandes M. et al. Skin and nail disorders in relation to chronic renal failure. Acta Derm Venereal (Stockh) 1974; 54:137

196. Nixon DW, Pirozzi D, York RM, et al. Dermatological changes after systemic cancer therapy. Cutis 1981; 27:181

197. Daniel CR III. Nail pigmentation abnormalities: An addendum. Cutis 1982; 30:364

198. Daniel CR III, Scher RK. Nail changes secondary to systemic drugs and ingestants. J Am Acad Dermatol 1984; 10:250

199. Scher RK. Yellow nail syndrome and half-and-half nail. Arch Dermatol 1987; 123:710

200. Leyden JJ, Wood MG. The half and half nail. Arch Dermatol 1972; 105:591

201. Stewart WK, Raffle EJ. Brown nail bed arcs and chronic renal disease. Br Med J 1972; 1:784

202. Bussels L, Kint A, Fernandes M, et al. Lesions cutaneous et unqueales dans l'insuffisance renale chronique. Arch Belg Dermatol Syphiligr 1972; 28:363

203. Gilkes JJH, Eady RAJ, Rees LH, et al. Plasma immunoreactive melanotrophic hormones in patients on maintenance haemodialysis. Br Med J 1075; 1:656

204. Lubach D, Strubbe J, Schmidt J. The half and half nail phenomenon in chronic hemodialysis patients. Dermatologica 1982; 164:350

205. Levitt JI. Creatine concentration of human fingernail and toenail clippings. Ann Intern Med 1966; 64:312

206. Saray Y, Seckin D, Gulec AT, et al. Nail disorders in hemodialysis and renal transplant recipients: a case-control study. J Am Acad Dermatol 2004; 50:197–202

207. Tercedor J, Lopez-Hernandez B, Rodenas JM, Serrano S. Nail diseases in hemodialysis patients: case-control study. Poster exhibit from the European Nail Society meeting 16 June 1997

208. Kelly MP, Kight MA, Castillo S. Trophic implications of altered body composition observed in or near nails of hemodialysis patients. Advances in Renal Transplant Surgery 1998; 5:241–251

209. Hwang SM, Lee SH, Ahn SK. Pincer nail deformity and pseudo-Kaposi's sarcoma: complications of an artificial arteriovenous fistula for haemodialysis. Br J Dermatol 1999; 141:1129–1132

210. Sarnow MR, Plotkin EL, Spinosa FA, Cohen R. Nail changes in the seropositive and seronegative arthritides. Clin Podiatr Med Surg 1989; 6:389

211. Lugo-Janer G, Sanchez JL, Santiago-Delpin E. Prevalence and clinical spectrum of skin disease in kidney transplant recipients. J Am Acad Dermatol 1991; 24:410

212. Maricq HR, Spencer-Green C, LeRoy EC. Skin capillary abnormalities as indicators of organ involvement in scleroderma (systemic sclerosis), Raynaud's syndrome and dermatomyositis. Am J Med 1976; 61:862

213. Minkin W, Rabhan NB. Office nail fold capillary microscopy using ophthalmoscope. J Am Acad Dermatol 1982; 7:190

214. Herd JK. Nailfold capillary microscopy made easy. Arthritis Rheum 1976; 19:1370

215. Ohtsuka T et al. Nailfold capillary abnormality and pulmonary hypertension in systemic sclerosis. Int J Dermatol 1997; 36:116–122

216. Monticone G, Colonna L, Palermi G, et al. Quantitative nailfold capillary microscopy findings in patients with acrocyanosis

compared with patients having systemic sclerosis and control subjects. J Am Acad Dermatol 2000; 42:787–790

217. Poszepczynska-Guigne E et al. Paraneoplastic acral vascular syndrome. Epidemiologic features, clinical manifestations, and disease sequelae. J Am Acad Dermatol 2002; 47:47–52

218. Fonollosa V et al. Morphologic capillary changes and manifestations of connective tissue diseases in patients with primary biliary cirrhosis. Lupus 2001; 10:628–631

219. Scher RK, Tom DWK, Lally EV, et al. The clinical significance of PAS-positive deposits in cuticle-proximal nail fold biopsy specimens. Arch Dermatol 1985; 121:1406

220. Ohtsuka T, Yamakage A, Tamura T. Image analysis of nail fold capillaries in patients with Raynaud's phenomenon. Cutis 1995; 56:215

221. Mannarino E, Pasqualini L, Fedeli F, et al. Nailfold capillaroscopy in the screening and diagnosis of Raynaud's phenomenon. Angiology 1994; 45:37–42

222. Maricq HR, Maize JC. Nailfold capillary abnormalities. Clin Rheum Dis 1982; 8:455

223. Ohtsuka T. The relation between nailfold bleeding and capillary microscopy abnormality in patients with connective tissue diseases. Int J Dermatol 1998; 37:23–26

224. Hamilton EBD. Nail studies in rheumatoid arthritis. Ann Rheum Dis 1960; 19:167

225. Michel C et al. Nail abnormalities in rheumatoid arthritis. Br J Dermatol 1997; 137:958–962

226. Tosti A. The nail apparatus in collagen disorders. Semin Dermatol 1991; 10:71

227. Jaizzo JL, Gonzalez EB, Daniels JC. Red lunulae in a patient with rheumatoid arthritis. J Am Acad Dermatol 1983; 8:711

228. Kint A, Herpe LV. Ungual anomalies in lupus erythematosus discoids. Dermatologica 1976; 153:298

229. Narehari SR, Srinivas CR, Kelkar SK. LE-like erythema and periungual telangiectasia among coffee plantation workers. Contact Dermatitis 1990; 22:296

230. Phelps RG, Fleischmajer R. Clinical, pathologic, and immuno-pathologic manifestations of the toxic oil syndrome. J Am Acad Dermatol 1988; 18:313

231. Garcia-Patos V, Bartralot R, Ordi J, Baselga E, Moragas JM, Castells A. Systemic lupus erythematosus presenting with red lunulae. J Am Acad Dermatol 1997; 36:834–836

232. Vaughn RY, Bailey JP, Field RS, et al. Diffuse nail dyschromia in black patients with SLE. J Rheumatol 1990; 17:640

233. Skowron R, Combemale P, Faisant M, Baran R. Functional melanonychia due to involvement of the nail matrix in systemic lupus erythematosus. J Am Acad Dermatol 2002; 47:S187–S188

234. Pallis M, Hopkinson N, Powell R. Nailfold capillary density as a possible indicator of pulmonary capillary loss in systemic lupus erythematosus but not in MLTD. J Rheumatol 1991; 18:1532

235. Su WPD, Perniciaro C, Robgers RS, White JW. Chilblain lupus erythematosus (lupus pernio): clinical review of the Mayo Clinic experience and proposal of diagnostic criteria. Cutis 1994; 53:395

236. Thiers BH, Dobson RL. Westwood Western Conference on clinical dermatology. J Am Acad Dermatol 1980; 3:651

237. Caputo R, Cappio F, Rigorri C, et al. Pterygium inversum unguius. Arch Dermatol 1993; 129:1307

238. Norton LA. The nail. Lecture presented at Nail and Hair Symposium sponsored by Columbia University, September 1989

239. Odom RB, Stein KM, Maibach HI. Congenital painful aberrant hyponychium. Arch Dermatol 1974; 110:89

240. Shikano Y, Mori S, Kitajima Y. Detection of scleroderma with capillaroscopic abnormalities of nailfolds. Int J Dermatol 1996; 35:857

241. Caputo R, Prandi G. Pterygium inversum unguium. Arch Dermatol 1973; 108:817

242. Drake L, Goodman TB. Pterygium inversum unguium. Society transactions. Arch Dermatol 1976; 112:255

243. Nogita T, Yamashita H, Kawashima M, Hidano A. Pterygium inversum unguis. J Am Acad Dermatol 1991; 24:787

244. Fleischmajer R. Unusual nail findings. Lecture presented at the meeting of the American Dermatological Society of Allergy and Immunology, New Orleans, September 1980

245. Sato S, Takehara K, Sama Y, et al. Diagnostic significance of nailfold bleeding in scleroderma spectrum disorders. J Am Acad Dermatol 1993; 28:198

246. Maricq HR. Capillary abnormalities, Raynaud's phenomenon, and systemic sclerosis in patients with localized scleroderma. Arch Dermatol 1992; 128:630

247. Barrow MV. The nails in multicentric reticulohistiocytosis. Arch Dermatol 1967; 95:200

248. Tani M, Hori K, Nakanishi T, et al. Multicentric reticulo-histiocytosis. Arch Dermatol 1981; 117:495

249. Sahin AA, Kaloncu AF, Selouk ZT, et al. Behçet's disease with half and half nail and pulmonary artery aneurysm (letter). Chest 1990; 97:1277

250. Greaves MS, Fieller NRJ, Moll JMH. Differentiation between psoriatic arthritis and rheumatoid arthritis: A biochemical and statistical analysis of fingernail amino acids. Scand J Rheumatol 1979; 8:33

251. Maeda K, Kawaquchi S, Niwa T, et al. Identification of some abnormal metabolites in psoriasis nail using gas chromatography-mass spectrometry. J Chromatogr 1980; 221:199

252. Rasmussen J. Childhood psoriasis in pediatric dermatology, dermavision. Videotape presented at the meeting of the American Academy of Dermatology, Evanston, IL, December 1982

253. Blockmans D, Vermylen J, Babhaers H. Nailfold capillaroscopy in connective tissue disorders in Raynaud's phenomenon. Acta Clin Belg 1993; 48:30

254. Gibson GE, Su WPD, Pittlekow MR. Antiphospholipid syndrome and the skin. J Am Acad Dermatol 1997; 36:970–982

255. Chanda JJ, Callen JP. Stevens–Johnson syndrome. Arch Dermatol 1978; 114:626

256. Wanscher B, Thormann J. Permanent anonychia after Stevens–Johnson syndrome. Arch Dermatol 1977; 113:970

257. Zaias H. Diseases of the nails. In: Demis J, Dobson RL, Crounse RB, eds. Clinical dermatology. New York: Harper & Row; 1974:1–5.

258. Wheeler GE, Barrows GH. Alopecia universalis, a manifestation of occult amyloidosis and multiple myeloma. Arch Dermatol 1981; 117:815

259. Leavell OW, Farley CH, McIntyre JS. Cutaneous changes in a patient with carbon monoxide poisoning. Arch Dermatol 1969; 99:429

260. Kahn G. Nail involvement in histiocytosis X. Arch Dermatol 1969; 100:699

261. Timpatanapong P, Hathirat P, Isarangkura P. Nail involvement in histiocytosis X. Arch Dermatol 1984; 120:1052

262. Holzberg M, Wade TR, Buchana ID, et al. Nail pathology in histiocytosis X. J Am Acad Dermatol 1985; 13:522

263. Harper JI, Staughton R. Histiocytosis X (letter). Cutis 1983; 31:493

264. Chesney PJ, Davis JP, Purdy WK, et al. Clinical manifestations of toxic shock syndrome. JAMA 1981; 246:741

265. Niemi KM, Kero M, Kanerva L, et al. Epidermolysis bullosa simplex. Arch Dermatol 1983; 119:138

266. Haber RM, Hanna W, Ramsey CA, et al. Hereditary epidermolysis bullosa. J Am Acad Dermatol 1985; 13:252

267. Main RA. Periodic shedding of the nails. Br J Dermatol 1973; 88:497

268. Palencia SI, Rodrigez-Peralto JL, Castano E, Vanaclocha F, Iglesias L. Lichenoid nail changes as sole external manifestation of graft vs. host disease. Int J Dermatol 2002; 41:44–45

269. Fujii K, Kanno Y, Ohgo N. Subungual hyperkeratosis due to sarcoidosis. Int J Dermatol 1997; 36:123–144

270. Kalb RE, Grossman ME. Pterygium formation due to sarcoidosis. Arch Dermatol 1985; 121:276

271. Wakelin SH, James MP. Sarcoidosis: nail dystrophy with or without underlying bone changes. Cutis 1995; 55:344

272. Ahmed I, Cronk JS, Crutchfield CE, Dahl MV. Myeloma-associated systemic amyloidosis presenting as chronic paronychia and palmodigital erythematous swelling and induration of the hands. J Am Acad Dermatol 2000; 42:339–342

273. Wong CK, Wang WJ. Systemic amyloidosis: a report of 19 cases. Dermatology 1994; 189:47–51

274. Dalziel KL, Telfer NR, Dawber RPR. Nail dystrophy in cutaneous T-cell lymphoma. Br J Dermatol 1989; 120:571

275. Wilson AGM, Cotter FE, Lowe DG, et al. Mycosis fungoides in childhood: an unusual presentation. J Am Acad Dermatol 1991; 25:370

276. de Berker D, Lever RK, Windebank K. Nail features in Langerhans cell histiocytosis. Br J Dermatol 1994; 130:523–527

277. Lynch PJ. Cutaneous signs of systemic malignancy. In: Sams WM, Lynch PJ, eds. Principles and practice of dermatology. New York: Churchill-Livingstone; 1996:739–746

278. Parameswara YR, Chinnappaiah RP. Onychomadesis associated with pemphigus vulgaris. Arch Dermatol 1981; 117:759

279. Akiyama C, Sou K, Furuya T, et al. Paronychia. A sign heralding an exacerbation of pemphigus vulgaris. J Am Acad Dermatol 1993; 29:494

280. Richards B. A radium fingernail polish. Wall Street Journal, 19 September 1983:72

281. Horan MA, Puxty JA, Fox RA. The white nails of old age (neopolitan nails). J Am Geriatr Soc 1982; 30:734

282. Fischer VE. Subunguale verkalkungen. Fortschr Rontgenstr 1982; 137:580

283. Wong RC, Ellis CN. Physiological skin changes in pregnancy. J Am Acad Dermatol 1984; 10:929

284. Hansen U, Haersley T, Knudsen B, Jacobson GK. Erythema elevation diutinum: case report showing an unusual distribution. Cutis 1994; 53:124

285. Basuck PJ, Scher RK. Onychomycosis in graft versus host disease. Cutis 1987; 40:237

286. Noppakun N, Swasdikul D. Reversible hyperpigmentation of skin and nails with white hair due to vitamin B12 deficiency. Arch Dermatol 1986; 122:896

287. Barth JH, Telfer MB, Dawber RPR. Nail abnormalities and autoimmunity. J Am Acad Dermatol 1988; 18:1062

288. Wieselthier JAS, Koh HK. Sezary syndrome: diagnosis, prognosis, critical review of options. J Am Acad Dermatol 1990; 22:381

289. Tosti A, Fanti PA, Varotti C. Massive lymphomatosis nail involvement in Sezary syndrome. Dermatologica 1990; 181:162

290. Simon CA, Su WPD, Chin-Yang L. Subungual leukemia cutis. Int J Dermatol 1990; 29:636

291. Lassoued K, Picard C, Danon F, et al. Cutaneous manifestations associated with gamma heavy chain disease. J Am Acad Dermatol 1990; 23:988

292. Harrison PV, Khunti K, Morris JA. Psoriatic nails, joints and autoimmunity (letter). Br J Dermatol 1990; 122:569

293. Novice F, ed. Handbook of genetic skin disorders. Philadelphia: WB Saunders; 1994

294. Yaghmai R et al. Overlap of dyskeratosis congenital with Hoyeraal–Hreidarsson syndrome. J Pediatr 2000; 136:390–393

295. Swensson O. [Pachyonychia congenital. Keratin gene mutation with pleiotropic effect]. Hautarzt 1999; 50:483–490

295a. Bongers EM, Knoers NV [from gene to disease; the nail-patella syndrome and the LMXIB gene]. Ned Tijdschr Geneeska. 2003 Jan 11; 147(2):67–9

296. Bardaro T, et al. Two cases of misinterpretation of molecular results in incontinentia pigmenti, and a PCR-based method to discriminate NEMO/IKKgamma gene deletion. Hum Mutat 2003; 21:8–11

297. Berlin AL, Paller AS, Chan LS. Incontinentia Pigmenti: a review and update on the molecular basis of pathophysiology. J Am Acad Dermatol 2002; 47:169–187

298. Adeniran A, Townsend PL, Peachey RD. Incontinentia Pigmenti (Bloch-Sulzberger syndrome) manifesting as painful periungual and subungual tumors. J Hand Surg [Br] 1993; 18:667–669

299. Nicolaou N, Graham-Brown RA. Nail dystrophy, an unusual presentation of incontinentia pigmenti. Br J Dermatol 2003; 149:1286–1288

# 16

# Systemic Drugs

## Philip R Cohen, C Ralph Daniel III and Richard K Scher

## Key Features

1. Antibiotics, antimalarials, chemotherapeutic agents, ingestants and poisons may cause a variety of nail changes
2. Drugs may alter different parts of the nail unti: matrix, nail bed, nail folds, hyponychium or a combination of all these
3. Photonycholysis is associated with antibiotic use

Systemic drugs and ingestants can produce nail abnormalities.[1–252] Asymptomatic growth rate changes and pigmentation abnormalities are the most common changes. Other changes vary from transient nail shedding to permanent nail deformities.[68,70]

The nail abnormalities that occur are frequently part of a symptom complex that includes additional mucosal or cutaneous changes – especially other keratinizing epithelium such as hair. However, the nail manifestations are often the only apparent finding. Therefore, it is important to be aware of these changes because: (1) nails are of cosmetic importance to the patient, (2) nail changes may be the initial manifestation of an unsuspected systemic problem, (3) nail changes may be an early feature of a serious drug-induced adverse reaction, (4) awareness of medication-associated nail changes can prevent the subsequent initiation of improper nail-directed therapy from being instituted, and (5) the practitioner shall be able to reassure the patient of the etiology of their drug-induced or ingestant-related nail changes.[68]

We have grouped these agents into different classes based on either the properties of the drug, the features of the nail changes, or both: antibiotics (Table 16.1), antimalarials (Table 16.2), cancer chemotherapeutic agents (Table 16.3), ingestants and poisons (Table 16.4), and miscellaneous drugs (Table 16.5).[68–70] Drug-induced nail changes may occur as an anecdotal finding or as a well-recognized, albeit uncommon, adverse side effect. Although all 20 nails may be involved, changes are often more readily observed on the nails of the thumbs and great toes, and on the fingernails, than on the toenails.[68]

**TABLE 16–1. Nail changes secondary to antibiotics**

| ANTIBIOTIC | NAIL CHANGE |
|---|---|
| Cephalexin[19,192] | Acute paronychia |
| Cephaloridine[17,80] | Onychomadesis, photoonycholysis |
| Chloramphenicol[17,69,178,203] | Photoonycholysis |
| Chlortetracycline[17,178] | Photoonycholysis |
| Cloxacillin[17,80] | Onychomadesis, photoonycholysis |
| Dapsone[186] | Beau's lines |
| Demethylchlortetracycline (demeclocycline, declomycin)[17,26,27,43,78,126,183] | Onycholysis with subungual discoloration, pain, photoonycholysis |
| Dicloxacillin[213] | Shore nails (transverse leukonychia and onychomadesis following drug-induced erythroderma) |
| Doxycycline (vibramycin)[17,45,53,105,244,246,252] | Nail discoloration: brownish-yellow or uniform dark purple, pain, photoonycholysis, splinter hemorrhages |
| Fluoroquinolones[17] | Photoonycholysis |
| Minocycline[7,17,59,68,96,133,159,164,171,173,188,198,243,244] | Blue–black or blue–gray or metallic dark blue discoloration, diffuse pigmentation, longitudinal pigmented bands, periungual hyperpigmentation, pain, photoonycholysis |
| Oxytetracycline[17] | Pain, photoonycholysis |
| D-penicillamine[68,192] | Absence of lunula, longitudinal ridges, onychoschizia |
| Penicillin (anaphylaxis)[47,49] | Onychomadesis |
| Roxithromycin[72] | Diffuse pigmentation (light to dark brown) |
| Sulfonamides[192] | Beau's lines, paronychia, partial leukonychia, photoonycholysis |
| Tetracycline hydrochloride[17,41,83,88,109,110,119,127,132,145,200,206,217] | Brittle nails, longitudinal pigmented bands, onycholysis, onycholysis with bluish residue, onychoschizia, pain, photoonycholysis, splinter hemorrhages, yellow–brown discoloration, yellow lunulae (with fluorescence) |

**TABLE 16–2.** Nail changes secondary to antimalarials

| ANTIMALARIAL | NAIL CHANGE |
|---|---|
| Amodiaquine[248] | Blue–brown nail bed, longitudinal pigmented bands |
| Camoquin (amodiaquine)[248] | Blue–gray fluorescence in ultraviolet light |
| Chloroquine[180,248] | Blue–brown nail bed, drug and desethylchloroquine detected in appreciable amounts in finger nail clippings up to 400 days after last oral dose, fluorescence in ultraviolet light |
| Mepacrine[248] | Discoloration: blue or brown, fluorescence yellow–green or white under Wood's light, longitudinal pigmented bands |
| Other antimalarials[12,248] | Discoloration: blue–gray or brown, longitudinal pigmented bands, transverse pigmented bands |
| Quinacrine[21,22,134,139,170,248] | Blue lunula, fluorescence of nails, nail dystrophy, nail shedding; transverse leukonychia (striate), transverse pigmented bands (blue–gray) |
| Quinine[17,221] | Photoonycholysis |

**TABLE 16–3.** Nail changes secondary to cancer chemotherapeutic drugs

| CANCER CHEMOTHERAPEUTIC DRUG | NAIL CHANGE |
|---|---|
| Actinomycin[235] | Diffuse pigmentation |
| Ametantrone[111] | Gray–blue nail |
| Anthracycline[48,167] | Mees' lines, transverse leukonychia |
| Asparaginase[212] | Transverse leukonychia |
| Azathioprine[93] | Slower linear growth |
| 3-Azido-3′-deoxythymidine[227] | Longitudinal pigmented bands |
| Bleomycin (intralesional)[82,95,168,192,251] | Cold-sensitive distal fingers, fingernail loss (and without regrowth in some patients), nail dystrophy, Raynaud's phenomenon |
| Bleomycin (systemic)[23,24,37,48,56,62,79,86,94,98,116,118,178,201,203,214,245] | Blue lunula, longitudinal pigmented bands, nail bed thickening, nail cuticle darkening, nail dystrophy, nail shedding, onycholysis, subungual hematoma or hemorrhage, transverse leukonychia, vascular activity pattern (tortuous or brushed capillaries and/or moderate loss of capillaries) on nail fold capillary microscopy |
| 5-Bromodeoxyuridine[163] | Yellow depressed horizontal bands (Beau's lines?) |
| Busulfan[48] | Longitudinal pigmented bands, transverse leukonychia |
| Capecitabine[49] | Leukonychia, nail dystrophy, onycholysis, onychomadesis |
| Carmustine[48] | Transverse leukonychia |
| Carboplatin[48,157] | Onycholysis, transverse leukonychia |
| Chlorambucil[191] | Onycholysis, transverse leukonychia (Muehrcke's lines) |
| Cisplatinum[25,48,135,152] | Beau's lines, longitudinal pigmented bands, periungual (nail fold) hyperpigmentation, nail shedding (transverse), transverse leukonychia |
| Cyclophosphamide (Cytoxan)[19,28,48,55,56,62,98,116,118,121,161,172,176,178,194,201] | Blue lunula, diffuse pigmentation, longitudinal pigmented bands, onycholysis, subungual hematoma or hemorrhage, transverse leukonychia, transverse pigmented bands, transverse blue band |
| Ciclosporin[55,93,113,181,226,239] | Faster linear growth, paronychia, periungual granulation tissue, Raynaud's phenomenon, slower linear growth, transverse blue band |
| Cytosine arabinoside (arabinosyl cytosine, ARA-C, cytarabine)[6,34,47,48,56,76,148,226] | Asymmetric lunula, Beau's lines, onychomadesis, periungual erythema, purple lunula, transverse leukonychia, transverse pigmented bands |
| Dacarbazine (DTIC)[48,56,176] | Blue lunula, diffuse pigmentation, transverse leukonychia |
| Dactinomycin[56] | Blue lunula |
| Daunorubicin[6,48,76,98,142,148,212,216] | Beau's lines, longitudinal pigmented bands, transverse leukonychia, transverse pigmented bands, transverse nail shedding |

**TABLE 16–3. (*Cont'd*) Nail changes secondary to cancer chemotherapeutic drugs**

| CANCER CHEMOTHERAPEUTIC DRUG | NAIL CHANGE |
|---|---|
| *Cis*-dichlorodiammineplatinum (II)[172] | Transverse pigmented bands |
| Docetaxel (taxotere)[57,118,129,152,187,192,234,237] | Beau's lines, diffuse pigmentation, hypopigmentation (diffuse), nail discoloration (irregular erythematous-brown, hemosiderin-like), nail ridging, nail thinning, onycholysis, onychomadesis, splinter hemorrhages, subungual hematoma or hemorrhage, subungual erythema, transverse leukonychia, transverse pigmented bands |
| Doxorubicin (adriamycin)[1,2,9,28,47,48,56,62,63,68,94,98,116,118,160,164,172,178,182,193,194,199,203] | Beau's lines, blue lunula, bluish nails, diffuse leukonychia, diffuse pigmentation, longitudinal pigmented bands, onycholysis, onychomadesis, red-brown nails, subungual hematoma or hemorrhage, subungual vesiculation, transverse leukonychia, transverse pigmented bands |
| Etoposide[25,47,48,62,118,172,179] | Beau's lines, onycholysis, onychomadesis, transverse leukonychia, transverse pigmented bands |
| Fludarabine[48] | Transverse leukonychia |
| 5-Fluorouracil (5-FU) (topical and systemic)[3,18,28,48,56,118,130,172,176,178,189,192,226] | Beau's lines, blue lunula, discoloration: blue or brown, diffuse pigmentation, leukonychia ('half-and-half' nail-like), longitudinal pigmented bands, nail bed thickening, nail dystrophy, onycholysis, pain, paronychia, photo changes, transverse leukonychia, transverse pigmented bands |
| Ftorafur (5-FU analog)[74] | Diffuse pigmentation |
| Hydroxyurea[10,41,56,79,102,112,131,144,198,236] | Atrophy, brittle nails, diffuse pigmentation, longitudinal pigmented bands, nail dystrophy, nail fold hyperpigmentation, onycholysis, onychoschizia, transverse pigmented bands |
| Idarubicin[34,48,56] | Purple lunula, transverse leukonychia, transverse pigmented bands |
| Ifosfamide[25,48] | Beau's lines, transverse leukonychia |
| Interferon-alpha[51,56] | Asymmetric lunula, Reiter's syndrome-like changes |
| Melphalan (alkeran)[48,98,178] | Longitudinal pigmented bands, transverse leukonychia |
| Mercaptopurine[13,55] | Nail shedding, transverse blue band |
| Methotrexate[3,34,48,55,75,118,176,192,240] | Acute paronychia, diffuse pigmentation, longitudinal pigmented bands, onycholysis, transverse leukonychia, transverse pigmented bands, transverse blue band |
| Mitomycin[118] | Onycholysis |
| Mitoxantrone[48,118,143,201,209,218] | Diffuse leukonychia, discoloration: black, blue, or red–brown, onycholysis, subungual hematoma, or hemorrhage, transverse leukonychia |
| Mustine hydrochloride[25] | Beau's lines |
| Nitrogen mustard[176] | Diffuse pigmentation, longitudinal pigmented bands |
| Nitrosoureas[176] | Diffuse pigmentation, longitudinal pigmented bands |
| Paclitaxel[118,157,191] | Finger-tip skin inflammation, hyponychial exudation, leukonychia, onycholysis, paronychia |
| Procarbazine[48] | Transverse leukonychia |
| Razoxane[229] | Beau's lines |
| Semustine[48] | Transverse leukonychia |
| Tegafur (5-FU analog)[151] | Longitudinal pigmented bands |
| Thiotepa[48] | Transverse leukonychia |
| Vinblastine[56] | Blue lunula |
| Vincristine[25,48,56,62,116,172,201,212,214] | Beau's lines, blue lunula, longitudinal pigmented bands, onycholysis, subungual hematoma or hemorrhage, transverse leukonychia, transverse pigmented bands |

**TABLE 16-4.** Nail changes secondary to ingestants and poisons

| INGESTANT/POISON | NAIL CHANGE |
| --- | --- |
| Acetyl salicylic acid[15] | Purpura |
| Aniline[66] | Discoloration: blue–violet |
| Arsenic[5,66,71,158,192,196] | Diffuse pigmentation, longitudinal pigmented bands, Mees' lines, onychomadesis, transverse leukonychia |
| Carbon monoxide[29,54,66,146] | Cherry-red nail bed and lunula, leukonychia, Mees' lines |
| Dinitro-orthocresol[56] | Yellow lunula |
| Diquat[56] | Hypertrophic nail, longitudinal pigmented bands, nail loss (permanent), soft nail, transverse leukonychia, transverse pigmented bands, yellow lunula |
| Fluoride (fluorosis)[30,66] | Longitudinal pigmented bands |
| Fluorine[226] | Beau's lines, brittle nails, onychorrhexis, transverse leukonychia |
| Heavy metals[11] | Increased nail plate coproporphyrin level after chronic exposure |
| Hydrogen selenide[4] | Transverse ridges |
| Lead poisoning[11,251] | Diffuse pigmentation, increased nail plate coproporphyrin level, leukonychia, onychomadesis, onychalgia |
| Mercury[13,29,32,209] | Acrodynia, discoloration: green–black, longitudinal pigmented bands, nail dystrophy, nail shedding |
| Paraquat[56,68] | Hypertrophic nail, nail loss (permanent), soft nail, transverse leukonychia, transverse pigmented bands, yellow lunula |
| Phosphorus[15] | Subungual hematoma or hemorrhage |
| Pilocarpine poisoning[192] | Transverse leukonychia |
| Polychlorinated biphenyls (PCBs)[230] | Diffuse pigmentation, ingrown nail, nail flattening |
| Selenium poisoning[46] | Nail shedding, transverse leukonychia |
| Silver[7,98,104,139] | Blue lunula, bluish nail bed, transverse blue–gray bands |
| Sulfhydrilic acid[15] | Subungual bluish color |
| Thallium[29] | Mees' lines, onychorrhexis |
| Trinitrotoluene (TNT)[66] | Purpura |
| Vinyl chloride[203,205] | Clubbing, nail fold changes, sclerodactyly |

The appearance of nail changes is preceded by the administration of the agent; however, the temporal association between discontinuation of the drug or ingestant and resolution of the agent-induced nail changes is variable – ranging from a few weeks to several months. The etiology for many of the drug-induced nail changes is a toxic effect of the agent. Yet, some of the nail alterations occur secondary to an alternative pathogenesis, such as deposition of the drug or a drug metabolite in the nail bed or nail plate.[65,68,70]

Systemic drugs can alter different parts of the nail unit: the nail matrix, the nail bed, the nail folds, the hyponychium, or some combination of these areas. Hence, the clinical manifestation of the drug-induced nail abnormality is usually related to the anatomic site that has been affected. When keratinocytes of the nail matrix are affected, nail changes may include alteration of nail growth rate, which are summarized in Table 16.6 (and caused by a drug-associated disturbance of cellular maturation), Beau's lines (transverse palpable depressions), nail brittleness and fragility, nail thinning, true transverse leukonychia (horizontal white bands) (Table 16.7), and onychomadesis (proximal nail shedding).[68,191,192]

Involvement of nail matrix melanocytes by systemic agents – possibly secondary to the drug's stimulation of these cells – can result in nail plate discoloration that appears as diffuse pigmentation or as pigmented (longitudinal and/or transverse) bands (Table 16.8), or both; occasionally, the pattern of pigmentation is significant, providing a clue to the cause. 'Idiopathic' or photo-induced onycholysis (distal nail shedding) (Table 16.9) and apparent leukonychia (see Table 16.7) may occur following drug-induced damage of the nail bed. Paronychia (inflammation of the nail folds) and periungual granulation tissue can result from drug-associated alteration of the periungual areas (Table 16.10); in addition, ingrown nails, malalignment of the nail plate, and contiguous nail plate dystrophy may occur.[17,68,191,192,230]

# ANTIBIOTICS

Several antibiotics have been implicated as drugs associated with nail changes (see Table 16.1). In general, when antibiotics affect the nail, they usually do so as part of a generalized drug eruption or hypersensitivity reaction. If a lesion, as a component of the drug eruption, is in the vicinity of the nail unit, one may see nail shedding and other nail deformities – depending on the part of the nail unit that is affected (Figs 16.1 and 16.2).

Antibiotics represent the majority of the medications associated with photo-onycholysis. Other groups of drugs for which subsequent photo-onycholysis has been reported include: angiotensin-converting enzyme inhibitors, drugs that act on the central nervous system, nonsteroidal anti-inflammatory drugs, psoralens (in combination with sunlight or ultraviolet A light), and other miscellaneous agents (see Table 16.9).[15–17,192] Baran and Juhlin[17] have defined four distinct types of photo-onycholysis based on the number of digits affected and the pattern of nail plate-nail bed separation (see Table 16.9).

**TABLE 16–5. Nail changes secondary to miscellaneous drugs** 181

| DRUG | NAIL CHANGE |
|---|---|
| Acebutolol (beta-blocker)[99] | Pincer nails (convex transverse over-curvature of nails with distal narrowing of the nail bed and lateral ingrowing of the nail) |
| Acetanilid[66,192] | Discoloration: purple, subungual hematoma or hemorrhage |
| Acetylsalicylic acid[192,226] | Subungual hematoma or hemorrhage, subungual purpura |
| Acitretin (see retinoids) | |
| Acridine derivatives[15] | Leukonychia, photoonycholysis |
| Acriflavine[15,17] | Photoonycholysis |
| Adrenocorticotropic hormone (ACTH)[9] | Pigmented banding |
| Allopurinol[213] | Shore nails (transverse leukonychia and onychomadesis following drug-induced erythroderma) |
| Amphetamines[50,184] | Drug and its metabolites detected in fingernails from drug user |
| Androgen[176] | Leukonychia ('half-and-half' nail-like) |
| Benoxaprofen[17,85,86,100,101,114,138,162,165,166,211] | Accelerated nail growth, painless photoonycholysis |
| Biotin[203] | Accelerated nail growth |
| Bucillamine[122] | Yellow nail syndrome |
| Buspirone[20] | Nail thinning |
| Calcium channel blockers[226] | Nail dystrophy |
| Cannabis (delta 9-tetrahydrocannabinol [THC])[149,184] | Drug and its metabolite detected in fingernails from cannabis users |
| Captopril[17,33,38,226] | Photoonycholysis |
| Carbamazepine[169] | Onychomadesis |
| Carotene[110,143] | Discoloration: yellow |
| Cetuximab (antiepidermal growth factor receptor antibody)[35] | Paronychia |
| Chlorazepate dipotassium[17,224] | Photoonycholysis |
| Chlorpromazine[7,17] | Discoloration: blue–gray to slate-gray, photoonycholysis |
| Chromium salts[15] | Discoloration: yellow ocher |
| Clofazimine[226] | Onycholysis, subungual hyperkeratosis |
| Cocaine (crack)[81,91,192,199,215] | Acrocyanosis, drug and its metabolites detected in postmortem finger nail and toe nail specimens, drug detected in postmortem nail specimens from a 3-month-old male who died from sudden infant death syndrome (resulting from prenatal drug exposure), paronychia |
| Codeine[213] | Shore nails (transverse leukonychia and onychomadesis following drug-induced erythroderma) |
| Corticosteroids[48,54,55,226] | Mees' lines, red lunula, transverse leukonychia, transverse pigmented bands, transverse blue band |
| Cysteine[203] | Accelerated nail growth |
| Dapsone (syndrome)[25,141] | Beau's lines |
| Diazepam[184] | Detected in fingernails from abusers |
| Dicyanodiamide[68] | Discoloration: brownish |
| Dimercaptosuccinic acid[232] | Nail dystrophy |
| Dinitrophenol[15] | Discoloration: yellow |
| Diphenylhydantoin[106,125] | Anonychia, diffuse pigmentation, hypoplasia, longitudinal pigmented bands, nail dystrophy |
| Divalproex sodium (Depakote)[40] | Yellow transverse bands that progressed to yellow discoloration of the entire nail plate |
| Emetine chlorhydrate[66] | Leukonychia (variable) |
| Enalapril[192] | Photoonycholysis |
| Ethanol (alcohol abuse)[54] | Red lunula |
| Etretinate (see retinoids) | |
| Fluconazole[129,184] | Detected in nails from patients treated for onychomycosis; longitudinal pigmented bands (involving only onychomycotic diseased fingernails) |
| Fluoroquinolones[14] | Photoonycholysis |
| Gefitinib (epidermal growth factor receptor tyrosine kinase inhibitor)[64,175] | Paronychia, periungual granulation tissue |
| Gelatin[203] | Accelerated nail growth |
| Gemfibrozil (Lopid)[137] | Longitudinal pigmented bands |

**TABLE 16–5.** (*Cont'd*) Nail changes secondary to miscellaneous drugs

| DRUG | NAIL CHANGE |
|---|---|
| Gold salts[66] | Discoloration: brown (variable), longitudinal pigmented bands, onychomadesis |
| Haloperidol[184] | Detected in nails from psychiatry patients on stable maintainance doses of the drug |
| Heparin[226] | Slow growth, transverse red band |
| Icodextrin[17] | Photoonycholysis |
| Indinavir[3,191,192,228,241] | Ingrown toenail, lateral nail fold changes (erythema, edema and seropurulent exudation) paronychia, periungual granulation tissue |
| Indomethacin[17] | Longitudinal pigmented bands, photoonycholysis |
| Infliximab[61] | Transverse pigmented bands |
| Isotretinoin (see retinoids) | |
| Itraconazole[184,192] | Accelerated nail growth, longitudinal striations (nail beading) detected in nails from patients treated for onychomycosis |
| Ketoconazole[15] | Longitudinal pigmented bands, splinter hemorrhages |
| L-dopa[203] | Accelerated nail growth |
| Lamivudine[3,192,228] | Ingrown toenail, lateral nail fold changes (erythema, edema and seropurulent exudation) paronychia, periungual granulation tissue |
| Lithium carbonate[49,77,117,202] | Discoloration: from golden-yellow to normal color, nail dystrophy, onychomadesis, psoriasis changes |
| Masoprocol (Actinex)[108] | Discoloration: grayish staining |
| Melanin stimulating hormone (MSH)[9,76] | Pigmented banding |
| Metoprolol[97,99] | Beau's lines |
| Methionine[203] | Accelerated nail growth |
| Mycophenolate[117] | Onycholysis |
| Opiates (codeine, hydrocodone, 6-monoacetylmorphine, and morphine)[81,184] | Detected in postmortem toenail specimens |
| Oral contraceptive (Norinyl 1 [norethindrone and mestranol])[39,178,226] | Accelerated growth rate, photoonycholysis, reduced splitting and chipping |
| Parathyroid extract[140] | Lunula necrosis |
| Peloprenoic acid[68] | Nail fragility |
| D-penicillamine[31,73,120,192,226] | Beau's lines, discoloration: orange (transient), onychoschizia, subungual hematoma or hemorrhage, transverse ridges, yellow nail syndrome changes (growth arrest and yellow, thick nails with transverse ridges) |
| Phenindione[66,139,177] | Blue lunula, discoloration: gray (diffuse) |
| Phenobarbital[115] | Nail hypoplasia |
| Phenolphthalein[56,140,155,192,214] | Blue lunula, dark gray lunula, nail dystrophy, paronychia, yellow nail syndrome |
| Phenothiazine[66,177,207,226] | Discoloration: brown or gray to violet, longitudinal pigmented bands, photoonycholysis |
| Phenylephrine hydrochloride (Neo-Synephrine)[226] | Purpura (nail bed) |
| Polychlorinated biphenyls (PCB)[15] | Brown-gray lines |
| Practolol (beta-blocker)[99,140,178,190,192,203,226] | Erythema (blotchy and subungual), onycholysis (psoriasis-like), peculiar over-curvature of nail plate with painful pincer effect (narrowing) of the distal nail bed, photoonycholysis, ridging, subungual hyperkeratosis |
| Propanolol (beta-blocker)[99,247] | Onycholysis, psoriasis-like changes: Beau's lines, discolorations, erythema (subungual), longitudinal splitting, nail dystrophy, onycholysis, pitting, ridging, thickening |
| Psoralen (5-methoxypsoralen, 8-methoxypsoralen, or trimethylpsoralen with sunlight or UVA)[17,156,174,242,249] | Diffuse pigmentation, longitudinal pigmented bands, photoonycholysis, splinter hemorrhages |
| Retinoids (acitretin, etretinate, and isotretinoin)[42,49,87,128,140,192,208,238] | Beau's lines, brittle nails, granulation tissue, ingrown nails, nail dystrophy, nail friability, nail shedding, pain, paronychia, onychomadesis, onychorrhexis, onychoschizia, periungual granulation tissue |
| Salbutamol[192,226] | Erythema (periungual), paronychia |
| Senna (chronic use and long-term diarrhea)[150] | Finger clubbing |

## TABLE 16–5. (*Cont'd*) Nail changes secondary to miscellaneous drugs

| DRUG | NAIL CHANGE |
|------|-------------|
| Sulfonamide[192] | Transverse leukonychia |
| Sodium hypochlorite[60] | Onycholysis |
| Tamoxifen citrate (nonsteroidal antiestrogen)[56] | Red lunula |
| Terbinafine[184] | Detected in nails from patients treated for onychomycosis |
| Thiazide (diuretics)[17] | Photoonycholysis |
| Timolol (beta-blocker)[18,84] | Discoloration: brown and symmetric, longitudinal pigmented bands |
| Trazodone[153] | Leukonychia |
| Trypaflavine[15] | Photoonycholysis |
| Vitamin A (large doses)[140] | Brittle nails, nail dystrophy |
| Warfarin sodium[83,147,192] | Discoloration: purple, nail bed hemorrhages |
| Zidovudine (azidothymidine, AZT, retrovir)[8,41,44,52,56,89,191,195,198,204,226,231,241] | Blue lunula, diffuse pigmentation, ingrown nail, longitudinal pigmented bands, paronychia, slow growth, transverse pigmented bands |

## TABLE 16–6. Systemic drugs associated with alteration of nail growth rate

| SYSTEMIC DRUGS THAT DECREASE NAIL GROWTH RATE | SYSTEMIC DRUGS THAT INCREASE NAIL GROWTH RATE |
|-----------------------------------------------|-----------------------------------------------|
| Chemotherapeutic agents | Benoxaprofen |
| Cyclosporin | Biotin |
| Gold salts | Calcium |
| Heparin | Cysteine |
| Lithium | Fluconazole |
| Methotrexate | Gelatin |
| Retinoids | Itraconzole (pulse therapy) |
| Sulfonamides | Levodopa (L-dopa) |
| Zidovudine (Azidothymidine [AZT], Retrovir) | Methionine |
| | Oral contraceptives |
| | Retinoids |
| | Terbinafine |
| | Vitamin D |

## TABLE 16–7. Systemic drugs associated with leukonychia

| TRUE LEUKONYCHIA | APPARENT LEUKONYCHIA |
|------------------|----------------------|
| Arsenic (transverse leukonychia) | Androgens (half-and-half nails) |
| Chemotherapeutic agents (transverse leukonychia) | Emetine (white nails) |
| Cortisone (transverse leukonychia) | Chemotherapeutic agents (half-and-half nails, Muehrcke's lines) |
| Fluorine (punctate leukonychia and transverse leukonychia) | Penicillamine (leukonychia) |
| Pilocarpine (transverse leukonychia) | |
| Retinoids (transverse leukonychia) | |
| Sulfonamides (transverse leukonychia) | |
| Trazodone (transverse leukonychia) | |

## TABLE 16–8. Systemic drugs associated with pigmented bands[a]

| LONGITUDINAL PIGMENTED BANDS | TRANSVERSE PIGMENTED BANDS |
|------------------------------|----------------------------|
| Antimalarials (amodiaquine, mepacrine) | Antimalarials (quinacrine) |
| Arsenic | Cancer chemotherapeutics[c] |
| Cancer chemotherapeutics[b] | Diquat |
| Diphenylhydantoin | Infliximab |
| Diquat | Paraquat |
| Fluoride | Silver |
| Gemfibrozil | Zidovudine (azidothymidine) |
| Gold salts | |
| Indomethacin | |
| Ketoconazole | |
| Mercury | |
| Minocycline | |
| Phenothiazine | |
| Psoralens (5-methoxypsoralen, 8-methoxypsoralen, trimethylpsoralen) | |
| Sulfonamides | |
| Tetracycline | |
| Timolol | |
| Zidovudine (azidothymidine) | |

[a]'Pigmented bands' have been described in patients who had elevated levels of adrenocorticotrophic hormone (ACTH) and melanin stimulating hormone (MSH).
[b]These include: 3-azido-3′-deoxythymidine, bleomycin, busulfan, cisplatinum, cyclophosphamide, daunorubicin, doxorubicin, 5-fluorouracil, hydroxyurea, melphalon, methotrexate, nitrogen mustard, nitrosourea, vincristine.
[c]These include: cyclophosphamide, cytosine arabinoside, daunorubicin, cis-dichlorodiammineplatinum (II), docetaxel, doxorubicin, etoposide, 5-fluorouracil, hydroxyurea, idarubicin, methotrexate, vincristine.

| TABLE 16–9. Systemic drugs associated with photoonycholysis[a] |
| --- |

### Angiotensin converting enzyme (ACE) inhibitors

Captopril
Enalapril

### Antibiotics

Cephalosporins: cephaloridin
Chloramphenicol
Fluoroquinolones
Penicillins: cloxacillin
Tetracyclines: chlortetracycline, demethylchlortetracycline, doxycycline, minocycline, oxytetracycline, tetracycline hydrochloride

### Central nervous system acting drugs

Chlorazepate dipotassium
Chlorpromazine

### Nonsteroidal anti-inflammatory drugs

Benoxaprofen
Indomethacin

### Other drugs

Acridine derivatives
Acriflavine
Icodextrine
Oral contraceptives
Practolol
Quinine
Thiazide diuretics
Trypaflavine

### Psoralens[b]

5-methoxypsoralen
8-methoxypsoralen
Trimethylpsoralen

[a]Baran and Juhlin[17] have defined four distinct types of drug-induced photoonycholysis: (1) type I involves several fingers (and the separating part of the nail plate is half-moon-shaped and concave distally with a pigmentation of variable intensity and shows a well-demarcated proximal border); (2) type II involves only one finger (and a well-defined circular notch is present, which opens distally and has a brownish hue proximally); (3) type III involves several fingers (and there is initially a round yellow staining that turns reddish after 5–10 days); and (4) type IV usually involves several fingers (and there are bullae under the nails).
[b]Drug in combination with sunlight or ultraviolet A light.

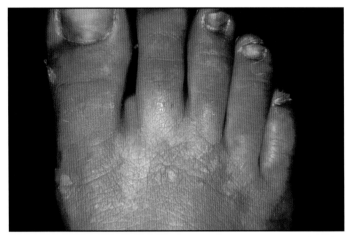

FIGURE 16–1. Phototoxic reaction to tetracycline hydrochloride. Opaque nails and onycholysis with nail shedding developed later (from ref. 66, used with permission).

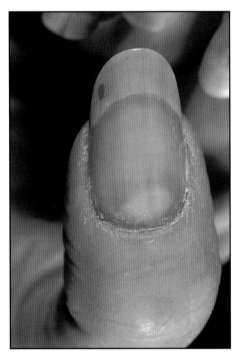

FIGURE 16–2. Hyperpigmented nail, including longitudinal pigmented band, in a patient on minocycline therapy (from ref. 69, used with permission).

Photo-onycholysis may accompany but often follows a cutaneous photosensitivity reaction, and usually appears after two or more weeks of drug exposure. Less commonly, it may appear in the absence of photosensitivity reaction in the skin. Photo-onycholysis is usually asymptomatic and may occur as part of Segal's triad: sequentially occurring photosensitivity, nail discoloration, and onycholysis. However, photo-onycholysis-associated onychodynia has been described in patients with drug-induced onycholysis resulting from either tetracycline derivatives or psoralens and ultraviolet A light.[17]

Photo-onycholysis results after ultraviolet light combines with by-products of the drug and energy is released or cellular maturation is changed.[68] Subsequently, the bond between the nail plate and nail bed is broken – possibly with accompanying pain and splinter hemorrhages – and onycholysis occurs. Less commonly, photo-onycholysis has been described to occur spontaneously.[107,185] Some safeguards that may be implemented to avoid or minimize drug-induced photo-onycholysis include taking the medication at bedtime, using opaque nail polish, using a combination oxybenzone PABA-containing sunscreen with a sun protection factor of at least 15, judicious sun exposure, and patient education.[68]

The tetracyclines have often been reported to cause medication-induced alteration of the nails (see Table 16.1). Demethyl-chlortetracycline and doxycycline are more likely to produce

TABLE 16–10. Systemic drugs associated with periungual granulation tissue and/or paronychia

| DRUG | PARONYCHIA | PERIUNGUAL GRANULATION TISSUE |
|---|---|---|
| **Amphetamines[192]** | | |
| Cocaine | X | |
| **Antibiotics[19,192]** | | |
| Cephalexin | X | |
| Sulfonamides | X | |
| **Cancer chemotherapeutics[157,178,192,240]** | | |
| 5-Fluorouracil | X | |
| Methotrexate | X | |
| Paclitaxel | X | |
| **Cathartics[192]** | | |
| Phenolphthalein | X | |
| **Epidermal growth factor receptor inhibitors[35,64,175]** | | |
| Cetuximab | X | |
| Gefitinib | X | X |
| **HIV antiretrovirals[3,191,192,204,228,241]** | | |
| Protease inhibitors | | |
| Indinavir | X | X |
| Lamivudine | X | X |
| Pyrimidine nucleoside analogue | | |
| Zidovudine (azidothymidine) | X | |
| **Miscellaneous[113,181,192,226,239]** | | |
| Salbutamol | X | |
| Cyclosporin | X | X |
| **Retinoids[191,192,208,238]** | | |
| Acitretin | X | X |
| Etretinate | X | X |
| Isotretinoin | X | X |

photosensitivity reactions than the other tetracyclines; phototoxicity, mediated by ultraviolet B light, is the cause of the vast majority of these changes.[68] Ultraviolet A light may also be involved but less commonly. With the tetracyclines, onycholysis – preceded by 1 to 4 weeks by pain – is encountered most commonly. Splinter hemorrhages and pigmentation changes are less common. Tetracyclines may also cause onycholysis that is not photomediated.[127,132]

Minocycline may cause drug-induced discoloration of the nail bed, nail plate, or periungual region.[59,164] A nail matrix biopsy in a patient with periungual hyperpigmentation and longitudinal pigmented bands secondary to minocycline showed findings similar to a benign lentigo, suggesting stimulation of melanocytes with subsequent increased melanin production resulting from the use of minocycline.[68] Dermatoscopic evaluation of the affected nails shows homogenous, longitudinal gray lines on a gray background.[198,225] Elemental analysis of nail clippings from the dis-

colored area, from another minocycline-treated patient with pigmented nail plates, showed the presence of iron.[96]

## ANTIMALARIALS

Antimalarials may cause nail changes (see Table 16.2). They are stored in the nails for a long period of time after being taken; in an individual receiving chloroquin for malaria prophylaxis, the drug was detected in appreciable amounts from his fingernail clippings up to 400 days after the last dose (Table 16.11).[180] The most common antimalarial-induced nail change is various kinds of pigmentation patterns (Fig. 16.3). The specific composition of the pigment remains to be determined. Deposits of hemosiderin and melanin have been observed and a melanin-antimalarial complex has been speculated.[68,226,248] Other changes, such as quinine-associated photo-onycholysis, may also occur.

**TABLE 16–11.** Systemic drugs detected in nail specimens

### Antifungals[184]

Fluconazole
Itraconazole
Terbinafine

### Antimalarials[180]

Chloroquine

### Central nervous system acting agents[50,81,90,91,149,184]

Amphetamines[a]
Diazepam
Cannabis (delta 9-tetrahydrocannabinol [THC])
Cocaine analytes[b]
Haloperidol
Opiates[c]

### Poisons[67,71]

Arsenic

[a]Amphetamine, methamphetamine, methylenedioxyamphetamine (MDA), methylenedioxymethamphetamine (MDMA).
[b]Anhydroecgonine methyl ester, benzoylecgonine, cocaine, cocaethylene, ecgonine ethyl ester, ecgonine methyl ester, norbenzoylecgonine, norcocaethylene.
[c]Codeine, hydrocodone, 6-monoacetylmorphine, morphine.

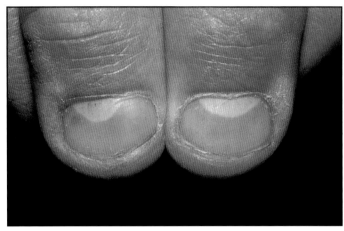

FIGURE 16–4. Asymmetric lunula in a 39-year-old Hispanic man with severe nodulocystic acne and chronic myelogenous leukemia receiving long-term therapy consisting of interferon alpha and cytosine arabinoside [cytarabine (ara-C)] (from ref. 56, used with permission).

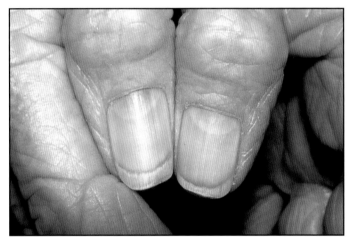

FIGURE 16–5. Red lunula on thumb nails of a 69-year-old White woman receiving tamoxifen for breast cancer (from ref. 56, used with permission).

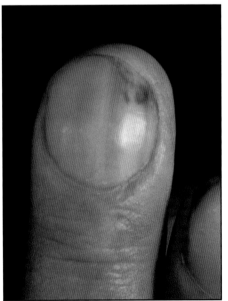

FIGURE 16–3. Longitudinal pigmented band appearing after antimalarial Plaquenil therapy was begun (the patient had porphyria cutanea tarda and also mild clubbing) (from ref. 69, used with permission).

# CANCER CHEMOTHERAPEUTIC AGENTS

Cancer chemotherapeutic drugs affect nails (see Table 16.3). The most common manifestations of chemotherapy-related nail changes are slower nail growth rate (see Table 16.6), asymptomatic pigmentation changes (see Tables 16.7 and 16.8) and nail shedding.[47,93,116,192,193,210,220] The two agents most likely to affect

the nails are cyclophosphamide and doxorubicin.[68,193] After patients have been treated with combination cancer chemotherapy, it is common to see subungual hemorrhage under the first and second toes – either occurring spontaneously or as a result of trauma.[223] Occasionally, chemotherapeutic agents can be associated with changes in the shape (Fig. 16.4) or color (Figs 16.5 and 16.6) of the lunula.[56]

The administration of antineoplastic agents can cause Beau's lines and onychomadesis.[47,116,191,192] Beau's lines are transverse nail plate grooves. When the horizontal depression involves the whole thickness of the nail plate and divides it into two parts, proximal shedding of the nail plate (onychomadesis) may occur. Beau's lines and onychomadesis result from a transient arrest of the nail matrix mitotic activity; when drug-induced, these nail changes are often dose-related and recurrent following re-administration of the drug.

Cancer chemotherapy-associated changes in nail pigment include either darkening of the nail plate or whitening of the nail plate or both.[65,192] Dark discoloration of the nails may present as diffuse hyperpigmentation, longitudinal bands, and/or transverse bands (see Table 16.8); these changes are more common in heavily pigmented individuals and matrix melanocyte stimulation is probably responsible. In patients with hydroxyurea-induced longitudinal pigmented bands, dermatoscopy of the affected nail showed a grayish coloration of the background and the presence of thin longitudinal gray lines with regular thickness, spacing, coloration, and absence of parallelism disruption.[198,225]

Whitening of the nail can present as a single horizontal white band, multiple transverse white bands, or confluent white discoloration of the nail.[48,103,192] Typically, there is a horizontal white nail plate band that corresponds to each course of chemotherapy that the patient has received (Fig. 16.6). Transverse leukonychia often presents as an isolated nail finding; alternatively, it can be associated with chemotherapy-induced Beau's lines (Fig. 16.7).[57,58]

Chemotherapy-induced leukonychia can be either true or apparent (see Table 16.7).[48,192] True leukonychia refers to the whitish discoloration of the nail plate following damage to the distal nail matrix keratinocytes; there is subsequent impairment of

their normal keratinization with retention of the cell nuclei within the nail plate. Reflection of the light results in the affected portion of the nail plate being white and opaque instead of transparent.

Chemotherapy-associated transverse leukonychia frequently appears as one or several horizontal white nail plate bands. They are typically 1 mm to 2 mm wide, although they can be wider. The bands often have smooth borders with a rounded distal edge similar in contour to the distal lunula, tend to be homogeneous, and usually extend across the entire breadth of the nail plate. As transverse leukonychia reflects simultaneous damage to the matrices of all of the nails, the horizontal white bands are usually located on the same site of each nail and each band corresponds to a course of cancer therapy.[48,192] The bands of transverse leukonychia present almost like a diary. After measuring the distance from the proximal nail fold to the leading edge of the abnormality, it is possible to estimate when the chemotherapy was given because fingernails grow at a rate of about 0.1 mm to 0.15 mm per day.

In oncology patients with chemotherapy-induced transverse leukonychia, neither a particular class of chemotherapeutic drug nor a specific drug combination is more frequently associated with these nail changes.[48,192] However, cyclophosphamide, doxorubicin, and/or vincristine were used in more than half of the antineoplastic regimens received by patients who developed antineoplastic therapy-associated transverse leukonychia.[48] New bands of chemotherapy-induced true transverse leukonychia stop appearing once the causative agent or agents are discontinued. Subsequently, there is growth of normal proximal nail plate and the existing white horizontal nail plate bands clear.

Apparent leukonychia occurs secondary to an abnormality of the nail bed.[48,191,192] In contrast to the normal nail, in which the nail bed appears pink due to its rich vascularization and is visible through the transparent nail plate, a white discoloration of the nail is observed in apparent leukonychia. In patients with chemotherapy-associated apparent leukonychia, the altered nail color may be the result of drug-induced abnormalities of the nail blood flow.

Chemotherapy-associated apparent leukonychia can also present as either half-and-half nails or Muehrcke's lines.[48,191,192] In half-and-half nails, the distal one-third to one-half of the nail maintains its normal color or is reddish or brown and the proximal

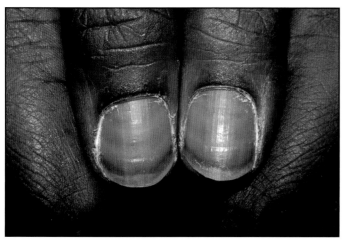

FIGURE 16–6. Purple lunula on thumb nails of a 37-year-old Black woman that appeared after she began idarubicin and cytosine arabinoside [cytarabine (ara-C)] for her refractory anemia with excess blasts; white horizontal bands of transverse leukonychia correspond to each of her cycles of chemotherapy (from ref. 56, used with permission).

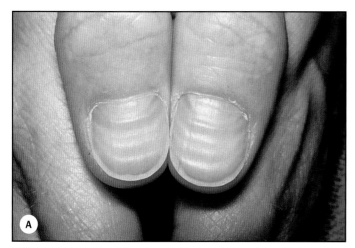

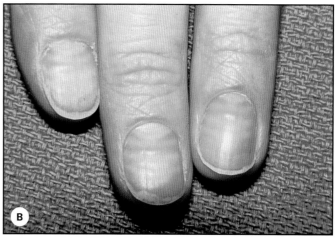

FIGURE 16–7. The Beau's lines (acquired horizontal ridges of the nail plate) and transverse leukonychia (horizontal white bands) present on the thumb nails (A) and finger nails (B) of a 36-year-old White man with stage IV non-small-cell lung cancer correspond to each of the courses of docetaxel (Taxotere) that he received (from refs 57 and 58, used with permission).

nail appears white, obscuring the lunula. Muehrcke's lines appear as two (or occasionally multiple) transverse pale to opaque non-palpable white bands that are parallel to the lunula, that are separated by a band of normal-appearing (usually pink) nail bed, and that do not migrate distally with nail growth. Although Muehrcke's lines may be observed in oncology patients who are receiving chemotherapy or who have previously been treated with antineoplastic agents, they are most commonly observed in individuals whose serum albumin is less than or equal to 2.2.

Similar to true transverse leukonychia caused by antineoplastic agents, drug-induced apparent leukonychia is asymptomatic, does not require any local treatment, and usually spontaneously resolves following discontinuation of the associated chemotherapeutic medication.[48,192] However, in contrast to true drug-induced transverse leukonychia in oncology patients, digital compression causes fading of Muehrcke's lines in patients with chemotherapy-related apparent leukonychia.[191]

Onycholysis has been reported in patients receiving chemotherapy. The drugs most frequently associated with distal nail plate shedding are anthracyclines and taxols. Some of the antineoplastic drugs that have been observed to cause onycholysis include doxorubicin, mitoxantrone, cyclophosphamide, etoposide, bleomycin, methotrexate, docetaxol, and paclitaxel (especially when the latter is given as a prolonged weekly course).[118]

Several modes of pathogenesis, not necessarily mutually exclusive, have been postulated as the mechanism for chemotherapy-induced onycholysis: (1) hyponychium hyperpigmentation (secondary to nail matrix melanocyte stimulation) and reduced nail growth, (2) drug-induced subungual hyperkeratosis and splinter hemorrhages in the nail bed with subsequent onycholysis, (3) subungual hemorrhagic bullae after the nail bed epithelium has been completely destroyed by the agent, (4) loss of nail bed-nail plate adhesion following chemotherapy-associated nail bed epithelium damage and subsequent epidermolysis, and (5) enhanced vulnerability of the chemotherapy treated patient's hyponychium to ultraviolet A radiation (sunlight) exposure.[118]

With regards to hyponychial vulnerability to ultraviolet radiation in oncology patients who have been treated with antineoplastic agents, ultraviolet radiation is focused on the hyponychium because the nail acts as a convex lens. Also, it is interesting that concurrent skin reactions occurred only in the immediate proximity to the hyponychium in a majority of patients with onycholysis. It is possible that radiation recall or reactivation of ultraviolet-induced erythema may play a role in the development of onycholysis in cancer patients who are being treated with chemotherapy and are exposed to ultraviolet radiation.[55,116] Other anatomic features that might contribute to potentiating the susceptibility of the hyponychium to ultraviolet radiation in patients receiving antineoplastic agents include the relative deficiency of stage IV melanosomes and the absence of horny keratinocytes, sebaceous glands, and the stratum granulosum.[118]

Cancer chemotherapy-associated onycholysis improves over several months once the inducing agent has been discontinued. However, the detached nail plate does not re-adhere; therefore – if the nail plate has not shed spontaneously – the distal free edge of the nail should be clipped. Soaking the effected distal digits in mild antiseptic solutions and applying topical antibiotic ointment are helpful to prevent secondary microbial colonization. Protective measures to diminish exposure of the distal digits to the sun – especially in patients receiving anthracyclines and taxanes – may even prevent onycholysis. Some of these barrier techniques to prevent sun exposure are using artificial nail, gloves, and opaque adhesive strapping.[118]

Dermatologists frequently prescribe methotrexate and topical 5-fluorouracil. Methotrexate usually causes only nail pigmentation changes and slower nail growth rate. It has more recently been reported to cause paronychial changes.[63,192] Numerous nail changes have also been described in patients who have received either systemic or topical 5-fluorouracil (see Table 16.3).

# INGESTANTS AND POISONS

Ingestants and poisons can cause various nail changes (see Table 16.4). Arsenic can cause a variety of nail changes, including Mees' lines. We had the opportunity to see a patient who was hospitalized for neurologic problems.[67] She had transverse white bands. Mees' lines were suspected, based on her clinical picture. Nail and hair clippings were collected and evaluated for arsenic content (see Table 16.11).[67,71] Elevated levels of arsenic were found and additional investigation revealed that the patient, as well as her father (who by then was deceased), had been poisoned with arsenic by her mother. Because fingernails grow about 0.1 mm to 0.15 mm per day, we were able to estimate the timing of the insult that caused the Mees' line by measuring the distance from the cuticle to the leading edge of the Mees' line (Fig. 16.8).

Cyanide poisoning has occurred in children from the ingestion of a cosmetic nail polish remover.[92,154]

# MISCELLANEOUS DRUGS

Nail changes have also been observed in association with several other drugs (see Table 16.5). Psoralens and retinoids are of particular interest to dermatologists. Psoralens, when activated by ultraviolet A radiation (sunlight), may cause photoonycholysis, splinter hemorrhages, tenderness, and nail pigmentation.[17,156,174,242,249] Other medications, such as nonsteroidal anti-inflammatory drugs, can also cause photo-onycholysis (see Table 16.9, Fig. 16.9).

Retinoids, especially in larger dosages, may cause brittle nails, nail dystrophy, paronychia, ingrowing nails, and other changes.[42,49,87,128,140,192,208,238] In addition to retinoids, other drugs can cause periungual inflammation or acute paronychia (see Table 16.10). Paronychia appears to be a typical adverse effect associated

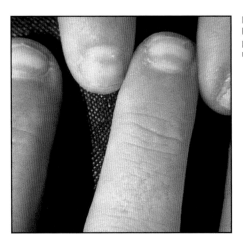

**FIGURE 16-8.** Mees' lines secondary to arsenic poisoning (from ref. 69, used with permission).

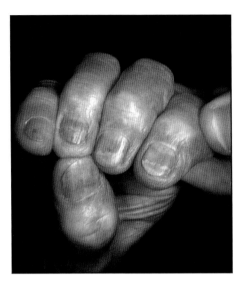

FIGURE 16–9.
Benoxaprofen-induced
onycholysis (from ref. 69,
used with permission).

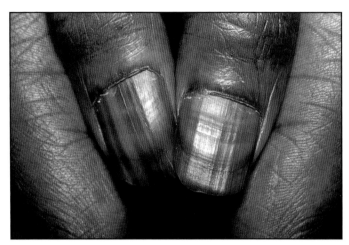

FIGURE 16–10. Longitudinal and horizontal pigmented bands on the thumb nails of an HIV-infected Black man who has been receiving zidovudine. Blue lunula also appeared after initiation of antiviral therapy (from ref. 56, used with permission).

with HIV antiretroviral therapy; other types of medications that can induce paronychial changes of the nail folds include amphetamines, antibiotics, cancer chemotherapeutics, cathartics, cyclosporin, epidermal growth factor receptor inhibitors, and salbutamol.

Drug-induced periungual granulation tissue has been observed after treatment with inhibitors of epidermal growth factor receptors, protease inhibitors (for HIV infection), and retinoids (see Table 16.10). For all of these medications, the clinical presentation (consisting of red friable tissue and papules extending from the nail folds) and histologic features (consisting of a proliferation of small endothelial-lined vessels surrounded by a dermal inflammatory infiltrate composed predominantly of neutrophils) are similar. However, depending on the associated drug, the nail change is either referred to as a periungual granulation (following gefitinib therapy),[64,175] pseudopyogenic granulomas (following indinavir or lamivudine therapy),[3,191,192,228,241] or pyogenic granulomas (following acitretin, etretinate, or isotretinoin therapy).[191,192,208]

In addition to antibiotics, antimalarials, antineoplastics, and poisons, pigmented bands have also been caused by several other systemic drugs (see Table 16.8, Fig. 16.10).[65,66] The clinical differential diagnosis of drug-induced nail pigmentation – particularly longitudinal pigmented bands – includes subungual melanoma. Dermatoscopic evaluation of nails in patients with nail pigmentation from hydroxyurea, minocycline, or zidovudine showed homogenous thin longitudinal gray lines (of regular color, spacing, and thickness without disruption of parallelism) on a gray background. These dermatoscopic features were similar to those observed in ethnic-type pigmentation of the nail and ungual lentigos. However, the dermatoscopic findings of drug-induced nail pigmentation were significantly different from those observed from subungual melanoma.[198,225]

Systemic exposure to certain drugs can be confirmed by their detection in the patient's nails (see Table 16.11).[50,67,71,81,90,91,149,180,184] Some of these drugs are also associated with visual nail changes: Mee's lines following arsenic exposure, nail bed pigmentation after chloroquin therapy, and resolution of dermatophyte-associated leukonychia during and subsequent to treatment with antifungal agents (such as fluconazole, itraconazole, and terbinafine). Nail clippings can also be used to verify consumption of agents that act on the central nervous system when there is suspicion of drug abuse or doping; these include amphetamines, diazepam, cannabis, cocaine, haloperidol, and opiates (see Table 16.11). In addition, forensic toxicology can utilize nail clippings to evaluate for these substances when death caused by drug overdose is suspected.[184]

Nail malformations in newborns may be caused if certain drugs were taken by the mother during pregnancy. Anticoagulants and anticonvulsants can be teratogenic and interfere with the nail development of the fetus. In addition to alcohol abuse, carbamazepine, dilantin (also referred to as hydantoin or phenytoin), phenobarbital, trimethadione, and warfarin can be associated with nail hypoplasia (which is often accompanied by malformation of the distal digits) when there is intrauterine exposure to these agents. Newborns with hyperconvex nails and long thin digits have been observed following treatment of their mothers with valproic acid (sodium valproate) during pregnancy.[191,192]

## REFERENCES

1. Adrian RM, Hood AF, Skarin AT. Mucocutaneous reactions to antineoplastic agents. CA Cancer J Clin 1980; 30:143
2. Alagaratnam TT, Choi TK, Ong GB. Doxorubicin and hyperpigmentation. Aust NZ J Surg 1982; 52:531
3. Alam M, Scher RK. Indinavir-related recurrent paronychia and ingrown toenails. Cutis 1999; 64:277–278
4. Alderman LC, Bergin JJ. Hydrogen selenide poisoning: an illustrative case with review of the literature. Arch Environ Health 1986; 41:354
5. Althause TL, Gunther L. Acute arsenic poisoning. JAMA 1929; 92:2002
6. Anderson LL, Thomas DE, Berger TG, Vukelja SJ. Cutaneous pigmentation after daunorubicin chemotherapy. J Am Acad Dermatol 1992; 26:255–256
7. Angeloni VL, Salasche SJ, Ortiz R. Nail, skin, and scleral pigmentation induced by minocycline. Cutis 1987; 40:229–233
8. Antoni AM, Mallolas J, Gatell J, et al. Zidovudine-induced nail pigmentation. Arch Dermatol 1988; 124:1570
9. Arakawa S, Takamatsu T, Imashuku S, Kusunoki T. Plasma ACTH and melanocyte-stimulating hormone in nail pigmentation. Arch Dis Child 1978; 53:249–258
10. Aste N, Fumo G, Contu F, Aste N, Biggio P. Nail pigmentation caused by hydroxyurea: report of 9 cases. J Am Acad Dermatol 2002; 47:146–147

11. Badcock NR. Detection of poisoning by substances other than drugs: a neglected art. Ann Clin Biochem 2000; 37:146–157
12. Bailin PL, Matkaluk RM. Cutaneous reactions to rheumatological drugs. Clin Rheum Dis 1982; 8:493
13. Baker H. Drug reactions. In: Rook A, Wilkinson DS, Ebling FJG, eds. Textbook of dermatology. 3rd edn. Oxford: Blackwell Scientific; 1979:1111–1140
14. Baran R, Brun P. Photoonycholysis induced by the fluoroquinolones pefloxacine and ofloxacine. Dermatologica 1986; 173:185
15. Baran R, Dawber RPR, Richert B. Physical signs. In: Baran R, Dawber RPR, de Berker DAR, et al., eds. Baran and Dawber's diseases of the nails and their management. 3rd edn. Oxford: Blackwell Scientific; 2001:48–103
16. Baran R, Juhlin L. Drug-induced photo-onycholysis: three subtypes identified in a study of 15 cases. J Am Acad Dermatol 1987; 17:1012
17. Baran R, Juhlin L. Photoonycholysis. Photodermatol Photoimmunol Photomed 2002; 18:202–207
18. Baran R, Laugier P. Melanonychia induced by topical 5-fluorouracil. Br J Dermatol 1985; 112:621–625
19. Baran R, Perrin C. Fixed-drug eruption presenting as an acute paronychia. Br J Dermatol 1991; 125:592–595
20. Barnhart ER. Physicians' desk reference. Oradell, NJ: Medical Economics Inc; 1989
21. Barr JF, Subungual pigmentation following prolonged atabrine therapy. US Navy Med Bull 1944; 43:924
22. Bauer F. Quinacrine hydrochloride drug eruption (tropical lichenoid dermatitis). J Am Acad Dermatol 1981; 4:239
23. Bellmunt J, Knobel H, Navarro M, Jolis L. Nailfold capillary microscopy and bleomycin-induced vascular toxicity [letter]. Cancer Investigation 1990; 8:641
24. Bellmunt J, Navarro M, Morales S, et al. Capillary microscopy is a potentially useful method for detecting bleomycin vascular toxicity. Cancer 1990; 65:303–309
25. Ben-Dayan D, Mittelman M, Floru S, Djaldetti M. Transverse nail ridgings (Beau's lines) induced by chemotherapy. Acta Haematol 1994; 91:89–90
26. Bethell HJN. Photo-onycholysis caused by demethylchlortetracycline. Br Med J 1977; 2:96
27. Bettley FR, Samman PD. Photo-onycholysis. Proc Roy Soc Med 1974; 67:600
28. Bianchi L, Iraci S, Tomassoli M, et al. Coexistence of apparent transverse leukonychia (Muehrcke's lines type) and longitudinal melanonychia after 5-fluorouracil/adriamycin/cyclophosphamide chemotherapy. Dermatology 1992; 185:216–217
29. Birmingham DJ. Cutaneous reactions to chemicals in dermatology. In: Fitzpatrick TB, Eisen AZ, Wolf K, et al., eds. Dermatology in general medicine. 2nd edn. New York: McGraw-Hill; 1979: 995–1006
30. Bisht DB, Singh SS. Pigmented bands on nails: a new sign of malnutrition. Lancet 1962; 1:507
31. Bjellerup M. Nail changes induced by penicillamine. Acta Derm Venereol (Stockh) 1989; 69:339
32. Bockers, M, Wagner R, Oster O. Nail dyschromia as the leading symptoms in chronic mercury poisoning caused by a cosmetic bleaching preparation. Z Hautkr 1985; 15:821
33. Borfders JV. Captopril and onycholysis. Ann Intern Med 1986; 105:305
34. Borecky DJ, Stephenson JJ, Keeling JH, Vukelja SJ. Idarubicin-induced pigmentary changes of the nails. Cutis 1997; 59:203–204
35. Boucher KW, Davidson K, Mirakhur B, et al. Paronychia induced by cetuximab, an antiepidermal growth factor receptor antibody. J Am Acad Dermatol 2002; 47:632–633
36. Bovednmyer DA. Cold-sensitive fingers from bleomycin. Schoch Lett 1984; 34:31
37. Bronner AK, Hood AF. Cutaneous complications of chemotherapeutic agents. J Am Acad Dermatol 1983; 9:645
38. Brueggemeyer CD, Ramirez G. Onycholysis associated with captopril. Lancet 1984; 1:1352
39. Bryden JP. Contraceptive pill-induced porphyria cutanea tarda presenting with onycholysis of fingernails. Postgrad Med J 1976; 52:535
40. Buka R, Hille R, McCormack P. Yellow nail pigmentation following depakote therapy. J Drugs Dermatol 2003; 2:545–547
41. Cakir B, Sucak G, Haznedar R. Longitudinal pigmented nail bands during hydroxyurea therapy. Int J Dermatol 1997; 36:236–237
42. Campbell JP, Grekin RC, Ellis CN, et al. Retinoid therapy is associated with excess granulation tissue responses. J Am Acad Dermatol 1983; 9:708
43. Carter WI. Disorders of the nails. Br Med J 1966; 2:1198
44. Cather JC, Cohen PR. Human immunodeficiency virus (unit 14-25). In: Demis DJ, Thiers BH, Burgdorf WHC, Raimer SS, eds. Clinical dermatology, 26th revision. Philadelphia: JB Lippincott Company; 1999:1–39
45. Cavens TR. Onycholysis of the thumbs probably due to a phototoxic reaction from doxycycline. Cutis 1981; 27:53–54
46. Centers for Disease Control. Morbidity and mortality report. JAMA 1984; 251:1938
47. Cetm M, Utas S, Unal A, Altmbas. Shedding of the nails due to chemotherapy (onychomadesis) [letter]. J European Acad Dermatol Venereol 1998; 11:193–194
48. Chapman S, Cohen PR. Transverse leukonychia in patients receiving cancer chemotherapy. South Med J 1997; 90:395–398
49. Chen G-Y, Chen Y-H, Hsu MML, et al. Onychomadesis and onycholysis associated with capecitabine [letter]. Br J Dermatol 2001; 145:521–522
50. Cirimele V, Kintz P, Mangin P. Detection of amphetamines in fingernails: an alternative to hair analysis. Arch Toxicol 1995; 70:68–69
51. Cleveland MG, Mallory SB. Incomplete Reiter's syndrome induced by systemic interferon alpha treatment. J Am Acad Dermatol 1993; 29:788
52. Cockerell CJ, Cohen PR. Cutaneous manifestations of HIV infection. In: Tyring SK, ed. Cutaneous manifestations of viral disease. New York: Marcel Decker, Inc.; 2002:307–395
53. Coffin SE, Puck J. Painful discoloration of the fingernails in a 15-year-old boy. Pediatr Infect Dis J 1993; 12:702–703, 706
54. Cohen PR. Red lunulae: case report and literature review. J Am Acad Dermatol 1992; 26:292–294
55. Cohen PR. Cancer chemotherapy-associated mucocutaneous reactions. In Pazdur R, ed. Medical oncology: a comprehensive board review (from the University of Texas MD Anderson Cancer Center and from the journal Oncology). Huntington, New York: PRR; 1993:491–500
56. Cohen PR. The lunula. J Am Acad Dermatol 1996; 34:943–953
57. Cohen PR. New onset nail abnormalities (cancer chemotherapy-induced Beau's lines [acquired horizontal ridges of the nail plate] and transverse leukonychia [horizontal white nail bands]). (Dermatology Clinic). The Clinical Advisor 2003; 6 (4):40–43
58. Cohen PR. New onset nail abnormalities (cancer chemotherapy-induced Beau's lines [acquired horizontal ridges of the nail plate] and transverse leukonychia [horizontal white nail bands]). (Dermatology Dx). Cortlandt Forum 2003; 16 (12):33, 37
59. Cohen PR, Tschen JA. What caused the extensive cutaneous pigmentation? (minocycline-induced cutaneous pigmentation) (Derm Dx). Skin & Aging 2003; 11 (7):94–96
60. Coskey RJ. Onycholysis from sodium hypochloride. Arch Dermatol 1974; 109:96
61. Cunha AP, Resende C, Barros L, et al. Transverse melanonychia caused by the use of infliximab to treat refractory pyoderma gangrenosum. (P23-28). J European Acad Dermatol Venereol 2002; 16 (Suppl 1):250
62. Cunningham D, Gilchrist NL, Forrest GJ, Soukop M. Onycholysis associated with cytotoxic drugs. Br Med J 1985; 290:675–676
63. Curran CF. Onycholysis in doxorubicin-treated patients (letter). Arch Dermatol 1990; 126:1141
64. Dainichi T, Tanaka M, Tsuruta N, et al. Development of multiple paronychia and periungual granulation in patients treated with gefitinib, an inhibitor of epidermal growth factor receptor. Dermatology 2003; 207:324–325
65. Daniel CR III. Nail pigmentation abnormalities. Dermatol Clin 1985; 3:431–443
66. Daniel CR III, Osment LS. Nail pigmentation abnormalities: their importance and proper examination. Cutis 1980; 25:595

67. Daniel CR III, Piraccini BM, Tosti A. The nail and hair in forensic science. J Am Acad Dermatol 2004; 50:258–261

68. Daniel CR III, Scher RK. Nail changes secondary to systemic drugs and ingestants. In: Scher RK, Daniel CR III, eds. Nails: therapy, diagnosis, surgery. 2nd edn. Philadelphia: WB Saunders; 1997: 251–262

69. Daniel CR III, Scher RK. Nail changes secondary to systemic drugs or ingestants. J Am Acad Dermatol 1984; 10:250–258

70. Daniel CR III, Scher RK. Nail changes caused by systemic drugs or ingestants. Dermatol Clin 1985; 3:491–500

71. Dawber RPR, de Berker DAR, Baran R. Science of the nail apparatus. In: Baran R, Dawber RPR, de Berker DAR, et al., eds. Baran and Dawber's diseases of the nails and their management. 3rd edn. Oxford: Blackwell Scientific; 2001:1–47

72. Dawn G, Kanwar AJ, Dhar S. Nail pigmentation due to roxithromycin. Dermatology 1995; 191:342–343

73. Degowin EL, Degowin RL. The nails. In: Degowin EL, Degowin RL, eds. Bedside diagnostic examination. 2nd edn. New York: Macmillan; 1969:644–653

74. Del-Pozo LJ, Vilalla J, Jimeno M, et al. Skin and ungual pigmentation caused by Ftorafur. Med Cutan Ibero Lat Am 1990; 18:78

75. Delaunay M. Effets cutanes indesirables de la chemiotherapie antitumorale. Ann Dermatol Venereol 1989; 116:1989

76. deMarinis M, Hendricks AW, Stoltzner G. Nail pigmentation with daunorubicin therapy. Ann Intern Med 1978; 89:516–517

77. Don PC, Silverman RA. Nail dystrophy caused by lithium carbonate. Cutis 1988; 41:19

78. Douglas AC. The deposition of tetracycline in human nails and teeth: a comparison of long-term treatment. Br J Dis Chest 1963; 57:44

79. Dunagin WG. Clinical toxicity of chemotherapeutic agents: dermatologic toxicity. Semin Oncol 1982; 9:14

80. Eastwood JB, Cutis JR, Smith EKM, DeWardener HE. Shedding of nails apparently induced by the administration of large amounts of cephaloridine and cloxacillin in two anephric patients. Br J Dermatol 1969; 81:750

81. Engelhart DA, Lavin ES, Sutheimer CA. Detection of drugs of abuse in nails. J Analytical Toxicology 1998; 22:314–318

82. Epstein E. Persisting Raynaud's phenomenon following intralesional bleomycin treatment of finger warts. J Am Acad Dermatol 1985; 13:468

83. Feder W, Auerback R. 'Purple toes': an uncommon sequela of oral coumarin drug therapy. Ann Intern Med 1961; 55:911

84. Feiler-Ofry V, Godel V, Lazar M. Nail pigmentation following timolol maleate therapy. Ophthalmologica 1981; 182:153

85. Fenton D. Side effects of benoxaprofen. BMJ 1982; 284:1631.

86. Fenton DA, English JS, Wilkinson JD. Reversal of male-pattern baldness, hypertrichosis and accelerated hair and nail growth in patients receiving benoxaprofen. Br Med J 1982; 284:1228

87. Ferguson MM, Simpson NB, Hammersley N. Severe nail dystrophy associated with retinoid therapy. Lancet 1983; 2:974

88. Frank SB, Cohen HJ, Minkin W. Photoonycholysis due to tetracycline hydrochloride and doxycycline. Arch Dermatol 1971; 103:520

89. Furth PA, Kazakis AM. Nail pigmentation changes associated with azidothymidine (zidovudine). Ann Intern Med 1987; 107:350

90. Garside D, Goldberg BA. Forensic and medicolegal issues. In: Hordinsky MK, Sawaya M, Scher RK, eds. Atlas of hair and nails. New York: Churchill Livingstone; 2000:227–232

91. Garside D, Ropero-Miller JD, Goldberger BA, et al. Identification of cocaine analytes in fingernail and toenail specimens. J Forensic Sci 1998; 43:974–979

92. Geller RJ, Ekins BR, Iknoion RC. Cyanide toxicity from acetonitrile-containing false nail remover. Am J Emerg Med 1991; 9:268

93. Geyer AS, Onumah N, Uytendaele H, Scher RK. Modulation of linear nail growth to treat diseases of the nail. J Am Acad Dermatol 2004; 50:229–234

94. Giacobetti R, Esterly NB, Morgan ER. Nail hyperpigmentation secondary to therapy with doxorubicin. Am J Dis Child 1981; 135:317

95. Gonzalez FU, Gil MDCC, Martinez AA, et al. Cutaneous toxicity of intralesional bleomycin administration in the treatment of periungual warts [letter]. Arch Dermatol 1986; 122:974–975

96. Gordon G, Sparano BM, Iatropoulos MJ. Hyperpigmentation of the skin associated with minocycline therapy. Arch Dermatol 1985; 121:618–623

97. Graeber CW, Lapkin RA. Metoprolol and alopecia. Cutis 1981; 28:633

98. Granstein RD, Sober AJ. Drug and heavy metal-induced hyperpigmentation. J Am Acad Dermatol 1981; 5:1

99. Greiner D, Schofer H, Milbradt R. Reversible transverse overcurvature of the nails (pincer nails) after treatment with a β-blocker. J Am Acad Dermatol 1998; 39:486–487

100. Griest MC, Norins AL. Benoxaprofen: a new arthritis medication that causes phototoxicity [letter]. J Am Acad Dermatol 1982; 5:689

101. Griest MC, Ozois II, Ridolfo AS, et al. The phototoxic effects of benoxaprofen and their management and prevention. Eur J Rheumatol Inflamm 1982; 5:138

102. Gropper CA, Don PC, Sadjadi MM. Nail and skin hyperpigmentation assoiated with hydroxyurea for polycythemia vera. Int J Dermatol 1993; 32:731

103. Grossman M, Scher RK. Leukonychia: review and classification. Int J Dermatol 1990; 29:535–541

104. Gulbranson SH, Hud JA Jr, Hansen RC. Argyria following the use of dietary supplements containing colloidal silver protein. Cutis 2000; 66:373–374, 376

105. Gventer M, Brunetti VA. Photo-onycholysis secondary to tetracycline: a case report. J Am Podiatric Med Assoc 1985; 75:658–660

106. Hanson JW, Smith DW. The fetal hydantoin syndrome. J Pediatr 1975; 87:285

107. Hario T. Spontaneous photo-onycholysis. J Dermatol (Tokyo) 1988; 15:540

108. Hart M. Grey staining of fingernails and flat wear with Actinex. Schoch Letter 1993; 43:34

109. Hatch DJ, Pascente RW. Photo-onycholysis associated with tetracycline: a case report and literature review. J Am Podiatry Assoc 1978; 68:172–177

110. Hendricks AA. Yellow lunulae with fluorescence after tetracycline therapy. Arch Dermatol 1980; 116:438–440

111. Hendrix JD, Greer KE. Cutaneous hyperpigmentation caused by systemic drugs. Int J Dermatol 1992; 31:458

112. Hernandez-Martin A, Ros-Forteza S, de Unamuno P. Longitudinal, transverse, and diffuse nail hyperpigmentation induced by hydroxyurea. J Am Acad Dermatol 1999; 40:333–334

113. Higgins EM, Hughes JR, Snowden S, et al. Cyclosporin-induced periungual granulation tissue. Br J Dermatol 1995; 132:829–830

114. Hindson C, Daymond T, Diffey B, et al. Side effects of benoxaprofen. Br Med J 1982; 284:1368

115. Holder M, Mijewski F, Lenard HG. Hypoplasie der Nagel und Endphalangen als Folge Pranataler Barbiturat Exposition. Monatsschr Klinderheilkd 1990; 138:34

116. Hood AF. Cutaneous side effects of cancer chemotherapy. Med Clin North Am 1986; 70:187–209

117. Hooper JF. Lithium carbonate and toenails. Am J Psychiatr 1981; 138:1519

118. Hussain S, Anderson DN, Salvatti ME, et al. Onycholysis as a complication of systemic chemotherapy: report of five cases associated with prolonged weekly paclitaxel therapy and review of the literature. Cancer 2000; 88:2367–2371

119. Ibsen HH, Andersen BL. Photo-onycholysis due to tetracycline-hydrochloride. Acta Derm Venereol (Stockh) 1983; 63:555–557

120. Ilchyshyn A, Vickers CFH. Yellow nail syndrome associated with penicillamine therapy. Acta Derm Venereol (Stockh) 1983; 63:554–555

121. Inalsingh CHA. Melanonychia after treatment of malignant disease with radiation and cyclophosphamide [letter]. Arch Dermatol 1972; 106:765–766

122. Ishizaki C, Sueki H, Kohsokabe S. Yellow nail induced by bucillamine. Int J Dermatol 1995; 34:493

123. Jacob CI, Patten SF. Nail bed dyschromia secondary to docetaxel therapy. Arch Dermatol 1998; 134:1167–1168

124. James WD, Odom RB. Chemotherapy-induced transverse white lines in the fingernails. Arch Dermatol 1983; 119:334
125. Johnson RB, Goldsmith LA. Dilantin digital defects. J Am Acad Dermatol 1982; 5:191
126. Kahn G, Legg JK. Recrudescence of acute photosensitivity following short-term steroid therapy. Arch Dermatol 1971; 103:94–97
127. Kanwar AJ, Singh OP. Onycholysis secondary to tetracycline hydrochloride. Cutis 1979; 23:657
128. Kaplan RP, Russell DH, Lowell NJ. Etretinate therapy for psoriasis: clinical response, remission times, epidermal DNA and polyamine responses. J Am Acad Dermatol 1983; 8:95
129. Kar HK. Longitudinal melanonychia associated with fluconazole therapy. Int J Dermatol 1998; 37:713–720
130. Katz ME, Hansen TW. Nail plate-nail bed separation: an unusual side effect of systemic fluorouracil administration. Arch Dermatol 1979; 115:860
131. Kennedy RJ, Smith LR, Goltz RW. Skin changes secondary to hydroxyurea therapy. Arch Dermatol 1975; 111:183
132. Kestel JL Jr. Tetracycline-induced onycholysis unassociated with photosensitivity [letter]. Arch Dermatol 1971; 106:766
133. Kestel JL. Photo-onycholysis from minocycline. Cutis 1981; 28:53
134. Kierland RR, Sheard C, Mason HL, et al. Fluorescence of nails from quinacrine hydrochloride. JAMA 1946; 13:809
135. Kim KJ, Chang SE, Choi JH, et al. Periungal hyperpigmentation induced by cisplatin. Clin Exp Dermatol 2002; 27:118–119
136. Kirkham N, Holt S. Nail dystrophy after practolol. Lancet 1976; 2:1137
137. Klein ME. Linear lateral black nail discoloration after months on Lopid. Schoch Letter 1990; 40:29
138. Kligman AM, Kaidbey KH. Photosensitivity to benoxaprofen. Eur J Rheumatol Inflamm 1982; 5:124
139. Koplon BS. Azure lunulae due to argyria. Arch Dermatol 1966; 94:333
140. Krebs A. Drug-induced nail disorders. Praxis 1981; 70:1951
141. Kromann NP, Vilhelmen R, Stahl D. The dapsone syndrome. Arch Dermatol 1982; 118:531
142. Kroumpouzos G, Travers R, Allan A. Generalized hyperpigmentation with daunorubicin chemotherapy. J Am Acad Dermatol 2002; 46:51–53
143. Kumar L, Kochipillae A. Mitoxantrone induced hyperpigmentation (letter). NZ Med J 1990; 103:55
144. Kuong YL. Hydroxyurea-induced nail pigmentation. J Am Acad Dermatol 1996; 35:275
145. Lasser AE, Steiner MM. Tetracycline photo-onycholysis. Pediatrics 1978; 61:98–99
146. Leavell UW, Farley CH, McIntyre JS. Cutaneous changes in a patient with carbon monoxide poisoning. Arch Dermatol 1969; 99:429
147. Lebsack CA, Weilbert RT. 'Purple toes' syndrome. Postgrad Med 1982; 71:81
148. Lemez P. Transverse nail ridgings (Beau's lines) induced by chemotherapy – a dose-dependent phenomenon. Acta Haematol 1994; 92:212–213
149. Lemos NP, Anderson RA, Robertson JR. Nail analysis for drugs of abuse: extraction and determination of cannabis in fingernails by RIA and GC-MS. J Analytical Toxicology 1999; 23:147–152
150. Levine D, Goode AW, Wingate DL. Purgative abuse associated with reversible cachexia, hypogammaglobulinemia and finger clubbing. Lancet 1981; 1:919 (cited by the Editors 'Finger clubbing associated with purgative abuse', Modern Medicine 1981; 153)
151. Llistosella E, Codina A, Alvarez R, et al. Tegafur-induced acral hyperpigmentation. Cutis 1991; 48:205
152. Llombart-Cussac A, Pivot X, Lacassagne CA, Spielmann M. Docetaxel chemotherapy induces transverse superficial loss of the nail plate. 1997; 133:1466–1467
153. Longstreth GF, Herhman J. Trazodone-induced hepatotoxicity and leukonychia. J Am Acad Dermatol 1985; 13:149
154. Losek JD, Rock AL, Boldt RR. Cyanide poisoning from a cosmetic nail remover. Pediatrics 1991; 88:337
155. Lubach D, Marghescu S. Yellow-nail syndrome durch D-penizillamin. Hautzart 1979; 30:547
156. MacDonald KJ, Ead RD. Longitudinal melanonychia during photochemotherapy. Br J Dermatol 1986; 114:395
157. Mackay-Wiggan J, Nair KG, Halasz CLG. Onycholysis associated with pacitaxel. Cutis 2003; 71:229–232
158. Madorsky DD. Arsenic in dermatology. J Assoc Milit Dermatol 1977; 3:19
159. Mallon E, Dawber RPR. Longitudinal melanonychia induced by minocycline [letter]. Br J Dermatol 1994; 130:794–795
160. Manalo FB, Marks A, Davis HL Jr. Doxorubicin toxicity: onycholysis, plantar callus formation, and epidermolysis. JAMA 1975; 233:56–57
161. Markenson AL, Chandra M, Miller DR. Hyperpigmentation after cancer chemotherapy. Lancet 1975; 2:128
162. McCormack LS, Elgart ML, Turner ML. Benoxaprofen-induced photo-onycholysis. J Am Acad Dermatol 1982; 7:678
163. McCuaig, Ellis CN, Greenberg HS, et al. Mucocutaneous complications of intraarterial 5-bromodeoxyuridine and radiation. J Am Acad Dermatol 1989; 21:1235
164. Meyerson MA, Cohen PR, Hymes SR. Tongue hyperpigmentation associated with minocycline therapy. Oral Surg Oral Med Oral Pathol Oral Radiol Endod 1995; 79:180–184
165. Mikulaschek WM. An update on long-term efficacy and safety with benoxaprofen. Eur J Rheumatol Inflamm 1982; 5:206
166. Mikulaschek WM. Long-term safety of benoxaprofen. J Rheumatol 1984; 7:100
167. Miles DW, Rubens RD. Images in clinical medicine: transverse leukonychia. N Engl J Med 1995; 333:100
168. Miller RAW. Nail dystrophy following intralesional injections of bleomycin for a periungual wart. Arch Dermatol 1984; 120:963–964.
169. Mishra D, Singh G, Pandey SS. Possible carbamazepine-induced reversible onychomadesis. Int J Dermatol 1989; 28:460.
170. Modny C, Barondess JA. Nail pigmentation secondary to quinacrine. Cutis 1973; 11:789.
171. Mooney E, Bennet RG. Periungual hyperpigmentation mimicking Hutchinson's sign associated with minocycline administration. J Dermatol Surg Oncol 1988; 14:1011–1013
172. Morris D, Aisner J, Wiernik PH. Horizontal pigmented banding of the nails in association with adriamycin chemotherapy. Cancer Treatment Reports 1977; 61:499–501
173. Morrow GL, Abbott RL. Minocycline-induced scleral, dental, and dermal pigmentation. Am J Opthalmol 1998; 125:396–397
174. Naik RPC, Singh G. Nail pigmentation due to oral 8-methoxypsoralen. Br J Dermatol 1979; 100:229
175. Nakano J, Nakamura M. Paronychia induced by gefitinib, an epidermal growth factor receptor tyrosine kinase inhibitor. J Dermatol 2003; 30:261–262
176. Nixon DW, Pirozzi D, York RM, et al. Dermatologic changes after systemic cancer therapy. Cutis 1981; 27:181
177. Norton LA. Disorders of the nails. In: Moschella SL, Pillsbury DM, Hurley HJ, eds. Dermatology. Philadelphia: WB Saunders; 1975:1222–1235
178. Norton LA. Nail disorders. J Am Acad Dermatol 1980; 2:451
179. Obermair A, Vavra N, Kurz C, et al. Letter to the editor [letter]. Gynecologic Oncol 1995; 57:436
180. Ofori-Adjei D, Ericsson O. Chloroquine in nail clippings [letter]. Lancet 1985; 2:331
181. Olujohungbe A, Cox J, Hammon MD, et al. Ingrowing toenails and cyclosporin. Lancet 1993; 342:1111
182. Orr LE, McKernan JF. Pigmentation with doxorubicin therapy [letter]. Arch Dermatol 1980; 116:273
183. Orentreich N, Harber LC, Tromovitch TA. Photosensitivity and photo-onycholysis due to demethylchlortetracycline. Arch Dermatol 1971; 83:68
184. Palmeri A, Pichini S, Pacifici R, Zuccaro P, Lopez A. Drugs in nails: physiology, pharmacokinetics and forensic toxicology. Clin Pharmacokinet 2000; 38:95–110
185. Parodi A, Guarrera M, Rebora A. Spontaneous photo-onycholysis. Photodermatology 1987; 4:160
186. Patki AH, Mehta JM. Dapsone induced erythroderma with Beau's lines. Lepr Rev 1989; 60:274

187. Pazdur R, Kudelka AP, Kavanagh JJ, et al. The taxoids: paclitaxel (taxol) and docetaxel (taxotere). Cancer Treatment Reviews 1993; 19:351–386

188. Pepine M, Flowers FP, Ramos-Caro FA. Extensive cutaneous hyperpigmentation caused by minocycline. J Am Acad Dermatol 1993; 28:292–295

189. Perlin E, Ahlgren JD. Pigmentary effects from the protracted infusion of 5-fluorouracil. Int J Dermatol 1991; 30:43

190. Pines A, Olchousky D, Bregman J, et al. Finger clubbing associated with laxative abuse. J South Med 1983; 76:1071

191. Piraccini BM, Iorizzo M, Tosti A. Drug-induced nail abnormalities. Am J Clin Dermatol 2003; 4:31–37

192. Piraccini BM, Tosti A. Drug-induced nail disorders: incidence, management and prognosis. Drug Safety 1999; 21:187–201

193. Pratt CB, Shanks EC. Hyperpigmentation of nails from doxorubicin. [letter] JAMA 1974; 288:460

194. Priestman TJ, James KW. Adriamycin and longitudinal pigmented banding of fingernails [letter]. Lancet 1975; 1:1337–1338

195. Prose NS, Abson KG, Scher RK. Disorders of the nails and hair associated with human immunodeficiency virus infection. Int J Dermatol 1992; 31:453–457

196. Quecedo E, San Martin O, Febrer MI, et al. Mees' lines. Arch Dermatol 1996; 132:350

197. Rault R. Mycophenolate-associated onycholysis. [letter] Ann Intern Med 2000; 133:921–922

198. Ronger S, Trouzet S, Ligeron C, et al. Dermatoscopic examination of nail pigmentation. Arch Dermatol 2002; 138:1327–1333

199. Rojas AR. Pigmentation de unas por doxorrubicina. Dermatol Esp 1978; 3:37

200. Rothstein MS. Onycholysis through phototoxicity [letter]. Arch Dermatol 1977; 113:520–521.

201. Roussou P, Ilias I, Foufopoulou E. Onycholysis after chemotherapy in a patient with lymphoma [letter]. Acta Derm Venereol (Stockh) 1998; 78:303

202. Rudolph RI. Lithium-induced psoriasis of the fingernails. J Am Acad Dermatol 1992; 26:135

203. Runne U, Orfanos CE. The human nail. Curr Probl Dermatol 1981; 9:102

204. Russo F, Collantes C, Guerrero J. Severe paronychia due to zidovudine-induced neutropenia in a neonate. J Am Acad Dermatol 1999; 40:322–324

205. Rycroft RJG, Baran R. Occupational abnormalities and contact dermatitis. In: Baran R, Dawber RPR (eds). Diseases of the nails and their management. 2nd edn. Oxford: Blackwell Scientific; 1994: 35–80

206. Sanders CV, Saenz RE, Lopez M. Splinter hemorrhages and onycholysis: unusual reactions associated with tetracycline hydrochloride therapy. South Med J 1976; 69:1090–1092

207. Santanove A. Pigmentation due to phenothiazines in high and prolonged doses. JAMA 1965; 191:263 (cited by Granstein RD, Sober AJ. Drug- and heavy metal-induced hyperpigmentation. J Am Acad Dermatol 1981; 6:1)

208. Saurat JH, Lefranca H, Geiger JM. European experience with acitretin in psoriasis and various disorders of keratinization. Poster presented at the Annual Meeting of the American Academy of Dermatology, San Francisco. 8 December 1993

209. Scheithauer W, Ludwig H, Kotz R, Depisch D. Mitoxantrone-induced discoloration of the nails. Eur J Cancer Clin Oncol 1989; 25:763

210. Schwartz RA, Vickerman CE. Muerke's lines of the fingernails. Arch Intern Med 1979; 139:242

211. Shedden WIH. Side effects of benoxaprofen. Br Med J 1982; 284: 1630

212. Shelley WB, Humphrey GB. Transverse leukonychia (Mee's lines) due to daunorubicin chemotherapy. Pediatr Dermatol 1997; 14: 144–145

213. Shelley WB, Shelley ED. Shoreline nails: sign of drug-induced erythroderma. Cutis 1985; 35:220–222, 224

214. Shetty MR. Case of pigmented banding of the nail caused by bleomycin. Cancer Treatment Reports 1977; 61:501–502

215. Skopp G, Potsch L. A case report on drug screening of nail clippings to detect prenatal drug exposure. Therapeutic Drug Monitoring 1997; 19:386–389

216. Slee PHTL. Images in clinical medicine: nail changes after chemotherapy. N Engl J Med 1997; 337:168

217. Smith ZS, Scheen SR, Allen JD, et al. Argyria. Arch Dermatol 1981; 117:595

218. Speechly-Dick ME, Owen ERTC. Mitozantrone-induced onycholysis. Lancet 1988; 1:113

219. Sulis E, Floris G. Nail pigmentation following cancer chemotherapy. A new genetic entity? Eur J Cancer 1980; 16:1517–1519

220. Susser WS, Whitaker-Worth DL, Grant-Kels JM. Mucocutaneous reactions to chemotherapy. J Am Acad Dermatol 1999; 40:367–398

221. Tan SV, Berth-Jones J, Burns DA. Lichen planus and photo-onycholysis induced by quinine (letter). Clin Exp Dermatol 1989; 14:335

222. Thomas G, Fournier L, Garnier R, et al. Nail dystrophy and dimercaptosuccinic acid. J Toxicol Clin Exp 1987; 7:285

223. Thomsen K. Nail changes after chemotherapy. In Burgdorf WHC, Katz SI, eds. Dermatology progress and perspectives. New York: Parthenon Publishers; 1993:372

224. Torras H, Mascaro JM Jr, Mascaro JM. Photo-onycholysis caused by clorazepate dipotassium. J Am Acad Dermatol 1989; 21:1304

225. Tosti A, Argenziano G. Dermoscopy allows better management of nail pigmentation. Arch Dermatol 2002; 138:1369–1370

226. Tosti A, Baran R, Dawber RPR. The nail in systemic diseases and drug-induced changes. In: Baran R, Dawber RPR, de Berker DAR, et al., eds. Baran and Dawber's diseases of the nails and their management. 3rd edn. Oxford: Blackwell Scientific; 2001:223–329

227. Tosti A, Gaddoni G, Fanti PA, et al. Longitudinal melanonychia induced by 3¢azidodeoxythymidine. Dermatologica 1990; 180:217

228. Tosti A, Piraccini BM, D'Antuono A, et al. Paronychia associated with antiretroviral therapy. Br J Dermatol 1999; 140:1165–1168

229. Tucker WFG, Church RE, Hallam R. Beau's lines after razoxane therapy for psoriasis. Arch Dermatol 1984; 120:1140

230. Urabe H, Asahi M. Past and current dermatological status of yusho patients. Am J Industr Med 1984; 5:5

231. Valance A, Lebrun-Vignes B, Descamps V, et al. Icodextrin cutaneous hypersensitivity. report of 3 psoriasiform cases. Arch Dermatol 2001; 137:309–310

232. Valencia ME, Pikntado V, Lavilla P, Aguado A: Ungual blue striae, HIV and zidovudine: What is their etiology? [letter]. Rev Clin Esp 1989; 185:167

233. Van Belle SJP, Dehou M-F, De Bock V, Volckaert A. Nail toxicity due to the combination adriamycin-mitoxantrone [letter]. Cancer Chemother Pharmacol 1989; 24:69–70

234. Vanhooteghem O, Andre J, Vindevoghel A, et al. Docetaxel-induced subungual hemorrhage. Dermatology 1997; 194:419–420

235. Vaughn RY, Bailey JP, Field RS, et al. Diffuse nail dyschromia in black patients with systemic lupus erythematosus. J Rheumatol 1990; 17:640

236. Vomvouras S, Pakula AS, Shaw JM. Multiple pigmented bands during hydroxyurea therapy. an uncommon finding. J Am Acad Dermatol 1991; 24:1016

237. Von Hoff DD, McCullough ML, Kuhn J, et al. Acute cutaneous reactions to docetaxil, a new chemotherapeutic agent. Arch Dermatol 1995; 131:202

238. Voorhees JJ, Orfanos CE. Oral retinoids. Arch Dermatol 1981; 117:418

239. Wakelin SH, Emmerson RW. Excess granulation tissue development during treatment with cyclosporin. Br J Dermatol 1994; 131: 147–148

240. Wantzin GI, Thomsen K. Acute paronychia after high-dose methotrexate therapy. Arch Dermatol 1983; 119:623

241. Ward HA, Russo GC, Shrum J. Cutaneous manifestations of antiretroviral therapy. J Am Acad Dermatol 2002; 46:284–293

242. Weiss E, Sayegh-Carreno. Puva induced pigmented nails. Int J Dermatol 1989; 28:188

243. Welsch MJ, Elston DM. Pigmentation due to minocycline [photo quiz]. Cutis 2001; 67:371–374

244. Wolfe ID, Reichmister J. Minocycline hyperpigmentation: skin, tooth, nail, and bone involvement. Cutis 1984; 33:457–458

245. Yogoda A, Mukherji B, Young C, et al. Bleomycin: an antitumor antibiotic. Ann Intern Med 1972; 77:861

246. Yong CKK, Prendiville J, Peacock DL, et al. An unusual presentation of doxycycline-induced photosensitivity. Pediatrics 2000; 106:131 (e13). Online. Available: www.pediatrics.org/cgi/content/full106/1/e13

247. Zaias N. The nail in health and disease. 2nd edn. Norwalk, CT: Appleton & Lange; 1990:169

248. Zaias N, Baden HP. Disorders of nails. In: Fitzpatrick TB, Eisen AZ, Wolf K, et al., eds. Dermatology in general medicine. 2nd edn. New York: McGraw-Hill; 1979:418–436

249. Zala L. Photo-onycholysis induced by 8-methoxypsoralen. Dermatologica 1977; 154:203

250. Zamora-Quezeda JC. Muscle and skin infarction after free-basing cocaine (crack). Ann Intern Med 1988; 108:564

251. Zhu WY, Xia MY, Huang SD, Du D. Hyperpigmentation of the nail from lead deposition. Int J Dermatol 1989; 28:273

252. Zuehlke RL. Papular doxycycline photosensitivity. Arch Dermatol 1973; 108:837–838

# 17 Tumors of the Nail Apparatus

## Antonella Tosti, Bertrand Richert and Massimiliano Pazzaglia

## Key Features

1. A tumor is a circumscribed neoformation
2. The growth pattern is often changed due to anatomical reasons
3. Biopsy is mandatory to distinguish the nature of the tumor
4. MRI/Echo/X-ray are helpful for the diagnosis

## Rx ⊙ TREATMENT

- Treatment is frustrating in certain tumors because of recurrences
- Surgery is often the best treatment, but not always the treatment of choice

## WARTS

## Key Features

* Periungual hyperkeratotic papules
* Hyperkeratosis of the cuticle
* Think of squamous cell carcinoma in recalcitrant lesions

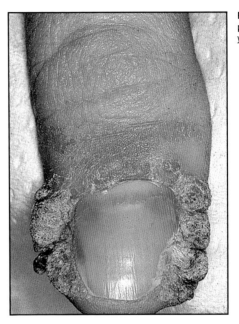

FIGURE 17–1. Extensive periungual warts in a young renal recipient.

These are the most common tumor involving the nail unit. They are caused by various human papillomavirus. They present as hyperkeratotic papules showing a rough surface. Most commonly they are located on the nail folds (proximal and lateral) but sometimes extend to the nail bed with associated onycholysis. Fissuring of the hyperkeratosis may be painful. Distortion of the nail plate is exceptional. **Nail biting enhances spreading on other fingernails.** Warts are very common and hard to treat in the immunosuppressed, particularly in organ-transplant recipients (Fig. 17.1).

The most significant lesion from which warts need to be distinguished is epidermoid carcinoma (Bowen's disease) (Tables 17.1 and 17.2).

Biopsy is mandatory in any longstanding wart in adults, warts resistant to proper therapy, and warts in immunocompromised patients, to rule out epidermoid carcinoma (Bowen's disease).

| TABLE 17–1. Periungual wart: differential diagnosis |
| --- |
| Squamous cell carcinoma |
| Fibrokeratoma |
| Subungual horn |
| Exostosis |
| Tuberculosis cutis verrucosa |
| Amyloidosis |
| Verrucous epidermal naevus |

| TABLE 17–2. Periungual wart: diagnosis pitfall |
| --- |
| Bowen's disease |

## Treatment

Treatment is often frustrating. It will depend on the number of lesions, location, duration, age, and immunologic status of the patient. It should also be cost-effective for such a benign condition. Most warts remit spontaneously, but a wide range of therapies is available, including keratolytics combined with abrasion, cryo-surgery, bleomycin puncture, imiquimod, laser therapy, interferon and immunotherapy using sensitization to diphencyprone, or naturally acquired immune sensitivity to pathogens.[1]

195

# PYOGENIC GRANULOMA

## Key Features

* Bleeding angiomatous nodule
* Periungual or subungual
* Often follows traumas, multiple lesions may be caused by drugs

Pyogenic granuloma is a benign vascular tumor, mostly seen in the early decades, usually presenting as a rapidly evolving, solitary, sessile or polypoid vascular nodule prone to ulceration or hemorrhage. Its precise pathogenesis remains unclear. Location on the nail apparatus is a common finding: Pyogenic granuloma formation is most commonly due to trauma on the fingernails; the nail-plate–lateral-sulcus interaction is responsible for their arising on the toenails. The lateral nail fold is the only part of the whole integument where a hard structure meets the skin. On the toes, this interaction is greatly increased by the weight of the body and footwear, which enhance the penetration of keratin spicules from the nail in the soft tissues of the lateral nail fold. Improper nail trimming is also a triggering factor. The pyogenic granuloma may fill the lateral nail sulcus, and sometimes covers the lateral third of the nail plate or becomes epithelialized at times. When located subungually it generates onycholysis and oozing. Pain is almost absent, even if the lesion is very prominent (Fig .17.2), except when infection occurs.

Several systemic drugs have been responsible for pyogenic granulomas in the lateral nail sulcus: indinavir,[2] retinoids,[3] ciclosporin, lamivudine, capecitabine, cetuximab. Cast immobilization and friction from footwear have been reported as causing pyogenic granulomas (Table 17.3).

## Treatment

Treament consists in curettage or $CO_2$ laser vaporization of the lesion under local anesthesia. In ingrowing toenail resulting from improper nail trimming, curettage must be completed by the resection of the offending spur. Drug-induced pyogenic granulomas are prone to recurrence and should be gently treated with a combination of antibiotic and potent steroid ointment in association with compressive dressings for several weeks or until drug discontinuation. Histological examination is mandatory in all cases in order to rule out amelanotic melanoma.

# GLOMUS TUMOR

## Key Features

* Severe pain
* Cold sensitivity
* Subjective symptoms contrast with minimal clinical signs

Glomus tumor can occur anywhere on the body but up to 75% are found in the hand, and the vast majority are located on the fingertips. It arises from the neuromyoarterial glomus cells of the nail bed dermis. **Amazingly, this condition is encountered in females around 45 years old in almost 90% of cases. The triad of pain, cold intolerance, and pin-point tenderness is highly suggestive of the condition.** Subjective symptoms typically exceed clinical signs. Pain is the leading symptom; it may be excruciating and irradiating proximally. Exquisite tenderness may be elicited by sharp probing directly over the tumor thus allowing its accurate location. Cold intolerance is associated in most but not all cases. Sometimes the tumor may be seen through the nail plate as a small reddish or bluish spot of several millimeters (Fig. 17.3) or present as a longitudinal erythronychia with distal notching. Differential diagnosis includes all causes of painful nail such as epidermal implantation cyst, subungual horn, osteoid osteoma, neuroma, and foreign body.

X-rays may reveal slight cortical erosion in about half of the cases. MRI is the best imaging technique for demonstrating the tumor (Table 17.4).[4]

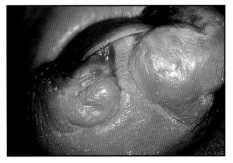

FIGURE 17–2. Very prominent pyogenic granuloma extending under the nail plate. No pain was associated.

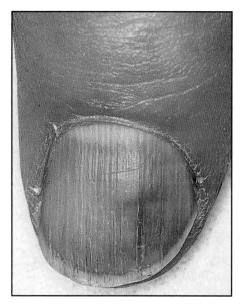

FIGURE 17–3. Glomus tumor presenting as a very painful bluish spot of the nail bed.

---

TABLE 17–3. Pyogenic granuloma: diagnosis pearls

Trauma
Ingrowing toenail
Drug-induced pyogenic granuloma
Histological examination of the specimen to rule out
   amelanotic melanoma

| TABLE 17–4. Glomus tumor: diagnosis pearls |
|---|
| Pain |
| Cold intolerance |
| Exquisite tenderness elicited by probing |
| MRI |

| TABLE 17–5. Subungual exostosis: diagnosis pearls |
|---|
| Lateral distal subungual tumor lifting the nail plate |
| Great toenail |
| Young patient |
| Porcelain white tumor with running telangiectasias on its surface |
| X-rays show the bony proliferation |

## Treatment

Treatment is the surgical removal of the tumor. Recurrence of symptoms is indicative of incomplete excision or presence of satellite lesions. MRI appears to be very helpful in those instances.

## EXOSTOSIS/ENCHONDROMA

### Key Features

* Subungual hard nodule
* Toenails commonly affected
* X-ray diagnostic

Subungual exostosis is a benign tumor of trabecular bone with a cap of fibrocartilage; whether subungual enchondroma is a different entity is not clear. It mostly occurs in children and young adults, in whom periosteum activity is intense. It is most commonly found on the great toes but involvement of the lesser toenails or the fingernails may be observed. Trauma may be implicated in some cases.

The suggestive clinical presentation is a distal lateral subungual tumor lifting the nail plate, with or without subsequent onycholysis, sometimes emerging from beneath the hyponychium. Pain is missing most of the time. A porcelain white subungual tumor with telangiectasias running on its surface is a diagnostic pearl (Fig. 17.4). In some rare instances the clinical features are less typical, mimicking other conditions such as paronychia, ingrowing toenail, subungual wart, epidermoid cyst, amelanotic melanoma, subungual calcification, onychoclavus, Bowen's disease, or pyogenic granuloma.

Diagnosis is confirmed by standard X-rays that demonstrate the bony proliferation (Table 17.5).

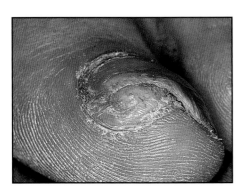

FIGURE 17–4. Subungual exostosis. Note the telangiectasias running on the surface of the tumor.

## Treatment

Treatment is the removal of the tumor under local anesthesia[5] and full aseptic conditions. There is a 10% relapse rate following surgery and children are more prone to relapse than adults.

## ONYCHOCLAVUS

Onychoclavus has also been referred to as either a subungual heloma or a subungual horn. This represents a hyperkeratotic process in the distal nail bed caused either by anatomic abnormalities or mechanical changes in foot function. Old patients are most often concerned. It typically occurs beneath the great toenail and presents as a painful distal onycholysis. Clipping of the detached nail reveals the horn (Fig .17.5). In some instances it may appear as a distal black spot (intraepidermal hemorrhages) through the nail plate. Pain is common on pressure (Table 17.6).

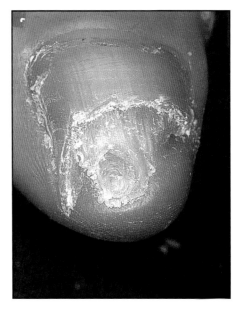

FIGURE 17–5. Onychoclavus exposed after partial nail avulsion.

| TABLE 17–6. Onychoclavus: diagnosis pearls |
|---|
| Old patient |
| Orthopedic and/or mechanical abnormalities of the forefoot |
| Painful distal onycholysis of the great toenail |
| Partial nail avulsion reveals the horn |

## Treatment

Removal of the hyperkeratotic process immediately alleviates the pain. This must be completed by prevention of recurrence by eliminating the causes (modification of footwear, inner soles, protective pads).[6]

## PSEUDOMYXOID CYST (SYNONYMS: GANGLION CYST, DIGITAL MYXOID PSEUDOCYST)

### Key Features

* Proximal nail fold swelling with possible periodic fluid drainage
* Nail plate depression and grooves
* MRI diagnostic

This entity is highly connected with osteoarthritis, especially in women. Location on the fingers is most common; involvement of the toes is possible. Anatomically, it represents the collection of gelatinous material in a cavity within connective tissue, in connection with the distal interphalangeal joint (DIJ) and lacking epithelial lining.[7] Magnetic resonance imaging demonstrates a communication between the cyst and the DIJ in more than 80% of cases.[8] Clinical features depend on the location of the cyst:

* Located on the proximal nail fold, half way between the DIJ and the cuticle, it presents as a skin-colored, smooth-surfaced, translucent, dome-shaped swelling, with a greater or lesser tendency to spontaneous discharge.
* Located more distally beneath the proximal nail fold, it faces a longitudinal groove on the nail plate due to compression of the cyst on the matrix. This gutter may exhibit transverse grooves of various depths acknowledging for the successive swelling and discharge episodes of the cyst (Fig. 17.6).
* Location beneath the nail matrix is unusual and produces several nail dystrophies such as red-blue lunula, proximal lamellar splitting, nail fissure or even pincer nail (Table 17.7).

## Treatment

Many treatments have been proposed for the condition but best results are obtained with surgery. The aim of the technique is to obliterate the duct between the DIJ and the cyst either by a ligature or by local fibrosis secondary to surgery (flap or graft).

For patients not willing to undergo surgery two other simple techniques are recommended:

* Injection of 0.2 mL sclerosing agents such as 1% tetradecyl sodium after puncture and expression of the jelly-like material. The procedure may have to be repeated 2 to 4 times at 6-week intervals.[9]
* Repeated puncture of the cyst followed by compressive dressings for several weeks may sometimes be helpful. This technique is most suitable for submatricial myxoid cyst. It may be repeated several times before embarking on matricial surgery.[10]

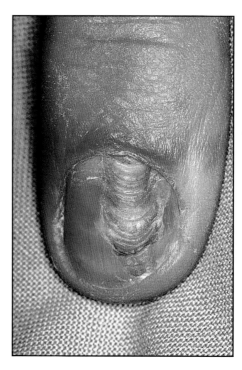

FIGURE 17–6. Pseudomyxoid cyst of the proximal nail fold. The facing gutter on the nail plate results from compression on the matrix. Transverse grooves of various depth account for the swelling and discharging episodes of the cyst.

TABLE 17–7. Pseudomyxoid cyst: diagnosis pearls

Skin-colored, dome-shaped, translucent tumor
Location on the proximal nail fold
Gutter facing the tumor
Needle puncture releases a crystal clear thick jelly

## FIBROKERATOMAS (AND KOENEN TUMORS)

### Key Features

* Periungual/subungual filiform growth
* Nail plate furrow
* Possible sign of tuberous sclerosis (Koenen's tumors)

The acquired digital fibrokeratoma (FK) is a benign fibroepithelial growth of unknown origin. Localization in the nail apparatus is common. FKs are usually unique, more common in men over 50 years old and do not resolve spontaneously (Fig. 17.7). Trauma has often been considered as a trigger of this overgrowth but some reports suggest a hamartomatous origin. They are pinkish elongated tumors often associated with a hyperkeratotic tip.

Clinical features depend on the location of the tumor:

* Developed from the ventral aspect of the proximal nail fold it causes a longitudinal depression on the nail plate due to compression on the underlying matrix. The tumor may be hardly visible as it may be covered by the proximal nail fold. Otherwise it rests within the gutter.

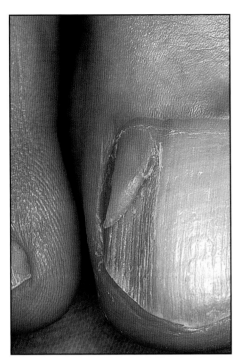

FIGURE 17-7. Fibrokeratoma emerging from under the proximal nail fold and lying in a longitudinal gutter. Note the hyperkeratotic tip.

TABLE 17-9. Implantation epidermoid cyst: diagnosis pearls

History of trauma
Vicinity of a scar
Whitish nodule

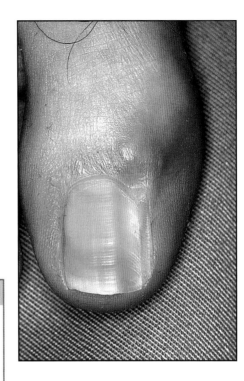

FIGURE 17-8. Implantation cyst compressing the matrix with a resultant longitudinal groove. Note the scar on the lateral side of the proximal nail fold acknowledging for prior surgery.

TABLE 17-8. Fibrokeratoma: diagnosis pearls

Elongated, pink tumor emerging from under the proximal nail fold
Tumor facing a gutter
Hyperkeratotic tip
When multiple, rule out tuberous sclerosis

- Originating from the dermis beneath the nail matrix it may be responsible for permanent nail dystrophy (even after excision of the tumor).
- Originating from the nail bed it pushes up the nail plate creating a prominent ridge. Subungual filamentous tumors are probably a very thin variant of that type (Table 17.8).

Differential diagnosis of FK include: true fibromas, pseudomyxoid cyst, Koenen's tumors, dermatofibrosarcoma, fibrosarcoma, eccrine poroma, pyogenic granuloma, verruca vulgaris, cutaneous horn, keloid, Bowen's disease. Koenen's tumors are present in 50% of tuberous sclerosis cases. They usually appear during puberty and grow in size and number. Fibrokeratomas, fibrous dermatofibromas (true fibromas) and Koenen's tumors are considered part of the same pathologic process.[11] Treatment is surgical.

## IMPLANTATION EPIDERMOID CYST

Epidermoid cysts (synonyms: keratin or squamous cyst) in the tip of the digits are most commonly secondary to trauma, sometimes years earlier, or surgery, with implantation of epidermis into subcutaneous tissue or even into the bone.

When located in the proximal nail fold, an implantation cyst may produce a smooth longitudinal gutter on the nail plate. Deeper implantation may produce enlargement of the tip of the digit, with subsequent clubbing or even pincer nail.[12] Pain may arise second-

ary to bone erosion. Diagnosis is obvious when the lesion is located in the vicinity of a scar, whether surgical or traumatic (Table 17.9). Traction on both lateral sides of the lesion may reveal the whitish color of the cyst through the skin (Fig. 17.8). For suspicious lesions, X-rays will show distortion of the cortical bone.

Lesions on the proximal nail fold may suggest myxoid cyst. Exostosis, glomus tumor and osteoid osteoma should be ruled out in case of pain with or without enlarging of the fingertip.

Treatment is surgical.

## NAIL MATRIX NEVI

### Key Features

* Longitudinal melanonychia with 'illusory' pigmentation of the overlying proximal nail fold (pseudo-Hutchinson's sign)
* More common in childhood; pigmentation may fade with age
* Dermoscopy is useful

Nail matrix nevi are rare and most frequently affect the fingernails, especially the thumb.

They are usually seen in children (see p. 242). Nail matrix nevi often appear as a band of longitudinal melanonychia or sometimes can totally involve the nail. Congenital nevi can also involve the nail fold and the hyponychium.

TABLE 17–10. Nail matrix nevi: diagnosis

Dermoscopy: regular pattern of longitudinal lines
Pathology

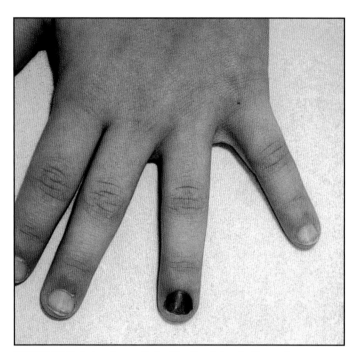

FIGURE 17–9. Dark melanonychia involving the whole nail with pseudo-Hutchinson's sign. The lesion was excised and the pathology revealed a junctional nevus.

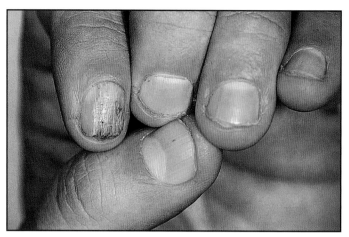

FIGURE 17–10. Onychomatricoma. The nail shows a longitudinal band of yellow thickening.

TABLE 17–11. Onychomatricoma: diagnosis pearls

Diffuse or partial nail thickening
Multiple holes in the thickened nail plate free margin
Nail plate over-curvature

The color of the band varies from light brown to black. In children the pigmentation frequently fades over the years. This does not indicate regression of the nevus but only reduced melanin production (Table 17.10).

Dark bands of melanonychia are often visible through the overlying nail fold, producing a pseudo-Hutchinson's sign (Fig. 17.9).

Most nail matrix nevi are junctional nevi. The rate of progression of nail matrix nevi to melanoma is not known but is probably exceptional.

## Treatment

The treatment of choice is still debated.

Surgical excision is a possible justified measure but only in adult life.

## ONYCHOMATRICOMA

Onychomatricoma is a benign tumor of the nail matrix first described by Baran and Kint in 1992.[13] The tumor is in our experience not rare despite the limited number of cases reported in the literature.[14]

Onychomatricoma affects most commonly the fingernails of middle-aged individuals and has never been reported in children.

The nail presents a longitudinal band of thickening or a diffuse thickening of the nail plate, which is transversally over-curved. The affected nail plate is white–yellow in color and often shows longitudinal ridging and proximal splinter hemorrhages (Fig. 17.10).

At the frontal view the tumor has a very characteristic picture because the nail plate shows multiple holes in its thickened free margin (Table 17.11). These correspond to longitudinal hollows that contain the digitating tumor, which perforate the nail plate. The tumor growth is quite slow and usually painless.

Histologically, the tumor consists of multiple fibroepithelial projections that perforate the nail plate. The tumor epithelium resembles the matrix epithelium with absence of a granular layer.

## Treatment

Surgical excision is the treatment of choice. The gross anatomy of the nail plate after excision suggests the diagnosis, showing the multiple cavities that perforate the nail plate.

## BOWEN'S DISEASE

### Key Features

* Localized longitudinal thickening with transverse over-curvature
* Multiple longitudinal hollows
* Holes in the distal nail

### Key Features

* More common in middle-aged males
* Verrucous lesion
* Melanonychia, inflammation, and crusting

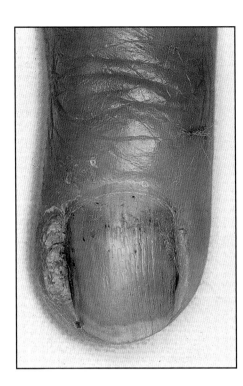

FIGURE 17–11. Bowen's disease. Wart-like periungual lesions associated with melanonychia.

| TABLE 17-12. Bowen's disease: differential diagnosis |
| --- |
| Warts<br>Paronychia<br>Melanoma |

Bowen's disease of the nail is uncommon and usually arises from the nail bed or the nail folds. It usually affects the fingernails of middle-aged individuals, especially males. The 1st, 2nd, and 3rd fingers of the left hand are most frequently affected.

Predisposing factors include HPV infection, radiodermatitis, exposure to arsenic or pesticides, and dyskeratosis congenita.

The clinical presentation is variable, depending on the anatomical location of the tumor:[15]

• Most commonly the affected digit shows periungual verrucous hyperkeratotic lesions resembling viral warts (Fig. 17.11). Ulceration may occur.
• In other cases the tumor only produces periungual erythema, hyperkeratosis and fissuring with a picture that resembles chronic dermatitis. Inflammation of the nail folds may mimic paronychia (Table 17.12).
• Subungual lesions produce onycholysis and nail destruction.
• Melanonychia is a common feature of Bowen's disease, and in some patients the tumor only produces melanonychia associated with mild nail bed hyperkeratosis or with nail plate fissuring.

Involvement of more than one nail may rarely occur.

Progression from in situ carcinoma to invasive squamous cell carcinoma occurs in up to 15% of cases.

## Treatment

Surgical ablation is the most common therapeutic modality but Mohs' micrographic controlled surgery is the treatment of choice, ensuring complete eradication of the tumor in over 90% of cases.

# SQUAMOUS CELL CARCINOMA

### Key Features

* Nodular ulcerated lesion
* Nail plate destruction
* Bone involvement may occur

Squamous cell carcinoma is the most common malignant tumor of the nail and usually affects the fingernails of middle-aged males.

Predisposing factors include chronic radiodermatitis and HPV infection. HIV-positive patients are especially susceptible to developing HPV associated squamous cell carcinoma.[18]

HPV types 16, 34, and 35 can be detected in more than 60% of cases of nail squamous cell carcinoma and possible transmission of HPV from genital lesions is suggested by several studies. Using hybridization techniques, similar HPV genomes were detected in the uterine cervical neoplasia and squamous cell carcinoma of the same patient.

The tumor usually presents as a slow-growing periungual or subungual nodule that ulcerates and bleeds (Fig. 17.12). Paronychia is commonly associated. Subungual lesions produce onycholysis and nail plate destruction.

Less commonly, squamous cell carcinomas appear as verrucous hyperkeratotic lesions that look like a viral wart.

Longstanding lesions are associated with bone involvement in up to 60% cases.

The lesion is painless until the growth is extensive. Radiological evaluation is necessary to exclude bone involvement, but it is

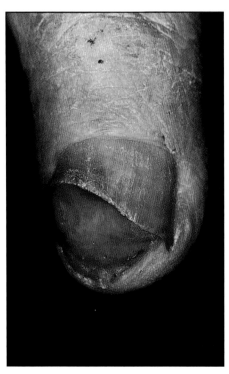

FIGURE 17–12. Squamous cell carcinoma presenting as a subungual bleeding nodule.

---

**TABLE 17–13. Bowen's disease: differential diagnosis**

Always biopsy long-lasting periungual warts
Explore the nail bed in unexplained onycholysis
Take an X-ray in patients with periungual/subungual nodules
Look for genital HPV infections in patients with fingernails with squamous cell carcinoma

---

important to keep in mind that radiography can be misleading since inflammatory reaction or pressure can induce bone abnormalities (Table 17.13).[19]

Metastasis and death from squamous cell carcinoma of the nail are extremely rare.

## Treatment

Mohs' surgery is the treatment of choice, especially for periungual and subungual squamous cell carcinoma without bone involvement where the cure rate approaches 96%.[20]

Amputation is necessary when the bone is affected.

## KERATOACANTHOMA

### Key Features

* Painful subungual nodule
* Rapid growth
* Osteolysis at X-ray

Keratoacanthoma of the nail is a rare tumor that usually affects the first three fingers of middle-aged individuals. The tumor often has a very rapid growth and a destructive behavior, with invasion and destruction of the bone.

Predisposing factors include traumas and possibly HPV infections, even though the latter are rarely detected.[21] Multiple and familial cases have been reported. Patients with incontinentia pigmenti may develop multiple subungual keratoacanthoma at a young age.

Keratoacanthoma is usually painful and may arise from the nail bed or the nail folds. The pain is initially intermittent but then increases in intensity and duration:

* Nail bed lesions cause painful onycholysis, which can be associated with digital erythema and swelling.
* Periungual lesions cause painful paronychia, which can be associated with exudation of keratinous or purulent material.

Spontaneous regression of keratoacanthoma of the nail is uncommon.

Features useful for differential diagnosis between keratoacanthoma and squamous cell carcinoma are reported in Table 17.14.

## Treatment

Most lesions can be treated with local excision and curettage. Mohs' microsurgery reduces the risk of recurrences and permits optimal cure. Systemic retinoids can be prescribed for prevention.

## CARCINOMA CUNICULATUM (VERRUCOUS CARCINOMA)

### Key Features

* Rapidly growing verrucous nodule
* Almost exclusively in the foot
* Bone resorption

Carcinoma cuniculatum is a rare, low-grade variant of squamous cell carcinoma characterized by a local aggressive clinical behavior but a low potential for metastasis.

The tumor presents as a rapidly growing verrucous nodule. Inflammation, purulent discharge and ulceration are common as well as bone involvement and destruction.

## Treatment

Surgical excision. Amputation is necessary in cases with involvement of the bone.

## MELANOMA

### Key Features

* Longitudinal melanonychia with pigmentation of the periungual tissues (Hutchinson's sign)
* Thumb most frequently affected with nail plate destruction
* Amelanotic in 25% of cases
* Dermoscopy is useful

Nail melanoma is rare in Caucasians, where it accounts for 0.7 to 3.5% of all melanomas. However, its relative incidence in non-Caucasians is much higher, accounting for 17 to 23% of melanomas in people of Japanese and Chinese ancestry and for 25% in Afro-Americans.[22]

It may occur at any age but it is exceptional in children.

The thumb and the big toe are most frequently affected. Although trauma is often referred to before the onset of nail melanoma, its role as a causative factor is unknown.

Nail melanoma may arise from the nail matrix or the nail bed where silent melanocytes are present. **It is amelanotic in about 25% of cases** (Fig. 17.13). Clinical presentation depends on the site of origin.

**Nail matrix melanoma usually causes a pigmentation of the nail plate (longitudinal melanonychia). This is the first symptom of nail melanoma in up to 76% of cases.** The color of the band is usually, but not necessarily, dark, and differential diagnosis with other causes of longitudinal melanonychia is often impossible on a clinical basis (Fig. 17.14). Features that should arouse suspicion of nail melanoma are reported in Table 17.15.

Hutchinson's sign describes the presence of a pigmentation of the proximal or lateral nail folds and/or the hyponychium and represents the clinical sign of the radial growth phase of nail

**TABLE 17–14.** Features useful for differential diagnosis between keratoacanthoma and squamous cell carcinoma

|  | **SQUAMOUS CELL CARCINOMA** | **KERATOACANTHOMA** | **CARCINOMA CUNICULATUM** |
| --- | --- | --- | --- |
| Growth | Months/years | Weeks | Months |
| Pain | Usually absent | Severe | Usually absent |
| HPV DNA | Usually present | Usually absent | Usually absent |
| X-ray | Osseous invasion | Pressure erosion | Osseous invasion |

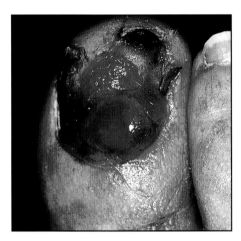

FIGURE 17–13. Amelanotic melanoma of the nail bed.

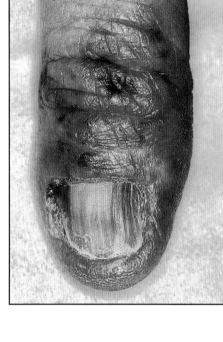

FIGURE 17–15. Nail melanoma. The periungual skin shows patchy hyperpigmentation (Hutchinson's sign). The lesion had been present for 3 years.

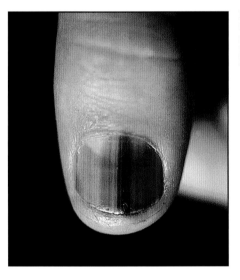

FIGURE 17–14. Nail melanoma. The affected nail shows multiple dark pigmented bands with blurred margins.

The role of dermoscopy in the diagnosis of nail melanoma is still not established and up to now it should not be considered a substitute for biopsy in the differential diagnosis of doubtful cases of longitudinal melanonychia.[24] Dermoscopy patterns suggestive for nail melanoma include the association of brown pigmentation of the background with longitudinal brown to black lines irregular in coloration, spacing, thickness, and parallelism.[25]

Nail bed melanoma causes a subungual nodule that is often not pigmented and closely resembles a pyogenic granuloma. Onycholysis is usually the presenting sign. Nail bed ulceration and bleeding occur when the tumor grows.

An A B C D E F rule for early detection of subungual melanoma has recently been proposed (Table 17.16).[26]

The prognosis of nail melanoma is poor, with the 5-year survival rate ranging from 16 to 87%, depending on the different series. This is due to the fact that diagnosis is usually delayed as compared with skin melanoma and also to the fact that the biologic behavior of nail melanoma is usually aggressive.

**TABLE 17–15.** Symptoms that should rise a clinical suspicion of melanoma

Dark band with blurred margins
Proximal portion of the band wider than its distal portion
Nail plate thinning and fissuring
Presence of periungual pigmentation (Hutchinson's sign)

melanoma (Fig. 17.15). Although Hutchinson's sign is not exclusive of melanoma, its presence requires a biopsy. It is important to distinguish Hutchinson's sign from the pseudo-Hutchinson's sign, which is due to the fact that very dark bands are visible by transparency through the cuticle.[23]

## Treatment

Local/proximal interphalangeal joint amputation is advisable in most cases. Higher amputation does not seen to reduce the incidence of recurrence or improve patient survival.

**TABLE 17–16. ABCDEF rule of for nail melanoma**

**A  Age**

Range 20–90 years
Peak 5th–7th decades
Race: African–American, Native American, Asian

**B  Band (nail band)**

Pigment (brown–black)
Breadth (3 mm)
Border (irregular/blurred)

**C  Change**

Rapid increase in size/growth rate of nail band
Lack of change: Failure of nail dystrophy to improve despite
    adequate treatment

**D  Digit involved**

Thumb > hallux > index finger
Single digit > multiple digits
Dominant hand

**E  Extension**

Extension of pigment to involve proximal or lateral nail fold
    (Hutchinson's sign) or free edge of nail plate

**F  Family or personal history**

Of previous melanoma or dysplastic nevus syndrome

# DIGITAL METASTASIS

## Key Features

* Patients with lung and genitourinary tumor
* Pseudo-inflammatory digital swelling is often misdiagnosed as acute paranychia

Digital metastasis to the bone of the distal phalanges can occur in patients with lung and genitourinary tumor.

Digital metastasis most often produces pseudo-inflammatory digital swelling and may be misdiagnosed as acute paronychia.

# REFERENCES

1. Tosti A, Piraccini BM. Warts of the nail unit: surgical and non-approaches. Dermatol Surg 2001; 27:235–239
2. Bouscarat F, Bouchard C, Bouhour D. Paronychia and pyogenic granuloma of the great toes in patients treated with indinavir. New Engl J Med 1998; 338:1776–1777
3. Pronck LC, Vasey P, Sparreboom A, et al. A phase I and pharmaco-kinetic study of the combination of capecitabine and doxetacel in patients with advanced solid tumors. Br J Cancer 2000; 83:22–29
4. Drapé JL, Idy-Peretti S, Goettmann S, et al. Subungual glomus tumors: evaluation with MR imaging. Radiology 1995; 195:507–505
5. de Berker DAR, Langtry J. Treatment of subungual exostoses by elective day case surgery. Br J Dermatol 1999; 140:915–918
6. Cohen PR, Scher RK. Geriatric nail disorders: diagnosis and treatment. J Am Acad Dermatol 1992; 26:521–531
7. de Berker DAR, Lawrence CM. Treatment of myxoid cysts. Dermatol Surg 2001; 27:296–299
8. Drapé JL, Idy Perreti I, Goettman S. MR imaging of digital mucoid cysts. Radiology 1996; 200:531–536
9. Audebert C. Treament of mucoid cysts of fingers and toes by injections of sclerosants. Dermatol Clinics 1989; 7:179–182
10. Goettman S, de Berker S, Baran R. Subungual myxoid cysts: clinical manifestations and response to therapy. J Am Acad Dermatol 2002; 46:394–398
11. Baran R, Perrin C, Baudet J, Requena L. Clinical and histological patterns of dermatofibromas of the nail apparatus. Clin Exp Dermatol 1994; 19:31–35
12. Baran R, Broutard JC. Epidermoid cyst of the thumb presenting as a pincer nail. J Am Acad Dermatol 1989; 19:143–144
13. Baran R, Kint A. Onychomatrixoma. Filamentous tufted tumour in the matrix of a funnel-shaped nail: a new entity (report of three cases). Br J Dermatol 1992; 126:510–515
14. Tosti A, Piraccini BM, Calderoni O, et al. Onychomatricoma: report of three cases, including the first recognized in a colored man. Eur J Dermatol 2000; 10:604–606
15. Sau P, McMarlin SL, Sperling LC, Katz R. Bowen's disease of the nail bed and periungual area. A clinicopathologic analysis of seven cases. Arch Dermatol 1994;130:204–209
16. Laffitte E, Saurat JH. Recurrent Bowen's disease of the nail: treatment by topical imiquimod (Aldara). Ann Dermatol Venereol 2003;130:211–213
17. Wong T-W, Sheu H-M, Lee J, et al. Photodynamic therapy for Bowen's disease (squamous cell carcinoma in situ) of the digit. Dermatologic Surgery 2001; 27: 452–456
18. Tosti A, La Placa M, Fanti PA, et al. Human papillomavirus type 16-associated periungual squamous cell carcinoma in a patient with acquired immunodeficiency syndrome. Acta Derm Venereol 1994; 74:478–479
19. McHugh RW, Hazen P, Eliezri YD, Nuovo GJ. Metastatic periungual squamous cell carcinoma: detection of human papillomavirus type 35 RNA in the digital tumor and axillary lymph node metastases. J Am Acad Dermatol 1996; 34:1080–1082
20. Zaiac MN, Weiss E. Mohs micrographic surgery of the nail unit and squamous cell carcinoma. Dermatol Surg 2001; 27:246–251
21. Baran R, Tosti A, De Berker D. Periungual keratoacanthoma preceded by a wart and followed by a verrucous carcinoma at the same site. Acta Derm Venereol 2003; 83:232–233
22. Thai KE, Young R, Sinclair RD. Nail apparatus melanoma. Austral J Dermatol 2001; 42:71–81
23. Baran R, Kechijian P. Hutchinson's sign: a reappraisal. J Am Acad Dermatol. 1996; 34:87–90
24. Tosti A, Argenziano G. Dermoscopy allows better management of nail pigmentation. Arch Dermatol 2002; 138:1369–1370
25. Ronger S, Touzet S, Ligeron C, et al. Dermoscopic examination of nail pigmentation. Arch Dermatol 2002; 138:1327–1333
26. Levit EK, Kagen MH, Scher RK, et al. The ABC rule for clinical detection of subungual melanoma. J Am Acad Dermatol 2000; 42:269–274

# 18

# Occupational Nail Disorders

## Antonella Tosti and Massimiliano Pazzaglia

## Key Features

1. Distribution of nail abnormalities consistent with occupational activity
2. Nail symptoms consistent with work-related exposure
3. Temporal relationship between exposure and onset of nail symptoms
4. Nail clippings can be utilized to evaluate worker's exposure to chemicals and toxics

## Rx ◗ TREATMENT

- Avoid mechanical/chemical/physical trauma
- Consider temporary discontinuation of work

The fingernails are very important tools for certain occupations. Nail fragility, nail thickening, and onycholysis may considerably reduce ability to manipulate small objects and can be a serious handicap to, for example, jewelers and musicians.

## NAIL CLIPPINGS IN THE DIAGNOSIS OF OCCUPATIONAL DISORDERS

Drugs and chemical and biological substances accumulate in the nails, where they can be detected and measured[1] (Table 18.1).

Nail clippings can therefore be utilized to evaluate workers' exposure to chemicals and toxics. Levels of nickel and chromate in fingernail clippings reflect occupational exposure to these metals. A nickel content greater than 8 µm/g is considered an indication of occupational exposure to nickel unless the subject has a hobby

TABLE 18-1. Chemicals which can be detected in nail clippings

| |
| --- |
| Nickel |
| Nicotine/cotinine |
| Arsenic |
| Cadmium |
| Chromium |
| Copper |
| Lead |
| Mercury |
| Silver |
| Thallium |
| Zinc |

with obvious nickel exposure.[2] Heavy metal poisoning can also be diagnosed utilizing nail clippings.[3]

## OCCUPATIONAL NAIL DISORDERS

Occupational nail disorders include nail abnormalities caused by occupation, and nail disorders which are worsened by occupational factors.

Diagnosis of a nail disorder as occupational requires the recognition of specific clinical symptoms, identification of a causal substance and determination of the probability of exposure in a given work environment.

Certain nail disorders are more likely than others to have an occupational or environmental etiology; these include koilonychia, paronychia, nail fragility, nail discoloration, foreign body granulomas, and Raynaud's phenomenon.

The occupational history is crucial and should include a chronology of all previous employment, as well as the current job description. Criteria for diagnosing occupational nail disorders are reported in Table 18.2.

Occupational nail disorders are usually classified according to the occupational substance that is responsible for the development of the nail abnormalities (Table 18.3). However, more than one noxa is often involved in most cases.[4]

TABLE 18-2. Criteria for diagnosing occupational nail disorders

| |
| --- |
| Clinical history consistent with nail symptoms |
| Known or highly suspected workplace exposure to potential noxious substances |
| Nail symptoms consistent with work-related exposure |
| Temporal relationship between exposure and onset of nail symptoms |
| Non-occupational exposure excluded as probable cause |

TABLE 18-3. Occupational entities responsible for the development of nail disorders

| |
| --- |
| Mechanical |
| Chemical |
| Physical |
| Infections |

# OCCUPATIONAL NAIL DISORDERS CAUSED BY MECHANICAL AND/OR CHEMICAL AGENTS

Traumatic nail disorders are observed in manual workers and are a consequence of repetitive trauma to the nail matrix and/or the nail plate; several nail symptoms may be present in the different nails or even in the same nail. Chemicals handled by the workers usually contribute to the development of, or aggravate the nail changes.

Nail disorders caused by traumas and/or chemicals will by discussed according to the nail symptoms.

## Koilonychia

**Key Features**

* Thinned concave nails (spoon appearance)
* 1st, 2nd, and 3rd fingers of the dominant hand are most affected
* Frequently associated with other nail signs

The nail plate is thinned and flattened and shows a 'spoon-like' appearance due to eversion of the lateral margins. The nail plate surface is frequently stained and may present mild abnormalities. Mild subungual hyperkeratosis is often associated (Fig. 18.1). Koilonychia is a consequence of repeated micro trauma and/or contact with chemicals that soften the nail plate, including mineral oil, alkali or acid, organic solvents, and keratolytic agents.

Occupational koilonychia usually involves the 1st, 2nd, and 3rd fingers and is more evident on the dominant hand; it is often more marked on the distal portion of the nail plate.

Differential diagnosis of occupational koilonychia is reported in Table 18.4.

Occupational koilonychia of the toenails is rare and caused by repetitive pressure and friction in people working barefoot. It has been described in rickshaw pullers and in people working barefoot in wet, alkaline mud.[5]

Occupations that have been most commonly associated with koilonychia are reported in Table 18.5:

* Dentists: Koilonychia of the 1st and 2nd fingers is associated with longitudinal grooves and results from mechanical traumas due to surgical instruments.
* Construction workers: Koilonychia is often associated with contact dermatitis of the proximal nail fold and subungual hyperkeratosis (cement nails[6]).
* Mushroom-growers: Koilonychia is associated with longitudinal splitting and splinter hemorrhages due to repeated rubbing of the nails against heavy plastic bags.[7]
* Butchers: Koilonychia is associated with onycholysis.[8]
* Cabinet makers: Koilonychia involves the thumb, index and middle fingers and is both traumatic and chemical due to the organic solvents utilized to clean the metal accessories of finished furniture.[9]
* Hairdressers: Koilonychia is caused by exposure to thioglycolates utilized for permanent waving.[10] It is often associated with nail pigmentation from hair dyes.

**TABLE 18–4. Differential diagnosis of occupational koilonychia**

| OCCUPATIONAL | IRON DEFICIENCY | PHYSIOLOGICAL |
|---|---|---|
| Usually fingernails | Usually fingernails | Usually toenails |
| Mild subungual hyperkeratosis | Nail fragility | Children |
| Staining of the nail plate | | |
| Mild superficial abrasion | | |
| More marked on the 1st, 2nd and 3rd fingers | | |

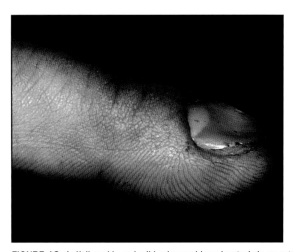

FIGURE 18–1. Koilonychia and mild subungual hyperkeratosis in an automotive worker.

**TABLE 18–5. Occupations associated with koilonychia**

**Fingernails**

Dentists
Glass workers
Construction workers
Mushroom growers
Cabinet makers
Butchers
Oil burner repairers
Automotive workers
Slaughterhouse workers

**Toenails**

Rickshaw pullers
People working barefoot in the mud

# Leukonychia Vera

## Key Features

* Punctate, striate or diffuse
* Repetitive traumas to the proximal nail plate
* Distal nail matrix damage

Occupations involving repetitive traumas to the proximal nail plate can damage keratinization of the dorsal matrix and cause striate or punctate leukonychia.[11]

# Nail Fragility

## Key Features

* Wet working conditions
* Occupational contact with solvents and solutions can modify the keratin content of the nail plate
* Different nail signs in the same patient

Nail fragility is common in occupations that involve frequent hand washing, including doctors, nurses, and hairdressers (Table 18.6). Women are more predisposed than men to develop brittle nails when working in wet conditions.[12]

Occupational contact with solvents can modify the keratin content of the nail plate, break the amino acid chains, and dehydrate the superficial layers.

Traumas significantly contribute to the nail plate damage and produce a fragility that is limited to a portion of the nail (Fig. 18.2).

Nail fragility manifests with several nail plate abnormalities that may be associated in the same nail or in different nails of the same patient (Table 18.7).

## Onychorrhexis

The nail plate is fragile and shows longitudinal ridging and fissuring. A recent study showed that onychorrhexis was very common among workers exposed to gasoline (62.3%), which is used as a solvent in many industries, e.g. rubber, plastic, and paint manufactures, and mechanical repair. Onychorrhexis is possibly a consequence of a reduction of the lipid content in the nail produced by gasoline.[13]

| TABLE 18-6. Occupations associated with nail fragility |
| --- |
| Medical personnel |
| Nurses |
| Chemical personnel |
| Photographers |
| Painters |
| Hairdressers |
| Bartenders |
| Dishwashers |
| Food handlers |

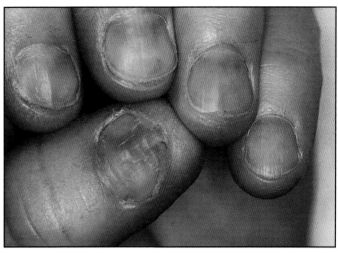

FIGURE 18-2. Occupational nail fragility in a dentist. Onychoschizia and thinning are more evident on the 1st and 2nd fingers of the dominant hand.

| TABLE 18-7. Symptoms of nail fragility |
| --- |
| Onychorrhexis |
| Onychoschizia |
| Nail plate erosions |
| Nail plate abrasion |
| Distal splitting |

Severe onychorrhexis with rough nails resembling twenty-nail dystrophy has been associated with judo due to grabbing of the nails against tissue.

## Onychoschizia

Lamellar exfoliation of the distal nail plate is common in workers exposed to water detergents and solvents. It has also been reported in professional swimmers.

## Nail plate erosions

Superficial nail erosions may occur as a consequence of mechanical traumas in manual workers. These differ from pits because the nail plate defects are larger in size, superficial, and irregular in shape. The borders of the erosions often show a black–brown staining (Fig. 18.3).

## Nail plate abrasion

Repetitive friction of the nail plate against hard surfaces induces nail plate abrasion. This may be limited to a side of the nail, such as in guitar players and pottery workers (Fig. 18.4).

Repetitive mechanical brushing of the dorsal nail plate on a hard surface may cause a marked triangular area of thinning of the nail plate extending from the middle nail to the distal margin, which shows a wedge-shaped incision (Fig. 18.5). We observed these nail abnormalities in tailors who utilize the dorsum of their nails to smooth the cloth while sewing.

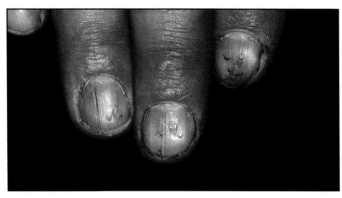

FIGURE 18-3. Nail plate erosions in a mechanical worker.

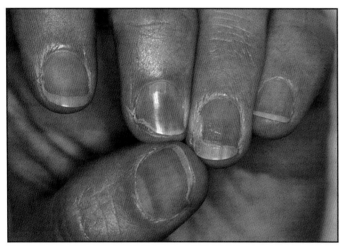

FIGURE 18-4. Occupational nail fragility in a viola player. The nail abnormalities are restricted to the 1st, 3rd, and 4th nails of the dominant hand.

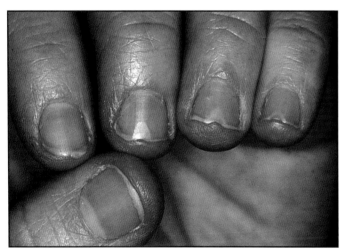

FIGURE 18-5. Occupational nail fragility in a tailor. The distal nail plate shows a triangular area of thinning due to repetitive brushing of the nail on the cloth.

Triangular worn-down nails are usually limited to the 2nd to 5th fingers of the dominant hand. Similar nail abnormalities may occur as a consequence of habit tic (rubbing the fingernails) or compulsive washing ('bidet' nails in a woman obsessed by personal hygiene).[14]

## *Distal splitting*

Distal nail splitting can result from repeated occupational trauma to the nail plate free margin. This occurs, for instance, in paint scrapers.

# Onycholysis

## Key Features

* Distal nail plate detachment
* May be associated with paronychia
* Nail bed commonly colonized by bacteria or fungi

Detachment of the nail plate from the nail bed may be a consequence of traumas or be caused by chemicals.

Traumatic onycholysis occurs in occupations that involve strong mechanical stress to the distal nail plate (Table 18.8). Onycholysis is more marked in the central portion of the nail and often associated with hemorrhages. The thumb is usually not affected.

Traumatic onycholysis of the fingernails is more commonly observed in butchers, slaughterhouse workers (Fig. 18.6), chicken-processing workers, and in workers lifting heavy bags. Traumatic onycholysis of the toenails can occur in athletes and dancers and most frequently affects the big toe, often bilaterally.

Chemical onycholysis results from chemical injury to the nail plate to nail bed adhesion and is favored by exposure to a wet environment and organic solvents. It usually starts from the distal and lateral sides of the nails and may be associated with paronychia.

Microorganisms, such as yeasts and *Pseudomonas* species, frequently colonize the onycholytic space; these cause green discoloration. Black pigmentation caused by *Proteus mirabilis* has been reported in workers exposed to metals that react with the hydrogen sulfide produced by the bacteria to form metal sulfides that blacken the nails.[15]

TABLE 18-8. Occupations associated with onycholysis

### Fingernails

Butchers
Slaughterhouse workers
Chicken processing workers
Bartenders
Food handlers
Dishwashers
Hairdressers
Gardeners
Floriculturists
Fishermen
Nail salon workers (manicurists)

### Toenails

Athletes
Dancers

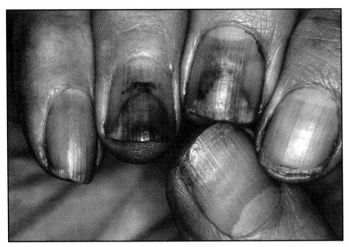

FIGURE 18-6. Traumatic onycolysis associated with nail plate hemorrhages in a slaughterhouse worker.

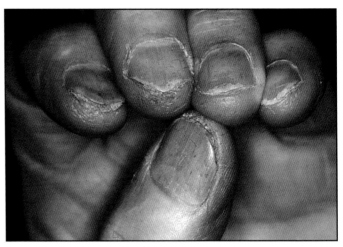

FIGURE 18-7. Nail bed hyperkeratosis and yellow discoloration in a construction worker exposed to chromium salts.

Acute onycholysis can occur after exposure to strong irritants such as sodium hypochlorite, detergent enzymes, thioglycolates in depilatories, and hydrofluoric acid. Painful onycholysis is a typical sign of hydrofluoric acid burns, which frequently involve the subungual areas. This chemical has a very high toxicity and usually reaches the fingertips through pinholes in the rubber gloves.[16] Development of onycholysis may be preceded by blue–green discoloration of the distal nail plate.

Penetration of foreign bodies under the nail plate can cause inflammation and pain. This can be seen in hairdressers because hair fragments easily penetrate under the nail plate or in the periungual folds. However, subungual hair implantation mostly occurs in nails already affected by onycholysis or other abnormalities.[17]

Allergic contact dermatitis of the hyponychium may also cause onycholysis (allergic onycholysis). This is usually seen in occupations involving mechanical traumas to the digits in association with exposure to sensitizers, as the nail bed is usually protected from the environment. Allergic onycholysis is rare and has been reported from color developers, quaternium 15, anaerobic acrylic sealants, and metacrylates in chemically-cured sculptured nails. Professional tulip and *Alstromeria* growers may also develop allergic onycholysis in association with fingertip eczema (tulip finger).[18]

Fishermen may develop a periungual and fingertip dermatitis with onycholysis caused by sea worms used as bait.[19]

## Hyperkeratosis of the Nail Bed

### Key Features

* Nail thickening
* Nail bed involvement by psoriasis or onychomycosis

Hyperkeratosis of the nail bed can be caused by repetitive pressure, trauma, and friction. It is most commonly seen in association with irritative or allergic contact dermatitis (Figs 18.7 and 18.8). It can also be a sign of occupational psoriasis.

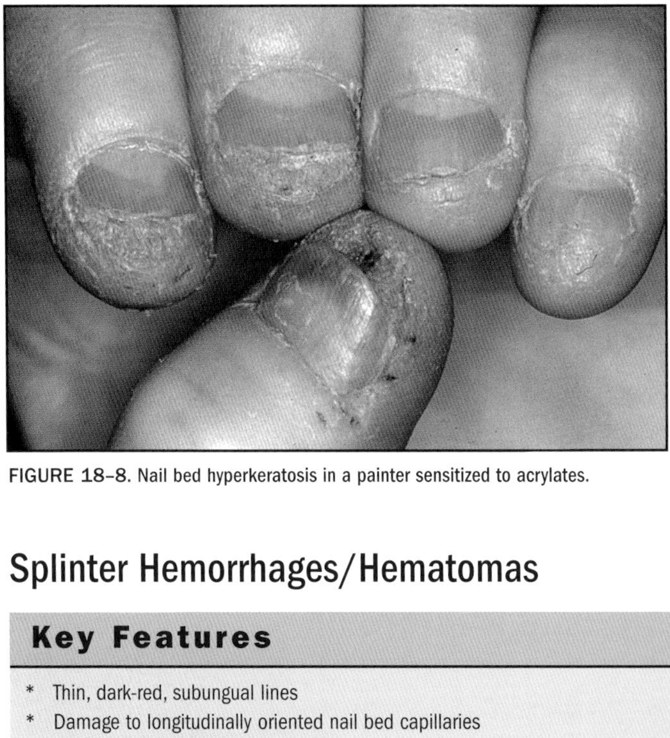

FIGURE 18-8. Nail bed hyperkeratosis in a painter sensitized to acrylates.

## Splinter Hemorrhages/Hematomas

### Key Features

* Thin, dark-red, subungual lines
* Damage to longitudinally oriented nail bed capillaries
* Big toe more frequently affected

Sports-related traumas can cause fingernail splinters, which have been reported in golfers and in frisbee or cricket players.[20] Mountain climbers can develop proximal splinter due to altitude. Gardening and playing percussion instruments are also associated with splinter hemorrhages (Fig. 18.9).

Subungual hematomas and hemorrhages of the toenails are common in dancers and athletes, especially in tennis, soccer or squash players and joggers; onycholysis is often associated (Fig. 18.10). The big toe is more frequently involved in tennis players, the 2nd and 3rd toes in soccer or squash players, and the 4th and 5th toes in joggers or runners. Workers wearing shoes with steel toe-caps may develop subungual hematomas, especially when the boots do not fit the foot correctly.

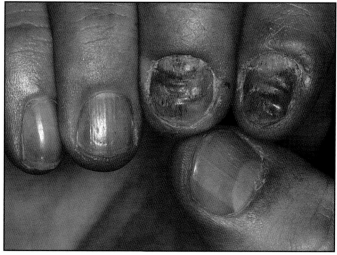

FIGURE 18-9. Splinter hemorrhages and nail plate abnormalities in a gardener.

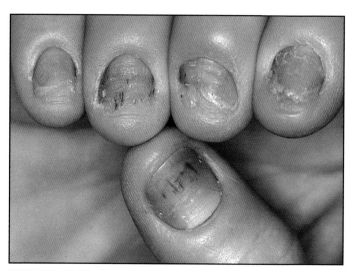

FIGURE 18-11. Allergic contact paronychia due to thiuram compounds.

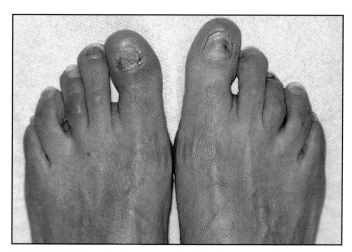

FIGURE 18-10. Subungual hematoma and nail bed hemorrhages in a squash player.

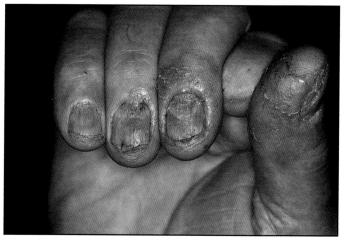

FIGURE 18-12. Chronic paronychia, splinter hemorrhages, and allergic onycholysis in an agricultural worker.

# CHRONIC PARONYCHIA

## Key Features

* Avoid moisture, contact irritants, and cuticular trauma
* *Candida* species and bacteria colonization is a secondary phenomenon
* Most commonly affects the 1st, 2nd, and 3rd digits of the dominant hand

Chronic paronychia is a common nail disorder that affects housewives, dishwashers, farmers, and other workers involved in wet occupations (Fig. 18.11).

Chronic paronychia results from an impairment of the epidermal barrier of the proximal nail fold. It usually follows mechanical or chemical traumas that damage the cuticle, especially exposure to water and/or irritative compounds. The condition is maintained by penetration of irritant and allergenic environmental agents, which cause an inflammatory reaction of the nail fold and matrix. Inflammation impairs nail fold keratinization and prevents

formation of a new cuticle. *Candida* species and bacteria colonization is a common secondary phenomenon.

Chronic paronychia most commonly affects the 1st, 2nd, and 3rd digits of the dominant hand. The fingers show mild erythema and swelling of the proximal nail fold with absence of the cuticle.

The nail plate may present transverse grooves and discoloration of the lateral margins due to *Pseudomonas* colonization; onycholysis may be associated.[21]

Most cases of chronic paronychia are caused by irritants, including soaps, detergents, and oils. Frictional paronychia can occur in musicians, such as pianists and harp or violin players (see chapter 10).

In some occupational groups, irritative paronychia is complicated by the penetration of small particles of organic or inorganic materials in the proximal nail fold. These include fragments of hair or thorns, metallic dust, fiberglass particles etc. Foreign bodies aggravate the inflammatory reaction but granulomatous infiltration is rare.

Contact allergy is uncommon and most frequently caused by rubber compounds and mineral oil additives (Fig. 18.12).

In occupational food handlers, chronic paronychia may be caused by an immediate hypersensitivity reaction to food. Patients complain of worsening of the periungual inflammation and itching immediately after handling raw food ingredients. This variety of chronic paronychia is most commonly seen in bartenders, restaurant helpers, and in workers who handle raw vegetables and fish.[22]

Paronychia due to immediate hypersensitivity to placenta extracts has been reported in veterinarians.

# NAIL DISCOLORATION (see Chapter 7)

### Key Features

* Exogenous staining of the nail plate
* Mee's lines as a sign of occupational exposure to arsenic and thallium poisoning but may be caused by many systemic insults

Occupational nail discoloration is almost always caused by exogenous staining of the nail plate due to exposure to local agents and is localized to the fingernails. Exceptions to this rule are rare and include silver intoxication (generalized argyria), nail discoloration due to methahemoglobinemia, Mee's lines due to occupational poisoning from arsenic or thallium, and brown discoloration of the nail fold in hemochromatosis.

## Exogenous staining

The discoloration does not fade with pressure and its proximal border follows the shape of the proximal nail fold.

**YELLOW** A white–yellow discoloration of the nails is seen in workers exposed to pesticides including paraquat, diquat, and dinitrocresol. The color changes do not affect the whole nail plate but appear as transverse bands involving two or more nails. Severe and long-term exposure to these pesticides can produce onycholysis and even loss of the nails.

Exposure to chromium salts causes an ochreous discoloration.

Textile dyes can cause a yellow discoloration of the nails.

Yellow staining of the nails and the palms is common in workers exposed to 4,4′-methylenedianiline, which is used as a curing agent in the epoxy industry. Because this chemical has hepatotoxic and potentially carcinogenic effects, workers with the yellow staining require strict follow-up and observation.[23]

**ORANGE/RED** Contact with hair dyes causes nail discoloration ranging from orange to brown. This is very common in hairdressers (Fig. 18.13). Henna pigmentation is usually orange-red.

Other chemicals that may cause orange/brown nails include glutaraldehyde, picric acid, and hydroquinone. Burnt sugar, roasted coffee, and nicotine can also induce brown nail discoloration.

**PURPLE** Gold potassium cyanide can cause a purple/brown discoloration of the fingernails associated with onycholysis.

**BLACK** A brown–black discoloration of the nails due to tannin is common in workers who handle fresh walnuts to make nocino liquor and in workers handling dark woods such as ebony and mahogany (Fig. 18.14).

Vintners may also have black nails caused by the tannin in red grapes and wine.

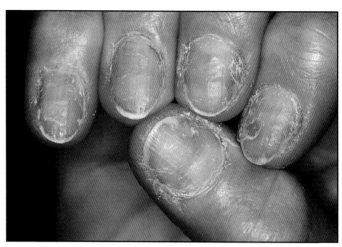

FIGURE 18–13. Nail fragility and discoloration in a hairdresser.

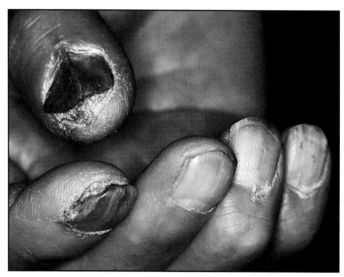

FIGURE 18–14. Black discoloration due to dark wood and marked subungual hyperkeratosis in a cabinet maker.

A black discoloration of the fingernails may occur in riflemen and hunters due to contact with gunpowder. Silver nitrite also causes black pigmentation. Photographers and printers may develop black nails due to exposure to hydroquinone salts.

# Foreign Body Granulomas

### Key Features

* Most commonly affect the nail bed or the hyponychium
* Painful onycholysis in the affected digit

Foreign body granulomas most commonly affect the nail bed or the hyponychium and may be caused by a large variety of organic and inorganic materials, including hair, vegetable thorns, animal shells or spines, and fragments of metal, plastic, or glass. The affected digit develops painful onycholysis.

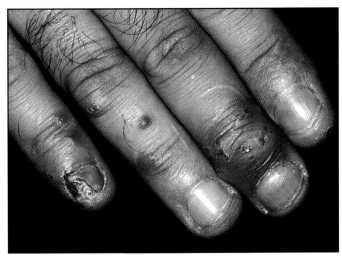

FIGURE 18–15. Foreign body granulomas due to sea urchins in a fisherman.

Granulomas of the proximal nail fold are less common and produce paronychia. Sea urchins and prickly pears may also cause granulomas of the nail[24] (Fig. 18.15).

## Raynaud's Phenomenon/Digital Ischemia

### Key Features

* Typical of workers using vibrating or drilling tools
* Carpal tunnel syndrome is often associated

Raynaud's phenomenon and digital ischemia are observed in workers using vibrating or drilling tools for many years. The use of pneumatic drills and chainsaws is associated with a high risk of vibration syndrome.

Carpal tunnel syndrome has also been associated with prolonged use of vibrating tools occurring in up to 20% of forestry workers.[25] Carpal tunnel syndrome with ischemic lesions and acroosteolysis can occur in manual workers who neglect their neurological signs for many years (Fig. 18.16).

Symptoms include paresthesia, shortening of the digits due to bone resorption, nail plate thinning and discoloration, nail bed hyperkeratosis, ulceration and crusting.

## CLUBBING

### Key Features

* Typical sign of acute silicosis and asbestosis
* Scleroderma-like changes and acrosteolysis can also occur

Finger clubbing is a typical sign of acute silicosis and asbestosis; it has also been reported in coal workers' pneumoconiosis. Traumatic clubbing has been described in karateka (karate practitioners).

Clubbing-like nail changes in the fingers have been observed in vinyl chloride disease. Scleroderma-like changes and acrosteolysis can also occur (see Chapter 15).

## OCCUPATIONAL NAIL DISORDERS CAUSED BY PHYSICAL AGENTS

### Ionizing Radiation

Chronic radiodermatitis can be an occupational hazard for radiologists, dentists, and veterinarians. The affected digits show periungual erythema and telangiectasia, nail thinning, onychorrhexis, and nail bed hemorrhages. Longitudinal melanonychia may occur as a consequence of melanocyte activation. The development of wart-like lesions requires a biopsy to exclude Bowen's disease or squamous cell carcinoma (Fig. 18.17).

### Microwaves

Beau's lines and onychomadesis have been reported in two snack bar employers who had used the same microwave oven; this was probably due to a defective oven.[26]

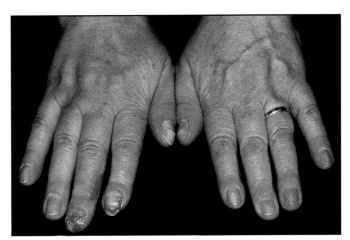

FIGURE 18–16. Digital ischemia to carpal tunnel syndrome in a manual worker.

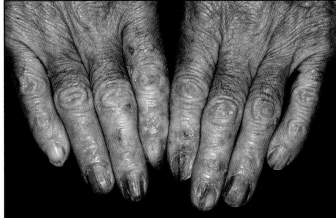

FIGURE 18–17. Chronic radiodermatitis in a veterinarian.

## INFECTIOUS NAIL DISORDERS

It is mandatory that healthcare workers avoid wearing artificial nails or nail polish during working time. Bacteria always colonize under the nail – natural or artificial – and the use of artificial nails and nail polish discourages vigorous hand washing. Chipped nail polish, nail polish worn longer than 4 days, and artificial nails can all increase the number of colony-forming units of bacteria that remain on the fingertips after hand washing and surgical hand scrub. Certain bacteria (e.g. *Serratia*, *Acinobacter*) can be recovered only from nurses with artificial nails, thus making these nurses a risk for susceptible patients.[27]

Some occupations are at risk of contracting infectious nail disorders (Table 18.9, Fig. 18.18).

| TABLE 18-9. Occupations at risk of infectious nail disorders | |
| --- | --- |
| *Mycobacterium tuberculosis* | Pathologists, morgue attendants |
| *Mycobacterium marinum* infection | Aquarium workers |
| Blastomycosis | Pathologists |
| Onychomycosis | Coal miners, soldiers, swimmers, steel/furnace workers |
| Periungual warts | Meat and fish handlers |
| Herpetic whitlow | Doctors, nurses |
| Milker's nodules | Agricultural workers |
| Human orf | Agricultural workers |
| Erysipeloid | Meat and fish handlers |

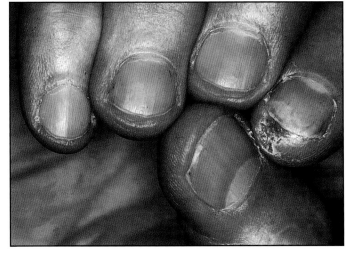

**FIGURE 18-18.** Mycobacteriosis due to *Mycobacterium marinum* in an aquarium worker.

## Onychomychosis

Nail fungal infections are encouraged by occlusive shoes and a humid environment. An increased prevalence of toenail onychomychosis from dermatophytes was recently reported in swimmers. *Candida* species are frequently isolated from the proximal nail fold of patients with chronic paronychia (see chapters 10 and 12).

## Warts

Certain occupations are susceptible to the occurrence of periungual warts; for instance up to 23% of handlers of meat, fish, and poultry develop warts in the periungual region (butchers' warts). Animals cannot contract butchers' warts because HPV are highly host specific; humans are not infected by other animal papillomaviruses, although they are favored by continuous skin maceration. Papillomaviruses 7 or 2 are commonly isolated in butchers' warts.[28]

## Herpes Simplex Infection

Digital primary and recurrent HSV-1 infections are not uncommon in doctors and nurses. Dentists, pathologists, and laboratory technicians are especially susceptible for infection that may involve the nail, producing acute paronychia.

## NAIL DISORDERS WORSENED BY OCCUPATIONAL FACTORS

### Psoriasis

Pressure, trauma, and friction caused by occupational procedures may cause or aggravate psoriasis. Psoriatic onycholysis can be aggravated by the penetration of environmental particles present in the working environment; this is, for instance, seen in hairdressers who frequently carry hair fragments in the onycholytic area. Arthropathic involvement can also be worsened by occupations that produce continuous traumas to interphalangeal joints.[29]

### Trachyonychia

Trachyonychia can be a considerable handicap for manual workers because the nails are thin, brittle, and easily break with repetitive mechanical traumas. Staining of the nail plate from environmental dyes may be a major feature.

### Lichen Planus

Traumas can worsen nail lichen planus through the Koebner phenomenon and the disease can be caused or activated by occupational procedures.

**TABLE 18–10. Nail symptoms by occupations**

## Nail salon workers

| | |
|---|---|
| Fingertip dermatitis | Raynaud's phenomenon |
| Periungual dermatitis | Paresthesia of the digits |
| Onycholysis | Respiratory hazards[30] |

## Hairdressers

| | |
|---|---|
| Onycholysis | Subungual hair implantation |
| Paronychia | Nail brittleness |
| Koilonychia | Nail pigmentation |

## Athletes

Subungual exostosis: Dance
Nail brittleness: Swimming
Onychorrhexis: Judo
Leukonychia: Karate
Beau's lines/onychomadesis: Soccer, dance, jogging
Onycholysis: Soccer, jogging
Onychomychosis: Swimming
Splinter hemorrhages: Fingernails (golf and frisbee)
Subungual hematoma: Soccer, squash: 1st, 2nd, 3nd toes
Subungual hemorrhages: Tennis: 1st toe; jogging, running: 2nd, 4th, 5th toes
Clubbing: Karate
Worn-down nails: Karate

## Agricultural workers

Koilonychia
Splinter hemorrhages
Onycholysis (tulip finger)
Chronic paronychia
Discoloration (pesticides, tannin)
Digital ischemia (forestry workers)
Milker's nodules
Human orf
Bowen's disease, squamous cell carcinoma (exposure to pesticides)

## Food handlers

Koilonychia
Nail fragility
Onycholysis
Chronic paronychia
Discoloration (burnt sugar, roasted coffee, tannin)
Periungual warts
Erysipeloid

## Medical personnel

Nail fragility
Paronychia
Chronic radiodermatitis
Warts
HSV infections
Tuberculosis
Blastomycosis
Nail discoloration (silver nitrate, glutaraldehyde)
Hyperkeratosis of the nail bed (dentists)

# REFERENCES

1. Gerhardsson L, Englyst V, Lundstrom NG, et al. Cadmium, copper and zinc in tissues of deceased copper smelter workers. J Trace Elem Med Biol. 2002; 16:261–266
2. Kristiansen J, Christensen JM, Henriksen T, et al. Determination of nickel in fingernails and forearm skin/stratum corneum. Analytica Chimica Acta 2000; 403:265–272
3. Daniel R, Tosti A, Piraccini BM. The nail and hair in forensic science J Am Acad Dermatol 2004; 50:258–261
4. Peters K, Gammelgaard B, Menné T. Nickel concentrations in fingernails as a measure of occupational exposure to nickel. Contact Dermatitis 1991;25: 237–241
5. Dolma T, Norboo T, Yayha M, et al. Seasonal koilonychia in Ladakh. Contact Dermatitis 1990; 22:78–80
6. Hagman JH, Ginebri A, Mordenti C, et al. Treatment of occupational koilonychia with tazarotene gel. Acta Derm Venereol 2003; 83:296–297
7. Schubert B, Minard JJ, Baran R, et al. Onychopathy of mushroom-growers. Ann Dermatol Venereol 1977; 104:627–630
8. Mayer-Hammes, Quadripur SA. Occupational koilonychia. Hautarzt 1983; 34: 577–579
9. Ancona-Alayon A. Occupational koilonychia from organic solvents. Contact Dermatitis 1975; 1:367–369
10. Alanko K, Kanerva L, Estlander T, et al. Hairdresser's koilonychia. Am J Contact Dermatol 1997; 8:177–178
11. Honda M, Hattori S, Kayama L, et al. Leukonychia striae. Arch Dermatol 112; 1976:1147
12. Lubach D, Beckers P. Wet working conditions increase brittleness of nails, but do not cause it. Dermatology 1992; 185:120–122
13. Jia X, Xiao P, Jin X, Shen G, et al. Adverse effects of gasoline on the skin of exposed workers.Contact Dermatitis 2002; 46:44–47
14. Baran R, Moulin G. The bidet nail: a French variant of the worn-down nail syndrome. Br J Dermatol 1999; 140:377
15. Qadripur SA, Schauder S, Schwartz P. Black nails caused by Proteus mirabilis. Hautarzt 2001; 52:658–661
16. Shewmaker W, Anderson BG. Hydrofluoric acid burns: a report of a case and review of the literature. Arch Dermatol 1979; 115:593
17. de Berker D, Dawber R, Wojnarowska F. Subungual hair implantation in hairdressers. Br J Dermatol 1994; 130:400–401
18. Goh CL. Allergic contact dermatitis and onycholysis from hydroxylamine sulphate in colour developer. Contact Dermatitis 1990; 22:109
19. Angelini G, Giglio G, Filotico R, Vena GA. Dermatite da contatto con Nereis diversicolor. In: Dermatologia in poster. Ayala F, Balato N (eds). Naples, Cilag SpA, 1989:35–37
20. Ryan AM, Goldsmith LA. Golfer's nails. Arch Dermatol 1995; 131:857–858
21. Tosti A, Piraccini BM. Paronychia. In: Amin S, Lahti A, Maibach HI (eds). Contact urticaria syndrome. New York, CRC Press, 1977:267–278
22. Tosti A, Guerra L, Morelli R, et al. Role of foods in the pathogenesis of chronic paronychia. J Am Acad Dermatol 1992; 27:706
23. Cohen SR.Yellow staining caused by 4,4'-methylenedianiline exposure. Occurrence among molded plastics workers. Arch Dermatol 1985; 121:1022–1027
24. Haneke E, Tosti A, Piraccini BM. Sea urchin granuloma of the nail apparatus: report of 2 cases. Dermatology 1996; 192:140–142
25. Diba VC, Holme SA, Savage R, Mills CM. Bilateral nail dystrophy associated with vibrating tool use. Br J Dermatol. 2003; 148:173–174
26. Brodkin RH, Bleiberg J. Cutaneous microwave injury. A report of two cases. Acta Derm Venereol 1973; 53: 50–52
27. Saiman L, Lerner A, Saal L, et al. Banning artificial nails from health care settings. Am J Infect Control 2002; 30:252–254
28. Tosti A, Piraccini BM. Warts of the nail unit: surgical and non-surgical approach. Dermatol Surg 2001; 27:235–238
29. Kanerva L, Estlander T. Occupational post-traumatic psoriasis. Contact Dermatitis 2001; 44:317–318
30. Gallagher F, Gaubert D, Hale M. Respiratory hazards of 'nail sculpture.' Br Med J 2003; 327:1050

# 19

# Disorders of the Nail Unit due to Podiatric Biomechanical Considerations

## Bryan C Markinson, Justin Wernick and Richard C Gibbs

## Key Features

1. Toenail pain is one of the most common reasons for seeking podiatric care
2. Structural deformities of the feet and toes, and the resulting repetitive trauma, may be the primary cause of toenail dystrophies or deformities, which may or may not be painful
3. Biomechanical foot problems can explain the majority of structural toe deformities
4. Biomechanical foot problems and resulting structural deformities can also intensify the symptomatology of primary nail diseases such as psoriasis and onychomycosis
5. The degree of rigidity or flexibility of structural deformities plays a significant role in determining the severity of resulting toenail problems

## Rx  TREATMENT

- Be mindful of any structural issues when evaluating toenail problems
- Painful primary nail pathology, as in onychomycosis or psoriasis, may not fully respond to conventional treatment if structural deformities and trauma are not addressed
- Shoe modifications, nail debridement, prescription nail softeners, and custom orthotics can all play a role in palliative management of toenail problems complicated by biomechanical issues
- Techniques of toenail surgery (permanent or not) and osseous surgery may offer options for definitive treatments of toenail problems complicated by biomechanical issues

For the purposes of this chapter, let us first define what we mean by the 'nail unit', as well as the full breadth of the scope of 'biomechanics'. When using the designation 'nail unit' we are speaking of the nail plate; nail bed; the medial, lateral, and proximal nail folds; and the most distal part of the bed, the hyponychium. 'Biomechanical' refers not only to normal and abnormal gait patterns but also to those deformities that may result and that may produce stress and repeated microtrauma to the nail unit. It is also important to evaluate footwear, which, in combination with faulty biomechanics, can produce toenail disorders. Some medical conditions, predominantly those involving the rheumatologic system, can produce deformity due to soft tissue changes or limitation of motion due to joint degradation, which may impact on toenail disease. Neuropathy, predominantly from diabetes, and neuromuscular disorders result in abnormal gait and can cause abnormal stresses on the nail unit. Some foot or toe deformities may result from prior injury such as sprains and fractures, and may produce toenail problems. Finally, it is also important to understand that faulty foot mechanics during gait may, and often do, determine what the impact of trauma and rheumatologic disease might be in the long term.

## NORMAL FUNCTION OF THE FOOT

The primary purpose of the foot is to perform specific dynamic functions at different phases of the gait cycle (Fig. 19.1). The total gait cycle is the time from heel contact of one foot until the next heel contact of that same foot. Initially, as the foot hits the ground, it is required to: (1) react to terrain that is often uneven and (2) absorb shock by allowing increased knee flexion. The pedal mechanism allowing these movements occurs at the subtalar and midtarsal joints (Fig. 19.2) and is called pronation. Pronation is a complex motion that takes place at several joints of the foot, moving the sole plantarward and lowering the arch.

Pronation (the contact phase of gait) occupies the first 27% of the gait cycle and allows for 'unlocking' of the foot. It is this unlocking mechanism that alters the structure of an otherwise rigid bony foot, creating a more flexible structure that is perfect for the purposes of adjusting to an uneven surface. Once the forefoot contacts the ground, the opposite limb then leaves the ground and swings past the planted limb. The planted foot then undergoes change in its architecture, moving from a flexible to a more rigid structure, thus providing stabilization for the total body as it swings over the support limb. This midstance phase occupies 40% of the gait cycle.

Once the body weight has been stabilized over the support limb, the terminal event in the stance phase of the gait cycle, called propulsion, takes place. This action occupies the last 30 to 40% of the cycle and is initiated when the opposite limb strikes the ground and the planted heel lifts from the surface, thrusting the body weight forward onto the forefoot. During this phase, the foot must be stable to balance the body solely on a small plantar area as it thrusts forward.

This propulsive phase allows transfer of the body weight from the support limb to the opposite limb, which is then in contact with the ground. This motion occurs mainly at the subtalar joint by supination. In supination, a complex motion involving several joints in the foot, the plantar surface of the foot moves dorsally, raising the arch.

The three phases (contact, midstance, and propulsion) that compose the stance or weight-bearing phase of gait occupy approximately 60% of the total gait cycle and occur in approximately 0.6 second. The orderly transfer of body weight is essential for the normal propulsive sequence and for the efficient distribution of body weight from one area of the foot to the next.

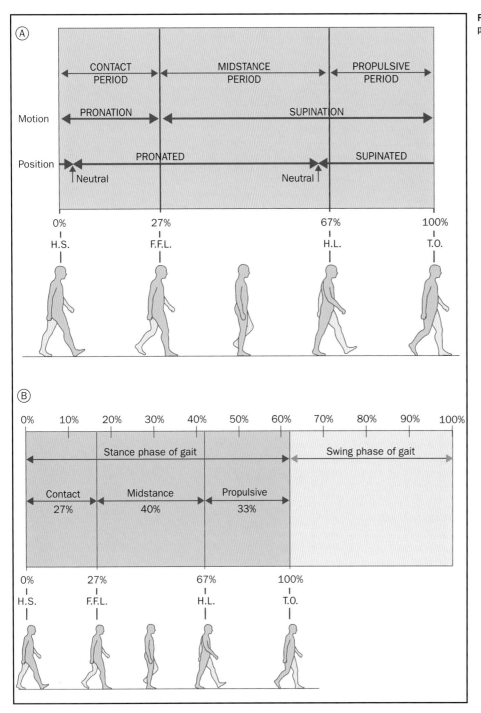

FIGURE 19–1. Gait cycle (from ref. 2, used with permission).

To summarize, it is apparent that for normal foot function, the foot has to be both flexible and rigid at appropriate times during gait. If this is not the case, instability and deformity may result.

## ABNORMAL FUNCTION OF THE FOOT

The aforementioned gait motions take place in a segmental and sequential manner, requiring specific time periods for each phase to occur. If these motions are interfered with, the foot is delayed in changing from its adaptive flexible structure to a more rigid one.[1] In that event, the supinatory phase, during which the foot is locked into a rigid propulsive lever, occurs much later in the cycle. As a result of this delay, the foot structure is still in a weakened and partially flexible state and is not prepared to accept the increase in the reactive force of the ground. This increased force reacts against the individual's body weight and eventually alters and deforms the osseous and muscular alignment, creating deformity.[2] Poorly fitting shoes can contribute to this deformity because the ground strikes the shoe first, exaggerating the reactive force. Because these events occur in the final stage of propulsion, the digits bear most of the

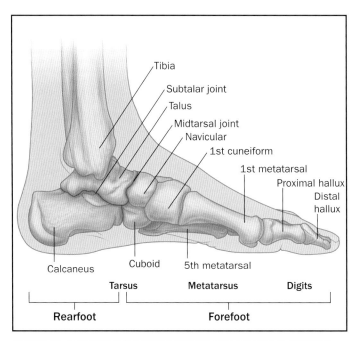

FIGURE 19-2. Diagram of foot showing anatomic parts important in locomotion.

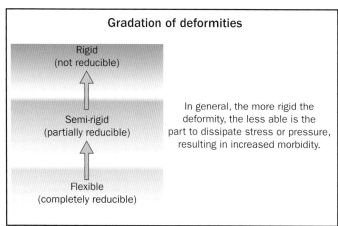

FIGURE 19-3. Gradation of acquired deformities.

deforming forces. These deforming forces, inflicted thousands of times per day over a period of time, traumatize the nail and nail tissue and cause damage and distortion.

Abnormal biomechanics of the limb resulting in abnormal timing mechanisms may be due to ligamentous laxity and to congenital and acquired deformities. Acquired deformities may be secondary to disease or abnormal development or to trauma, including that inflicted by shoes. In conclusion, therefore, abnormal biomechanics may produce deformities, and deformities may be responsible for abnormal biomechanics.

## Congenital Deformities

Congenital deformities (that are severe, untreated, or do not reduce on their own with maturity) such as bowlegs (tibia vara) or flat feet (pes valgus) may directly alter the function of the foot so that prolonged pronation occurs, increasing instability in the forefoot. As far as the toes go, certain angular deformities of the digits present at birth but not severe enough to need intervention may be destined to contribute to toenail disorders in adulthood.

## Acquired Deformities

Diseases such as poliomyelitis can cause talipes equinus, a deformity in which the foot is plantar flexed, forcing the patient to walk on the toes without touching the heel to the ground. The deformed foot resembles a horse's hoof. Limb length discrepancies resulting from diseases such as scoliosis may prematurely load the forefoot with the body weight, damaging the feet and nails. Specific disease processes such as arthritis, diabetes, or neuromuscular problems can also alter normal biomechanics, resulting in disturbances of the gait cycle.

Developmental problems such as inward or outward malpositions of the heel and forefoot can result in disruption of the pronation–supination sequence, leading to instability of the forefoot at propulsion.

Deformities such as hallux valgus, hallux rigidus, under- and overlapping toes, and contracted digits can result.

Shoes can be a factor in distorting normal biomechanics. The height of the heel, the shape and design of the last, the construction of the shoe itself (particularly the toe box), and the material used can place excessive pressure on the nail unit, resulting in nail problems.

Additionally, the flexibility of the resultant toe deformities is a factor in determining the severity of the nail unit disturbance, illustrated by the chart above (Fig. 19.3).

## DEFINITIONS OF COMMON DIGITAL DEFORMITIES

- Common bunion or hallux valgus (Fig. 19.4): This is a deviation of the great toe towards the second toe and the plantar surface of the toe is turned away from the midline of the body.

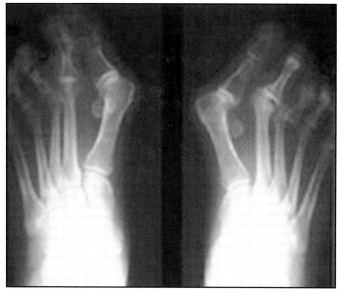

FIGURE 19-4. Radiograph of both feet demonstrating hallux valgus deformity.

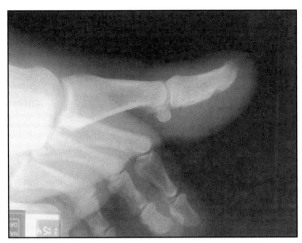

FIGURE 19-5. Early hallux limitus with mild extension of the interphalangeal joint. Note the presence of a sesamoid in the joint.

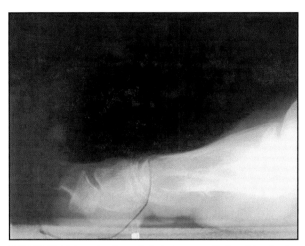

FIGURE 19-7. Lateral radiograph depicting severe flexion of the distal interphalangeal joint causing tip of nail unit to be traumatized.

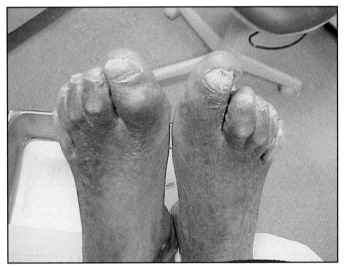

FIGURE 19-6. Patient with multiple semi-rigid hammertoes. Note mycotic nail changes whose causation may have been contributed to by constant trauma at the tips of the toes.

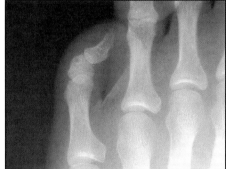

FIGURE 19-8. Radiograph depicting the underlapping 5th toe as well as the rotation of the distal phalanx, orienting the lateral nail fold plantarward and causing it to be weight bearing.

Table 19.1 outlines common congenital or acquired deformities and the nail disorders associated with them.

## THERAPY

### Biomechanical Therapy

The biomechanical factors that contribute to the faulty function of the foot should be assessed. Common assessment techniques include comprehensive static biomechanical examination, weight-bearing X-ray series, and visual gait analysis. Computerized gait analysis can contribute information to the decision-making process.

Once a proper assessment has been made, a functional orthotic device may be indicated (Fig. 19.9). A functional orthosis is a mechanical device made of various moldable materials and worn in a shoe to create more normal leg and foot motions. It captures the contour of the individual's foot in its anatomic neutral position, a position that is most efficient for a particular individual, and maintains this relationship. By effectively maintaining true osseous angular relationships, the orthosis permits more efficient locomotion by restoring the normal anatomic relationships of bones.

The continual deforming forces that help create hallux valgus, hammer toes, and underlapping and overlapping toes can be eliminated or reduced with proper treatment. Continuing a particular treatment and having patients wear proper shoes can actually prevent or eliminate the pathologic process.

- Hallux limitus/rigidus (Fig. 19.5): This is a loss of motion of the first metatarso-phalangeal joint, causing extension at the hallux interphalangeal joint.
- Contracted toes: There are three main types of digital contracture – hammer toe, mallet toe, and claw toe. The hammer toe (Fig. 19.6) is most common and is characterized by a flexion contracture at the proximal interphalangeal joint.
- The mallet toe (Fig. 19.7) is characterized by a flexion deformity at the distal inter-phalangeal joint.
- The claw toe is characterized by flexion deformity at both the proximal and distal inter-phalangeal joints.

Underlapping or overlapping toes may be congenital or may result from soft tissue disruption at the lesser metatarso-phalangeal or interphalangeal joints. The 5th toe is most commonly affected, and the underlapping or overlapping is usually accompanied by a rotational deformity as well (Fig. 19.8).

TABLE 19–1. Biomechanically induced onychial diseases and suggested therapy

| BIOMECHANICAL ABNORMALITY | RESULTANT ONYCHODYSTROPHY | THERAPY |
|---|---|---|
| Common bunion (hallux valgus) the hallux is shifted and rotated toward the 2nd toe | Hypertrophic nail – caused by abnormal pressure of the distal nail - of the hallux against the shoe | 1. Periodic reduction and debridement of the nail plate.<br>2. Change to a shoe with a high toe box<br>3. If severe hypertrophy, permanent removal of all or a portion of the nail plate |
| | Onychocryptosis – caused by the lateral nail margin of the hallux being pushed against the 2nd toe because of the abducted position of the hallux | Surgical removal of the offending portion of the nail plate and perhaps destruction of a portion of the nail matrix |
| | Subungual hematoma – caused by the shoe's pressure on the hallux nail, which overalps on the hallux nail, which overlaps the adjacent toe. | 1. Relief of pressure from the hematoma by cutting back the nail periodically<br>2. Surgical removal of the exostosis.<br>3. Change to a shoe with a high toe box. |
| | Long-term pressure might eventually cause subungual exostosis. Hypertrophic nail usually accompanies or is subsequent to hematoma | |
| | *Note*: All of these conditions generally improve with realignment of the hallux. Therefore, a comprehensive surgical procedure to realign the first metatarsal-hallucal mechanism or a functional orthotic device with or without the surgical procedure may be indicated | |
| Hallux rigidus – motion is lost in the first metatarsal phalangeal joint, excessive motion at the interphalangeal joint and a dorsiflexed position of the distal phalanx | Hypertrophic nail plate and subungual hyperkeratosis – caused by the distal phalanx and nail plate contacting the dorsal and distal surface of the toe box, resulting in recurrent microtrauma | 1. Periodic reduction of the nail<br>2. Permanent removal of the nail<br>3. Surgical procedure to reestablish motion in the first metatarsal phalangeal joint and use of an orthotic device to maintain proper function |
| Contracted toes (hammertoes) – the muscles that control the digits are shortened, resulting in a buckling of the toes | Subungual hyperkeratosis and hypertrophic lesser nail plate caused by the distal phalanx applying direct pressure into the sole of the shoe | 1. Periodic reduction of the nail plate and subungual tissue<br>2. Permanent removal of the offending nail plate<br>3. Sometimes a shoe with a longer and higher toe box will help, as will use of softer lining material<br>4. Surgical procedure to straighten the toe |
| Overlapping and underlapping toes – severe dislocation of a toe, resulting in toes resting on top of or below one another | Hypertrophic nail plate and subungual bleeding caused by pressure on the nail plate directly from the toe above or, in the case of an overlapping toe, pressure from the toe box of the shoe | 1. Periodic reduction of the nail plate and subungual hyperkeratosis<br>2. Permanent removal of the nail<br>3. Broad and deep toe box<br>4. Surgical procedure to realign the digits |
| Rotated toe – the 5th toe is rotated so that the individual walks on the lateral portion of the nail plate | Onychoclavus – pressure from the shoe continues to traumatize the nail bed, resulting in hypertrophy and eventual cornification and heloma development; most often found in the nail groove itself. *Note*: Might be associated with hallux valgus deformity | 1. Periodic debridement of cornified tissue<br>2. Change offending shoe if the problem persists<br>3. Surgical removal of the lateral nail plate, nail groove, and osseous condyle of the underlying area<br>4. Plastic surgery to derotate the 5th toe |
| Shoe-induced biomechanical abnormality – the shoe directly causes distorted growth of toenails | Onychogryphosis – pressure from the shoe encourages abnormal growth of toenails, tennis toe, pincer toenails | 1. Periodic reduction of the nail plate and subungual hyperkeratosis<br>2. Permanent removal of the nail<br>3. Sometimes a shoe with a longer and higher toe box will help, as will use of softer lining material |

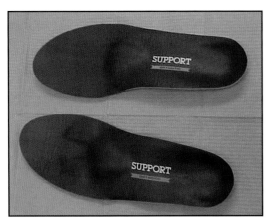

FIGURE 19–9. Example of orthotics.

## Minor Surgical Therapy

Minor surgery can sometimes reduce the signs and symptoms directly related to the nail condition. It may require the periodic reduction and debridement of the nail plate and subungual tissue. Total or partial removal of a nail plate may be necessary, either permanently or temporarily.

## Major Surgical Therapy

The objective of podiatric surgical procedures is to realign the malpositioned digits, restoring proper function and position. By placing a digit and its associated metatarsal in proper alignment before propulsion, the recurrent deforming forces are neutralized. Nail dystrophies often respond once the concomitant pressure is relieved. If there is permanent nail matrix damage, certain nail changes will not be affected by the surgical procedure. The surgeon must judge whether a specific nail condition may require an extensive surgical procedure.

In conclusion, the abnormal function of a foot in gait and its consequences can be the prime mechanism causing nail disorders. Recognizing the underlying factors and implementing the proper treatment plan can be very effective in restoring normal nail tissue.

## REFERENCES

1. Wernick J, Langer S. A practical manual for a basic approach to biomechanics. Deer Park, NY, Langer Acrylic Laboratory, 1972
2. Root M, Weed J, Orien W. Normal and abnormal function of the foot – clinical biomechanics, vol. 2. Los Angeles, Clinical Biomechanics Corporation, 1977

# 20 Nail Cosmetics: The Benefits and Pitfalls

Phoebe Rich and C Ralph Daniel III

## Key Features

1. Nail cosmetic materials can result in contact allergic or irritant reactions in a periungual location and at distant sites such as eyelids
2. Cutting or excessive manipulation of cuticles is not recommended because this practice sets the stage for paronychia and infections
3. When visiting nail salons, clients should bring their own instruments or be certain that the implements are adequately sterilized

## Rx ⊙ TREATMENT

- When allergic contact dermatitis is suspected, the cosmetic material should be removed and appropriate patch testing performed.
- Allergic reactions to acrylic artificial nail materials present as dermatitis in periungual location in contrast to allergic reaction to nail polish ingredients (TSFR), which occurs more commonly on the face, neck, and eyelids.
- Artificial nail use should be minimized in medical settings such as operating rooms.

The adornment and grooming of fingernails and toenails is an enormous industry, with over US$6 billion spent annually at nail salons in the US alone. The beneficial effects of nail cosmetics to beautify the nails are professed by millions of women. Uniform, smooth, glossy nails are highly desirable in our culture. Since earliest times, women have been adorning their nails and staining them with dyes and pigments to enhance their beauty. For many women, a biweekly trip to the nail salon is a beauty ritual as fixed as monthly hairdresser appointments. Manicures, pedicures, artificial nail extensions, and enhancements are the most popular nail salon rituals. Fortunately, most women have very few problems with nail cosmetics and salon services. Although the absolute rate of nail salon problems is difficult to calculate, the rate appears to be no higher than for hair salon problems of allergy and infections.

Many women use nail cosmetics to disguise and conceal nail imperfections and unsightly dystrophies. Lacquer-based nail enamel and ridge fillers help smooth the surface of ridges of aging, pitting, and onychorrhexis. Nail polish will cover splinter hemorrhages and discoloration from various sources, nail bed psoriasis, and onycholysis, although the latter may be worsened by the use of nail polish. Artificial nail enhancement can disguise nail shape abnormalities such as shortened thumbs (racquet nails) and nail plate surface irregularities and dystrophy. Acrylic nail overlays help people who habitually bite or pick at their nails and those with habit tic disorder by reminding the patient to avoid the bad habit of picking cuticles and manipulating the proximal nail fold.

Nail cosmetic use may or may not be helpful in the management of brittle, soft, splitting, or damaged nails. Whereas the dehydrating effect of nail polish removers can exacerbate brittle nails, a layer of nail polish can be helpful in strengthening and protecting fragile nails by providing an external shell that is flexible and durable. Polish may help hydrate the nail by sealing in moisture that would otherwise evaporate. It is most helpful in soft and weak nails because several layers of polish will add a protective veneer on the surface of the nail.

Problems of nail cosmetics are divided into those related to nail cosmetic ingredients and those related to the procedures, processes, and instruments that are used to beautify and groom fingernails and toenails.

## NAIL SALON PROCEDURES AND PROCESSES

The actual process of grooming and enhancing the appearance of the natural fingernails and toenails requires the use of multiple instruments and materials. The potential problems associated with nail care can occur in the professional nail salon as well as in the home as people perform these procedures themselves. The processes of manicure and pedicure follow logical sequential steps (Table 20.1). Implements, clippers, nail files, electric drills, and credo blades are some of the tools used by nail technicians in the processes of grooming and applying enhancements to the fingernails and toenails. These implements can injure delicate paronychial tissue and, if not properly cleaned, result in the spread of infectious agents.

## Potential Negative Effects of Nail Cosmetics and Salon Services

Although millions of women visit nail salons and use nail cosmetics with absolutely no adverse reactions or problems, there are potential problems that need to be recognized, diagnosed, and managed. Adverse outcomes can be related to the specific ingredients used in nail products or to the techniques and procedures performed in nail salons (Table 20.2).

## MATERIALS USED IN NAIL COSMETICS

Nail polish, also called nail enamel and nail lacquer, is the liquid that is brushed on the nail plate to add shine and color. Nail polish contains ingredients that make the product hard and strong (film former, nitrocellulose), improve adhesion (resins), flexibility (plasticizers), viscosity (solvents), colorants, and suspending agents.

**TABLE 20-1.** The steps and procedures used in manicures, pedicures and application of nail enhancements

## The process of a manicure and a pedicure

1. Nail polish, if present, is removed from nails with nail polish remover on saturated cotton ball
2. Nails are soaked in fingerbowl or footbath to soften the nail and cuticle
3. The nails are cleaned with a brush and sometimes an orange stick under the free edge of nail
4. Cuticle remover is applied and the cuticles are removed by nipping, pushing with nippers or metal cuticle pushers (nonendorsed step)
5. Stained nails are bleached with a solution of 6% hydrogen peroxide
6. The nails may be buffed at this point
7. Cuticle oil is applied and massaged into the cuticle
8. Nails are shaped and beveled by filing the undersurface of the free edge
9. The nail plate is cleaned to remove oil
10. Nail basecoat, nail polish and topcoat are applied and allowed to dry

## Process of applying plastic nail tips

1. Wash and buff nails to remove shine
2. Apply antiseptic dehydrator with a cotton tip orangewood stick
3. Apply adhesive (cyanoacrylate glue) to prepared nail plate
4. Apply the plastic tip and press for 5–10 seconds
5. Apply additional adhesive along the line where the plastic tip attaches to the nail plate for strength (not recommended due to skin contact)
6. Shape nails and apply desired finish

## Process for applying nail wrap

1. Initial steps same as for tips except small trimmed pieces of silk, linen or fiberglass fabric are glued to the nail plate Additional nail glue is applied over the surface and allowed to dry
2. Shape and finish nails as desired

## The process of acrylic nails

1. Nails prepared as above to accept the product
2. Nail forms, disposable or metal forms are positioned in the client's digit taking care to align the form in the natural arch of the nail
3. Primer is applied
4. Dip a small brush into liquid monomer and then into the powder polymer and rotate the brush to pick up a ball of powder
5. Apply this wet ball of product to the tip of the nail over the sculpture form. Repeat the application over the other parts of the nail and spread the material to the cuticle
6. Allow the material to harden, then smooth and shape with a file and polish as desired

## Process of acrylic nail fills

1. As the nail grows, a gap develops between the proximal portion of the acrylic nail and the nail folds. Filling this gap with more acrylic product is necessary every 2 weeks
2. Remove polish, clean nails, apply primer as above
3. File the proximal ridge in the acrylic nail to feather

## Process of photo bonded nail application

1 Prepare nails as above
2 Apply primer base to nail and harden by exposure to UV light
3 Apply building layer on top of the base later and polymerize by exposing to light
4 Apply top layer and expose to light again
5 Remove tacky residue film from surface of the nail with acetone or other solvent
6 Finish nails as desired

**TABLE 20–2. Types of nail cosmetic problems**

| PROBLEMS FROM NAIL COSMETIC INGREDIENTS | TYPE OF PROBLEM | SYMPTOMS | CAUSATIVE AGENTS |
|---|---|---|---|
| Nail polish | Contact allergy, contact irritant | Itching at distant site (face), onycholysis, paronychia | TSFR<br>Nickel beads solvents |
| | Yellow staining | Yellow nail plate | Dye in nail polish |
| | Fragility, granulation, brittle | White friable crumbling on the surface, fragility | Solvents, base coat, prolonged use of polish |
| Nail enhancements: acrylic sculptured nails, UV photobonded nails, silk or linen wrap | Allergic contact dermatitis | Itching, red, scaling around nails, onycholysis | Acrylates: methyl methacrylates, ethyl methacrylates, 2-hydroxyethylacrylate, (tri)ethylene glycol dimethacrylate, 5 ethyl cyanoacrylate, others |
| Nail hardeners | Irritant allergic | Burning , paresthesias, onycholysis | Formaldehyde |
| Cuticle remover | Irritant | Paronychia | Sodium, potassium hydroxide |
| **Problems from nail techniques and procedures** | | | |
| Traumatic injury | Cut, break in skin from sharp instruments | Cutting cuticle, pushing, prodding under free edge of nail | Sharp instruments<br>Poor technique, traumatic injury to cuticle |
| Infections | Skin infections, paronychia, subungual abscess, secondary infection of onycholysis and paronychia | Red tender inflamed skin, scaling, hyperkeratosis of nail bed | Bacteria – staphylococcus, streptococcus, pseudomonas<br>Fungus – candida, dermatophyte<br>Virus – HPV, HSV, others<br>Instrument transmission |
| Trauma and injury to the nail unit by drills and files | Thinning of the nail plate, cutting of paronychial tissue by electric drills | Thin weak nail plate.<br>Fissures, abrasions, around and under nail plate | Electric drills, files |

The major problem with allergy occurs with toluene sulfonamide formaldehyde resin, also called tosylamide resin. This ingredient is found primarily in salon polishes rather than the consumer-purchased brands.

Nail polish remover contains solvents that dissolve the nail polish, most often acetone and acetate. These solvents dehydrate the nail plate and overuse leads to onychoschizia and brittleness.[12]

Cuticle remover is a cream that contains sodium hydroxide or potassium hydroxide, which is intended to dissolve the keratin of the cuticle so it can be removed from the nail plate. Cuticle removers are irritants; moreover the cuticle is protective and should not be removed.

Nail enhancements and extensions are materials that are applied over natural nails or plastic tips glued to the natural nails to strengthen and lengthen nails. These are of three types:
1. Wraps, which consist of a piece of silk, linen or fiberglass that is glued on the nail with cyanoacrylate glue.
2. Sculptured nails, which are formed on the natural nail or plastic tip with a powder polymer and liquid monomer. The acrylic sculpting material is formed and extended past the free edge of the nail.
3. Photo-bonded acrylic gel products, which are applied as a thick gel and hardened under a UV light.

Most problems associated with nail cosmetic ingredients are due to contact irritant and allergic reactions. Allergic sensitization occurs when material comes in contact with skin and elicits a type IV hypersensitivity reaction. There may be itching or burning around the nails from acrylate monomer in nail enhancement, which may come in contact with the paronychial skin prior to the rapid polymerization of the product. The highly sensitizing methyl methacrylate (MMA) has been largely replaced by the ethyl methacrylate (EMA) and other acrylate compounds, which are less sensitizing. Ethyl methacrylates readily polymerize and rapidly react with multifunction methacrylates to form a highly cross-linked polymer. These cross-linked polymers are not reactive and, although EMA is a sensitizer, it is not a potent one. EMA monomer is short lived in the course of artificial fingernail application so the primary sensitization hazard occurs when the skin is inadvertently exposed to the non-reacted EMA monomer. Thus it is important to avoid contact with skin.[3] Kuppola et al. determined that the best screening allergen for nail enhancement acrylate allergy is ethyl methacrylate, to which 91% of patients in their series reacted.[4] Cyanoacrylate glue used to glue plastic tips and fabric on nails can cause allergic sensitization.[5]

Pruritic dermatitis on the eyelids, neck and face is sometimes seen in allergic contact dermatitis to nail cosmetic ingredients such as toluene sulfonamide formaldehyde resin (TSFR) in nail polish. The contact dermatitis associated with TSFR is usually on the neck, face, and eyelids as the nail polish continues to harden as the solvent slowly evaporates over 24–36 hours after application. Many ingredients, including acrylates, are used in nail extensions, and nickel beads are found in nail polish; these can result in potential allergic reactions (see Table 20.2, Figs 20.1 and 20.2).

Yellow staining of the nail can occur when nail polish is worn for a prolonged period, particularly deeply colored polishes (Fig. 20.3). Rough striations on the surface of the nail plate result in friability of the surface. **This appears as white surface striations and patches, which have been called keratin granulations by Baran[6]** (Fig. 20.4). This condition is similar in appearance to white superficial onychomycosis, in which there is superficial crumbling of the surface of the nail plate due to a dermatophyte.

Many nail cosmetic preparations act as contact irritants and can result in or exacerbate onycholysis (Fig. 20.5) and chronic paronychia. Avoiding these contact irritants by using gloves and avoiding known irritants as described by Daniel is crucial.[7]

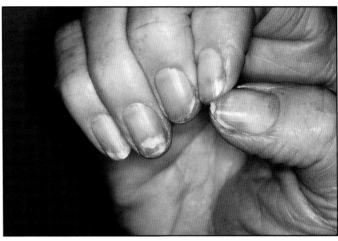

FIGURE 20-3. Yellow staining of the nail is often the result of wearing a deep-colored polish for a prolonged period.

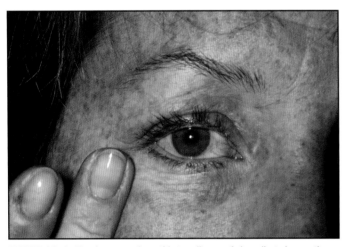

FIGURE 20-1. Allergic contact dermatitis to nail cosmetic ingredients is sometimes seen on the eyelids, neck, and face.

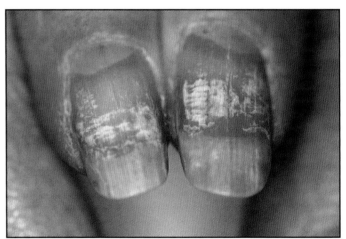

FIGURE 20-4. Keratin granulations – similar in appearance to white superficial onychomycosis.

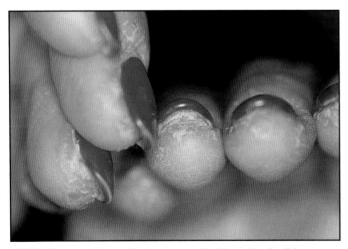

FIGURE 20-2. Acrylates in nail extensions and nickel beads in nail polish are among the ingredients that can cause allergic reactions.

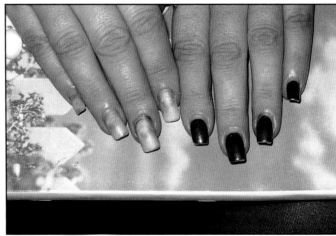

FIGURE 20-5. Nail cosmetic preparations can act as a contact irritant and can result in or exacerbate onycholysis.

# PROBLEMS ASSOCIATED WITH NAIL COSMETIC PROCEDURES AND TECHNIQUES

Traumatic and infectious nail salon incidents are related to breaks in the cutaneous barrier through which microorganisms gain access. The portal of entry may be induced by manicure procedures that cut or nip cuticle, shave callous, and probe around and under nail with sharp metal or wooden instruments, all practices that should be discouraged. These small breaches in the integrity of the skin around the nail become easily infected with staphylococcus or streptococcus, resulting in an acute paronychia or subungual abscess (Fig. 20.6). The incidence of infection rate is unknown but many anecdotal cases have been reported. Poor sanitation of implements in the salon is a factor in the spread of infection.

Nail enhancements that are excessively long can result in traumatic injuries to the nail bed. The strong shell of product on the nail surface prevents the bending or breaking of the nail when injured and results in traumatic separation of the nail bed and nail plate (Fig. 20.7).

Although the nail plate is dead, the practice of filing or even buffing the surface of the nail plate damages, thins, and weakens the nail. It is perfectly safe to file the free edge of the nail but the surface of the nail should not be filed. Excessive manipulation of the cuticle can cause punctate leukonychia in the nail plate (Fig. 20.8). By following the advice set out in Table 20.3, patients could avoid many of the problems associated with use of nail cosmetics.

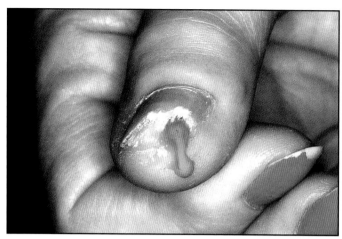

FIGURE 20-6. Breaks in the cutaneous barrier that become infected can result in a subungual abscess such as this one.

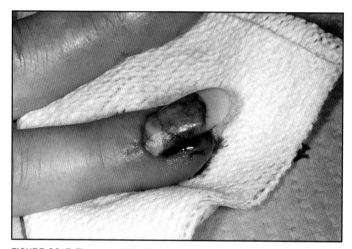

FIGURE 20-7. The strong shell of product on the surface of nail enhancements prevents the bending or breaking of the nail when injured and can result in traumatic separation of the nail bed and nail plate.

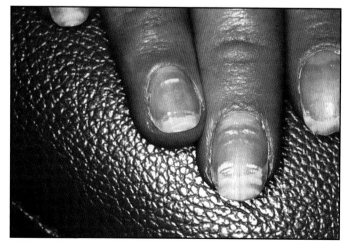

FIGURE 20-8. Punctate leukonychia, which can be caused by excessive manipulation of the cuticle.

**TABLE 20-3. Patient information on safe use of nail products in salons**

1. Be certain that your nail technician and nail salon are licensed
2. Wash hands before any nail salon services
3. Do not allow your cuticles to be cut. The cuticle seals and protects the nail and should remain intact
4. Ask about sanitization and sterilization in the salon. Look for cleanliness in the salon
5. Bring your own instruments, particularly files and other items that can not be sterilized
6. If you experience any itching or burning after a service, it could signal a reaction to an ingredient. Remove the product and see your doctor
7. Allergy to nail polish can show up on the face and eyelids and neck, whereas allergy to acrylic nails usually appears around the nails
8. Keep nail extensions short to minimize trauma
9. Do not allow the technician to file the surface of the nail plate in preparation for extensions and do not over-buff the nails, which will weaken them
10. Wear gloves for all wet work chores to protect the manicure and help prevent infections associated with artificial enhancements
11. If you experience a nick or cut during a salon procedure, seek medical attention to avoid infections

# CONTROVERSIES IN NAIL COSMETICS

## Nail Salon Safety and Infections

There are no data on the prevalence of infections following services in a nail salon. Although many salons take nail sanitation very seriously and practice careful techniques, there are still many salons that do not. When implements such as nail files and clippers are used on multiple clients without proper disinfection between clients, there is a real risk of spread of infectious particles from person to person. (Fig. 20.10). The risk of spread of infectious disease is increased significantly if the integrity of the skin is breached by practices such as cutting the cuticle, filing and shaving (credo blade) callous during pedicure, and the presence of skin disease such as eczema or chapping or trauma. Theoretically, infectious fungal, bacterial, or viral particles can be transmitted from client to client.[8]

Different US States vary significantly in the requirements for State licensure of technicians. Some require continuing education and specify the number of hours of training before taking a certifying exam. With over 250,000 salons in the US, it is difficult for State inspectors to police and standardize sanitation practices in salons. Staphylococcus, streptococcus, fungi, viral warts, and other pathogens can theoretically be transmitted by salon instruments and practices that do not follow adequate precautions.

A study of 120 nail salons in Ontario, Canada, concluded that infection-control procedures need to be established for nail salons.[9] In this study, almost all nail technicians reused most instruments, even if that was not the manufacturer's intent; ethyl alcohol was the most common disinfectant used. About 90% of the nail technicians were immunized against hepatitis B but none used gloves for procedures.

Two separate incidents of lower extremity furunculosis caused by rapidly growing mycobacteria that contaminated whirlpool footbaths used for pedicures have been reported. One salon in Watsonville, California, was found to have *Mycobacterium fortuitum* in footbaths after nearly 100 women had had pedicures at that salon.[10,11]

Inadequately cleaned instruments, inadequate skin disinfection, and lack of universal precautions in nail salons represent a disaster waiting to happen when blood-borne pathogens are present. Viral warts and dermatophyte spread are made possible by reuse of contaminated implements used for filing and cutting callous on the feet during a pedicure.

## How Safe is a Nail Salon as a Workplace?

Nail technicians spend long hours in their salon applying nail products to their clients' nails. Salons must follow National Institute for Occupational Safety and Health (NIOSH) and OSHA guidelines and have material safely data sheets (MSDS) for the materials that they use in the salon.[12]

Not all salons are well ventilated. Organic vapors (ethyl methacrylate, toluene, butyl acetate) and dust from filings of acrylics were measured from six salons and concentrations ranged from 0.4 to 15.6 parts per million. Health questionnaires from 20 nail technicians and 20 controls in the salons were questioned about symptoms experienced and the only statistically significant health effect noted was throat irritation. Also noted, but not statistically significant, were symptoms of dizziness, drowsiness, skin irritation, and trembling of hands.[13]

The neuropsychological performance of nail technicians who were exposed to neurotoxic organic solvents and methacrylate chemicals was evaluated. Cognitive and neurosensory effects of occupational exposure to these substances were evaluated by psychologic, neuropsychologic, and neurosensory tests. The results showed that nail technicians performed more poorly than controls on tests of attention and processing speeds. No significant differences were observed in memory, fine motor coordination, or depression. The researchers concluded that exposure to low-level neurotoxicants common in nail salons might result in mild cognitive and neurosensory changes that are similar to those observed among solvent-exposed workers in other settings.[14]

In 1990, six cases of physician-diagnosed occupational asthma in cosmetologists working with artificial fingernails prompted the Colorado Department of Health to request the assistance of NIOSH researchers in the evaluation and control of nail salon technician exposure. The Center for Disease Control and Prevention and NIOSH recommended the use of flood hoods and filters to minimize the exposure of technicians to toxic materials used in nail salons.[15]

A recent study has suggested concern about the plasticizer dibutyl phthalate in nail polish, which is teratogenic at high doses in rats.[16] Two cosmetic companies – Procter & Gamble and Estee Lauder – are removing dibutyl phthalate from their nail polish in the lines of Max Factor, Cover Girl, Clinique, and Mac.

## Should Nail Cosmetics and Enhancements be Banned in Healthcare Settings?

Numerous case reports support the potential hazards of artificial nails in the healthcare setting.[17,18,19] In some medical settings, artificial nails have harbored pathogens that led to surgical complications or infections.[20] This has led the Association of Operating Nurses to recommend that surgical personnel keep their nails short and unadorned.[18]

A recent report by Gupta et al. described an outbreak of *Klebsiella* infection in a neonatal intensive care unit (NICU). They found that the longer the stay in the NICU, and therefore the more contact with healthcare workers who wore artificial fingernails, the more significant the likelihood of developing infections. Their conclusion is that healthcare workers should avoid artificial fingernails.[21]

Three patients with postlaminectomy deep wound infections due to *Candida albicans* were linked to a single operating room technician who was scrubbed-in on all three cases. The infections were found to be caused by identical *Candida* (isolated by gel electrophoresis). The single operating room technician who scrubbed-in on these cases wore artificial fingernails during the 3-month period of the infected laminectomy cases and *C. albicans* was isolated from her throat.[21]

A case report from the Cornea Service, Wills Eye Hospital, Philadelphia, described a *Pseudomonas*-infected corneal ulceration related to an artificial fingernail injury. Presumably, the *Pseudomonas*-infected acrylic nail inoculated the corneal ulcer with the bacteria during an inadvertent abrasion of the eye.[23]

Although there are no universal mandates, most hospitals have policies regarding the use of nail cosmetics in the operating room.

# REFERENCES

1. Kechijian P. Nail polish removers. Are they harmful? Semin Dermatol 1991; 10:26
2. Scher RK. Cosmetics and ancillary preparation for the care of the nails. J Am Acad Dermatol 1982; 6:523
3. Cosmetic Ingredient Review Expert Panel. Amended final report on the safety assessment of ethyl methacrylate. Int J Toxicol 2002; 21 (Suppl 1):63–79
4. Koppula SV, Feldman, JH, Storrs, FJ. Screening allergens for acrylate allergy to artificial nails. Am J Contact Dermatitis 1995; 6:78
5. Kanerva L. Estlander T. Allergic onycholysis and paronychia caused by cyanoacrylate nail glue, but not by photobonded methacrylates nails. Eur J Dermatol 2000; 3:223–225
6. Baran R. Cosmetics: care and adornment of nails. In: Baran R, Maibach H, eds. London, Martin Duntz, 1994
7. Daniel CR, Daniel MP, Daniel J, et al. Managing simple chronic paronychia and onycholysis with ciclopirox 0.77% lotion and an irritant avoidance regimen. Cutis 2004; 73:81–85
8. Sekula SA. Nail salons can be risky business. Arch Dermatol 2002; 138 (3):414–415
9. Johnson, IL, Dwyer, JJ, Rusen ID, Shanin R. Survey of infection control procedures at manicure and pedicure establishments in North York. Can J Public Health 2001; 92 (2):134–137
10. Winthrop KL, Albridge K, South D, et al. The clinical management and outcome of nail salon-acquired *Mycobacterium forituium* skin infections. Clin Infect Dis 2004; 38 (1):38–44
11. Winthrop,KL Abrams M, Yakrus M, et al. An outbreak of furunculosis associated with footbaths at a nail salon. New Engl J Med 2002; 346 (18):1366–1371
12. Anonymous. Controlling chemical hazards during the application of artificial fingernails. National Insititue for Occupational Safety and Health (NIOSH), May 2001:509–511
13. Hiipakka D, Samimi B. Exposure of acrylic fingernail sculptors to organic vapors and methacrylate dusts. Am Ind Hyg Assoc 1987; 48 (33):230–237
14. LoSasso GL, Rapport, JL, Axelrod BN. Neuropsychological symptoms associated with low-level exposure to solvents and (meth)acrylates among nail technicians. Neuropsychiatr Neuropsychol Behav Neurol 2001; 14 (3):183–189
15. Spencer AB, Estill CF, McCammon JB et al. Control of ethyl methacrylate exposures during the application of artificial fingernails. Centers for Disease Control and Prevention/National Institute for Occupational Safety and Health, Cincinnati, OH 45226-1998, USA. Am Ind Hyg Assoc J 1997; 58 (3):214–218
16. Ema M, Kurosaka R, Amano H, Ogawa Y. Comparative developmental toxicity of *n*-butyl benzyl phthalate and di-*n*-butyl phthalate in rats. Arch Environ Contam Toxicol 1995; 2:223–228
17. Saiman L, Lerner A, Saal L. Banning artificial nails from health care settings. Am J Infect Control 2002; 30 (4):252–254
18. Beesley J. Artificial nails should not be worn in the operating room theatre. Br J Periop Nursing 2001; 8:336
19. Arrowsmith VA, Maunder JA, Sargent RJ, Taylor R. Removal of nail polish and finger rings to prevent surgical infection. Cochrane Database System Rev 2001; CD003325
20. Saiman L, Lerner A, Saal L, et al. Banning artificial nails from health care settings. Am J Infect Control 2002; 30 (4):252–254
21. Gupta A, Della-Latta P, Todd B, et al. Outbreak of extended-spectrum beta-lactamase-producing *Klebsiella pneumoniae* in a neonatal intensive care unit linked to artificial nails. Infect Control Hosp Epidemiol 2004; 3:210–215
22. Parry MF, Grant B, Yukna M, et al. Candida osteomyelitis and diskitis after spinal surgery: an outbreak that implicates artificial nail use. Clin Infect Dis 2001; 32 (3):352–357
23. Parker AV, Cohen EJ, Arentsen JJ. Pseudomonas corneal ulcers after artificial fingernail injuries. Am J Ophthalmol 1989; 107 (5):548–549

# 21 Pediatric Diseases

## Antonella Tosti and Bianca Maria Piraccini

### Key Features

1. Some nail diseases have a predilection for children
2. Nail abnormalities in children are frequently reversible but may be responsible for functional and aesthetic malformations
3. Several nail dystrophies are only of cosmetic importance but others may be important signs of systemic and genetic diseases

### Rx ● TREATMENT

- Not all diseases require treatment because of a spontaneous improvement with age
- Treat disorders in case of possible scarring

Nail growth rate in children is comparable to the values observed in young adults. The fastest values of nail growth (0.15 mm/day) are reached between the ages of 10 and 14 years.

At birth, the length of the fingernails is related to the newborn gestational age, with premature children often showing a short nail plate with a pseudo-anterior ingrowing appearance. The nails of premature infants also have a slower growth rate than those of at-term newborns.

The thickness and breadth of the nail plate increase rapidly from birth to the second year of life.

**It is important to trim the fingernails a few days after birth because they are sharp and might scratch the skin and the eyes.**

## NAIL DISORDERS IN CHILDREN

Nail disorders in children can be congenital or acquired. Table 21.1 lists nail disorders in children according to the most common age of onset.

### Anonychia/Micronychia[2]

Possible causes of partial or total absence of the nails are reported in Table 21.2.

Partial or total absence of the nail plate can be a consequence of teratogens taken during pregnancy. Drugs that most frequently cause nail hypoplasia include anticonvulsants and warfarin.

*Nail–patella syndrome* is an autosomal dominant disorder due to mutations in the LMX1B gene, where nail abnormalities are associated with bone and renal disorders. The nails are absent or hypoplastic. Nail hypoplasia can be limited to the thumb or involve several or all fingers. The severity of the hypoplasia, which

| TABLE 21–1. Nail disorders according to possible age of onset | |
|---|---|
| Newborn-infant[1] | Anonychia/micronychia |
| | Genetic disorders: |
| |    epidermolysis bullosa |
| |    pachyonychia congenita |
| |    ectodermal dysplasias |
| |    dyskeratosis congenita |
| | Beau's lines/onychomadesis |
| | Koilonychia |
| | V-shaped ridging |
| | Periungual pigmentation |
| | Congenital malalignment |
| | Congenital hypertrophy of the lateral nail folds |
| | Distal nail embedding |
| | Fingernail ingrowing with pyogenic granuloma |
| | *Veillonella* infection |
| Children | Paronychia |
| | Herpetic whitlow |
| | Blistering distal dactilitis |
| | Nail biting |
| | Punctate leukonychia |
| | Total/subtotal leukonychia |
| | Ingrown toenails |
| | Parakeratosis pustolosa |
| | Trachyonychia |
| | Alopecia areata |
| | Lichen planus |
| | Psoriasis |
| | Onychomycosis |
| | Melanonychia |
| | Tumors: |
| |    warts |
| |    Koenen's tumors |
| |    subungual exostoses |
| |    pyogenic granulomas |
| |    hemangiomas |
| |    histiocytosis X |
| |    juvenile xanthogranuloma |

is more marked on the radial side of the digit, usually decreases from the 1st to the 5th fingernail (Fig. 21.1). A triangular-shaped lunula is also a feature. In children, about one-third of patients have only involvement of the thumbs and one-third of both thumbs and index. Toenails are affected in about 14% of cases.

TABLE 21-2. Causes of anonychia – micronychia

Amniotic bands
Dermolytic epidermolysis bullosa
DOOR syndrome (deafness-onycho-osteodystrophy-mental retardation)
Ectodermal dysplasias
Iso-Kikuchi syndrome
Isolated
Nail–patella syndrome
Teratogens (drugs, alcohol)

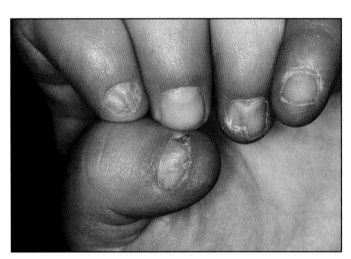

FIGURE 21-1. Nail patella syndrome: micronychia and koilonychia. The nail abnormalities are more severe on the thumb and index finger.

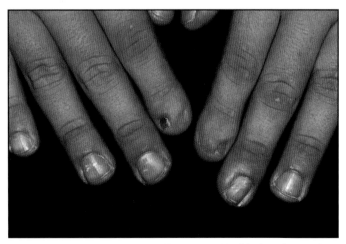

FIGURE 21-2. Iso-Kikuchi syndrome: Bilateral anonychia of the index finger and emionychogryphosis of the 3rd left finger.

The diagnosis is best confirmed by the presence of iliac horns at pelvis X-ray.

*Iso-Kikuchi syndrome* is also known as congenital onychodysplasia of the index finger. One or both index fingers show micronychia or absence of the nail. The hypoplastic nail plate is often thickened or deformed (emionychogryphosis) (Fig. 21.2). Other fingers may occasionally be involved.

At lateral projections, X-ray of the affected finger shows a typical Y-shaped bifurcation of the distal phalanx.

# GENETIC DISORDERS

## Epidermolysis Bullosa (EB)

### Key Features

* Nail abnormalities may be the first symptom of the disease
* Periungual/subungual blistering
* Nail thickening/shortening
* Pterygium/nail atrophy

This is a family of 23 genetic skin disorders. Nail involvement is frequent in all types of EB (Table 21.3).[3-5] Nail abnormalities may be the first or the only symptom of the disease. In fact, they may precede the development of skin blistering as in the 'late onset' junctional EB (JEB), or be an isolated finding as in some families with dominant dystrophic EB (DEB) or epidermolytic EB (EEB). Trauma undoubtedly contributes to nail dystrophy and, for this reason, the great toenails are often severely affected. The nail abnormalities are quite similar in all types of EB and their severity usually parallels the severity of the skin lesions.

### Clinical features

*Pachyonychia*: the nail plate is shortened, thickened and yellow in color (Fig. 21.3). Onycholysis and nail bed hemorrhages are frequently associated (Fig. 21.4). The nail abnormalities may affect several nails or be limited to the great toenails. In fingernails, pachyonychia is often associated with pincer nail deformity (EEB, DEB, JEB).

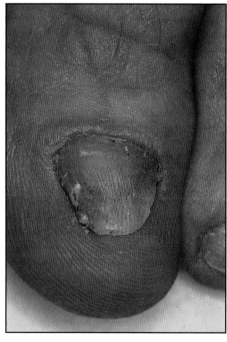

FIGURE 21-3. Pachyonychia of the great toenail in a patient with Dowling–Meara epidermolytic epidermolysis bullosa.

TABLE 21–3. Classification of epidermolysis bullosa

| TYPES | SUBTYPES | FREQUENCY OF NAIL INVOLVEMENT | NAIL SIGNS |
|---|---|---|---|
| EEB (epidermolytic EB) | Weber–Cockayne; AD | 10–25% | Onychomadesis with normal regrowth, pachyonychia |
| | Koebner; AD | 50% | Onychomadesis with normal regrowth, pachyonychia |
| | Dowling-Meara; AD | >75% | Onychomadesis, pachyonychia, onychogryphosis, pincer nails |
| | With muscular dystrophy; AR | 50% | Onychomadesis, anonychia, pachyonychia |
| | Superficialis; AD* | >75% | |
| JEB (junctional EB) | Herlitz; AR | >75% | Pachyonychia, exuberant granulation tissue, anonychia |
| | Non-Herlitz; AR | >75% | Anonychia |
| | With pyloric atresia; AR* | | Nail thinning and atrophy |
| DEB (dermolytic EB) | Dominant dystrophic; AD | >75% | Onychomadesis, pachyonychia, onychogryphosis |
| | Hallopeau–Siemens; AR | >75% | Anonychia |
| | Non-Hallopeau–Siemens; AR | >75% | Anonychia |
| | Transient bullous dermolysis of the newborn; AD/AR* | 25–50% | Onychomadesis |
| | Inversa; AR* | >75% | Pachyonychia of the toenails |

AD, autosomal dominant; AR, autosomal recessive; * rare subtype

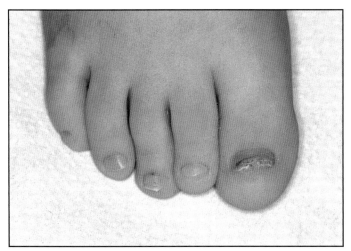

FIGURE 21–4. Pachyonychia and nail bed hemorrhages in a child with dominant dystrophic epidermolysis bullosa.

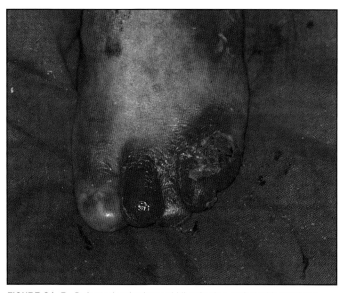

FIGURE 21–5. Periungual and subungual blistering in a patient with junctional epidermolysis bullosa.

*Onychogryphosis*: the nail is thickened, opaque, and yellow with an oyster-like appearance due to an exaggerated growth in the upward and lateral directions. The dystrophy is usually limited to the great toenails (EEB, JEB).

*Nail blistering* (Fig. 21.5): periungual or subungual bullae produce hemorrhagic onycholysis and hemorrhagic paronychia with onychomadesis. Nail shedding may be followed by regrowth of normal or dystrophic nails (EEB, JEB) or produce loss of the nails (JEB, DEB).

*Nail erosions with granular tissue* (Fig. 21.6): the nail plate is absent and the distal digit covered by granulation tissue producing a drumstick appearance of the digit (JEB).

*Nail atrophy*: the nail plate is very thin, brittle and short. Nail changes result from nail matrix damage due to repetitive blistering (DEB).

*Anonychia*: nail loss due to scarring is common in autosomic recessive DEB and fusion of the digits with a mitten-hand appearance is typical of the Hallopeau–Siemens subtype.

# Pachyonychia Congenita

## Key Features

* Thickened and extremely hard nails
* All digits involved
* Palmoplantar keratoderma

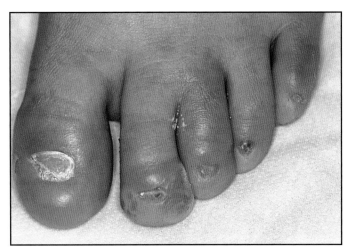

FIGURE 21-6. Nail loss and erosions in junctional epidermolysis bullosa (JEB).

**TABLE 21-5.** Causes of nail thickening

| DISEASE | CLUES FOR DIFFERENTIAL DIAGNOSIS |
|---|---|
| Chronic mucocutaneous candidiasis | Periungual inflammation |
| Ectodermal dysplasias | Short/hypoplastic nail plate |
| Epidermolysis bullosa | Hemorrhages/blisters |
| Pachyonychia congenital | Massive thickening/upward growth |
| Psoriasis | Pitting/salmon patches |
| Traumas | Hemorrhages/hematoma |

**TABLE 21-4.** Pachyonychia congenita subtypes

| TYPES | CLUE FOR DIAGNOSIS | MUTATION |
|---|---|---|
| Jadassohn–Lewandowsky | Palmoplantar keratoderma Follicular keratosis Oral leukokeratosis | Krt 6a/16 |
| Jackson–Lawler | Steatocystoma multiplex Hair abnormalities Hoarseness Natal teeth | Krt 6b/17 |
| Pachyonychia congenita tarda | Onset in adulthood | 2B helical domain Krt 16 |

# Ectodermal Dysplasias

## Key Features

* Presence of hair and/or teeth defects
* Nail thickening/shortening
* Nail hypoplasia

Nail abnormalities are a distinctive sign of ectodermal dysplasias and represent a criterion for classification of this condition (Table 21.6). In general, there are no clues for diagnosing any particular type of ectodermal dysplasias on the nail symptoms. The nail abnormalities can be distinguished into two main types: (1) the nails are small, short and present a thickened nail plate (Fig. 21.8), and (2) the nails are hypoplastic, thin, and fragile.

# Dyskeratosis Congenita

The nails show lichenoid changes with longitudinal ridging, splitting, and even pterygium formation.

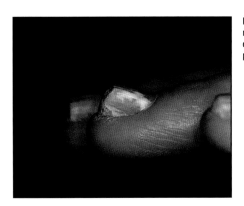

FIGURE 21-7. Massive nail thickening and over-curvature in a patient with pachyonychia congenita.

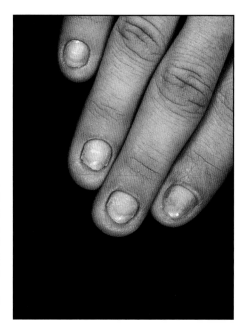

FIGURE 21-8. Hydrotic ectodermal dysplasia. The nails are short and thick.

Nail abnormalities are a constant feature of all types of pachyonychia congenita and develop during childhood (Table 21.4). All the 20 nails are thickened, very difficult to trim, darkened, and have an increased transverse curvature (Fig. 21.7). Nail thickening is a consequence of nail bed hyperkeratosis and is more evident on the distal half of the nails, which have an upward angling. The thumb and index finger are more severely affected. Development of nail thickening may be preceded by nail bed erythema.

Differential diagnosis includes other diseases that produce nail thickening (Table 21.5).

### TABLE 21-6. Ectodermal dysplasias

| TYPES | NAILS | ASSOCIATED DERMATOLOGICAL FEATURES |
|---|---|---|
| Hydrotic ectodermal dysplasia (Clouston syndrome); AD | Thick, short | Palmoplantar keratosis Alopecia |
| Hypohydrotic ectodermal dysplasia (Christ–Siemens-Touraine); XR | Thin, fragile | Alopecia |
| Ankyloblepharon–ectodermal defects–cleft lip and palate (AEC, Hay–Wells syndrome) (Rapp–Hodgkin syndrome); AD | Thin, brittle, hypoplasia | Cicatricial alopecia |
| Ectodactyly–ectodermal dysplasia–cleft lip and palate (EEC) | Small, thin, brittle | Sparse blond hair |

AD, autosomal dominant; XR, X-linked recessive

## Beau's Lines

### Key Features

* Transverse depressions
* Most often traumatic
* Involvement of multiple digits may indicate systemic causes

Beau's lines appear as transverse depressions of the nail plate surface, which migrate distally with the nail growth and indicate a temporary interruption of the mitotic activity of the proximal nail matrix.

In newborns, Beau's lines of most or all nails may be visible after the 4th week of life and are probably due to the stress of adapting to extrauterine life. **They are quite common, occurring in up to 25% of healthy newborns.**

In children, multiple Beau's lines may occur after exanthematic infections or other systemic diseases (Fig. 21.9). Beau's lines limited to 1 or few nails are usually due to mild traumas or to inflammatory periungual conditions (Table 21.7).

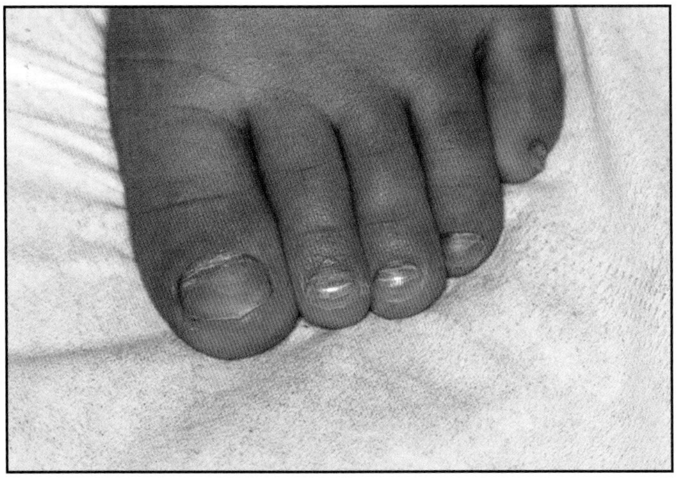

### TABLE 21-7. Causes of Beau's lines - onychomadesis

| MOST/ALL NAILS | FEW NAILS |
|---|---|
| Acrodermatitis enteropathica | Congenital malalignment |
| Drugs | Paronychia |
| High fever | Trauma |
| Kawasaki disease | |
| Mouth-hand-foot disease | |
| Measles | |
| Stevens–Johnson syndrome | |

## Onychomadesis (Nail Shedding)

### Key Features

* Proximal detachment of the nail
* Most often traumatic
* Involvement of multiple digits suggests systemic causes or strong contactants

It follows severe insults producing complete arrest of nail matrix activity. The nail plate detaches from the proximal nail fold with the formation of a transverse whole thickness sulcus.

Onychomadesis limited to one or a few digits is usually caused by traumatic or inflammatory disorders that affect the matrix. Involvement of most or all nails indicates systemic causes (Fig. 21.10 and see Table 21.7).

## Koilonychia (Spoon Nails)

### Key Features

* Thinned concave nails
* Physiological in children
* Toenail most commonly affected

FIGURE 21-9. Beau's line of toenails in child with Kawasaki disease

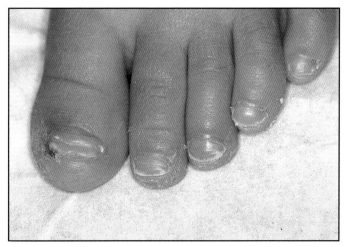

FIGURE 21–10. Onychomadesis of several toenails in mouth-hand-foot disease.

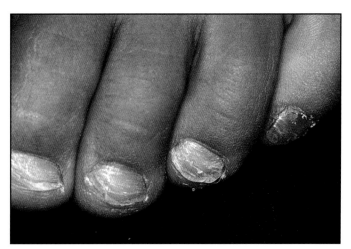

FIGURE 21–11. Koilonychia and onychoschizia of the toenails in an infant.

Transitory koilonychia is a physiological phenomenon in children, most commonly affecting the toenails, especially the great toe. The condition is caused by the fact that the nails of small children are thin and soft. The nail plate is flat and spoon shaped due to upward eversion of its lateral edges.

Marked brittleness with onychoschizia is often evident (Fig. 21.11). Lateral embedding may occur and produce transitory mild nail ingrowing. Koilonychia regresses spontaneously when the nails thicken with age.

## V-shaped Ridging (Chevron Nails; Herringbone Nails)[6]

### Key Features

* All fingernails affected
* Superficial longitudinal ridges that cross the nail plate surface diagonally
* Spontaneous improvement with age

Children's fingernails often show superficial longitudinal ridges that cross the nail plate surface diagonally from the lunula to the distal margin, forming a typical V-shaped pattern. The nail is otherwise normal. The condition often affects all the fingernails and regresses spontaneously with aging. It is possibly a consequence of incomplete formation of the central portion of the dorsal matrix.

## Periungual Pigmentation

### Key Features

* Light-brown to ochre pigmentation
* More evident between 2 and 6 months
* Declines before the age of 1 year

This is a prominent feature of dark skinned newborns but has recently been reported as a common transitory phenomenon in Caucasian people.[7] The dorsal aspect of the distal digit shows a light-brown to ochre pigmentation. The pigmentation is more evident between the ages of 2 and 6 months and declines before the age of 1 year.

## Congenital Malalignment Of The Great Toenail[8]

### Key Features

* Lateral deviation of the nail plate
* Often bilateral
* Nail ingrowing frequent

This common condition is characterized by lateral deviation of the nail plate with respect to the longitudinal axis of the distal phalanx. Congenital malalignment is possibly caused by an abnormality in the ligament that connects the matrix to the periosteum of the distal phalanx. The condition is often bilateral. The pressure caused by the lateral nail fold alters the growth of the nail plate. The affected nail is often thickened and transversally over-curved with onycholysis. Multiple Beau's lines and onychomadesis may occur as signs of nail matrix damage (Fig. 21.12). Congenital malalignment is often complicated by nail ingrowing that most commonly involves the external portion of the lateral nail fold.

The condition improves spontaneously in most cases, but may persist into adulthood.

## Congenital Hypertrophy Of The Lateral Nail Fold[9]

### Key Features

* Hypertrophic lateral nail fold
* Big toenail most commonly affected
* Newborns/infants

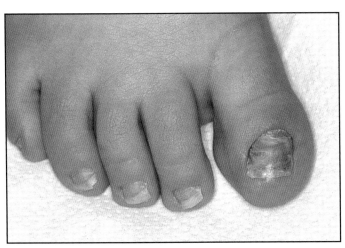

FIGURE 21–12. Onycholysis and onychomadesis in a child with congenital malalignment of the great toenail.

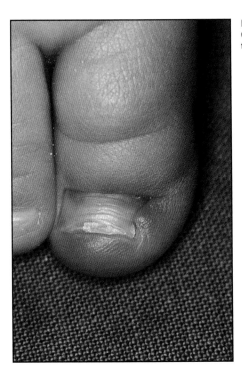

FIGURE 21–13. Congenital hypertrophy of the lateral nail fold.

This condition affects the hallux, often bilaterally, and usually appears at birth or shortly thereafter. The lateral nail fold is hypertrophic and forms a dome-shaped lip that partially covers the nail plate (Fig. 21.13).

Congenital hypertrophy of the lateral nail fold is usually asymptomatic but may be complicated by lateral ingrowing, which typically affects the medial side of the nail with acute inflammation and pain. Congenital malalignment and koilonychia may be associated. Congenital hypertrophy of the lateral nail fold usually improves with age.

## Rx ☉ TREATMENT

- Conservative with topical steroids and antibiotics in case of inflammation
- Surgical excision is usually not necessary

## Distal Nail Embedding

### Key Features

* Congenital hypertrophy of the distal pulp
* Resolves spontaneously in most cases

This results from a congenital hypertrophy of the distal pulp and usually becomes evident when the child starts wearing shoes. It resolves spontaneously in most cases.

## Fingernail Ingrowing with Pyogenic Granuloma

### Key Features

* Lateral ingrowing of several fingernails
* Consequence of the grasp reflex
* Disappears before the 4th month of age

Lateral ingrowing of several fingernails with paronychia and pyogenic granulomas is probably not rare in infants as a consequence of the grasp reflex.[10] Lateral ingrowing is caused by penetration of the lateral edge of the fingernail into the soft tissues that are easily penetrated due to bone immaturity. The lateral nail fold is inflamed and may show small pyogenic granulomas.

The condition regresses spontaneously when the grasp reflex disappears before the 4th month of age.

## Rx ☉ TREATMENT

- Topical antibiotics to prevent infections
- Give something soft to grasp to decrease pressure to the soft tissues

## *Veillonella* Infection

The Gram-negative *Veillonella* may cause subungual abscesses of one or several fingernails in newborns. Epidemics have occurred in special care baby units.

## Paronychia

*Acute paronychia*

### Key Features

* Bacteria are responsible for most cases
* Recurrences may suggest herpes simplex virus
* Compression of the nail fold may produce pus drainage

This is common in children and most frequently follows small traumas to the nails. Bacteria, such as *Staphylococcus aureus* and *Streptococcus pyogenes*, are responsible for most cases. The affected digit is swollen, red and painful (Fig. 21.14). Compression

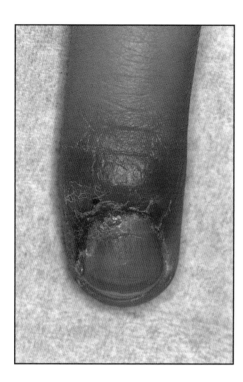

FIGURE 21-14. Acute paronychia.

colonize the proximal nail fold and contribute to inflammation. The affected digit shows mild inflammation and swelling of the proximal nail fold with loss of the cuticle.

## Rx ◑ TREATMENT

* Topical hydrocortisone and topical antifungals

## Herpetic Whitlow[11]

### Key Features

* Vesicular eruption
* Adenopathy and systemic symptoms can be associated
* Multiple digits can be involved

*Primary infection* with HSV 1 or HSV 2 can involve the finger and produce acute paronychia associated with a vesicular eruption. Adenopathy and systemic symptoms can be associated.

Most cases occur secondary to autoinfection with HSV gingivostomatitis. Thumb or finger sucking is a common mode of autoinfection in 1- to 3-year-old children. Multiple digits can be involved.

*Recurrent infections* are uncommon in children. The digit is painful and inflamed. Vesicles may be located in the nail bed and appear as an area of hemorrhagic onycholysis or be located in the ventral nail fold with acute paronychia.

Differential diagnosis with other vesiculopustular eruptions is reported in Table 21.8.

## Rx ◑ TREATMENT

* Oral acyclovir (<2 years: 100 mg 5 times a day for 5 days; >2 years: 200 mg 5 times a day for 5 days)

of the nail fold may produce pus drainage. Damage to the nail matrix is frequent with onychomadesis.

## Rx ◑ TREATMENT

* The abscess should be drained to avoid matrix compression.
* Systemic penicillinase-resistant antibiotics

### Chronic paronychia

### Key Features

* Frequent in finger sucking
* *Candida* species frequently colonize the proximal nail fold
* Absence of the cuticle and nail plate surface abnormalities

Chronic paronychia of the thumb is frequent in infants who suck their fingers. Paronychia is a consequence of maceration and irritation of the periungual tissues. *Candida* species frequently

## Blistering Distal Dactylitis[12]

### Key Features

* Group A β-hemolyic streptococci
* One or few fingers of children aged 2 to 16 years
* Painful blister with an erythematous base and a white purulent content in the distal volar pad

TABLE 21-8. Differential diagnosis of periungual vesico-bullous eruptions

| | BLISTERING DISTAL DACTYLITIS | IMPETIGO | HERPETIC WHITLOW | HALLOPEAU'S ACRODERMATITIS |
|---|---|---|---|---|
| Localization | Volar fat pad | Periungual tissues | Nail bed or periungual tissues | Nail bed or periungual tissues |
| Lesion | One large deep blister | Multiple superficial blisters | Multiple vesicles | Multiple pustules |
| Culture | Usually group A β-hemolytic streptococci | Staphylococci | HSV 1 or 2 | Sterile |
| Frequency | Rare | Common | Uncommon | Exceptional |

This condition, which is usually caused by infection by group A *β-hemolytic streptococci*, typically affects one or a few fingers of children aged 2 to 16 years. The distal volar fat pad develops a large, tense, painful blister with an erythematous base and a purulent white content. Uncommonly the blister extends dorsally to the nail folds.

*Staphylococci* may also cause the condition and, occasionally, both *staphylococci* and group A *β-hemolytic streptococci* are cultured from the lesion. Involvement of multiple fingers is suggestive for a staphylococcal infection.

## Rx ◗ TREATMENT

- Drainage of the blister.
- Penicillinase-resistant antibiotics are the treatment of choice

## Nail Biting

### Key Features

* Cuticle absent/proximal nail fold inflamed
* Nail plate surface abnormalities
* Melanonychia

**Nail biting is common in children and is usually not associated with psychological problems. It occurs in up to 60% of children and 45% of teenagers.** Nail biting in infants is exceptional and may be a sign of congenital absence of pain or Lesch–Nyhan syndrome.

Nail biters may just bite the distal nail plate or, more often, also damage the cuticle and periungual skin (perionychophagia). In this case nail matrix damage and infections may occur.

The nails are short, show an irregular margin and the hyponychium is visible. Distal splinter hemorrhages may be present. Periungual warts, especially in the cuticular area, are frequent.

Longitudinal melanonychia due to activation of nail matrix melanocytes is common as well.

Apical root resorption is a possible complication of nail biting.

## Rx ◗ TREATMENT

- Application of distasteful nail solutions

## Punctate Leukonychia

### Key Features

* Small opaque white spots
* Most often traumatic
* Distal nail matrix damage

Punctate leukonychia is characterized by small, opaque, white spots on the nail plate; these move distally with nail growth. These spots result from the presence of foci of parakeratotic cells within the ventral portion of the nail plate, which loses its transparency. The condition is caused by repetitive mild traumas that disturb distal nail matrix keratinization. The nail plate surface is normal.

The white spots may disappear before reaching the distal edge of the nail plate, as parakeratotic keratinocytes can mature within it.

There is no relationship between punctate leukonychia and the presence of calcium or oligoelements in the nail plate.

## Total/Subtotal Leukonychia[13]

### Key Features

* Nails are partially or totally milky white
* The discoloration does not fade with compression
* Deafness may be associated in some families

The condition is evident at birth or during childhood and often occurs in families. The nails appear partially or totally milky white and koilonychia may be associated. The discoloration does not fade with compression. In most cases the white discoloration extends from the lunula to the distal third of the nail that looks normal (Fig. 21.15). In some cases the discoloration is less homogeneous and the nail shows transverse or longitudinal bands of normal pink-color. Deafness may be associated with leukonychia in some families.

## Ingrown Toenails (Onychocryptosis)

### Key Features

* Congenital malalignment often present
* Painful inflammation of the lateral fold
* Growth of granulation tissue

Lateral ingrowing often occurs as a complication of congenital malalignment of the big toenail in children and adolescents. The condition is usually precipitated by improper nail trimming and trauma. Hyperhidrosis and daily use of occlusive shoes probably facilitate distal nail splitting with formation of small sharp spicules. The penetration of these spicules into the lateral nail fold

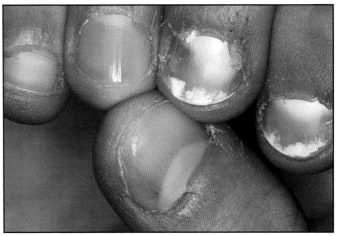

**FIGURE 21-15.** Subtotal leukonychia.

TABLE 21-9. Differential diagnosis of nail ingrowing

|  | HYPERTROPHY OF THE NAIL FOLD | CONGENITAL MALALIGNMENT | ONYCHOCRIPTOSIS | DISTAL NAIL EMBEDDING |
|---|---|---|---|---|
| Age | Infants | Infants | Adolescents | Infants |
| Site | Medial side of the great toenail | Lateral side of the great toenail | Medial or lateral sides | Distal pulp |
| Clue | Hypertrophy of the lateral nail fold | Lateral deviation of the nail plate | Inflammation; pyogenic granulomas of the lateral folds | Embedding of the nail margin in the distal pulp |
| Nail plate | Normal; koilonychia | Thickening; onycholysis; Beau's lines | Usually normal; irregular distal edges | Short; Beau's lines; koilonychia |

epithelium causes painful inflammation, growth of granulation tissue and nail fold hypertrophy.

Progression of the nail ingrowing can be divided into three stages:

- Stage I: Erythema, swelling and pain of the affected lateral nail fold.
- Stage II: Growth of granulation tissue (pyogenic granuloma) that emerges from the lateral nail fold. This is associated with pain and seropurulent exudation.
- Stage III: The embedded nail is surrounded by a hypertrophic nail fold that results from epithelialization of the granulation tissue.

Differential diagnosis of toenail abnormalities associated with nail ingrowing is based on age of onset, site of nail involvement and clinical features (Table 21.9).

## Rx TREATMENT

- First stage: Remove the embedded spicula. Topical antibiotics and podiatric care to avoid recurrences
- Second stage: Topical steroids and antibiotics to reduce the granulation tissue
- Third stage: Phenolization of the lateral horn of the matrix

# Parakeratosis Pustolosa[14]

## Key Features

* Exclusive of children, more common in females
* Usually limited to one digit, most commonly a finger
* Psoriasiform abnormalities
* Spontaneous regression with age

**Parakeratosis pustolosa is a nail condition exclusive of children and most frequently affects girls aged from 5 to 7 years.** The condition is usually limited to one digit, most commonly a finger, especially the thumb and the middle finger. The nail shows psoriasiform abnormalities with onycholysis and mild subungual hyperkeratosis (Fig. 21.16). The abnormalities are often more marked on one side of the nail. Mild pitting may be associated. The distal pulp may be normal or show mild erythema and scaling. Pustules are almost never seen.

**Parakeratosis pustolosa is a benign condition that usually regresses spontaneously when the child grows up.** Some children may develop a mild nail psoriasis afterwards. Differential diagnosis includes nail psoriasis and onychomycosis (Table 21.10).

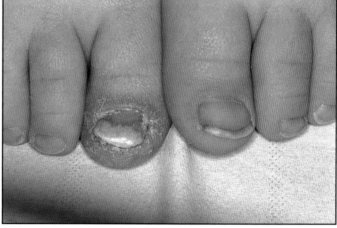

FIGURE 21-16. Parakeratosis pustolosa: Psoriasiform nail changes limited to the left big toe.

TABLE 21-10. Differential diagnosis of parakeratosis pustolosa

|  | PARAKERATOSIS PUSTOLOSA | PSORIASIS | ONYCHOMYCOSIS |
|---|---|---|---|
| Involved digit | One fingernail | Several fingers/toenails | One toenail |
| Prominent features | Onycholysis | Pitting | Hyperkeratosis |
| Frequency | Common | Uncommon | Rare |
| Associated skin lesions | Pulp scaling | Scalp/skin psoriasis | Tinea pedis |

## Rx ◑ TREATMENT

- Emollients and topical tretinoin 0.05%

# Trachyonychia (Twenty-nail dystrophy)[15]

## Key Features

* Nail roughness
* Several nails usually affected
* Benign course

Trachyonychia describes an abnormality of the nail plate surface that is rough due to excessive longitudinal ridging. The condition most commonly affects most or all nails and is idiopathic or associated with alopecia areata. Idiopathic trachyonychia is uncommon and almost exclusively seen in children.

Trachyonychia associated with alopecia areata occurs in up to 12% of children affected by the disease, especially those with alopecia totalis or alopecia universalis. This explains why the presence of trachyonychia is considered a negative prognostic factor in patients with alopecia areata.

The nails are thin, opaque and lusterless and give the impression of having been sandpapered in a longitudinal direction (vertically striated sandpapered nails; Fig. 21.17). Fragility of the superficial nail plate may be severe. Koilonychia is occasionally associated. Hyperkeratosis of the cuticle is often present.

A shiny, less severe, variety of trachyonychia results from a diffuse regular superficial pitting. Shiny trachyonychia is often associated with mottled erythema of the lunulae. In some patients opaque and shiny trachyonychia may coexist in different nails.

Idiopathic trachyonychia may be caused by lichen planus, psoriasis, and alopecia areata limited to the nails. In this last case the nail biopsy shows spongiotic changes of the nail epithelia.

Although trachyonychia has been reported in the literature in association with other diseases, such as ichthyosis vulgaris, vitiligo, atopic dermatitis, Down syndrome, selective IgA deficiency, and autoimmune disorders, this is only due to the fact that it often represents a symptom of alopecia areata, which can be limited to the nails for many years. The same applies for familiar and hereditary cases.

## Rx ◑ TREATMENT

- Trachyonychia is a benign condition that never causes nail scarring. The nail changes tend to regress spontaneously over the years. For this reason, trachyonychia does not need to be treated, especially in children
- Systemic or intralesional steroids improve the nail changes

# Alopecia Areata[16]

## Key Features

* Geometric pitting
* Trachyonychia

Up to 50% of children affected by alopecia areata (see p. 116) show nail abnormalities, which are more common and severe in alopecia totalis or alopecia universalis. Geometric pitting (Fig. 21.18) is typical as is trachyonychia. Beau's lines and onychomadesis may occur shortly after acute onset or relapse of hair loss.

# Lichen Planus[17]

## Key Features

* Nail thinning and fissuring
* Possible scarring outcome
* Biopsy mandatory for diagnosis

In children, nail lichen planus (see p. 112) is rare, but is more common than skin lichen planus. It is possibly underestimated due to reluctance to perform nail biopsies in children. It affects boys more frequently than girls and it is not usually associated with skin or mucosal signs of the disease.

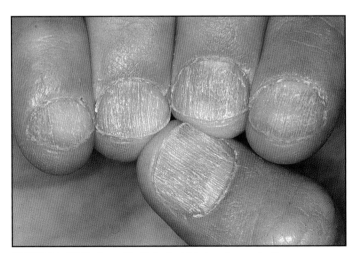

FIGURE 21–17. Trachyonychia: Vertically striated sandpapered nails.

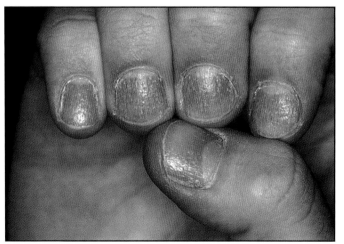

FIGURE 21–18. Geometric pitting in alopecia areata.

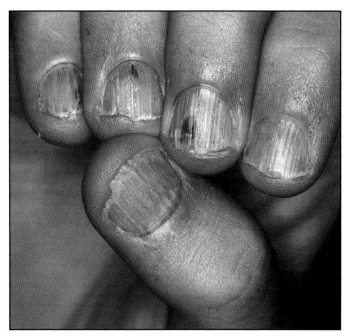

FIGURE 21-19. Typical nail lichen planus in a child. Note nail plate thinning, longitudinal fissuring and onycholysis.

Three different clinical presentations may be seen:

1. Typical nail lichen planus: The nail abnormalities are usually mild with nail thinning associated with longitudinal ridging and splitting. Nail bed involvement with distal onycholysis is often associated (Fig. 21.19). Severe onychorrhexis and pterygium are very rare.

2. Trachyonychia: The nail changes may be quite severe. The diagnosis of trachyonychia due to lichen planus cannot be made on a clinical basis but requires a nail biopsy. However, the benign course of trachyonychia makes this unnecessary.

3. Idiopathic atrophy of the nails: This is the rarest form of lichen planus, which occurs mostly in people of Asian descent. The nails are rapidly destroyed with or without pterygium formation (Fig. 21.20).

Autoimmune skin or systemic diseases are found in up to 30% of children with nail lichen planus.

## Rx TREATMENT

- Typical nail lichen planus: Systemic steroids (we use intramuscular triamcinolone acetonide 0.3-0.5 mg/kg/month)
- Trachyonychia: No treatment required
- Idiopathic atrophy of the nail: Treatment is useless because the nails are already destroyed

## Psoriasis

### Key Features

* Several nails affected
* Presence of large, deep and irregularly distributed pits
* Koebner phenomenon worsens nail symptoms

Nail involvement in children with psoriasis is less common than in adults, ranging from 7 to 39% in different studies. Psoriasis (see p. 105) limited to the nails is rare, as is pustular psoriasis.

Pitting is the most common symptom: pits are typically large, deep and irregularly distributed (Fig 21.21). Pits in the toenails, which are exceptional in adults, may occur. Toenails may also show onycholysis with erythematous border. Nail thickening due to subungual hyperkeratosis is uncommon.

## Rx TREATMENT

- Topical calcipotriol 0.005% cream, however, not consistently effective

## Onychomycosis

### Key Features

* Onychomycosis due to dermatophytes is extremely rare before the age of 6
* Tinea pedis is often associated
* *Candida* onychomycosis may occur in newborns and spontaneously resolve in a few months

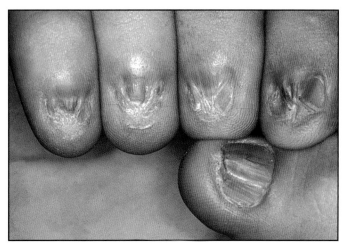

FIGURE 21-20. Idiopathic atrophy of the nails.

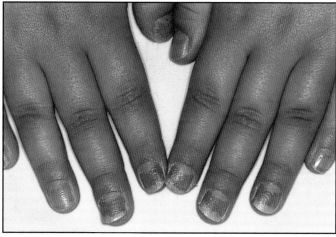

FIGURE 21-21. Nail psoriasis in a child.

### Dermatophytes

Onychomycosis due to dermatophytes is uncommon in children and extremely rare before the age of 6. Distal subungual onychomycosis (DSO) due to *T. rubrum* is the most common type and, as in adults, affects toenails more than fingernails (Fig. 21.22). White superficial onychomycosis (WSO) can be observed in prepubertal children, in whom it is due to *T. rubrum*. Clinically, it may look like a classical WSO or more frequently affect the nail plate more deeply and diffusely.[18] The nail is homogeneously white, opaque, and friable, resembling a proximal subungual onychomycosis (PSO) extending to the superficial nail plate. Involvement of the whole thickness of the nail plate depends on the fact that in children the nail plate is thin. Tinea pedis is often associated.

## Rx ◑ TREATMENT

- Terbinafine (weight <20 kg: 62.5 mg/day; weight 20–40 kg: 125 mg/day), 6 weeks for fingernails and 3 months for toenails
- Itraconazole (5 mg/kg/day as pulse treatment 1 week a month), 6 weeks for fingernails and 3 months for toenails

### Candida

Candidal onychomycosis may occur in healthy newborns and spontaneously resolve in a few months. Clinically the nails show an opaque milky white discoloration. Nail infection has been associated with contamination during delivery due to vaginal candidiasis of the mother.

Chronic mucocutaneous candidiasis (CMCC) often presents in childhood (Table 21.11). One or most nails may be affected with paronychia and nail plate crumbling and discoloration. Thickening of the periungual tissues produces a bulbous appearance of the fingers (Fig. 21.23). Differential diagnosis mainly involves psoriasis.

## Rx ◑ TREATMENT

- Itraconazole (200 mg/day as continuous treatment or 400 mg/day for 1 week a month) and fluconazole (50 mg/day or as pulse therapy at 300 mg/week) are effective in treating the nail changes, but recurrences are common. Duration of treatment is 6 weeks to 3 months

# Melanonychia[19-21]

### Key Features

* Most commonly due to a nail matrix nevus
* Pigmentation usually fades with age
* Nail melanoma is rare in children
* Dermoscopy is useful for diagnosis and follow-up

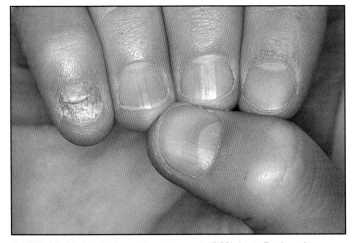

FIGURE 21–22. Distal subungual onychomycosis (DSO) due to *T. rubrum* in a child.

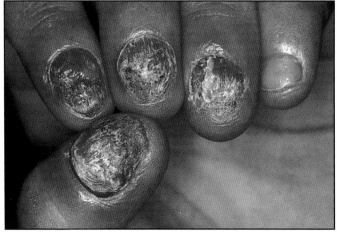

FIGURE 21–23. Chronic mucocutaneous candidiasis (CMCC): Severe nail thickening and crumbling associated with marked inflammation of the periungual tissues.

TABLE 21–11. Classification of chronic mucocutaneous candidiasis (CMCC)

| TYPE | INHERITANCE | CLINICAL/IMMUNOLOGICAL FEATURES |
|---|---|---|
| Without endocrinopathy | Recessive | Onset in childhood |
| With endocrinopathy | Recessive | Onset in childhood; endocrine diseases most frequently detected are hypoparathyroidism and hypoadrenalism |
| Without endocrinopathy | Dominant | Onset in childhood |
| With endocrinopathy | Dominant | Onset in childhood; associated with hypothyroidism |
| Sporadic CMCC | Unknown | Onset in childhood |
| CMCC with keratitis | Unknown | Onset in childhood; associated with keratitis |
| CMCC late onset | Unknown | Onset in adult life; associated with thymoma |

Melanonychia describes the presence of a longitudinally pigmented band of the nail plate that extends from the proximal nail fold to the distal margin. Longitudinal melanonychia is due to the presence of melanin within the nail plate and may be caused by activation or hyperplasia of the nail melanocytes, by nail matrix nevus or by nail matrix melanoma. The nail presents one or more longitudinal pigmented bands varying in color from light brown to black. The width of the band ranges from a few millimeters to the whole nail width (Fig. 21.24). Dark bands are often associated with pseudo-Hutchinson's sign, due to the fact that the dark nail plate pigmentation is visible through the transparent nail fold.

Almost all cases of longitudinal melanonychia in children are due to a nail matrix nevus.

Congenital nevi can also involve the nail folds and the hyponychium. The intensity of the pigmentation may vary in time and in children it is quite common to observe a gradual fading of the band. Fading of the pigmentation is not an indication of regression of the nevus. Thinning and fissuring of the pigmented nail plate may also occur. Pathologically, most of the nevi in children are junctional nevi. Dermoscopy shows a brown background and a regular pattern of the longitudinal lines, which are regular in thickness, spacing, coloration, and parallelism.

### Treatment

Management of longitudinal melanonychia in children is still discussed. Three possible options are the following:
- 'Wait and see': Nail melanoma in children is exceptional and excision of the band can be postponed to adolescence. Periodic follow-up with pictures and dermoscopy permits the detection of changes that may require intervention.
- Incisional biopsy is not considered a good approach because it does not allow examination of the whole lesion.
- Excisional biopsy is the treatment of choice for small bands that can be removed with a 3-mm punch. Excision of large nevi is associated with considerable morbidity and is not advisable as a routine approach.

## Tumors

### Key Features

- Tumors are rare in children, except for warts and pyogenic granulomas
- Think of tuberous sclerosis in case of periungual fibromas
- Surgical treatment is often necessary

*Periungual warts* are common in children and teenagers with a peak between the ages of 12 and 16 years. Nail biting facilitates occurrence and spreading of warts. Warts originate from the hyponychium or the proximal and lateral nail folds that possess a granular layer and may spread to invade the nail bed but not the matrix. They appear as hyperkeratotic papules on the proximal and lateral nail folds or as a diffuse hyperkeratosis of the cuticle. Subungual warts cause onycholysis that may sometimes have a linear pattern with splinter hemorrhages.

Warts often disappear spontaneously, especially in children. Differential diagnosis is reported in Table 21.12.

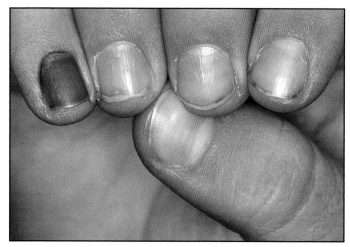

FIGURE 21–24. Melanonychia involving the whole nail in a 5-year-old child.

TABLE 21–12. Warts: clues for differential diagnosis

Bowen's disease – not reported in children
Fibrokeratoma – exceptional in children
Koenen's tumors – absence of hyperkeratosis
Onychopapilloma – not reported in children
Subungual exostosis – hard hyperkeratotic nodule. X-ray diagnostic

### Rx ◗ TREATMENT

- Aggressive approaches are unnecessary and may even cause enlargement of the wart
- Keratolytic agents are the best first-line treatment, especially for young children
- Topical immunotherapy with strong topical sensitizers (squaric acid dibutylesther or diphenylcyclopropenone) can be an option for multiple recalcitrant warts. The objective of treatment is to induce a mild contact dermatitis that causes wart regression through an immunological reaction[22]

*Koenen's tumors* (periungual fibromas) are rare in children. They should alert the suspicion of tuberous sclerosis and require a complete dermatological examination of the patient to detect other possible signs of the disease. Koenen's tumors occur in 50% of patients with tuberous sclerosis and usually develop after puberty. Fibromas may be single or multiple and the number of affected nails is variable. Periungual fibromas usually originate from the proximal nail fold and appear as a pink or flesh-colored growth. Compression of the nail matrix produces a longitudinal depression of the nail plate. Subungual filiform lesions may occur.

*Pyogenic granulomas* are common in children and usually follow a minor wound. They may occur in the lateral nail fold of nail biters. Possible causes of pyogenic granulomas in children are listed in Table 21.13.

*Subungual exostoses* are not uncommon in the big toe of teenagers, in whom they are frequently precipitated by traumas.

*Superficial hemangiomas* of the nails are very rare and usually become evident during the first year of life. Subungual location

**TABLE 21-13. Possible causes of pyogenic granulomas**

### Fingernails

Associated with lateral ingrowing in infants – grasp reflex
Associated with periungual wounds – nail biting
Associated with digital swelling – foreign body reaction
Associated with onychomadesis – mild peripheral nerve
    damage after cast wearing
Associated with nail erosions – epidermolysis bullosa

### Toenails

Associated with lateral ingrowing – stage II onychocryptosis

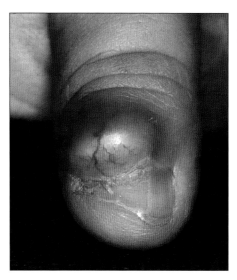

**FIGURE 21-26.**
Juvenile xanthogranuloma of the proximal nail fold.

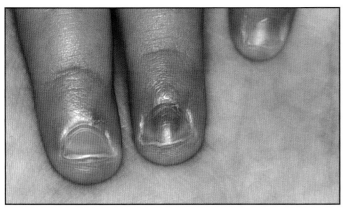

**FIGURE 21-25. Pseudoclubbing due to subungual superficial hemangioma.**

produces nail pseudoclubbing with a reddish discoloration (Fig. 21.25). Spontaneous regression occurs in a few years.[23]

*Hystiocytosis X.*[24] In Letterer–Siwe disease and in Hand–Schueller–Christian disease, nail involvement is common, with periungual and subungual pustules and hemorrhages. Paronychia with subungual purpura is highly suggestive for the diagnosis. Subungual lesions may destroy the overlying nail plate and, when localized in the nail matrix, may result in nail atrophy.

*Juvenile xanthogranuloma*[25] of the nail is rare and may be subungual and periungual. The nodular lesion has a typical yellow hue with teleangectasia (Fig. 21.26). Spontaneous regression is the rule.

## REFERENCES

1. Viseux V, Plantin P. L'ongle du nouveau-né et du nourrisson. Ann Dermatol Venereol 2003; 130:74–78
2. Rogers M. Nail manifestations of some important genetic disorders in children. Dermatologic Therapy 2002; 15:111–120
3. Fine JD, Eady RAJ, Bawer EA et al. Revised classification system for inherited epidermolysis bullosa: report of the second International Consensus Meeting on diagnosis and classification of epidermolysis bullosa. J Am Acad Dermatol 2000; 42:1051–1066
4. Bruckner-Tuderman L, Schnyder UW, Baran R. Nail changes in epidermolysis bullosa: clinical and pathogenetic considerations. Br J Dermatol 1995; 132:339–344
5. Tosti A, Piraccini BM, Scher RK. Isolated nail dystrophy suggestive of dominant dystrophic epidermolysis bullosa. Ped Dermatol 2003; 20:456–457
6. Zaiac MN, Glick BP, Zaias N. Chevron nail. J Am Acad Dermatol 1998; 38:773
7. Crespel E, Plantin P, Schoenlaub P et al. Hyperpigmentation of the distal phalanx in healthy caucasian neonates. Eur J Dermatol 2001; 11:120–121
8. Baran R, Bureau H, Sayag J. Congenital malalignment of the big toenail. Clin Exp Dermatol 1979; 4: 359–360

9. Piraccini BM, Parente G, Varotti E, Tosti A. Congenital hypertrophy of the lateral nail fold of the hallux: clinical features and follow up of seven cases. Pediatr Dermatol 2000; 17:348–351

10. Matsui T, Kidou M, Ono T. Infantile multiple ingrowing of the fingers induced by the grasp reflex - a new entity. Dermatology 2003; 205:25–27

11. Gill MJ, Arlette J, Buchan KA. Herpes simplex virus infections of the hand. J Am Acad Derm 1990; 22:111–116

12. Ney AC, English JC 3rd, Greer KE. Coexistent infections on a child's distal phalanx: blistering dactylitis and herpetic whitlow. Cutis 2002; 69:46–49

13. Bettoli V, Tosti A. Leukonychia totalis and partialis: a single family presenting a peculiar course of the disease. J Am Acad Dermatol 1986; 15:535

14. Tosti A, Peluso AM, Zucchelli V. Clinical features and long-term follow-up of 20 cases of parakeratosis pustulosa. Pediatr Dermatol 1998; 15:259–263

15. Tosti A, Piraccini BM. Twenty nail dystrophy. Curr Opin in Dermatol 1996; 3:83–86

16. Tosti A, Morelli R, Bardazzi F, Peluso AM. Prevalence of nail abnormalities in children with alopecia areata. Pediatr Dermatol 1994; 11:112–115

17. Tosti A, Piraccini BM, Cambiaghi S, Iorizzo M. Nail lichen planus in children: clinical features, response to treatment and long-term follow up. Arch Dermatol 2001; 137:1027–1032

18. Piraccini BM, Tosti A. White superficial onychomycosis: clinical and pathological study of 79 patients. Arch Dermatol, in press

19. Ronger S, Touzet S, Ligeron C, et al. Dermoscopic examination of nail pigmentation. Arch Dermatol 2002; 138:1327–1333

20. Goettmann-Bonvallot S, André J, Belaich S. Longitudinal melanonychia in children: a clinical and histopathologic study of 40 cases. J Am Acad Dermatol 1999; 41:17–22

21. Tosti A, Baran R, Piraccini BM, Cameli N, Fanti PA. Nail matrix nevi: a clinical and hystopathological study of 22 patients. J Am Acad Dermatol 1996; 34:765–771

22. Silverberg NB, Lim JK, Paller AS, Mancini AJ. Squaric acid immunotherapy for warts in children. J Am Acad Dermatol 2000; 42:803–808

23. Piraccini BM, Antonucci A, Neri I, Patrizi A, Tosti A. Congenital reddish pseudoclubbing of a fingernail due to subungual hemangioma. In press

24. deBerker D, Lever LR, Windebank K. Nail features in Langerhans' cell hystiocytosis. Br J Dermatol 1995; 130:523–527

25. Piraccini BM, Fanti PA, Iorizzo M, Tosti A. Juvenile xanthogranuloma of the proximal nail fold. Pediatr Dermatol 2003; 20:307–308

# 22 Nails In Older Individuals

## Philip R Cohen and Richard K Scher

### Key Features

1. Nail plate changes in the older patient include the following: Color, contour, histology, growth, surface, and thickness
2. Nail abnormalities in the older patient include: Brittle nails or problems due to faulty biomechanics and trauma
3. Infections include: Onychomycosis, bacterial infections, mycobacterial and spirochete infections, and mite and viral infections

Nail changes and nail disorders occur in older individuals, who comprise a large and rapidly growing segment of the population (Table 22.1).[1–4] As people age, the color, contour, histology, growth, surface, and/or thickness of their nail units may also change (Table 22.2).[3–11] In addition, acquired nail disorders in the older individuals may represent changes of the nail unit associated with aging and altered biomechanics, may be related to either concurrent dermatologic or systemic diseases and their treatments, or may be secondary to tumors of the nail and surrounding structures. Brittle nails, dystrophies secondary to faulty biomechanics and trauma, infections, onychauxis, onychoclavus, onychogryphosis, onychophosis, splinter hemorrhages, subungual hematomas, and subungual exostosis are some of the acquired nail

TABLE 22–1. Nail changes and nail disorders in older individuals

### Changes

Color
Contour
Histology
Linear growth
Surface
Thickness

### Disorders

Brittle nails
Faulty biomechanics and trauma
Infections
Onychauxis
Onychoclavus
Onychocryptosis
Onychogryphosis
Onychophosis
Splinter hemorrhages and subungual hematomas
Subungual exostosis

TABLE 22–2. Nail changes in older individuals

| CHARACTERISTIC | CHANGES |
|---|---|
| Color | Yellow to gray with a dull, opaque appearance |
| | 'Neapolitan' nails: nails with a loss of the lunula and a white proximal portion, a normal pink central band, and an opaque distal free edge |
| Contour | Increased transverse convexity |
| | Decreased longitudinal curvature |
| Histology | Nail plate keratinocytes: |
| | increased size |
| | increased number of pertinax bodies (keratinocyte nuclei remnants) |
| | Nail bed dermis: |
| | thickening of the blood vessels |
| | degeneration of elastic tissue |
| Linear growth | Decreases |
| Surface | Increased friability with splitting and fissuring |
| | Longitudinal furrows that are superficial (onychorrhexis) and deep (ridges) |
| Thickness | Variable: normal, increased, or decreased |

Republished with permission from Cohen PR, Scher RK. Geriatric nail disorders: diagnosis and treatment. J Am Acad Dermatol 1992; 26:521–531. Copyright 1992, Mosby-Year Book, Inc, St. Louis, Missouri.

disorders. The appropriate assessment and management of these onychologic concerns in older individuals is reviewed.

## NAIL CHANGES IN OLDER INDIVIDUALS

### Color

The color of the normal nail plate varies. The region of the nail plate overlying the lunula is white. The nail plate overlying the nail bed is pink. A slightly paler, pink–amber-tinged, onychodermal band is found on the nail plate overlying the area just prior to and including the hyponychium. Overlying the distal nail groove, the nail plate is white.

The color of the nail plate may change as individuals become older. The nails can be dull and opaque in appearance. Their color varies from shades of yellow to gray (Fig. 22.1). The lunula is often decreased in size or absent in older people.[12,13]

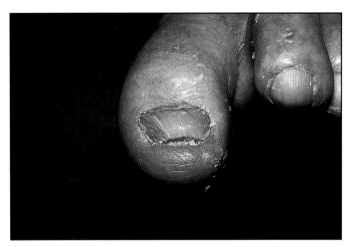

FIGURE 22-1. The great toenail of an 85-year-old man is yellow, thickened, and has an increased transverse convexity of the nail plate (republished with permission from Cohen PR. Nail dystrophies (photo quiz). Consultant 1998; 38:1995-2006)

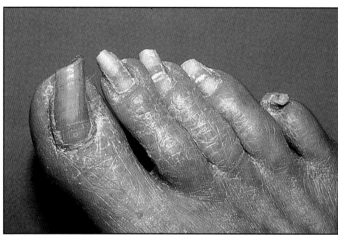

FIGURE 22-2. The transverse convexity of the great toenail is increased. The nail plate is yellow and thickened. Early changes of onychogryphosis are also present (republished with permission from Cohen PR, Scher RK. Nail changes in the elderly. Geriatric Dermatol 1993; 1:45-53. Copyright 1993, Hospital Publications, Inc, King of Prussia, Pennsylvania).

Horan et al. evaluated the fingernails and toenails of 258 individuals over the age of 70 years.[14] Loss of the lunula, a white appearance of the proximal portion of the nail, a more normal pink band, and an opaque free edge of the nail were observed in 19% of these patients. These nail changes were identical to those described by Lindsay[15] in patients with associated renal failure and similar to those observed by Terry[16] in patients with hepatic cirrhosis; however, none of the elderly individuals had evidence of renal or liver disease. Horan et al.[14] introduced the term 'Neopolitan nails' to describe these color changes of the nails in older individuals, because the three distinctive color bands on the nails were analogous to those of Neopolitan ice cream.

## Contour

The normal nail plate has a smooth surface and a double curvature: Longitudinal and transverse. However, in older individuals, the transverse convexity may increase and the longitudinal curvature may decrease (Fig. 22.2). In addition, nail plate flattening (platyonychia), nail plate spooning (koilonychia), 'ram's horn' deformity (onychogryphosis), and digit clubbing may develop as individuals age. Also, cutaneous or systemic diseases can result in modifications of the nail plate contour in older individuals (Fig. 22.3).[17-20]

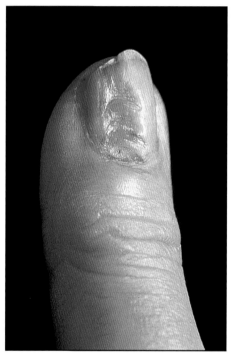

FIGURE 22-3. The normal fingernail contour is altered by focal mucinosis (a myxoid cyst) that presses against the proximal nail matrix and results in a groove in the nail plate (republished with permission from Cohen PR, Scher RK. Nail changes in the elderly. Geriatric Dermatol 1993; 1:45-53. Copyright 1993, Hospital Publications, Inc, King of Prussia, Pennsylvania).

## Histology

The nail unit consists of a cuticle, matrix, bed, hyponychium, plate, and surrounding proximal and lateral folds or perionychium. The distal skin on the dorsal digit forms the proximal nail fold. The cuticle extends from the proximal nail fold onto the nail plate. The nail matrix is present beneath the proximal nail fold and extends about 5 mm proximally. Melanocytes are present in the nail matrix: in greater number distally than proximally. However, neither the nail matrix nor the nail bed has a granular layer.

The nail matrix that extends distally beyond the proximal nail fold is clinically visualized as the lunula. The nail bed begins where the lunula ends. The nail bed extends distally to the hyponychium, which is located where the nail plate begins to separate from the underlying epithelium. The nail plate begins in the groove between the proximal nail fold and the matrix, continues over the entire nail bed, and ends slightly distal to the hyponychium. Normal ventral digital epidermis begins at the distal groove – a subtle depression that represents the end of the hyponychium.

Histologic changes in the nail plate and nail bed of older individuals have been described. There is thickening of the subungual blood vessels and alteration of the nail bed connective tissue characterized by degeneration of the elastic tissue. These changes in elastic tissue were most severe in the dermis beneath the pink nail bed, less marked beneath the lunula, and absent in the matrix area beneath the proximal nail fold. The alteration of elastic tissue in the nail bed is more pronounced than that observed in the adjacent paronychial skin. Diminished local blood supply may account for some of these changes.[21]

Nail plate keratinocyte morphology also changes with age: their size significantly increases as individuals became older. The number of pertinax bodies in the nail plate keratinocytes of older individuals also increases. These bodies, interpreted to be keratinocyte nuclei remnants, consist of perinuclear eosinophilic material and/or vacuolization.[22,23]

# Linear Growth

The linear nail growth rate varies among individuals and among digits. Normal fingernail growth can range from 1.8 mm to 4.5 mm per month; an average growth rate of the fingernails is 0.1 mm per day or 3.0 mm per month. Thus, it takes approximately 6 months for a fingernail to grow from the matrix to the free edge. Toenails grow at one-half to one-third the fingernail rate: 0.3 mm per day or 1.0 mm per month. Hence, it may take as long as 12 to 18 months for a toenail to grow from the cuticle to the distal free edge.[24]

In addition to aging, there are also many other factors that influence the linear nail growth rate (Table 22.3).[1,9,10,24] The rate of growth is proportional to the length of the digit and is more rapid on the dominant hand. Alterations in temperature, hormonal status, circulation, or activity can increase or decrease nail growth. Although certain dermatologic disorders that involve the nail unit may stimulate the growth rate, many systemic diseases or infections slow nail growth.

Aging tends to decrease the rate of linear nail growth. One study that evaluated thumbnails revealed that linear nail growth was most rapid in the first and second decades of life. The rate of nail growth subsequently decreased steadily thereafter.[11,25–27]

Another study measuring thumbnail growth in 257 individuals observed that the rate of linear nail growth increased not only during the first and second decades, but also well into the third decade of life. However, upon reaching the ninth decade of life, the linear nail growth rate had decreased by approximately 38% from the average linear growth rate of 0.9 mm per week during the third decade. Specifically, the linear nail growth rate decreased approximately 0.5% per year from 25 to 100 years of age. The rate of decrease was greater for women until the sixth decade and greater for men after the eighth decade; between the sixth and eighth decades, the rate of decreased nail growth was similar for both sexes.[28]

In a later study, the effect of aging on the rate of linear nail growth was evaluated in 171 people from 10 to 100 years of age. A multiple year biorhythm of nail growth rate was demonstrated. There were 7-year periods of slow decline of linear nail growth alternating with seven years periods of rapid decline.[10]

Individual investigators have also studied the linear nail growth rate on their own nails. During a 35-year period, Bean[11] observed that the average daily growth of his left thumbnail decreased from 0.123 mm a day at 32 years of age to 0.095 mm a day at 67 years of age. Similarly, Dawber[9] noticed a 10.4% decline in the rate of linear nail growth of his right index finger over a 12-year period.

In older individuals, decreasing linear nail growth can have important clinical significance. One setting where this may occur is the treatment of onychomycosis with systemic antifungals. In comparison to younger individuals with tinea unguium, the necessary duration of treatment in older patients is often much longer.[24]

---

**TABLE 22–3. Factors that influence linear nail growth rate**

## Factors increasing linear nail growth rate

Brittle nail syndrome
Daytime
Dominant hand (handedness)
Epidermolytic hyperkeratosis
Hyperpituitarism
Hyperthyroidism
Increased blood supply (arteriovenous shunt)
Localized trauma (nail biting, piano playing or typing)
Longer digits (third digit)
Males
Medications[a]
Morgagni–Stewart–Morel syndrome
Onycholysis
Periungual inflammation
Pityriasis rubra pilaris
Pregnancy
Premenstrual
Psoriasis
Regeneration after avulsion
Summer
Warmer temperatures
Youth

## Factors decreasing linear nail growth rate

Acute infection (fever, measles, mumps, pneumonia)
Aging
Antimitotic drug therapy
Chronic systemic diseases
Colder temperatures
Congestive heart failure
Decreased circulation (atherosclerosis, peripheral vascular disease)
Females
Hypothyroidism
Immobilization or paralysis of the digit
Laceration
Lichen planus
Malnutrition
Medications[b]
Night-time
Onychomycosis
Peripheral neuropathy (denervation)
Relapsing polychondritis
Shorter digits (first and fifth digits)
Smoking
Yellow nail syndrome
Winter

[a]Benoxaprofen, biotin, calcium, cysteine, fluconazole, gelatin, itraconazole (pulse therapy), levodopa (L-dopa), methionine, oral contraceptives, retinoids, terbinafine, vitamin D.
[b]Chemotherapeutic agents, cyclosporin, gold slats, heparin, lithium, methotrexate, retinoids, sulfonamides, zidovudine (azidothymidine [AZT], retrovir).

## Surface

Nail plate friability, splitting, fissuring, and superficial longitudinal striations (onychorrhexis) frequently develop in older individuals (Fig. 22.4). Deeper longitudinal lines (ridging) also become more numerous and pronounced in the elderly and have been described as 'sausage-shaped' ridges or 'sausage-link' ridges (Fig. 22.5). These surface changes, reflecting the relative depth of the indented grooves and the prominence of their adjacent projection ridges, may be localized or diffuse.[29]

Onychorrhexis or longitudinal ridging, rarely a functional problem for the older individual, may become a source of cosmetic concern. Daily buffing of the nail plates is a practical and safe treatment. The buffing agent can be a powder, a paste, or a cream containing waxes for enhancing nail surface gloss and finely ground pumice (particles of kaolin, precipitated chalk, silica, stannic acid, and/or talc) as an abrasive. The buffing agent is applied to each nail plate. Subsequently, each nail plate is polished with a chamois-covered buffer until it shines.[30]

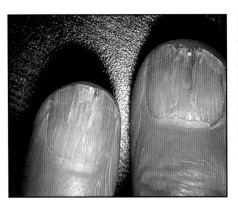

FIGURE 22–4. Friable nail plates with fissures, distal splitting, and superficial longitudinal striation (republished with permission from Cohen PR, Scher RK. Geriatric nail disorders: diagnosis and treatment. J Am Acad Dermatol 1992; 26:521–531. Copyright 1992, Mosby-Year Book, Inc, St. Louis, MO).

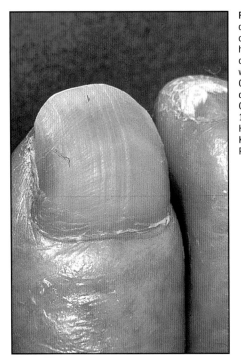

FIGURE 22–5. Multiple deep longitudinal ridges on a nail plate that also has increased longitudinal curvature (republished with permission from Cohen PR, Scher RK. Nail changes in the elderly. Geriatric Dermatol 1993; 1:45–53. Copyright 1993, Hospital Publications, Inc, King of Prussia, Pennsylvania).

## Thickness

The length of the nail matrix determines the thickness of the nail plate. The nail plate thickness varies with the sex of the individual and with each of the separate digits. The nail plate is approximately 0.6 mm thick in men and 0.5 mm thick in women. The nail plate of the thumb is the thickest and that of the little finger is the thinnest. For the remaining digits of the hand, the index finger is thicker than the middle finger, which is thicker than the ring finger.[3,4]

The thickness of the nail plate is normal, increased, or decreased in older individuals. One study found that the thickness of the left thumb nail increased rapidly during the first two decades of life and then more slowly thereafter; however, there was little change in the volume of nail growth per day as the patients aged because the increase in nail plate thickness counterbalanced the decrease in linear nail plate growth.[26] Another study observed a difference between the thickness of the fingernail plates and the toenail plates as a given individual ages: the fingernails often became soft and fragile whereas the toenails usually became thicker and harder.[18,31]

'Pachyonychia' refers to thickening of the entire nail plate, whereas 'onychauxis' describes localized nail plate hypertrophy. Pachyonychia and onychauxis can occur as idiopathic, age-associated, nail plate changes. However, they can also develop secondary to several conditions that may occur in older individuals.

Thickened nail plates may be cosmetically improved by daily buffing. Alternatively, the superficial surface of the thickened nail plate can be thinned mechanically by using an abrasive disc attached to an electric drill. Mechanical or chemical avulsion of the nails may be required when there is severe nail plate thickening (Table 22.4).[32–38] And, when it is necessary to prevent subsequent recurrences, concurrent destruction of the nail matrix may be performed.

## NAIL DISORDERS IN OLDER INDIVIDUALS

### Incidence

Nail abnormalities are frequently observed during the mucocutaneous examination of patients. Nail disorders that may occur in older individuals are summarized in Table 22.5. Although it is difficult to estimate the exact incidence of nail disorders in the elderly, some investigators have attempted to clarify the prevalence of onychodystrophy in this population.

A survey of skin problems and skin care regimens discovered that 12% of the 68 noninstitutionalized volunteers aged 50 to 91 years did not practice regular fingernail care. Only 34 of the 68 individuals cut their own toenails. Onychorrhexis (superficial longitudinal striations of the nail plate) was observed in 85% of these individuals.[5]

Foot problems in the elderly were evaluated in another study. The patients were aged 65 or older and encountered over a 3-year period in an outpatient foot clinic. Nail or skin problems were identified in 154 of 426 (36%) of these older individuals.[6]

Another study evaluated footwear in 274 consecutive elderly patients who were admitted to a geriatric medical unit during a 3-month period. Foot problems were identified in 106 patients. An associated nail disorder was present in 70% of these older individuals.[7]

**TABLE 22–4. Summary of chemical modalities for nail avulsion**

| REAGENT | COMMENTS |
|---|---|
| **Compound A:**<br>Urea 22.25%<br>Anhydrous lanolin 22.25%<br>White wax 5.50%<br>White petrolatum 50.00%<br>Total 100.00% | The normal skin was treated with tincture of benzoin and cloth adhesive tape. Compound A or B was generously applied to the nail plate; adhesive tape or plastic (vinyl) glove occluded the plastic film wrap that covered the ointment. The area was kept absolutely dry. |
| **Compound B:**<br>Urea 40.00%<br>Anhydrous lanolin 20.00%<br>White wax 5.00%<br>White petrolatum 35.00%<br>Total 100.00% | Results: (1) Average occlusion duration for successful avulsion was 9.4 days (range, 3-8) for Compound A and 7.2 days (range, 4-10) for Compound B. (2) Only the abnormal nail was affected[32] |
| Urea 40.00%<br>White beeswax (or paraffin) 5.00%<br>Anhydrous lanolin 20.00%<br>White petrolatum 25.00%<br>Silica gel type H 10.00%<br>Total 100.00% | New preparation used instead of Compounds A and B by the same investigators. Similar treatment protocol was used. After 7 days of occlusion, treated nail was removed without anesthesia followed by curettage of nail bed. Easily controlled, pinpoint bleeding occurred in 25% of patients[33] |
| Urea 20.00%<br>Salicylic acid 10.00%<br>Distilled water 15.00%<br>Aquaphor[a] 55.00%<br>Total 100.00% | Painless avulsion of nondystrophic nails occurred after a period of 2 weeks of occlusive application. This is a single detailed case report with reference to 3 additional patients whose nondystrophic nails were successfully treated[34] |
| Potassium iodide 50.00%<br>Anhydrous lanolin 45.50%<br>Iodochlorhydroxyquine 0.50%<br>Total 100.00% | 1500 onychomycotic finger- or toenails from 250 individuals were successfully removed by the patients themselves using this preparation[35] |
| Urea ointment 40.00%<br>Bifonazole cream 1.00% | Occlusive treatment was followed by antifungal cream alone. Mycologic cure rates of 60% to 90% were achieved[36–38] |

[a]Aquaphor contains 10% lanolin, 20% petrolatum, 30% mineral oil, and 40% water.

The prevalence of fingernail abnormalities was studied in randomly selected nondermatologic patients admitted to the departments of internal medicine and general surgery during a period of 2 years. The mean age of the 567 patients included was 73 years. White nails (apparent leukonychia), absence of lunula, and red lunula were the most common findings. Brittle nails, Terry nails, and subjective complaints of nail problems occurred more often in women than in men. Hematologic disease was found to be significantly associated with brittle nails and Terry nails; also gastrointestinal disease was noted to be significantly associated with onychocryptosis (pincer nails) and subjective complaints of nail problems.[13,39]

## Brittle Nails

Clinical features of brittle nails include excessive onychorrhexis (longitudinal ridging), onychoschizia (transverse splitting, lamellar separation, and/or horizontal layering) of the distal nail plate, trachyonychia (roughness) of the nail plate surface, and/or irregularity of the distal edge of the nail plate (Fig. 22.6). Individuals with brittle nails are unable to grow long nails because their nail plates are easily breakable, dry, soft, and weak. Also, their fragile and frayed nail plates tend to catch on things.

Brittle nails may be observed in older individuals. This might be because the nails of the elderly are drier than those of younger people and because of environmental factors due to the decelerated linear nail growth rate in older individuals. Approximately 20% of 1584 subjects in a recent study had brittle nails; specifically, brittle nails were present in 18 of 79 residents (23%) of an old people's home and 56 of the 161 individuals greater than 60 years of age (35%).[40]

In addition to aging, several endogenous and exogenous etiologies can cause impairment of either the nail plate or the nail matrix, with subsequent development of brittle nails. These include certain skin diseases and systemic disorders; for example, a recent study showed a significant association between brittle nails and hematologic disease.[13] Repetitive hydration and dehydration cycles, or evaporation of water in the nail plate, or excessive use of dehydrating agents (such as nail enamels and remover, and cuticle removers) can result in brittle nails. The normal water content of

**TABLE 22–5. Nail disorders in older individuals**

## Brittle nails

Clinical: excessive longitudinal ridging, horizontal layering (lamellar separation) of the distal nail plate, roughness (trachyonychia) of the nail plate surface, and/or irregularity of the distal edge of the nail plate

Therapy: eliminate exacerbating factors and rehydrate the nail plate, cuticle, and surrounding nail folds. Oral biotin may be useful. Weekly applications of nail enamel may be helpful when preliminary measures are unsuccessful or in extreme cases

## Faulty biomechanics and traumatic-induced onychodystrophies

Clinical: presents as onychauxis, onychoclavus, onychocryptosis, onychogryphosis, onychophosis, splinter hemorrhages, subungual exostoses, subungual hematoma, or subungual hyperkeratosis

Therapy: treatment of the underlying limb function and/or gait cycle abnormality, correction of the associated bony deformity, and/or use of a molded shoe or an orthotic insert

## Infections

Clinical: (1) onychomycosis (distal subungual, white superficial, proximal subungual, and *Candida*); (2) paronychia: (a) acute – the nail fold is red, tender, and contains pus; (b) chronic – the cuticle is absent and the nail fold is swollen and uncomfortable.

Treatment: (1) onychomycosis: (a) medical – topical or systemic antifungals; (b) surgical – nail avulsion; (2) paronychia: (a) acute – lancing, warm soaks, oral and/or topical antibiotics; (b) chronic – keeping the nail fold dry and applying topical antifungal and/or antiseptic agents; application of topical corticosteroids may also be helpful

## Onychauxis

Clinical: localized hypertrophy of the entire nail plate characterized by a hyperkeratotic, discolored, nontranslucent nail plate; subungual keratosis and debris are often present

Treatment: periodic partial or total debridement of the thickened nail plate: nail thinning using electric drills and burrs; nail avulsion chemically (40% urea paste) or surgically; and, if necessary, matricectomy chemically (phenol) or surgically

## Onychoclavus (subungual heloma, subungual corn)

Clinical: a sometimes painful, hyperkeratotic process that is most commonly located under the distal nail margin of the great toenail

Treatment: (1) removal of the lesion, and (2) prevention of recurrence by modifying the footwear and using protective pads or tube foam in order to eliminate the causative pressure

## Onychocryptosis (ingrown nail)

Clinical: the nail plate pierces the lateral nail fold and causes inflammation with or without accompanying granulation tissue, tenderness at rest, and pain on ambulation or with pressure to the digit

Treatment: (1) correcting predisposing factors and proper nail trimming, (2) elevation of the lateral nail border by placing a small wisp of cotton beneath the edge of the nail plate, (3) local care consisting of warm soaks and topical antibiotics, (4) surgical removal of the nail plate with or without partial or total ablation of the nail matrix, and/or (5) alternative modalities such as (a) liquid nitrogen spray cryotherapy or (b) an orthonyx technique using a stainless steel wire nail brace

## Onychogryphosis

Clinical: an exaggerated, oyster- or ram's horn-like, nail plate enlargement primarily only involving the great toenails

Treatment: (1) proper nail plate trimming and foot care by filing of the thickened nail plate using an electric drill and burr and removal of the subungual hyperkeratosis, and (2) nail avulsion with or without ablation of the nail matrix

## Onychophosis

Clinical: localized or diffuse hyperkeratotic tissue of varying degree that develops on the lateral or proximal nail folds, in the space between the nail folds and the nail plate, or even subungually

Treatment: (1) initially, debriding the hyperkeratotic tissue; (2) additional management may also include thinning of the nail plate, packing of the nail, or surgical intervention similar to that described for onychocryptosis

## Splinter hemorrhages

Clinical: idiopathic or trauma-induced lesions that are black in color and located in the middle or distal third of the nail

Treatment: avoidance of trauma

TABLE 22–5. (*Con'td*) Nail disorders in older individuals

## Subungual exostosis

Clinical: a benign tender bony proliferation, most commonly on the great toe, which usually produces hypertrophy of the entire nail
   bed such that the appearance of the nail is an 'inverted U' with incurvation of the medial and lateral aspects of the nail plate
Treatment: nail plate avulsion and aseptic removal of the excess bone

## Subungual hematomas

Clinical: (1) acute – recent hemorrhage may be red and painful; (2) chronic – older lesions with residual hematoma may appear
   dark blue and are usually non-tender
Treatment: (1) acute: (a) a roentgenogram if a fracture of the underlying phalanx is suspected, and (b) piercing the nail plate with
   either a needle or electric drill to relieve the underlying pressure; (2) chronic: if the patient cannot remember an associated
   traumatic incident, it may be necessary to rule out a pigmented lesion (melanoma) with microscopic evaluation of the nail plate
   and a biopsy specimen from the underlying nail matrix and/or nail bed

Republished with permission from Cohen PR, Scher RK. Nail changes in the elderly. Geriatric Dermatol 1993; 1:45–53. Copyright 1993, Hospital
Publications, Inc, King of Prussia, Pennsylvania.

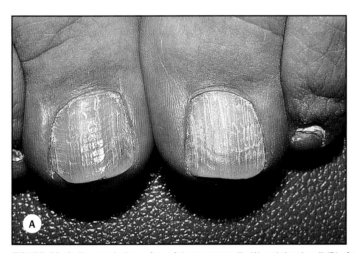 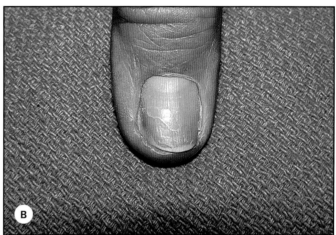

FIGURE 22–6. Changes in the surface of the great toenails (A) and thumb nail (B) of a 64-year-old woman with brittle nails. There is excessive longitudinal ridging (onychorrhexis), roughness (trachyonychia), and irregularity of the distal edge of the toenails (A). There is lamellar splitting of the distal nail plate (onychoschizia) of the thumb nail (B) (republished with permission from Cohen PR. Nail dystrophies (photo quiz). Consultant 1998; 38:1995–2006).

the nail plate is approximately 18% and varies between 10 and 30%. Brittle nails appear in dry environments, when the water content goes below 16%. In contrast, softness of the nail plate occurs in humid environments when the water content level of the nail plate is above 25%.[41,42]

The initial treatment of brittle nails involves the elimination of exogenous factors that may cause or exacerbate nail fragility. Hence, successful management of an existing brittle nail-associated systemic disorder may improve the onychodystrophy. When there is not a readily identifiable causative condition, precipitating habits and agents should be eliminated.

The next intervention for treating brittle nails is the inauguration of local measures to rehydrate the nail plate, cuticle, and surrounding nail folds. A moisturizer (such as 12% alpha hydroxy acid [lactic acid] lotion, mineral oil, phospholipid, or urea cream) should be applied after the nails have been soaked for 10 to 20 minutes in lukewarm water. Optimally, the moisturizing agent should be used under occlusion. For this purpose, light cotton glove liners or white cotton socks are excellent.

When preliminary measures for treating brittle nails are unsuccessful, or in extreme cases, the use of nail enamel may be helpful because it slows the evaporation of water from the nail plate. If a nail enamel is used, it should not be removed and reapplied more often than once a week. Although formaldehyde-containing lacquers may be used for intractable cases, some individuals may develop an allergic contact dermatitis or onycholysis. Hence, the potential possibility of these adverse sequelae makes treatment with formaldehyde-containing lacquers less appealing.

Oral agents have also been used to treat brittle nails. Statistically significant improvement of brittle nails occurred in 47 women who were treated orally with 10 mL colloidal silicic acid (Silicol) once daily for 90 days.[43] Oral biotin, a water-soluble B-complex vitamin has also been demonstrated to be an effective agent for the management of brittle nails.[44] The recommended daily oral biotin dose is 2.5 mg for 3 to 6 months; treatment for an average of 2 months is necessary before clinical improvement is observed.[45,46]

# Faulty Biomechanics and Trauma

Acute trauma to the nail unit can result in onychodystrophy. These nail dystrophies include clubbing, koilonychia (following frostbite or thermal burns), leukonychia, longitudinal melanonychia striata (Fig. 22.7), onycholysis, ridging and splitting of the nail plate, splinter hemorrhages, and subungual hematomas (with or without a fracture of the underlying digit).[47–52] Depending on the etiology, the nail changes may be temporary or permanent.

Chronic trauma to the nail unit can result from faulty biomechanics. The normal gait cycle is composed of a stance phase (60%) and a swing phase (40%); the stance phase is divided into contact, midstance, and propulsion periods.[53,54] Disease, abnormal development, or trauma can alter the normal biomechanical function of the limb and/or the gait cycle. Some of the bony deformities that can result in a biomechanical abnormality are listed in Table 22.6. The onychodystrophies observed in elderly patients secondary to faulty ambulatory biomechanics are summarized in Table 22.7 (Fig. 22.8).

Shoe-induced biomechanical abnormalities secondary to incompatibility between the foot, its digits, and the shoe can also result in trauma to the toenails and subsequent onychodystrophy. Onychauxis and onychogryphosis may develop from the abnormal growth of the toenails secondary to pressure from the shoes. Subungual hematoma and subsequent onycholysis of that nail may occur in individuals who wear rigid platform shoes or footwear that is too short, because of the repeated trauma to the nail unit during walking. Onychocryptosis and onychoclavus of the 5th toe may also be caused by inappropriate, poorly fitting footwear. In addition, if the distal nail plate becomes worn down by continually rubbing against the inside of the shoe, elderly patients may mistakenly interpret that their toenails do not grow.

Treatment of onychodystrophy secondary to biomechanical abnormalities should be directed toward: (1) the underlying bony abnormality, and (2) the elderly patient's foot care and footwear. Visual and arthritic difficulties are not uncommon in older individuals. These patients might not only have difficulty seeing their shoelaces but may also be unable to bend over and reach the shoes or tie the laces. Footwear with Velcro closures could be used

| TABLE 22-6. Bony deformities of the foot which can result in biomechanical abnormality and subsequent nail dystrophy | |
|---|---|
| **BONY DEFORMITY** | **COMMENT** |
| Digiti flexus | Contracted or hammer toes, in which the toes buckle since the muscles controlling the digits are shortened |
| Hallux rigidus | The distal phalanx is dorsiflexed and there is excessive motion of the interphalangeal joint secondary to a loss of motion in the metatarsal phalangeal joint of the great toe |
| Hallux valgus | Shifting and rotation of the great toe toward the second toe |
| Overlapping and underlapping toes | |
| Rotated fifth toe | The digit is oriented such that the person ambulates on the lateral portion of the nail plate |

instead of laced shoes. A molded shoe or an orthotic insert that conforms to the shape of the foot is helpful in the nonsurgical management of bony deformities. These modalities can provide adequate shoe fit by comfortably accommodating the existing deformity, by relieving pressure from the deformed joints, and by evenly distributing that pressure over the foot. Soft athletics shoes or sneakers are a less expensive (and less optimal) footwear alternative for elderly patients with bony deformities of the feet.

Other causes of chronic trauma to the nail unit include self-induced habits such as onychotillomania. Onychotillomania is an uncommonly described disorder in which the patient picks off pieces of the nail plate, nail bed, and/or nail folds. One elderly woman claimed that she was 'merely dissecting and removing tissue which had been destroyed by "minute organisms"'.[55]

Patients with onychophagia bite the free edge of their nails. They develop short, irregular nails that grow faster than normal. Features that may accompany onychophagia include periungual verruca, 'hang nails' (in which small, superficial portions of skin have split away from the lateral nail folds), and recurrent paronychia. In addition, leukonychia striata has been observed in individuals after they have pushed back their cuticles.

The management of patients with onychotillomania and onychophagia can be challenging. Application of distasteful preparations (such as 1% clindamycin, quaternary ammonium derivatives or 4% quinine in petrolatum) onto the nail folds may be helpful to discourage nail biting and chewing. Occlusive dressings can also aid as an adjunctive measure. However, referral of these individuals for psychiatric counseling and treatment should be considered.[55,56]

Habit tic deformity is another self-induced habit that results in chronic trauma to the nail plate. This condition involves the thumbnails and develops after the individual, consciously or inadvertently, rubs the central portion of the proximal nail fold of the thumb with the ipsilateral index fingernail. This onychodystrophy can be unilateral or bilateral. It appears as central transverse Beau's lines of the thumbnail plate. Spontaneous

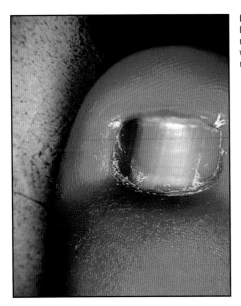

**FIGURE 22-7.** Longitudinal melanonychia striata that was caused by benign melanocytic hyperplasia.

**TABLE 22-7. Onychodystrophy secondary to faulty biomechanics**

### Onychauxis (nail plate hypertrophy)

Digiti flexus
Foot-to-shoe incompatibility
Hallux rigidus
Hallux valgus
Overlapping and underlapping toes

### Onychoclavus (subungual corn)

Digiti flexus
Foot-to-shoe incompatibility
Hallux valgus
Rotated fifth toes

### Onychocryptosis (ingrown toe nails)

Foot-to-shoe incompatibility
Hallux valgus

### Onychogryphosis

Foot-to-shoe incompatibility

### Subungual exostosis

Hallux rigidus
Hallux valgus

### Subungual hematoma

Foot-to-shoe incompatibility
Hallux rigidus
Hallux valgus
Overlapping and underlapping toes

### Subungual hyperkeratosis

Digiti flexus
Hallux rigidus
Rotated fifth toes

Modified and republished with permission from Cohen PR, Scher RK. Geriatric nail disorders: diagnosis and treatment. J Am Acad Dermatol 1992; 26:521–531. Copyright 1992, Mosby-Year Book, Inc, St. Louis, Missouri.

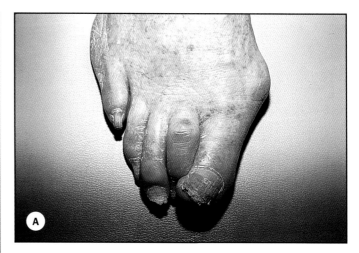

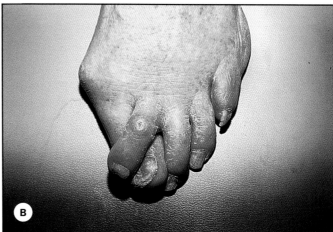

FIGURE 22-8. Above (A) and below (B) feet of a 75-year-old man with nail dystrophy of the great toenails secondary to bony deformities and resultant faulty ambulatory biomechanics. This patient's abnormal nails are caused by overlapping and underlapping toes (A and B), hallux valgus (the great toe is rotated and shifted toward the second toe) (A and B), and digiti flexus (buckling of the toe caused by shortening of the muscles that control the digit), also referred to as hammer toes or contracted toes (A) (republished with permission from Cohen PR. Nail dystrophies (photo quiz). Consultant 1998; 38:1995–2006).

resolution occurs if the patient stops injuring the corresponding nail matrix.[57]

Habit tic nail deformity should be distinguished from dystrophia unguium mediana canaliformis. Median nail dystrophy may occur on any fingernail but frequently involves those of the thumbs. It consists of an inverted fir-tree-like split or canal in the nail plate, which is slightly off-center. The nail plate dystrophy extends from the cuticle to the free edge of the nail.[58]

# Infections

## Onychomycosis

The nail structures may be the target of a primary infection or the innocent bystander secondarily involved in an infectious process localized to that area. Onychomycosis is more common in older individuals and frequently involves both toenails and fingernails. The diagnosis of onychomycosis may be confirmed by: (1) observing a fungal organism after a potassium hydroxide preparation has been performed, (2) culturing the organism from specimens taken (preferably) from the nail bed or (less optimally) from the nail plate, or (3) detecting fungi on (preferably periodic acid-Schiff stained) sections prepared from a biopsy specimen of the nail bed and nail plate.[25,59–61]

Many nail dystrophies clinically resemble onychomycosis. These include aging-associated nail changes, alopecia areata, chronic onycholysis, chronic paronychia, lichen planus, median nail dystrophy, pincer nail, onychogryphosis, psoriasis, subungual malignant melanoma, subungual squamous cell carcinoma, traumatic subungual hematoma, and yellow nail syndrome. Even in the presence of bonified onychomycosis, the potassium hydroxide preparation and the fungal culture may be negative. Therefore, a biopsy of the nail plate and underlying nail bed for histology, culture, or both may be necessary to definitively establish the presence of fungal organisms.[60,62]

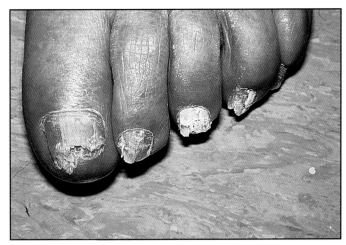

FIGURE 22–9. Distal subungual onychomycosis of the toenails from the left foot of a 94-year-old man. Tinea unguium-associated nail dystrophy includes nail plate discoloration, distal separation of the nail plate from the nail bed (onycholysis), distal nail plate splitting, and longitudinal ridges and furrows of the nail plate (republished with permission from Cohen PR. Nail infections (photo quiz) Consultant 1998; 38:2133–2147 and 2001; 41:805–817).

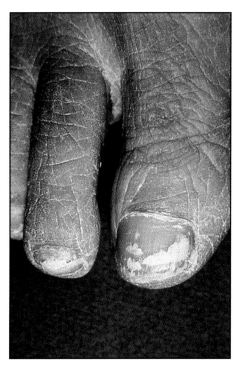

FIGURE 22–10. White superficial onychomycosis located on the surface of the toenails (republished with permission from Cohen PR, Scher RK. Geriatric nail disorders: diagnosis and treatment. J Am Acad Dermatol 1992; 26:521–531. Copyright 1992, Mosby-Year Book, Inc, St. Louis, MO).

An aging population is one of the factors that have contributed to the growing incidence of fungal nail infection. The fungal flora in 205 older individuals from Alexandria was evaluated. Onychomycosis was demonstrated in 64% of the people investigated: pathogenic yeast (10%), dermatophytes (3%), and saprophytic filamentous fungi (51%).[59,63]

Onychomycosis was also studied in 168 patients over 60 years of age who attended a chiropody clinic. Microscopic confirmation of tinea unguium was observed in 68 individuals (41%); however, the organism could not be cultured in 12% of these patients. Twenty of the remaining individuals (12%) were infected by dermatophytes and 42 (25%) were infected by molds.[64]

Onychomycosis has traditionally been divided into four types: (1) distal subungual onychomycosis (Fig. 22.9); (2) proximal subungual onychomycosis; (3) white superficial onychomycosis (Fig. 22.10); and (4) *Candida* onychomycosis. Two additional types of onychomycosis have recently been described: endonyx onychomycosis (in which neither nail bed hyperkeratosis nor onycholysis is present; fungal hyphae are present in the nail plate but not in the nail bed, and *Trichophyton soudanense* is the causative dermatophyte) and total dystrophic onychomysosis (which can either be a secondary manifestation representing the end stage of one of the other forms of onychomycosis or the primary manifestation in chronic mucocutaneous candidiasis). In addition, in the elderly, organisms previously considered to be saprophytic may also behave as nail pathogens: *Scytalidium dimidiatum* (previously called *Hendersonula toruloidea*), *Scytalidium hyalinum*, and *Scopulariopsis brevicaulis*.[25,65–67]

Distal subungual onychomycosis is the most common dermatophyte type. It is most often caused by *Trichophyton rubrum* and manifests clinically by subungual hyperkeratosis and uplifting of the nail plate (Fig. 22.11). In contrast, proximal subungual onychomycosis is the least common type of onychomycosis. In proximal subungual onychomycosis, the point of fungal entry is the proximal nail fold region and a white area extends distally from this site.[65–68]

White, superficial onychomycosis shows coalescing, opaque-to-white, islands of fungi on the surface of the toenails. *Trichophyton*

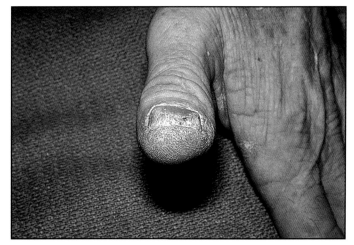

FIGURE 22–11. Distal subungual onychomycosis in an older man presenting as subungual hyperkeratosis of the left thumb nail (republished with permission from Cohen PR. Nail infections (photo quiz). Consultant 1998; 38:2133–2147 and 2001; 41:805–817).

*mentagrophytes* is usually the causative organism. Treatment merely requires scraping the fungi from the nail plate surface.[65–68]

There are several possible treatment alternatives for onychomycosis.[69] Topical therapy has minimal associated toxicity. As an individual therapeutic approach, topical treatments are helpful in containing fungal infections of the nail yet usually unable to cure onychomycosis. Topical agents are available in several galenical forms: creams, gels, lacquers, lotions, ointments, solutions, sprays, and tinctures.[68–74]

Once the decision has been made to treat fungal infection of the nail with a topically applied agent, the patient should apply the medication two to three times each day. Using topical antifungal medications under occlusion may help to expedite improvement.

The patient should be reevaluated approximately every 3 to 4 weeks. At each visit, the nail plate should be trimmed back and the underlying nail bed vigorously curetted. The anticipated duration of topical monotherapy for onychomycosis is typically prolonged (ranging from 6 to 12 months) – if not life long.[68,72–74]

Systemic therapies are often used to treat patients with onychomycosis. Treatment with griseofulvin and ketoconazole has been replaced by more effective and safer agents: terbinafine, itraconazole, and fluconazole. Fluconazole is most commonly dosed at 150 mg or 300 mg once weekly for 6 to 12 months for toenail dermatophyte infection.[68,74,75]

Itraconazole is a synthetic triazole. It exerts its antifungal activity by interfering with the synthesis of ergosterol (a component of fungal cell membranes). Itraconazole can be dosed daily or intermittently (pulse therapy). Daily treatment consists of 200 mg for 12 weeks in onychomycosis of the toenail and for 8 weeks in fingernail disease. Pulse therapy (200 mg twice daily for 1 week each month) is continued for 3 months in toenail tinea unguim and for 2 months in fingernail disease.[74,75]

Terbinafine is an allylamine. It inhibits squalene epoxidase; this results in both the inhibition of cell growth secondary to a deficiency of ergosterol and toxicity to the fungal cells secondary to the accumulation of squalene. Therapy consists of 250 mg daily; treatment duration is 6 weeks for fingernails and 12 weeks for toenails.[74,75]

Several reasons may preclude the use of systemic antifungals in elderly patients. The oral medications available for onychomycosis can have drug-associated adverse side effects – including potential interactions with other systemic drugs. Therefore, it is recommended to have a culture-confirmed diagnosis of onychomycosis prior to initiating therapy with these agents.

Nail avulsion may be a useful adjuvant therapy when the onychomycosis is limited to only one or two nails that are markedly dystrophic. Following removal of the infected nail, the course of antifungal therapy may be shortened, the duration of remission may be increased, and the opportunity to prevent recurrence of infection may be enhanced. In addition to dermatophyte nail infections, nail plate avulsion is also helpful in treating onychomycosis secondary to saprophytes.[69,76]

Nail avulsion may be performed nonsurgically (Table 22.4)[32–38] or surgically.[77] The advantages and disadvantages of using urea ointment for the chemical 'avulsion' of dystrophic nails are summarized in Table 22.8.[69] Surgical instruments or the carbon dioxide laser can be used for the surgical treatment of onychomycosis.[76]

## Bacterial infections

Inflammation of the nail folds may either be acute or chronic. Acute paronychia is erythematous, tender, and contains pus (Fig. 22.12). It is frequently caused by bacterial organisms such as *Staphylococcus aureus*. Occasionally, paronychia occurs in elderly individuals with protozoal (leishmaniasis) or viral infection (herpes simplex virus, orf, or cow pox) of the distal digit or who are receiving oral medications (such as retinoids, human immunodeficiency virus antiretrovirals, epidermal growth factor receptor inhibitors, ciclosporin, and certain chemotherapy agents). Initial treatment may require the lancing of a localized abscess. Oral antibiotics are often required. In addition, warm soaks to the area, followed by adequate drying and the application of an antibiotic such as 2% mupirocin ointment, can be used.[25,78–80]

| TABLE 22–8. Advantages and disadvantages of urea ointment for chemical nail avulsion |
| --- |

### Advantages

1. Nonsurgical method
2. Less expensive for the patient
3. Multiple abnormal nails can be treated in one session
4. Essentially a painless procedure
5. The procedure is without risk of hemorrhage or infection
6. The procedure is optimal for patients:
   with diabetes mellitus
   with vascular insufficiency
   with digital neuropathy
   receiving anticoagulants
   with immune suppression

### Disadvantages

1. Time consuming for the physician
2. Inconvenient to keep dressings absolutely dry for duration of occlusion (approximately 7 days)
3. Because commercial preparation is not available, the formulation must be compounded by a skilled pharmacist
4. The preparation has a 4 month to 6 month shelf life
5. Treatment failures secondary to:
   lack of gross nail dystrophy
   dressing inadequately occluded
   immersion of the dressing into water
   outdated urea preparation

Republished with permission from Cohen PR, Scher RK. Topical and surgical treatment of onychomycosis. J Am Acad Dermatol 1994; 31:S74–S77. Copyright 1994, Mosby-Year Book, Inc, St. Louis, Missouri.

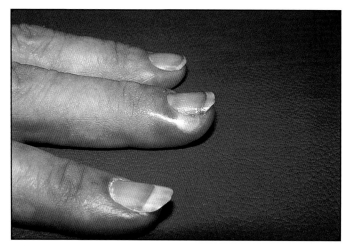

FIGURE 22–12. A painful erythematous pustule on the lateral nail fold of the right middle finger of an older woman with *Staphylococcus aureus*-associated acute paronychia (republished with permission from Cohen PR. Nail infections (photo quiz). Consultant 1998; 38:2133-2147 and 2001; 41:805-817).

Acute paronychia commonly only involves one nail. However, primary squamous cell carcinoma of the nail fold or a subungual metastasis from a primary visceral tumor can mimic an acute paronychia of a single nail. Alternative possibilities should be entertained when several nails are involved by what appears to be

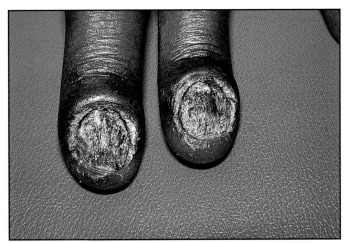

FIGURE 22–13. Chronic paronychia of the left third and fourth fingers of an older woman which resulted in hypertrophy of the proximal nail folds and total dystrophy of the nails (republished with permission from Cohen PR. Nail infections (photo quiz). Consultant 1998; 38:2133–2147 and 2001; 41:805–817).

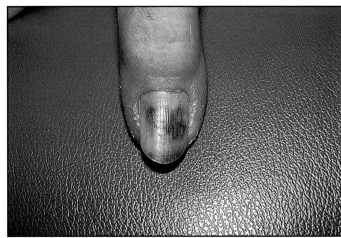

FIGURE 22–14. Green discoloration of the right thumb nail plate in an older woman whose onycholytic nail became colonized with *Pseudomonas aeruginosa* (republished with permission from Cohen PR. Nail infections (photo quiz). Consultant 1998; 38:2133–2147 and 2001; 41:805–817).

an acute paronychia. For example, subacute or chronic paronychial involvement of multiple nails secondary to one of chronic dermatitis, psoriasis vulgaris, or Reiter's disease can morphologically mimic an acute paronychia. In addition, chronic lymphocytic leukemia cutis involving eight fingers has masqueraded as chronic paronychia.[4,78,81]

Chronic paronychia appears as swollen, uncomfortable (but usually not painful) nail folds (Fig. 22.13). Often, there is a clear space that results from the loss of the cuticle and the creation of a patent proximal nail groove between the proximal nail fold and the nail plate. *Candida* species are commonly isolated from the proximal nail fold of patients with chronic paronychia. Occasionally, Gram-negative bacteria, such as *Proteus* or *Klebsiella* species, are also isolated. However, evidence continues to accumulate supporting the concept that chronic paronychia is an eczematous condition with a multifactorial etiology with secondary colonization by *Candida* or bacteria instead of a primary chronic fungal or bacterial infection. In comparison to acute paronychia, which rarely causes a nail plate deformity, multiple transverse ridges may be present secondary to repeated acute exacerbations in chronic paronychia.[25,78,82,83]

The optimal therapy for chronic paronychia is topical corticosteroid. It is also important to eliminate the predisposing cause or causes and to avoid exposure to contact allergens and irritants. In addition, avoiding nail trauma (by eliminating manipulation of the cuticle and nail fold), keeping the nails short, and wearing light cotton gloves under vinyl gloves when doing wet house work are helpful in the management of chronic paronychia. As the presence of *Candida* may contribute to the inflammation through a hypersensitivity mechanism, local or systemic antifungal treatment may enhance clinical improvement. Also, a topical antiseptic agent, such as 4% thymol in chloroform or alcohol, may be helpful to keep the area dry and free of bacteria and fungal colonization. If chronic hypertrophy of the proximal nail fold persists and is of significant concern to the patient, surgical removal is an alternative option.[25,78,82,83]

*Pseudomonas aeruginosa* may colonize nail plates that are onycholytic. The pyocyanin pigment of the bacteria provides the green discoloration of the nail plate (Fig. 22.14). After the onycholytic nail plate is cut away, local therapy is often successful.

For example, either an antiseptic or antibiotic such as 15% sulfacetamide, gentamicin, or chloramphenicol ophthalmic solution should be applied to the area three times a day.[3,4,25,84]

### Mycobacterial and spirochetal infections

Painful subungual abscess, paronychia, leukonychia, disappearing lunulae, pterygium, and traumatic dystrophy with nail plate thickening and ridging secondary to digital anesthesia have been observed in patients with leprosy who have *Mycobacteria leprae* infection that involves the nail.[85] Rarely, individuals with syphilis may present with nail lesions. Onychodystrophy observed in patients with this spirochetal infection includes clubbing, finger-tip chancre, fragility and thinning of the nail plate, koilonychia, loss of the nail plate substance only in the lunula area, onycholysis, and ulcerative paronychia.[86]

## Mite Infection

In older individuals with ordinary or crusted (Norwegian) scabies, subungual hyperkeratotic debris may harbor *Sarcoptes scabiei* (Fig. 22.15). Several reports have documented organisms in this location as the cause of persistent infestations or epidemics in the elderly and nursing home patients. Crusted scabies is more common in people who are not able to scratch, such as older individuals; in addition to subungual debris and hyperkeratosis, scabies-associated nail plate thickening and periungual plaques can be present (Fig. 22.16). Topical scabicides (such as 5% permethrin cream, 5–10% precipitated sulfur in petrolatum, 10% crotamiton cream or lotion, or 10–25% benzyl benzoate lotion) can be used to treat older individuals for scabies. However, it is important that the nail plates are cut short and that the fingertips be brushed with the scabicide. Scabies cures have also been demonstrated after one or two oral doses of 200 µg/kg of ivermectin, 1 to 2 weeks apart.[84,87–90]

## Viral Infections

Herpetic whitlow refers to a herpes simplex virus infection that involves the terminal digit and presents as painful inflammation of

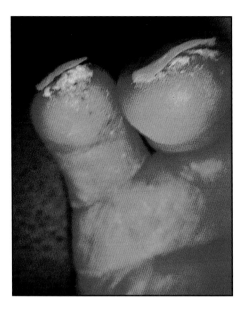

FIGURE 22-15. *Sarcoptes scabiei* mites were present in the subungual hyperkeratotic debris from this elderly patient living in a nursing home (republished with permission from Cohen PR, Scher RK. Geriatric nail disorders: diagnosis and treatment. J Am Acad Dermatol 1992; 26:521-531. Copyright 1992, Mosby-Year Book, Inc, St. Louis, MO).

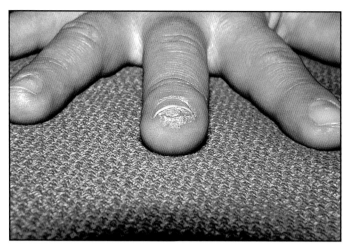

FIGURE 22-17. Subungual wart presenting as a hyperkeratotic lesion beneath the right middle finger distal nail plate (republished with permission from Cohen PR. Nail infections (photo quiz). Consultant 1998; 38:2133-2147 and 2001; 41:805-817).

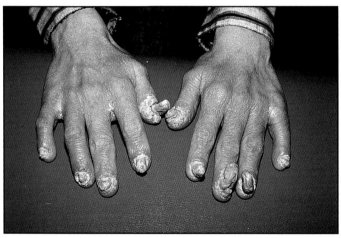

FIGURE 22-16. Nail plate thickening, subungual hyperkeratosis, and fissured plaques were observed on the distal digits of a man who had generalized pruritus and papulosquamous lesions on the remainder of his body. Skin scrapings taken from the periungual plaques contained *Sarcoptes scabiei* mites (republished with permission from Cohen PR. Nail infections (photo quiz). Consultant 1998; 38:2133-2147 and 2001; 41:805-817).

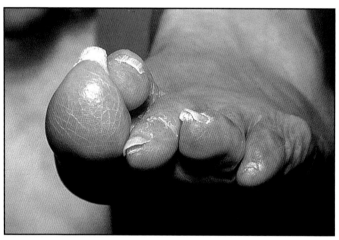

FIGURE 22-18. Localized hypertrophy of the nail plates of several digits (onychauxis) caused by faulty ambulatory biomechanics secondary to overlapping and underlapping of the toes (republished with permission from Cohen PR, Scher RK. Geriatric nail disorders: diagnosis and treatment. J Am Acad Dermatol 1992; 26:521-531. Copyright 1992, Mosby-Year Book, Inc, St. Louis, MO).

the proximal and lateral nail folds; in addition, verrucae can be subungual (Fig. 22.17). When the pustular lesion of an orf or cowpox infection occurs on the nail fold, an acute paronychia can also be mimicked. Human papillomavirus infections also involve the nail folds. Periungual warts are more common in children. However, they may be seen in elderly patients – especially those who are receiving immunosuppressive therapy. These lesions are often difficult to eradicate and may require more aggressive treatment modalities.[79,91,92]

## Onychauxis

Localized hypertrophy of the nail plate is referred to as onychauxis. When the entire nail plate is thickened, the term 'pachyonychia' is used. Onychauxis is characterized by hyperkeratotic, discolored

nails and by loss of translucency of the nail plate (Fig. 22.18). Subungual hyperkeratosis and debris are often also present.[3,93]

Elderly patients with onychauxis of one or two nails may be misdiagnosed as having tinea unguim because subungual hyperkeratosis is the most reliable sign for distal subungual onychomycosis. Therefore, in older individuals who present with onychauxis – especially when there is accompanying subungual hyperkeratosis – microscopic and/or culture confirmation of onychomycosis should be obtained prior to initiating antifungal therapy. When diagnosis of tinea is suspected and mycology is persistently negative, histologic evaluation of the nail plate (with or without the underlying nail bed) should be considered.[1]

Idiopathic onychauxis may be associated with aging; however, onychauxis can present as a component of several disorders that commonly occur in the geriatric population. Local complications of onychauxis include distal onycholysis, increased susceptibility to acquiring onychomycosis, and pain. Subungual ulceration and hemorrhage may also occur in elderly patients with onychauxis as a result of constant pressure of the hypertrophic nail on the underlying and surrounding tissues.[2]

Treatment for onychauxis involves periodic partial or total debridement of the thickened nail plate.[93] The nail plate can be thinned using electric drills and burrs. In older individuals, there are several potential advantages to using urea paste for partial or complete chemical avulsion of the nail (Table 22.8).[69] The hyperkeratotic nail plate can also be surgically removed. Removal of the nail plate may be followed by permanent ablation with either chemical (phenol) or surgical matricectomy when onychauxis is recurrent or associated with significant morbidity and local complications.[94]

## Onychoclavus

Onychoclavus is a hyperkeratotic process in the nail area. It has also been referred to as a subungual heloma, a subungual corn, or a subungual callus. It is most commonly located under the distal nail margin.[95]

Subungual heloma results from either an anatomic abnormality and/or a mechanical change in foot function. It is caused by repeated minor trauma with accompanying localized pressure on the distal nail bed and hyponychium. For example, when the toes are contracted in a patient with a hammer toe deformity, an 'end corn' may develop beneath the pulp of the toe just below the nail plate edge.[1]

The subungual corn typically occurs beneath the great toenail and appears as a dark spot under the nail plate; however, other toes may be affected. Applying pressure with a probe can elicit a circumscribed area of intense pain that corresponds to the location of the corn. In addition, the corn may cause elevation or splitting of the overlying nail plate.[2,95]

The differential diagnosis of an onychoclavus includes an epidermoid cyst, a distal subungual keratosis, a foreign body, a subungual filamentous tumor, a subungual melanoma, and a subungual exostosis (Fig. 22.19). Similar to a subungual foreign

body, an onychoclavus does not blanch with pressure. In contrast to a subungual exostosis, which is unchanged even after applying firm pressure, an onychoclavus will yield to slight pressure. A roentgenogram of the digit will readily identify the presence of an exostosis. Subungual exostosis or chondroma may be associated with a subungual corn; therefore, a radiologic examination may be useful in the elderly patient in whom an onychoclavus is suspected. A biopsy may be necessary when the clinical presentation suggests the possibility of a melanoma.[61,96]

Lesion removal and recurrence prevention are the therapeutic cornerstones for treating onychoclavus. The subungual heloma can be ennucleated by removing the corresponding section of nail plate and excising the hyperkeratotic tissue. If the corn is associated with an underlying bony abnormality, correction of the osseous lesion must also be performed. Recurrent onychoclavus can be prevented by eliminating the causative pressure. Modification of the footwear and protective pads or tube foam may be useful to reduce pressure to the distal toe area.[3,95]

## Onychocryptosis

Onychocryptosis is commonly referred to as ingrown nails. This condition results from the nail plate piercing the lateral nail fold. The nail and accompanying distal digit are often tender, usually unsightly, frequently functionally impaired, and typically predisposed to developing paronychia. Onychocryptosis can be extremely debilitating in older individuals.[97,98]

Over-curvature of the nail plate, subcutaneous ingrowing of the toenail, and hypertrophy of the lateral nail fold are the three major types of onychocryptosis which have been described (Fig. 22.20). Inflammation, tenderness at rest, and pain on ambulation or with pressure to the digit are the clinical features of onychocryptosis. Granulation tissue at the lateral nail fold may also be present (Fig. 22.21).

The most common causes of onychocryptosis are improper cutting of the nails and external pressure secondary to poorly fitting footwear. Abnormally long toes, hereditary conditions (congenital excessive convexity of the nail plate and congenital

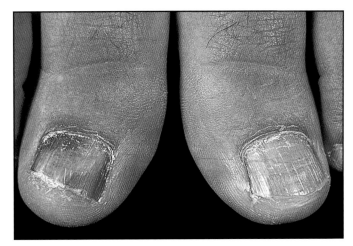

FIGURE 22–19. Although the distal subungual hyperkeratosis mimicked an onychoclavus, the melanocytic pigmentation of the proximal nail fold (positive Hutchinson sign) prompted a biopsy that revealed a subungual malignant melanoma (republished with permission from Cohen PR, Scher RK. Geriatric nail disorders: diagnosis and treatment. J Am Acad Dermatol 1992; 26:521–531. Copyright 1992, Mosby-Year Book, Inc, St. Louis, MO).

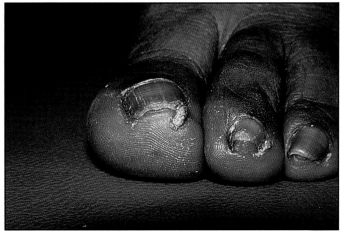

FIGURE 22–20. Onychocryptosis of the great toe and second toe of an older woman. The toes are tender at rest and painful when she walks or applies pressure to the distal digits or their nails (republished with permission from Cohen PR. Nail dystrophies (photo quiz). Consultant 1998; 38:1995–2006).

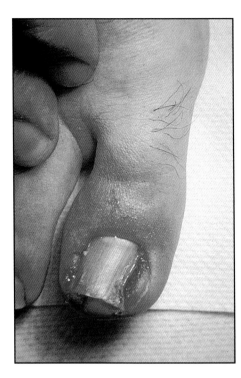

FIGURE 22–21. Recurrent onychocryptosis with subsequent periungual inflammation and granulation tissue (republished with permission from Cohen PR, Scher RK. Geriatric nail disorders: diagnosis and treatment. J Am Acad Dermatol 1992; 26:521–531. Copyright 1992, Mosby-Year Book, Inc, St. Louis, MO).

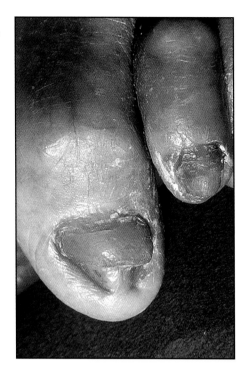

FIGURE 22–22. Partial regrowth of normal nail after previous nail plate avulsion for onychocryptosis secondary to severe over-curvature of the nail plate with painful constriction of the nail bed (pincer nail) (republished with permission from Cohen PR, Scher RK. Geriatric nail disorders: diagnosis and treatment. J Am Acad Dermatol 1992; 26:521–531. Copyright 1992, Mosby-Year Book, Inc, St. Louis, MO).

malalignment of the great toenail), hyperhidrosis, imbalance between the width of the nail plate and that of the nail bed, pointed-toed or high-heeled shoes, poor foot hygiene, and prominence of the nail folds are other etiologic factors. A study of hospitalized older individuals with fingernail abnormalities demonstrated that onychocryptosis was significantly associated with gastrointestinal disease. Nail fold width, degree of medial rotation, and nail thickness are features that may predispose older individuals to develop onychocryptosis.[13,76,99]

Onychocryptosis can be a devasting problem with significant morbidity – especially in an older individual with decreased sensation in the feet or toes secondary to an underlying systemic disease such as diabetes mellitus, peripheral vascular disease, or arteriosclerosis. These elderly individuals are often unaware that a problem exists because their neuropathy results in minimal pain. Consequently, they often do not present for treatment until more serious complications such as deep infection, osteomyelitis, or gangrene have occurred.[3,4]

Several therapeutic alternatives are available for the management of onychocryptosis. Correcting predisposing factors and proper nail trimming are prophylactic measures to prevent onychocryptosis. Cutting the distal nail plate straight across allows the corners of the nail plate to be beyond the distal edge of the lateral nail folds. This decreases the opportunity for onychocryptosis to develop.[25,76,99–102]

Conservative treatment of onychocryptosis involves placing a small wisp of cotton beneath the free edge of the lateral nail plate. This results in an elevation of the lateral border of the nail. As the nail subsequently grows out, its lateral edge does not penetrate into the soft tissue of the lateral nail fold.[25]

Warm soaks and topical antibiotics are local treatment modalities that can be helpful. Microbiologic and radiographic evaluation should be performed if bacterial infection of the skin or underlying bone is suspected. Systemic antibiotics are indicated when a secondary infection is present.[25]

More aggressive therapy is necessary for severe onychocryptosis or if the preliminary therapeutic measures have been unsuccessful. The condition may persist until the stimulus for inflammation is removed. This usually requires complete or partial avulsion of the ingrown nail and excision of the involved adjacent tissue (Fig. 22.22). Recurrence of ingrown toenails is observed for 60 to 80% of onychocryptosis patients treated only with partial or complete nail plate avulsion. For these individuals, partial or total ablation of the nail matrix is often necessary.[76,101]

A stainless steel wire nail brace has been used for flattening the nail plates with severe over-curvature that have caused onychocryptosis. The brace fits the over-curved nail exactly and maintains constant tension on the nail plate. Gradually, a series of adjustments are made. The nail plate is flattened painlessly within a 6-month period.[102]

Silicone gel sheeting has also been used for the management and prevention of onychocryptosis. The silicone is placed and loosely bandaged without pressure on the granulation tissue and exposed nail bed each day for 12 hours beginning 24 hours after partial nail plate excision with retention of the granulation tissue. After 4 months of daily treatment and an additional 10 months of observation, 12 of 14 patients (86%) had resolution of their onychcryptosis, reduction of their hypertrophic nail fold thickness, and no recurrence of the condition.[100]

Another initial treatment modality for patients with onychocryptosis is cryotherapy. Liquid nitrogen is sprayed on to an area that includes not only the granulomatous and infected tissue, but also the adjacent nail fold. A freeze time of 20 to 30 seconds is recommended. Oral aspirin (600 mg, three times daily for 3 days) and topical 0.05% clobetasol prioponate cream (twice daily) can minimize the immediate post-treatment inflammatory reaction.[99]

Liquid nitrogen spray cryotherapy for treating ingrown toenails resulted in complete resolution without recurrence during 13 to 18 months of follow-up in 24 of the 44 patients treated in this manner. Several of these individuals had previously been treated by nail avulsion and/or resection of the lateral nail plate and nail matrix. Loss of infection and granulation tissue were initially observed in the remaining 20 patients; however, recurrence developed within one to three months. Complete resolution, without recurrence during 14 months of follow-up, was demonstrated in 4 of 6 individuals from this latter group who were retreated with cryotherapy.[99]

Treating onychocryptosis with cryotherapy should be considered in older individuals with ingrown toenails. This technique is a simple, quick, and inexpensive outpatient procedure. It not only produced rapid pain relief, but also an acceptable cure rate.

## Onychogryphosis

Onychogryphosis is an exaggerated enlargement of the nail plate (Fig. 22.23). It most often only involves the great toenails. However, it may occur on the fingernails. Onychogryphosis is common in older individuals. This condition can also be observed in individuals who are homeless, have senile dementia, or are infirm.[3,103]

The primary predisposing factor for onychogryphosis is inadequate foot and nail care. This may be caused by self-neglect, the inability of an individual to cut his or her nails (due to immobility and/or failing eye sight), or insufficient professional nursing services. Secondary factors that can influence the development of onychogryphosis include continuous pressure and friction on the toenails due to improper footwear, a previous history of nail trauma, hypertrophy of the nail bed, biomechanical bony abnormalities such as hallux valgus, impairment of the vascular and neuronal system, and onychomycosis.[104]

Clinically, the shape of onychogryphotic nails appears 'oyster-like' or 'ram's horn-like'. The nail plate is typically uneven, thickened, and brown to opaque. Multiple transverse striations are often present. In addition, the underlying nail bed may also be hypertrophic (Fig. 22.24).[105]

Onychogryphosis is primarily caused by the patient permitting the nail to continue to grow without treatment. Some investigators have noted that the nail matrix in onychogryphosis produces the nail plate at uneven rates. The nail plate initially grows in an upward direction; subsequently, its growth is deviated laterally

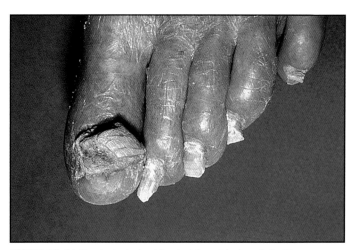

FIGURE 22–24. Onychogryphosis of the great toenail is characterized by an opaque, thickened nail plate with subungual hyperkeratosis and transverse striations in which there has been exaggerated growth in an upward and lateral direction (republished with permission from Cohen PR, Scher RK. Geriatric nail disorders: diagnosis and treatment. J Am Acad Dermatol 1992; 26:521–531. Copyright 1992, Mosby-Year Book, Inc, St. Louis, MO).

toward the other toes. Therefore, the direction of the nail deformity in this condition is determined not only by the pressure from the patient's footwear but also by whether the lateral or medial side of the nail plate grows more rapidly.[104]

Hemionychogryphosis clinically mimics onychogryphosis. It is a potential complication in patients with congenital malalignment of the great toenails – an inherited disorder in which the nail plate is deviated laterally with respect to the longitudinal axis of the distal phalanx of either one great toe or both halluces. Hemionychogryphosis can occur in older individuals in whom congenital malalignment of the great toenails persists into adulthood. In contrast to onychogryphosis, in which the abnormal nail growth is initially upward prior to its lateral deviation, the hypertrophic nail initially grows in a lateral direction in individuals with hemionychogryphosis.[106,107]

There are preventative, palliative, and aggressive treatments for onychogryphosis. Proper nail plate trimming and foot care will prevent the development of this condition, and can be done by someone else if an individual has poor eyesight or is otherwise unable to cut his or her own toenails.[104]

The medical status of the patient influences the decision between a conservative and a radical treatment approach for the onychogryphotic nail. In patients with peripheral vascular disease or diabetes mellitus, the pressure on the onychogryphotic nail can result in subungual gangrene. Conservative treatment for these individuals should initially include filing of the thickened nail plate using an electric drill and burr and removal of the subungual hyperkeratosis. Subsequently, the dystrophic nail should be periodically clipped and trimmed.[104]

More aggressive therapy is preferable for patients with a good vascular supply to the involved onychogryphotic toe. In these individuals, nail avulsion (with or without ablation of the nail matrix) should be performed. The nail can also be removed either by chemical nail destruction (using urea, potassium iodide, or salicylic acid) or surgical avulsion. When necessary, nail matrix ablation can be performed surgically (scalpel or carbon dioxide laser) or chemically (phenol or 10% sodium hydroxide).[76,94,104]

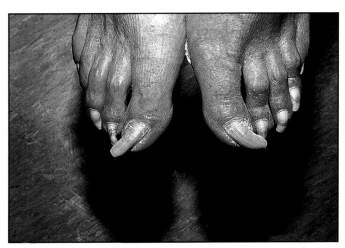

FIGURE 22–23. Exaggerated enlargement of the great toenails (onychogryphosis) of a 68-year-old man (republished with permission from Cohen PR. Nail dystrophies (photo quiz). Consultant 1998; 38:1995-2006).

# Onychophosis

Onychophosis refers to the localized or diffuse hyperkeratotic tissue that can develop on the lateral or proximal nail folds, in the space between the nail folds and the nail plate, or even subungually. This condition is common in older individuals. It mainly involves the first and fifth toes and results from repeated minor trauma to the nail plate. Nail fold hypertrophy, onychocryptosis, onychomycosis, and xerosis are some of the nail plate and adjacent soft tissue deformities that predispose the elderly to develop periungual hyperkeratotic tissue and subsequent onychophosis.[3]

Precautionary measures to prevent the development of onychophosis include wearing comfortable shoes and relieving any pressure exerted by the nail on the surrounding soft tissue. Once onychophosis is present, the initial treatment consists of debriding the hyperkeratotic tissue. Keratolytics can be used for debridement. For this purpose, 12% ammonium lactate, 6% to 20% salicylic acid preparations, or 20% urea preparations may be helpful. Emollients can also be helpful to maintain hydration and lubrication. Thinning of the nail plate, packing of the nail, or surgical intervention similar to that described for onychocryptosis are additional options that may be necessary in order to reduce further trauma to the nail.[1,2]

# Splinter Hemorrhages and Subungual Hematomas

Splinter hemorrhages were noted in 35 of 220 patients over 65 years of age who had been admitted to an acute geriatric ward. However, splinter hemorrhages occurred less often in elderly patients than in younger individuals. Nail trauma was the main cause for these lesions in older individuals. Many of these individuals used walking aids and had fingernail splinter hemorrhages on the hand that held the walking aid.[47–49,108,109]

Splinter hemorrhages have been observed in patients with various underlying systemic disorders. The splinter hemorrhages were usually red and found on the proximal third of the nail plate of individuals with systemic disorder-associated splinter hemorrhages. In contrast, the idiopathic or trauma-induced splinter hemorrhages usually observed in older individuals were typically black and located in the middle or distal third of the fingernail (Fig. 22.25).[47–49,108,109]

The clinical appearance and symptoms of a subungual hematoma vary with the age of the lesion. A recent hemorrhage is typically red and painful. If a fracture of the underlying distal phalanx is suspected, a roentgenogram of the digit may be necessary. An older lesion often appears dark blue, purple, or black and is not usually tender (Fig. 22.26).[47,50,109]

Idiopathic hemorrhage under the nail plate has been observed in older individuals. Trauma to the fingernail or toenail is the most common etiology in these patients. Subungual hemorrhage has also been described in elderly patients who are receiving anticoagulants.[47]

The differential diagnosis of subungual hematoma includes melanoma – especially when the older individual does not remember or associate a traumatic event with the subsequent subungual hematoma. As the nail plate grows, a pigmented lesion of the nail matrix or nail bed will persist. By contrast, a subungual hemorrhage will be replaced proximally by a normal-appearing nail plate (Fig. 22.27). Also, distal onycholysis and eventual

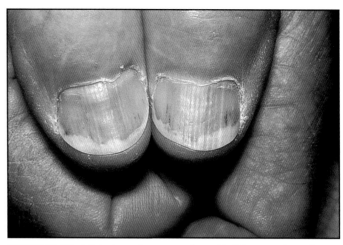

FIGURE 22–25. Splinter hemorrhages presenting as black linear streaks on the distal thumb nail plates of a 65-year-old man. Age-associated nail changes are also noted: superficial longitudinal striations (onychorrhexis) and deeper longitudinal lines ('sausage-shaped' ridging) (republished with permission from Cohen PR. Nail dystrophies (photo quiz). Consultant 1998; 38:1995–2006).

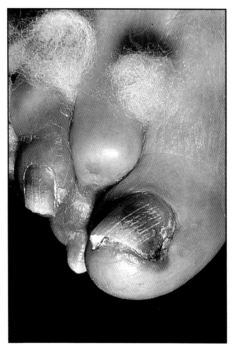

FIGURE 22–26. Several toes have subungual hematomas which were caused by altered pedal function secondary to bony deformities of the digits. Onychocryptosis and subungual hyperkeratosis have also developed (republished with permission from Cohen PR, Scher RK. Geriatric nail disorders: diagnosis and treatment. J Am Acad Dermatol 1992; 26:521–531. Copyright 1992, Mosby-Year Book, Inc, St. Louis, MO).

autoavulsion of the nail plate may occur in some patients with subungual hematoma. Microscopic evaluation of the nail plate and a biopsy specimen from the underlying nail matrix and/or nail bed should be considered when the diagnosis of subungual hematoma cannot be clinically established with certainty.[51,76,105]

Treatment of subungual hematoma may require subungual decompression. Prompt treatment of the hematoma will not only reduce pain significantly but also help to minimize further damage to the nail bed and nail matrix. This can be done by simple trephining of the nail plate to create one or more small holes that allow the compressed blood to be evacuated. Possible complications following decompression treatment may include onycholysis, transient and permanent nail deformity, and infection.[50,110,111]

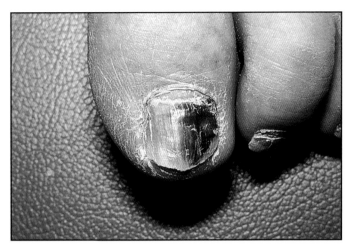

FIGURE 22–27. There is proximal shedding of the black-appearing nail plate from the great toe of this 59-year-old man. The pigmentation represents a subungual hematoma that is progressing distally; the area of pigmentation is gradually being replaced by normal nail plate (republished with permission from Cohen PR. Nail dystrophies (photo quiz). Consultant 1998; 38:1995–2006).

## Subungual Exostosis

Subungual exostosis is a benign tumor that most commonly occurs on the medial surface of the distal great toe (Fig. 22.28). It typically presents as a reactive hyperkeratotic nodule with secondary onychodystrophy of the overlying nail plate. Osseous bone with a fibrocartilage cap is observed histologically. The patient often seeks medical attention because of symptoms related to alteration of the surrounding soft tissue such as pain, paronychia, a pyogenic granuloma, or a callus.[4,112]

The majority of subungual exostoses occur in young adults. However, they have been described in older individuals. Less commonly, these lesions have appeared in children.[113]

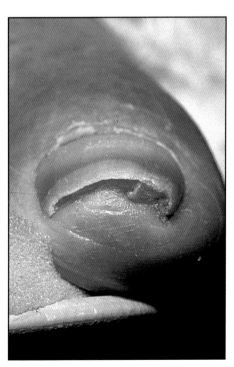

FIGURE 22–28. Radiographic examination confirmed that the incurvature of the medial and lateral aspects of this elderly patient's great toenail was caused by a subungual exostosis (republished with permission from Cohen PR, Scher RK. Geriatric nail disorders: diagnosis and treatment. J Am Acad Dermatol 1992; 26:521–531. Copyright 1992, Mosby-Year Book, Inc, St. Louis, MO).

Subungual exostosis occurs twice as often in women as in men. Nearly two-thirds of the patients had a history of preceding trauma localized to the involved digit. Subungual exostoses are typically solitary, acquired, and without a family history of similar lesions. Rarely, multiple subungual exostoses have been described in patients who have autosomal dominant multiple exostosis syndrome.[113,114]

The differential diagnosis of subungual exostosis includes benign and malignant tumors. Osteochondromas and enchondromas, two of the benign tumors that clinically mimic subungual exostoses, can usually be differentiated from exostoses based upon radiologic findings. The radiograph of a subungual exostosis usually shows a broad-based lesion of trabeculated bone with an expanding distal flare; the fibrocartilage cap is radiolucent and areas of calcification are absent. Distinguishing features of osteochondromas and enchondromas are a scalloped dome with a hyaline cartilage cap and a loculated medullary bone cyst with calcification, respectively.[76,112,113,115,116]

The treatment of subungual exostosis involves removal of the excess bone aseptically after the suspected diagnosis has been confirmed radiographically. Neither radiation nor simple cautery is effective in the management of subungual exostosis. After a local anesthetic block is given, the nail plate is avulsed and the exostosis is exposed via a longitudinal incision of the overlying nail bed. With a bone rongeur, chisel, or mastoid curet, the tumor is then separated from the underlying bone. To attempt to prevent local recurrence, the rough edges are chiseled flat and the tumor bed is saucerized by curettage to completely remove the lesion. Finally, the cutaneous wound is closed by suturing the nail bed and an impregnated paraffin gauze dressing is applied.[76,112,113,117]

## CONCLUSIONS

Age-associated nail changes in color, contour, histology, linear growth, surface, and thickness have been observed in older individuals. Age-related onychodystrophies that occur in the elderly include brittle nails, faulty biomechanics, trauma, infections, onychauxis, onychoclavus, onychocryptosis, onychogryphosis, onychophosis, splinter hemorrhages and subungual hematomas, and subungual exostosis. The ability to evaluate, diagnose, and manage the onychologic needs of older individuals can be enhanced by an awareness and understanding of the clinicopathophysiology of nail changes and disorders in this patient population.

## REFERENCES

1. Cohen PR, Scher RK. Geriatric nail disorders: Diagnosis and treatment. J Am Acad Dermatol 1992; 26:521–531
2. Cohen PR, Scher RK. Nail changes in the elderly. J Geriatr Dermatol 1993; 1:4553
3. Cohen PR, Scher RK. Aging (Chapter 16). In: Hordinsky MK, Saway M, Scher RK, eds. Atlas of hair and nails. New York, Churchill Livingstone, 2000:213–225
4. Cohen PR, Scher RK. The nail in older individuals. In: Scher RK, Daniel CR III, eds. Nails: therapy, diagnosis, surgery. 2nd edn, Philadelphia, WB Saunders, 1997:127–150
5. Beauregard S, Gilchrest BA. A survey of skin problems and skin care regimens in the elderly. Arch Dermatol 1987; 123:1638–1643
6. Hsu JD. Foot problems in the elderly patient. J Am Geriatr Soc 1971; 19:880–886

7. Finlay OE. Footwear management in the elderly care programme. Physiotherapy 1986; 72 (Apr):172–178
8. Scher RK. Nail surgery. Clin Dermatol 1987; 5 (4):135–142
9. Dawber R. The effect of immobilization on fingernail growth. Clin Exp Dermatol 1981; 6:533–535
10. Orentreich N, Markofsky J, Vogelman JH. The effect of aging on the rate of linear nail growth. J Invest Dermatol 1979; 73:126–130
11. Bean WB. Nail growth: thirty-five years of observation. Arch Intern Med 1980; 140:73–76
12. Cohen PR. The lunula. J Am Acad Dermatol, 1996; 34:943–953
13. Jemec GBE, Kollerup G, Jensen LB, Mogensen S. Nail abnormalities in nondermatologic patients: prevalence and possible role as diagnostic aids. J Am Acad Dermatol 1995; 32:977–981
14. Horan MA, Puxty JA, Fox RA: The white nails of old age (neapolitan nails). J Am Geriatr Soc 1982; 30:734–737
15. Lindsay PG. The half-and-half nail. Arch Intern Med 1967; 119:583–587
16. Terry R. White nails in hepatic cirrhosis. Lancet 1954; 1:757–759
17. Stone OJ. Clubbing and koilonychia. Dermatol Clin 1985; 3:485–490
18. Baran R. Nail care in the 'golden years' of life. Cur Med Res Opinion 1982; 7 (Suppl 2):95–97
19. Helfand AE. Nail and hyperkeratotic problems in the elderly foot. Am Fam Physician 1989; 39 (Feb):101–110
20. Gilchrist AK. Common foot problems in the elderly. Geriatrics 1979; 34 (Nov):67–70
21. Lewis BL, Montgomery H. The senile nail. J Invest Dermatol 1955; 24:11–18
22. Germann H, Barban W, Plewig G. Morphology of corneocytes from human nail plates. J Invest Dermatol 1980; 74:115–118
23. Fenske NA, Lober CW. Structural and functional changes of normal aging skin. J Am Acad Dermatol 1986; 15:571–585
24. Geyer AS, Onumah N, Uyttendaele H, Scher RK. Modulation of linear nail growth to treat diseases of the nail. J Am Acad Dermatol 2004; 50:229–234
25. Moossavi M, Scher RK. A hands-on guide to common nail disorders. Clin Advisor 2003; 6 (11):10–19
26. Hamilton JB, Terada H, Mestler GE. Studies of growth throughout the lifespan in Japanese: growth and size of nails and their relationship to age, sex heredity, and other factors. J Gerontol 1955; 10:401–415
27. Balin AK, Pratt LA. Physiological consequences of human skin aging. Cutis 1989; 43:431–436
28. Orentreich N, Scharp NJ. Keratin replacement as an ageing parameter. J Soc Cos Chem 1967; 18:537–547
29. Baran R, Dawber RPR. The nail in childhood and old age. In: Baran R, Dawber RPR, de Berker DAR, et al., eds. Baran and Dawber's diseases of the nails and their management. 3rd edn. Oxford, Blackwell Scientific, 2001:104–128
30. Scher RK. Cosmetics and ancillary preparations for the care of nails: composition, chemistry, and adverse reactions. J Am Acad Dermatol 1982; 6:523–528
31. Edelstein JE. Foot care for the aging. Physical Therapy 1988; 68:1882–1886
32. Farber EM, South DA. Urea ointment in the nonsurgical avulsion of nail dystrophies. Cutis 1978; 22:689–692
33. South DA, Farber EM. Urea ointment in the nonsurgical avulsion of nail dystrophies—a reappraisal. Cutis 1980; 25:609–612
34. Buselmeier TJ. Combination urea and salicylic acid ointment nail avulsion in nondystrophic nails: a follow-up observation. Cutis 1980; 25:397–405
35. Dorn M, Kienitz T, Ryckmanns F. Onychomycosis: experience with non-traumatic nail avulsion. Hautarzt 1980; 31:30–34
36. Hardjoko FS, Widyanto S, Singgih I, Susilo J. Treatment of onychomycosis with a bifonazole-urea combination. Mycoses 1990; 33:167–171
37. Hay RJ, Roberts DT, Doherty VR, et al. The topical treatment of onychomycosis using a new combination urea/imidazole preparation. Clin Exp Dermatol 1988; 13:164–167
38. Torres-Rodriguez JM, Madrenys N, Nicolas MC. Non-traumatic topical treatment of onychomycosis with urea associated with bifonazole. Mycoses 1991; 34:499–504
39. Cohen PR. Red lunulae: case report and literature review. J Am Acad Dermatol 1992; 26:292–294
40. Lubach D, Cohrs W, Wurzinger R. Incidence of brittle nails. Dermatologica 1986; 172:144–147
41. Scher RK. Brittle nails. Int J Dermatol 1989; 28:515–516
42. Scher RK, Bodian AB. Brittle nails. Semin Dermatol 1991; 10:21–25
43. Lassus A. Colloidal silicic acid for oral and topical treatment of aged skin, fragile hair and brittle nails in females. J Int Med Res 1993; 21:209–215
44. Hochman LG, Scher RK, Meyerson MS. Brittle nails: patient response to daily biotin supplementation. Cutis 1993; 51:303–305
45. Uyttendaele H, Geyer A, Scher RK. Brittle nails: pathogenesis and treatment. J Drugs Dermatol 2003; 2:48–49
46. Cohen PR. Coping with brittle nails (advisor forum: 63-3). Clin Advisor 2004; 7 (1):56.
47. Samman PD. Nail deformities due to trauma. In: Samman PD, Fenton DA, eds. The nails in disease. London, William Heinemann Medical Books, 1986:135–153
48. Gross NJ, Tall R. Clinical significance of splinter haemorrhages. Br Med J 1963; 2:1496–1498
49. Robertson JC, Braune ML. Splinter haemorrhages, pitting, and other findings in fingernails of healthy adults. Br Med J 1974; 4:279–281
50. Farrington GH. Subungual haematoma – an evaluation of treatment. Br Med J 1964; 1:742–744
51. Baran R, Kechijian P. Longitudinal melanonychia (melanonychia striata): diagnosis and management. J Am Acad Dermatol 1989; 21:1165–1175
52. Grossman M, Scher RK. Leukonychia: review and classification. Int J Dermatol 1990; 29:535–541
53. Wernick J, Gibbs RC. Pedal biomechanics and toenail disease. In: Scher RK, Daniel CR III, eds. Nails: therapy, diagnosis, surgery. Philadelphia, WB Saunders, 1990:244–249
54. Riccitelli ML. Foot problems of the aged and infirmed. J Am Geriatr Soc 1966; 14:1058–1066
55. Combes FC, Scott MJ. Onychotillomania: case report. Arch Dermatol 1951; 63:778–780
56. Tosti A, Piraccini BM. Treatment of common nail disorders. Dermatol Clin 2000; 18:339–348
57. Samman PD. A traumatic nail dystrophy produced by a habit tic. Arch Dermatol 1963; 88:895–896
58. van Dijk E. Dystrophia unguium mediana canaliformis. Dermatologica 1978; 156:358–366
59. Scher RK. Onychomycosis: a significant medical disorder. J Am Acad Dermatol 1996; 35:S2–S5
60. Daniel CR III, Elewski BE. The diagnosis of nail fungus infection revisited [editorial]. Arch Dermatol 2000; 136:1162–1164
61. Cohen PR, Scher RK. Nail disease and dermatology [commentary]. J Am Acad Dermatol 1989; 21:1020–1022
62. Lynde C. Nail disorders that mimic onychomycosis: what to consider. Cutis 2001; 68:8–12
63. Gad ZM, Youssef N, Sherif AA, et al. An epidemiologic study of the fungal skin flora among the elderly in Alexandria. Epidem Inf 1987; 99:213–219
64. English MP, Atkinson R. Onychomycosis in elderly chiropody patients. Br J Dermatol 1974; 91:67–72
65. Cohen PR. Onychomycosis. J Greater Houston Dental Soc 1997; 68 (9):22–23
66. Elewski BE. Onychomycosis: treatment, quality of life, and economic issues. Am J Clin Dermatol 2000; 1:19–26
67. Gupta AK. Types of onychomycosis. Cutis 2001; 68:4–7
68. Daniel CR III. Traditional management of onychomycosis. J Am Acad Dermatol 1996; 35:S21–S25
69. Cohen PR, Scher RK. Topical and surgical treatment of onychomycosis. J Am Acad Dermatol 1994; 31:S74–S77
70. Meyerson MS, Scher RK, Hochman LG, et al. Open-label study of the safety and efficacy of fungoid tincture in patients with distal subungual onychomycosis of the toes. Cutis 1992; 49:359–362
71. Meyerson MS, Scher RK, Hochman LG, et al. Open-label study of the safety and efficacy of naftifine hydrochloride 1 percent gel in patients with distal subungual onychomycosis of the fingers. Cutis 1993; 51:205–207

72. Cohen PR. Treatment of fungal nail infections (advisor forum). Clin Advisor, in press

73. Cohen PR. Bleaching out onychomycosis (advisor forum: 6:–7). Clin Advisor, 2004; 7(6):75.

74. Obadiah J, Scher R. Nail disorders: unapproved treatments. Clin Dermatol 2002; 20:643–648

75. Scher RK. Onychomycosis: therapeutic update. J Am Acad Dermatol 1999; 40:S21–S26

76. Alam M, Scher RK. Current topics in nail surgery. J Cutan Med Surg 1999; 3:324–335

77. Daniel CR III. Basic nail plate avulsion. J Dermatol Surg Oncol 1992; 18:685–688

78. Hochman LG. Paronychia: more than just an abscess [commentary]. Int J Dermatol 1995; 34:385–386

79. Stetson CL, Butler DF, Rapini RP. Herpetic whitlow during isotretinoin therapy. Int J Dermatol 2003; 42:496–498

80. Iftikhar N, Bari I, Ejaz A. Rare variants of cutaneous leishmaniasis: whitlow, paronychia, and sporotrichoid. Int J Dermatol 2003; 42:807–809

81. Cohen PR, Buzdar AU. Metastatic breast carcinoma mimicking an acute paronychia of the great toe: case report and review of subungual metastases. Am J Clin Oncol (CCT) 1993; 16:86–91

82. Daniel CR III, Daniel MP, Daniel CM, et al. Chronic paronychia and onycholysis: a thirteen-year experience. Cutis 1996; 58:397–401

83. Tosti A, Piraccini BM, Ghetti E, Colombo MD. Topical steroids versus systemic antifungals in the treatment of chronic paronychia: an open randomized double-blind and double dummy study. J Am Acad Dermatol 2002; 47:73–76

84. Cohen PR. Nail infections (photo quiz). Consultant 1998; 38:2133–2147 and 2001; 41:805–817

85. Patki AH, Mehta JM. Pterygium unguis in a patient with recurrent type 2 lepra reaction. Cutis 1989; 44:311–312

86. Kingsbury DH, Chester EC Jr, Jansen GT. Syphilitic paronychia: an unusual complaint [letter]. Arch Dermatol 1972; 105:458

87. Scher RK. Biopsy of nails. Subungual scabies. Am J Dermatopathol 1983; 5:187–189

88. Scher RK. Subungual scabies [letter]. J Am Acad Dermatol 1985; 12:577–578

89. Scoffle NN, Cohen PR. *Sarcopetes scabiei* (images in clinical medicine). New Engl J Med, in press

90. Orion E, Matz H, Ruocco V, Wolf R. Parasitic skin infestations II, scabies, pediculosis, spider bites: unapproved treatments. Clin Dermatol 2002; 20:618–625

91. Cohen PR. Tests for detecting herpes simplex virus and varicella-zoster virus infections. Dermatol Clin 1994; 12:51–68

92. Cohen PR. Herpesviruses: herpes simplex virus, varicella-zoster virus and cytomegalovirus [Section IV (Viruses), Chapter 18]. In: Lesher JL Jr., ed. An atlas of microbiology of the skin. Pearl River, NY, Parthenon Publishing, 1999:110–119

93. Bartolomei FJ. Onychauxis. Surgical and nonsurgical treatment. Clin Podiatr Med Surg 1995; 12:215–220

94. Baran R, Haneke E. Matricectomy and nail ablation. Hand Clin 2002; 18:693–696

95. Adams BB, Lucky AW. A center's callosities. Cutis 2001; 67:141–142

96. Cohen PR. A thumbnail sketch. (consultations & comments) Consultant 2002; 42:453–454

97. Ikard RW. Onychocryptosis. J Am Coll Surg 1998; 187:96–102

98. DeLauro TM. Onchocryptosis. Clin Podiatr Med Surg 1995; 12:201–213

99. Sonnex TS, Dawber RPR. Treatment of ingrowing toenails with liquid nitrogen spray cryotherapy. Br Med J 1985; 291:173–175

100. Aksakal AB, Ozsoy E, Gurer M. Silicone gel sheeting for the management and prevention of onychocryptosis. Dermatol Surg 2003; 29:261–264

101. Serour F. Recurrent ingrown big toenails are efficiently treated by $CO_2$ laser. Dermatol Surg 2002; 28:509–512

102. Dawber RPR, Baran R. Nail surgery. In: Samman PD, Fenton DA, eds. The nails in disease. London. William Heinemann Medical Books, 1986:194–206

103. Kouskoukis CE, Scher RK. Onychogryphosis. J Dermatol Surg Oncol 1982; 8:138–140

104. Mohrenschlager M, Wicke-Wittenius K, Brockow K, et al. Onychogryphosis in elderly persons: an indicator of long-standing poor nursing care? Report of one case and review of the literature. Cutis 2001; 68:233–235

105. Cohen PR. Nail dystrophies (photo quiz). Consultant 1998; 38:1995–2006

106. Cohen J, Scher RK, Pappert A. Congenital malalignment of the great toenails. Pediatr Dermatol 1991; 8:40–42

107. Cohen PR. Congenital malalignment of the great toe nails: case report and literature review. Pediatr Dermatol 1991; 8:43–45

108. Young J, Mulley G. Splinter haemorrhages in the elderly. Age and Ageing 1987; 16:101–104

109. Cohen PR. Nail disorders in athletes. The Sports Monthly (South County Sports Cover to Cover). The Woodlands, TX, 1999; 1(4:June):10.

110. Helms A, Brodell RT. Surgical pearl: prompt treatment of subungual hematoma by decompression. J Am Acad Dermatol 2000; 42:508–509

111. Meeks S, White M. Subungual haematomas: is simple trephining enough? J Accid Emerg Med 1998; 15:269–271

112. Young RJ III, Wilde JL, Sartori CR, Elston DM. Solitary nodule of the great toe. Cutis 2001; 68:57–58

113. Davis DA, Cohen PR. Subungual exostosis: case report and literature review. Pediatr Dermatol 1996; 13:212–218

114. Baran R, Bureau H. Multiple exostosis syndrome. J Am Acad Dermatol 1991; 25:333–335

115. Vine JE, Cohen PR. Renal cell carcinoma metastatic to the thumb: a case report and review of subungual metastases from all primary sites. Clin Exp Dermatol 1996; 35:923–927

116. Cohen PR. Metastatic tumors to the nail unit: subungual metastases. Dermatol Surg 2001; 27:280–293

117. Oliveira ADS, Picoto ADS, Verde SF, Martins O. Subungual exostosis: treatment as an office procedure. J Dermatol Surg Oncol 1980; 6:555–558

# 23 Basic and Advanced Nail Surgery (Part 1: Principles and Techniques)

Philippe Abimelec and Christian Dumontier

## Key Features

1. Knowledge of nail anatomy and medical history is crucial for successful nail surgery
2. The nail matrix forms the nail plate
3. Preoperative work-up – including mycology, X-ray, and medical/drug history – is important before nail surgery
4. Anesthesia can be achieved by several methods but most simple nail surgery can be performed with a distal block

Interest in the field of nail surgery is recent and growing; nail surgery has only recently been included in the core curriculum of US dermatology residents and two treaties entirely devoted to the subject have recently been published.[1,2]

Basic nail surgery is within the domain of the general dermatologist. Nail surgery requires a thorough knowledge of anatomy and good technical skills, and a dermatopathologist specialized in nail diseases. More advanced nail surgical techniques require collaboration between an orthopedic or plastic surgeon and the dermatologist. Careful clinical examination supplemented by suitable laboratory tests and imaging techniques should lead to a correct diagnosis and surgical management when it is suitable. Mastering nail surgery techniques is essential to effectively treat benign and malignant nail tumors as well as nail unit infections, congenital or post-traumatic nail deformity, and to reduce postoperative morbidity.

This chapter has been written by a hand surgeon and a dermatologist team, merging their efforts to transmit their experience in the field of nail surgery.

## PRINCIPLES IN NAIL SURGERY

## Preoperative Evaluation

### Surgical consultation

The preoperative consultation should assess all aspects of the planned surgical procedure. Surgical complications should be thoroughly reviewed with the patient, including short- and long-term postoperative nail dystrophies. It is vital to evaluate as accurately as possible the length of time for which healing might affect the use of hands and feet: Walking and working impediments can last for up to 1 month in the case of larger surgeries. Written, informed consent should be obtained from the patient before any surgical procedure. It is very helpful to have preoperative photographs of the nail.

### Preoperative assessment

Minor nail surgical procedures require a careful medical and medication history, bacterial and mycology studies if infection is suspected, and imaging (X-ray or MRI) of the affected digit if a subungual tumor is possible. Preoperative screening should take place before the larger nail surgery procedures that require regional anesthesia or intravenous sedation. Depending on the patient's age and medical history, the anesthesiologist will decide the preoperative assessment that is needed. Particular attention should be focused on distal neurovascular compromise (peripheral arteriopathy, Raynaud's phenomenon, diabetes), hemostasis (coagulopathy), and drug intake that may interfere with anesthetic drugs or coagulation (beta-blockers, phenothiazines, anticoagulants, aspirin, nonsteroidal anti-inflammatory drugs and blood thinners) as well as allergies (anesthetic drugs, latex, antibiotics). Perioperative monitoring and drug control of high-risk patients is especially important for diabetics, the immunocompromised, and subjects on anticoagulants. Although no evidence supports this practice,[3] some practitioners recommend an antibiotic injection before incision for operations that carry a higher risk of postoperative infection (osteitis, foot surgery[4]); we use preoperative antibiotic prophylaxis for patients whose mucous cysts have drained preoperatively.

## Surgical Setting

Nail avulsions, biopsies, and simple excisions are safely performed in the dermatologist's office under the same conditions as basic skin surgery procedures. Prepping is usually done with povidone iodine or a 0.5% chlorhexidine–alcohol preparation. Draping is conventional. We recommend that advanced nail surgery be performed in a surgical facility that meets orthopedic surgery standards. We generally advise surgical scrubbing of the patient's hand with a povidone iodine or chlorhexidine-impregnated surgical scrub, or soaking of the patient's foot in an antiseptic solution. Preparation and draping of the extremity prior to advanced nail surgery is standardized as for any orthopedic surgical procedure.

## Pain Management

Pain control requires perioperative interventions. The perioperative period extends from the preoperative day through the operation and into the postoperative recovery period. Preoperative measures include nonsteroidal anti-inflammatory medications and anxiolysis if necessary. Anesthetic creams prior to distal digital anesthesia may be valuable for children. The use of nerve blocks with long-acting anesthetics bupivacaine (Marcaine®), and ropivacaine (Naropin®) enhances postoperative analgesia for up to 24 hours after the surgery. The presence of an anesthesiologist is necessary for pre- and perioperative sedation, to perform nerve blocks (median, cubital, axillary or foot nerve blocks) or to manage painful postoperative procedures.

## Preoperative anxiolysis

Preoperative anxiolysis is not mandatory but offers numerous advantages. Benzodiazepines are the most widely used medication for anxiety relief; midazolam (Versed®) is favored because of its higher potency and shorter duration. Short-acting midazolam offers hypnotic, anxiolytic, and anterograde amnestic properties, which are advantageous because patients often do not remember the pain, associated with local nerve blocks.

## Anesthesia/sedation

**LOCAL AND REGIONAL ANESTHESIA** Depending on the procedure, and on personal preference, there is a choice of distal, proximal, or transthecal digital anesthesia, as well as a variety of regional blocks. Simple nail surgeries require only distal or proximal digital blocks.

**DISTAL NAIL BLOCKS** Distal digital anesthesias (Fig. 23.1) can be performed in different ways: distal digital block or distal digital anesthesia through the proximal nail fold and through the hyponychium. Plain 2% lidocaine is preferred but 1% also may also be used. Although lidocaine with epinephrine is safe for digital anesthesia,[5,6] it is not useful because exsanguination is necessary and sufficient. Very slow injections beginning with a dermal papule are necessary to minimize pain. A dental syringe and a 30-gauge needle are useful for this purpose; a 2 mL Luer lock and syringe are also adequate.

- *Distal digital block* (wing block): Offers an immediate and total nail unit anesthesia; the needle is inserted 2 to 3 mm proximal to the junction of the proximal and lateral nail fold. A dermal papule of anesthetic is done at the dorsal level, the needle is then directed vertically and the injection carried out along the lateral aspect of the digit. We inject 0.5 mL of anesthetic. The opposite side of the digit is anesthetized in the same way.
- *Distal anesthesia through the proximal nail fold (PNF)*: This is useful for anesthesia of the PNF, matrix and the proximal bed. The needle is inserted in the middle of the PNF; a dermal papule of anesthesia is carried out before penetrating the proximal nail plate and the matrix where most of the injection takes place. We inject 0.5 to 1 mL of anesthetic very slowly. We observe the lunula and nail bed blanching, which roughly indicates the territory of anesthesia.
- *Distal anesthesia through the hyponychium*: This is done more rarely because it is more painful. The territory of anesthesia may include the hyponychium, the bed, and most of the matrix. The needle is inserted in the lateral hyponychial area (to avoid the prominent distal phalangeal ungueal process) and directed horizontally in the nail bed while the anesthetic is injected. Here also, blanching roughly indicates the territory of anesthesia, which may include the hyponychium, the bed, and most of the matrix.

Distal anesthesia is helpful because it takes effect almost immediately. Because the major digital vessels and nerves are not transected, these techniques carry a low risk of neurovascular compromise. The subungual space is limited and nonexpandable.

Anesthetic injection induces compression hemostasis, which may be sufficient to realize most nail surgery. Injection under pressure is painful and should be carried out very slowly. It is easier to perform with a dental syringe. Limited territory of anesthesia should be anticipated for distal digital anesthesia through the PNF and hyponychium. Local infection and vasculopathy are contraindications of all distal techniques. Distal digital anesthesia is useful for most nonseptic surgery, especially when you need rapid onset of anesthesia. Distal digital nail unit blocks are seldom used for large nail surgery because they are painful and may cause swelling of the surgical field.

**PROXIMAL NAIL BLOCKS** Proximal digital blocks should not be performed as 'ring blocks'; more proximal blocks may be preferred to minimize vascular compromise. Plain 2% lidocaine is preferred. A 5 mL (fingers) or 10 mL (toes) syringe is used. The 30-gauge needle is introduced at the base of the digit where a dermal papule is realized. The needle is then slowly introduced along the lateral side of the digit/toe while slowly injecting the anesthetic. A larger amount of lidocaine is delivered around the dorsal and ventral digital nerves lying respectively near the palmar and dorsal aspects of the digit/toe. In adult patients, 1 mL (thumb) to 2 mL (big toe) of anesthetic are delivered around each collateral nerve. This proximal block should be avoided in case of infection. It is necessary to wait 10 to 15 minutes for anesthesia to take place.

**TRANSTHECAL DIGITAL ANESTHESIA** Transthecal digital anesthesia has been described by Chiu et al[7] as a new approach to achieve digital anesthesia by the use of the flexor tendon sheath to introduce anesthetics to the core of the digit. After a palmar percutaneous injection, the anesthetic diffuses to the dorsal digital nerves via centrifugal infusion through the flexor tendon sheath and by local diffusion around the puncture site.

This technique is indicated for distal anesthesia of the three central digits.[8] Infections and a hypocoagulating state are contraindications. A sterile technique is required; a 5-mL syringe mounted with 27-gauge needle is used. Plain 2% lidocaine is generally employed; bupivacaine may be used for long-lasting anesthesia. The hand is supinated to expose its palmar aspect, flexion and extension of the digit to be anesthetized give the opportunity to palpate the flexor tendon as it glides over the protuberance of the metacarpal head. Penetration of the skin with the 27-gauge needle is slightly distal to the metacarpophalangeal joint, through the subcutaneous tissue, down to the flexor tendon sheath (Fig. 23.2). The needle may be slightly withdrawn if the tendon is penetrated inadvertently. Intrathecal injection of 3 to 5 mL of anesthetic is performed and the patient feels the centrifugal inflow of anesthetics through the digit. Anesthesia is expected to occur in 7 to 8 minutes.[9] Transthecal digital anesthesia benefits include the need of a single prick, the absence of neurovascular compromise, and long-lasting anesthesia. No significant complications have been reported so far. The drawbacks of transthecal digital anesthesia include a painful palmar skin penetration and a localized, sometimes intense pain that may be prolonged for a few days after the procedure. Unreliable anesthesia of the 1st and 5th digits is a limitation of this technique.

**REGIONAL BLOCKS** For more advanced nail surgeries, the hand can be anesthetized effectively with radial, median, ulnar, or axillary blocks; anterior and posterior ankle blocks can be used for

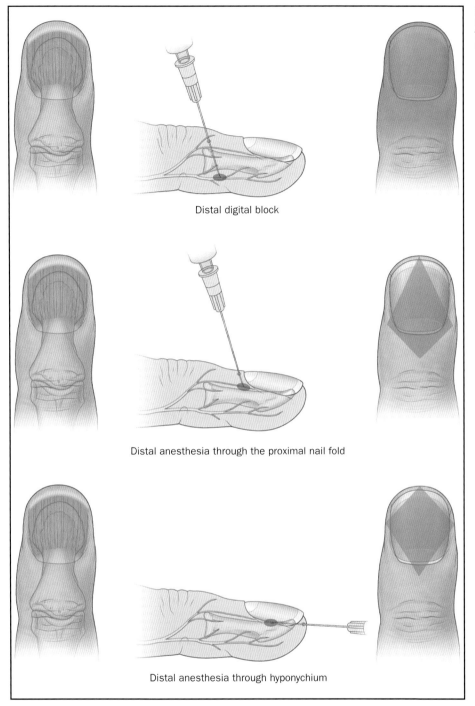

Distal digital block

Distal anesthesia through the proximal nail fold

Distal anesthesia through hyponychium

FIGURE 23–1. The three types of distal digital anesthesia: distal digital block, distal digital anesthesia through the proximal nail fold, and distal digital anesthesia through the hyponychium.

regional anesthesia for the foot, description of these techniques is beyond the scope of this review.[10]

Ropivacaine (Naropin™) and bupivacaine are the preferred local anesthetic agents for larger nerve blocks, whereas plain 2% lidocaine and/or bupivacaine are used for distal blocks. The newer long-acting amino-amide local anesthetic, ropivacaine, combines the anesthetic potency and long duration of action of bupivacaine with a toxicity profile intermediate between bupivacaine and lidocaine. Low concentrations of ropivacaine may produce clinically significant vasoconstriction.[11] It is now recognized that lidocaine with epinephrine is safe for digital anesthesia[5,6] but no study has evaluated the vasoconstrictive effects of ropivacaine on digital perfusion; we avoid its use for distal anesthesia.

## Preoperative sedation

Although the average patient does well with preoperative anxiolysis associated with regional anesthesia, patients undergoing advanced surgical procedures may require deeper conscious intravenous sedation (an anesthesiologist is required).

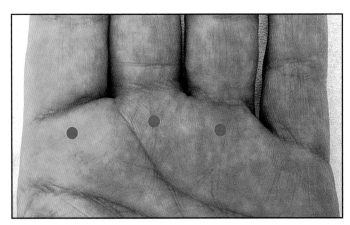

FIGURE 23–2. Transthecal digital anesthesia injection sites.

## Operative technique

Operative measures to alleviate postoperative pain include wound tension control. Wound tension should be kept as minimal as possible. Undermining should be done when necessary and the wound should be closed with a limited number of stitches to facilitate drainage. Openings should be made in the nail plate: at the base, the extremity, or laterally to ensure drainage.

## Postoperative analgesia

Postoperative measures rely on a pharmacological intervention. The analgesic should be chosen according to the anticipated level of pain (Table 23.1) and should be given at regular intervals depending on the drug elimination half-life and before the reappearance of the pain. Adaptation of analgesic strength levels and doses is necessary. In the absence of sedation, the physician should not hesitate to repeat the initial dose or to increase the analgesic level to achieve satisfactory pain relief.

Pain levels associated with nail surgery are variable. In our experience, surgical techniques that induce an intense level of pain are laterolongitudinal excisions; large nail bed, nail unit, or skin flaps; and total nail unit removal. Simple excisions and biopsies are moderately painful whereas avulsions and segmental matricectomies generate a low level of pain.

Initial drug choice depends on the expected level of pain. Step 1 refers to a low to moderate level of pain for which acetaminophen or nonsteroidal anti-inflammatory drugs are used. Step 2 refers to a moderate level of pain. Mild opioid narcotic analgesics are recommended at this step. They include: dextropropoxyphen, tramadol, dihydrocodeine, and opioid cyclooxygenase combinations such as acetaminophen + codeine or dextropropoxyphen. Step 3 refers to expected intense pain or pain that is not alleviated by step 2 measures. Narcotic analgesics used at this step are morphine and morphine derivatives. Initiation of therapy requires titration of the chosen analgesic to the optimal dose and interval with a nyctohemeral drug delivery. Painful procedures require step 2 or step 3 levels of analgesia from the onset. Side effects should be explained and prevented.

# Instruments

Most instruments used for nail surgery are not specific, including magnifying loupes and delicate instruments such as those used in plastic surgery. Adequate magnification is essential, Heine® or Zeiss® binocular loupes that magnify 2.5 to 3.5 times at 13 to 16 inches are adequate.

Delicate forceps are necessary to avoid crushing the small tissue specimens; delicate Adson models with one by two teeth or Castroviejo forceps are optimal. Double-prong Guthrie retractors are used for proximal nail fold retraction or nail bed/matrix tissue flaps. A delicate needle holder is required to secure fine suture material. Nail plate avulsions may necessitate some specific tools such as nail elevators, nail nippers or nail splitters. Lempert elevators 2- and 3-mm large (Fig. 23.3) are useful to perform partial avulsions for lateral matrix segmental phenolization. Their extremity is slightly bent to conform to the nail bed shape (see Fig. 23.3). The larger freer septum elevator is used for larger hemi- or total nail plate avulsions. When missing, the smooth side of the jaw of an opened Halstead or Mosquito forceps or the thin lateral external side of a blunt-tipped Stevens scissors may replace this instrument.

Straight 5-inch nail nippers may be used to section the nail plate during distal avulsions; double-action nail nippers are invaluable in cutting thick toenails, and our preferred model is the Ruskin bone-cutting forceps. The English anvil-action nail splitter (Fig. 23.4) is helpful for laterolongitudinal toenail avulsions. The lower blade of the instrument has a flat and smooth undersurface that glides along the nail bed atraumatically. As the anvil-like upper surface of the lower blade slides under the nail plate, the inferior cutting edge of the upper blade is placed over the nail plate. The spring action of the instrument allows it to cut through the thickest nail plate with ease.

Curved and blunt tipped scissors such as Stevens or Graddle are convenient to section thin nail plate. Nail-pulling forceps are seldom used because regular Halstead or Mosquito forceps or regular needle holders with teeth do their job efficiently. A bone curette is essential for matricectomies. We use them after

| | INTENSE | MODERATE | LOW |
|---|---|---|---|
| Avulsion | | | X |
| Phenolization | | | X |
| Biopsy | | | X |
| Shave excision | | X | |
| Fusiform longitudinal excision | | X | |
| Lateral longitudinal excision | X | | |
| Flaps | X | | |
| Nail unit graft | X | | |

TABLE 23–1. Pain in nail surgery

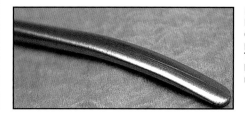

FIGURE 23–3. The Lempert elevator. Lempert elevator is useful to perform partial avulsion. Their extremity is slightly bent to conform to the nail bed shape.

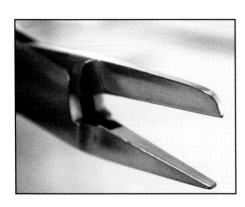

FIGURE 23-4. The English nail splitter. The lower blade has a flat and smooth undersurface, the upper having an inferior cutting edge. The spring action allows the ENS to cut through the thickest nail plate with ease.

laterolongitudinal avulsions to ensure lateral matrix horn removal. The Sprattor Brudon bone curette is our preferred model.

## Sutures

We prefer suturing all nail unit wounds to minimize scarring. Nonetheless, some basic nail surgical procedures do not require sutures; these include biopsies or excisions with diameter ≤3 mm. When skin approximation is needed, we use Ethicon sutures (Johnson & Johnson). Coated Vicryl rapide® (polyglactin 910) suture offers short-term wound support (7–10 days) and avoids the need for suture removal, which is often feared by nail surgery patients. Drawbacks are essentially a reduced tensile strength that is markedly visible when trans nail plate suturing is needed. We routinely used 4-0 (toenails) and 5-0 (fingernails) for latero-longitudinal excisions and to approximate proximal and lateral nail folds.

Nail epithelium approximation is performed with absorbable sutures. Undyed (clear) coated Vicryl® (polyglactin 910) suture or PDS II® (polydioxanone) synthetic absorbable suture are preferred for nail bed and nail matrix approximations. We use 6-0 for matrix suturing and 5-0 for nail bed. Vicryl® is preferred for its ease of knot tying, knot security, and knot sliding capabilities. Surgeons preferring monofilament sutures choose the PDS II® because of its pliability and extended wound support.

## Exsanguination and Hemostasis

A bloodless field is mandatory to perform nail surgery under optimal conditions. In minor nail surgery such as avulsions or simple nail biopsy, the assistant can apply pressure to the lateral digital arteries at the side of the digit for several minutes to facilitate short-term hemostasis, avoiding the need for a tourniquet. In larger nail surgical procedures, a bloodless field is achieved with a digital tourniquet or a pneumatic tourniquet applied to the limb after exsanguinations.

Except in special conditions (arterial trauma, amputation), no hemostasis is necessary for nail surgery. Bleeding is always abundant; a bulky dressing should be anticipated. Although bleeding may sometimes be a problem in the postoperative period, electrocoagulation should not be used to avoid nail tissue scarring that may be responsible for permanent nail dystrophy. Gentle pressure, overhead hand positioning and a bulky dressing are all that is needed in the vast majority of patients. Full-thickness grafts benefit from a tie-over dressing.

### Digital tourniquet

When the procedure is performed under local digital anesthesia, a digital tourniquet is placed at the base of the finger.[12] Digital tourniquets have been condemned on the basis of excessive pressure applied on the neurovascular bundles. It has been shown that rubber band and Penrose drain deliver high and unreliable pressure.[13] A sterile rubber glove finger whose tip has been removed may be stretched over the digit.[13] It has been shown that a rolled rubber glove whose size is equal to the patient's glove size delivers a reliable pressure under 500 mmHg.[13] The main disadvantage of the glove's finger technique is that the tourniquet can inadvertently be left in place at the end of surgery. When performing fingernail surgery, the use of a whole surgical glove offers (Fig. 23.5) a safer and reproducible digit exsanguination while providing a sterile surgical field. The whole glove cannot be forgotten during the dressing at the end of the procedure. When the glove's finger technique is used, we recommend securing a hemostat to the rubber band in order to prevent any accident; we also ask our nurse to control the tourniquet removal at the end of the procedure.

### Pneumatic tourniquet

When the patient has a digital infection or a distal vascular compromise (atherosclerosis, diabetes or Raynaud's phenomenon), a proximal pneumatic tourniquet is preferred. An awake patient will tolerate a pneumatic tourniquet for about 30 minutes; a forearm tourniquet is also adequate and may be better tolerated.[14] Longer procedures need adequate regional block or general anesthesia.

## Postoperative Dressings

We use a nonadherent dressing coated with petrolatum emulsion (Adaptic®) associated with an ointment or a cream that keeps the wound from drying and provides a good microenvironment for wound healing[15] (silver sulfadiazine, bacitracin, or mupirocin ointments). The first dressing is made with a sufficient number of large gauzes to absorb bleeding, which is always noticeable. A loose

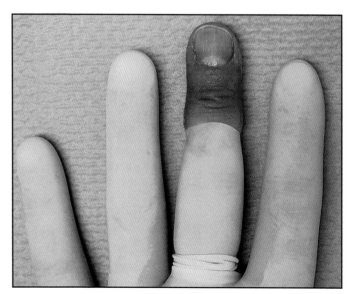

FIGURE 23-5. Surgical glove tourniquet.

bandage is then wrapped in an anatomic position and secured with adhesive tape. Postoperative forearm support is useful to avoid unnecessary digital trauma. Dermatologic surgeons commonly use antibiotic prophylaxis to prevent bacterial endocarditis. Although this practice is appropriate for high-risk patients when skin is contaminated, it is not recommended for noneroded, noninfected skin.[16] No evidence exists on the usefulness of prophylactic antibiotic administration with regard to noncomplex aseptic surgeries.[3]

The patient is generally seen at 48 hours for the second dressing; this is the time to control the wound as well as check the absence of hematoma, infection, and dehiscence. A daily dressing change is recommended for 10 to 30 days. Dressings should be changed at regular intervals according to the type of surgery (daily or every other day dressing change is usual) for 2 weeks.

## TECHNIQUES IN NAIL SURGERY

Although the surgical procedure should be tailored to each individual, we present some principles and techniques that will enhance the dermatosurgeon's results.

## Nail Unit Exposure

### Nail bed and matrix and exposures

NAIL PLATE AVULSIONS Avulsion of the nail plate, whether partial or total, is mandatory for nail bed or matrix approach. Different techniques are presented which can be tailored to individual needs.

*TOTAL NAIL PLATE AVULSION* Removal of the entire nail plate (Figs 23.6 and 23.7) is necessary when partial nail plate removal does not offer an appropriate approach to the structure that needs to be reached. When feasible, partial avulsions should be preferred because total nail plate removal may result in prolonged pain and secondary anterior nail plate embedding, which may be a problem for big toenails.

The nail plate is freed from its proximal nail fold attachments and then separated from the nail bed.

*NAIL PLATE, PROXIMAL NAIL FOLD SEPARATION* The large spatula of a Freer septum elevator is pushed back toward the cuticle and gently introduced under the proximal nail fold. Lateral gliding of the instrument liberates the proximal nail fold from its remaining nail plate attachments.

*NAIL PLATE, NAIL BED SEPARATION* The distal approach is generally preferred; the elevator is introduced under the nail plate at the level of the hyponychium and pushed gently but firmly toward the lunula where the resistance is reduced due to looser attachment. The elevator is withdrawn and moved a few millimeters laterally and the same procedure is repeated until all the nail plate is entirely detached.

In the case of exploration, simple excision or distal nail bed surgery it may not be necessary to remove completely the avulsed nail plate; the nail plate can be lifted (Fig. 23.8). In this case, the first step of the procedure is omitted (nail plate, proximal nail fold separation). The nail plate is separated from the nail bed as

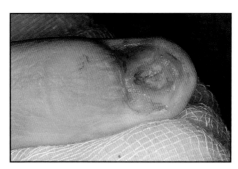

FIGURE 23–6. The large defect secondary to the tumor excision will be responsible for a secondary onycholysis.

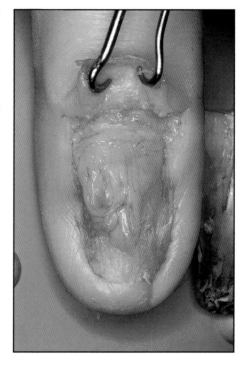

FIGURE 23–7. Onychomatricoma. Matrix approach exposes the multidigitated tumor.

explained and lifted up, the surgery performed and the nail plate positioned back in place and secured to the lateral nail folds.

A proximal approach is rarely needed (distal nail plate destruction or absence, nail bed tumefaction, distal nail thickening); once the proximal nail fold has been detached from the nail plate as seen previously, the elevator is gently pushed more proximally to come into contact with the most proximal part of the nail plate, the instrument is then reoriented downward to slide on its under surface, the instrument is then pushed in the direction of the hyponychium, detaching the nail plate from its nail bed attachment. This proximal technique is more difficult to perform and more traumatic than the distal technique.

A nail-pulling forceps, a standard Halstead hemostat, or the needle holder may be used to grasp and avulse the detached nail plate, the undersurface of which should be inspected.

*PARTIAL NAIL PLATE AVULSIONS[17]* Partial nail plate avulsion is a versatile procedure that may be performed in many different ways (Fig. 23.9).

*DISTAL AVULSIONS* Distal avulsions are used for the distal nail bed and hyponychial surgical approach. They may be central, lateral, or concern the distal half of the nail plate. Distal and

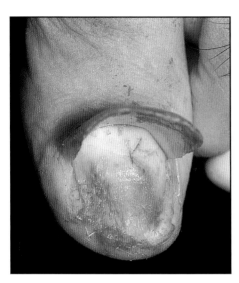

FIGURE 23–8. Nail plate is lifted up as a car cap to expose the tumor.

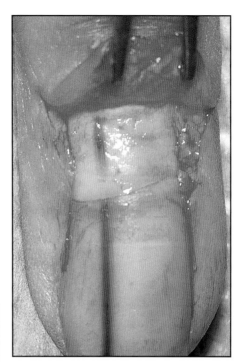

FIGURE 23–10. Junctional nevus. Proximal matrix exposed, showing the longitudinally oriented pigmented lesion.

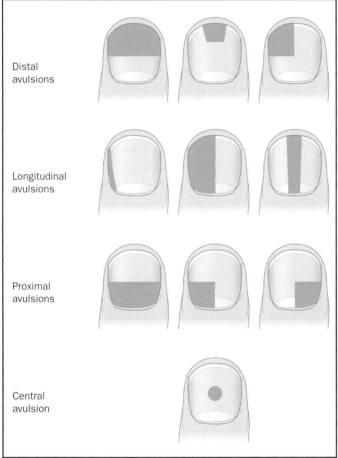

Distal avulsions

Longitudinal avulsions

Proximal avulsions

Central avulsion

FIGURE 23–9. Partial nail plate avulsion is a versatile procedure that may be performed in many different ways.

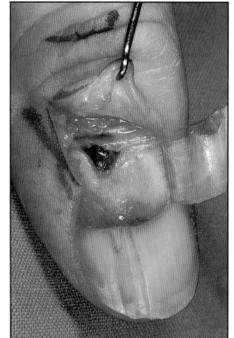

FIGURE 23–11. Matrix blue naevus. Proximal nail fold reflexion and proximal transversal nail plate avulsion are performed to give matrix access.

central quarter avulsion offers the opportunity to explore the distal nail bed, remove a foreign body, or perform a biopsy.

The portion of the nail plate to be avulsed is freed from its nail bed and attachment by inserting the nail elevator between the nail bed and the nail plate that is sectioned to the desired size with Stevens' scissors.

*PROXIMAL AVULSIONS* Proximal avulsions are used to expose the matrix; they may concern the whole proximal (Fig. 23.10), 1 : 3 or 1 : 2 of the nail plate or may be localized to a lateral portion (Fig. 23.11).

The nail plate is freed from its nail matrix and proximal nail fold attachment by inserting the nail elevator between the proximal nail fold and the nail plate, and then between the nail plate and the distal nail matrix laterally from the lateral nail sulcus at the level of the lunula. The nail plate is partially cut transversally with a Stevens' scissor and lifted up to perform the surgery (it may be a proximal hemi-avulsion or a proximal quarter avulsion). After the surgery, the nail plate is either removed or positioned back in place (in this case a 2-mm transversal recut may be needed).

*LONGITUDINAL AVULSIONS* Longitudinal avulsions may be used to expose nail bed or matrix in their lateral or central aspect (Fig. 23.12). It is possible to avulse from 15 to 80% of the lateral nail plate (Figs 23.12 and 23.13). The procedure is the same as described in total nail avulsion but limited to a narrow strip of nail plate. The nail plate is sectioned with a Stevens' scissor when the nail plate is thin (digit), with an English nail splitter for a toenail, or an anvil-action nail nipper for thick toenails. The nail plate is then removed with a Mosquito hemostat or a nail-pulling forceps.

*CIRCULAR AVULSIONS* Circular avulsions may be used for localized procedures of the central nail bed or distal matrix. This technique is useful to evacuate hematomas or remove foreign bodies such as metallic splinter or gravel that may have penetrated the nail plate. It may be used as nail bed or matrix approach before a 3-mm biopsy punch.

A 5-mm circular punch is used to drill the nail plate, which is removed as a lid.

Partial nail plate avulsion is a versatile procedure that may be performed in many different ways.

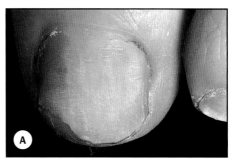

**FIGURE 23–12.** (A) Longitudinal avulsion to approach lateral nail bed (B) post-traumatic nail bed pyogenic granuloma is uncovered.

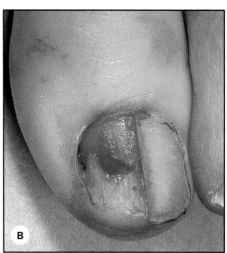

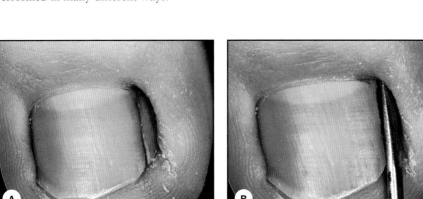

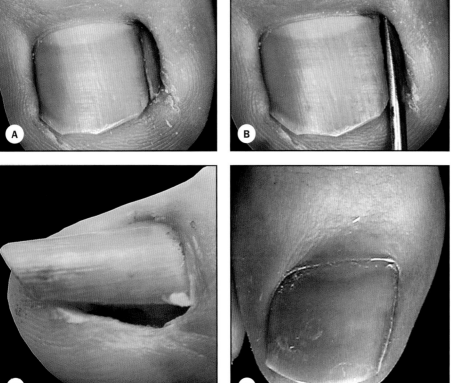

**FIGURE 23–13.** (A) Lateral nail plate section; (B) phenol application with a 3 mm large Lempert elevator; (C) lateral nail bed and matrix darkening after three phenol applications; note a tiny proximal leuconychia due to inadvertent phenol spill which will have no consequence: (D) result of a selective phenolization.

## Nail Plate Repositioning

After the surgery, the nail plate is positioned back as often as possible. Nail plate repositioning (NPR) is valuable because it protects the wound and the nail bed or matrix naturally and effectively for 3 to 12 postoperative weeks.

When the avulsed nail plate is put back in place, openings should be made at the base, extremity, or laterally, to ensure drainage (Fig. 23.14). In the case of matrix surgery, the proximal avulsed nail plate may be positioned back after a transversal recut, which offers the necessary opening drainage. Larger nail bed fusiform excisions may require large undermining and contra-lateral incisions in the lateral sulci. The nail plate is positioned back after an anterior triangular and/or lateral nail plate recut that facilitates postoperative drainage.

We avoid positioning the nail plate back when there is an infection, increased risk of surgical field contamination, and when we feel that there is a need for greater drainage.

### Total nail plate avulsion

After its removal, the plate is kept in povidone iodine. The nail plate is cut laterally (1 mm on each side) and proximally (3 to 4 mm) to facilitate postoperative drainage (see Fig. 23.14). The nail plate is then positioned back. One stitch is placed laterally on each side to secure the lateral nail plate to the lateral nail folds (Fig 23.14). The stitches are placed in the center of the lateral nail fold if the nail plate has been completely removed and placed distolaterally if the plate has just been lifted up. Another technique that is more appropriate in traumatology and nail reconstructive surgery avoids suture placement through the nail plate and bed. A longitudinal suture is placed in both lateral pulps and crossed over the nail plate in an X fashion (Fig. 23.15).

### Partial nail plate avulsion

After a proximal partial avulsion, the nail plate may be put back in place (Fig. 23.16). A proximal (3 to 4 mm) and a distal cut (1 mm) that ensure adequate drainage are done. The nail plate may then be sutured to the lateral nail fold with one stitch of 5-0 Vicryl rapide®.

## Nail Matrix Approach

Proximal nail matrix approaches necessitate proximal nail fold and nail plate reflections. The proximal nail fold is reflected by the mean of one (Figs 23.11 and 23.17) or two oblique incisions (Figs 23.7, 23.10 and 23.23) that are made at the angles of the proximal and lateral nail folds (Figs 23.11, 23.10 and 23.17). This technique was proposed by Kanavel in 1920.[18] An elevator is introduced under the nail fold to protect the undersurface from unnecessarily deep incisions. The incisions are directed toward the distal interphalangeal joint at the junction of the volar and dorsal skin. These incisions are made at an angle of 60° with the axis of the finger. This will not only avoid any inadvertent matrix incision that may lead to secondary nail plate dystrophy, but these incisions may be prolonged on the dorsum of the finger and be included in the design of dorsal rotation flaps. One incision may be sufficient for a proximolateral approach but two are needed to reflect completely the proximal nail fold. A proximal transversal nail plate avulsion is performed to give a complete access to the matrix (Figs 23.10 and 23.11). The nail fold is then retracted with skin

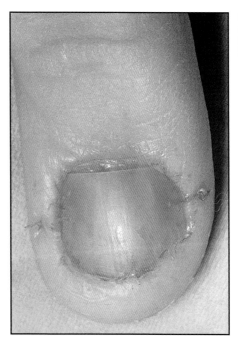
FIGURE 23–14. Nail plate repositioned and sutured to the lateral nail fold.

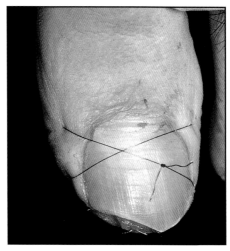
FIGURE 23–15. Nail plate repositioned with an X stitch.

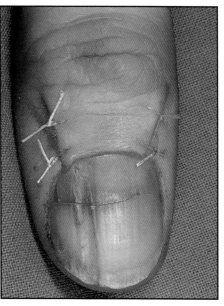
FIGURE 23–16. After completion of surgery, proximal nail fold incisions are sutured with 5-0 absorbable sutures.

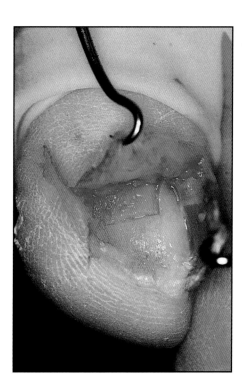

FIGURE 23-17. A shallow vertical incision is made with an eleven blade to circumscribe the lesion that will be shaved.

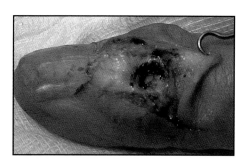

FIGURE 23-18. Cyst lining and its articular connection are colored by the methylene blue.

nail unit to finish at the opposite end (fish-mouth incision) or may be limited to one lateral nail fold. The latter approach may be used to excise subcutaneous tumors like glomus tumors or epidermal cysts, whereas fish-mouth incision is more appropriate to expose the dorsal phalanx to remove bony tumors (Fig. 23.19). The plane of dissection stands between the fat of the pulp and the nail bed dorsally. It is easier to begin the dissection in the pulp to reach the interphalangeal ligament.[19] This ligament protects the fine dorsal artery and nerve branches that innervate the nail bed. Collateral nerve and artery usually divide at the level of the DIP joint. Branches for the pulp should be left with the palmar edge of the incision.

hooks or sutures to expose the matrix. After completion of surgery, incisions are sutured with two stitches done with Vicryl rapide® 5-0 (Fig. 23.16). One stitch is placed at the very distal end of the incision to avoid unsightly nail fold retraction.

## Phalangeal and Subcutaneous Tissue Exposures

### Dorsal approach, the L incision

This technique is used to approach subcutaneous tissue of the dorsal phalanx. It may be used for digital myxoid pseudocyst excision.

The first incision is made at the angle of the proximal and one lateral nail fold until the distal interphalangeal crease (Fig. 23.18). The incision may be prolonged transversally over the distal interphalangeal (DIP) joint. Great care is necessary to avoid extensor tendon injury. The proximal nail fold may then be raised as a banner. The defect is closed with a corner stitch and two other separate 5-0 Vicryl rapide® stitches placed over the DIP and proximal to the PNF.

### Lateral approach and fish-mouth incision (Fig. 23.19)

These techniques are used to expose the phalanx, deep dermal nail bed, lateral or ventral subcutaneous tissue of the digit or toenail units.

As lateral approaches do not wound the nail bed or matrix, the theoretical risk of postoperative nail dystrophy is lessened. However, as small nerve branches are cut, persistent sensitive scars may be observed.

A lateral incision is made through the lateral nail fold at the level of the virtual line that separates the dorsal and the ventral skin. Depending on the need, the length of the incision line may vary greatly. The incision begins at the level of the distal interphalangeal crease or more distally, circumscribes completely the

## Biopsies

### Indications[20]

Nail biopsy is useful for the diagnosis and treatment of various nail diseases as well as for the prevention of potentially harmful or disfiguring conditions. Nail unit biopsy is an integral part of the dermatologist's armamentarium. Nail biopsy is indicated when careful medical history, clinical examination, and appropriate diagnostic tests (e.g. mycology, standard X-ray, MRI) fail to establish a precise diagnosis. The nail biopsy can be performed by a variety of techniques depending on the type and/or the nail unit localization. Any specific part of the nail unit (matrix, nail bed, bone, nail folds, pulp) may be sampled; nail semiology (Table 23.2) should dictate the preferred biopsy site. A nail unit biopsy that is performed using the nail surgery standards described in this chapter will not be very painful or leave unsightly scars; it should be performed wisely, as often as necessary.

A monodactylous onychopathy should always be suspected of being a tumor and sampled when a definite origin is not recognized.

The most frequent reasons to sample the nail unit are nail unit tumors (melanoma, squamous cell carcinoma, pyogenic granuloma, osteochondroma), inflammatory nail diseases (functional melanonychia, lichen planus, psoriasis), and onychomycosis.

### Localization

Nail semiology should be analyzed as critically as possible to sample the correct anatomical zone that is suspected of being at the origin of the symptomatology. When the origin is equivocal the whole nail unit may be sampled (lateral longitudinal biopsy).

NAIL BED Onycholysis, subungual hyperkeratosis, tumefaction, ulceration, tumor, pigmented macules, partial colored streaks, distal fissure, pain and distal nail plate destruction may indicate a nail bed origin.

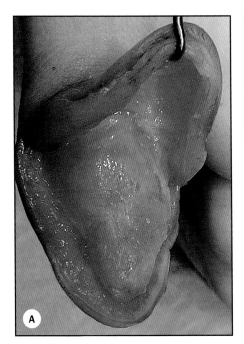 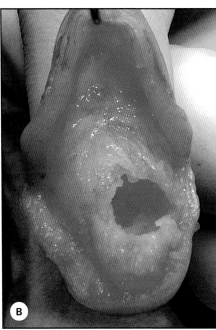

FIGURE 23–19. (A) The bony tumor (chondroma) is exposed by a fish-mouth incision; (B) the large tumor defect.

TABLE 23-2. Anatomical origin of nail signs and symptoms

| | MATRIX | NAIL BED | NAIL PLATE | PROXIMAL NAIL FOLD | BONE |
|---|---|---|---|---|---|
| Onycholysis | | X | | | X |
| Subungual hyperkeratosis | | X | | | X |
| Ulceration | | X | | X | |
| Pachyonychia | X | X | X | | |
| Dyschromia: | X | X | X | X | X |
|   macular | X | X | X | | X |
|   longitudinal | X | X | | X | |
| | Total | Partial | | Total | |
| Onychomadesis | X | | | X | X |
| Nail surface alterations | X | | | X | |
| Trachyonychia | X | | | X | |
| Fissure | X | X | | X | |
| | Deep/full thickness | Distal | | Superficial | |
| Pits | X | | | X | |
| Onychorrhexis | X | | | X | X |
| Longitudinal nail groove | X | | | X | |
| Transversal nail groove | X | | | X | |
| Nail destruction | X | X | X | | X |
| Dorsal pterygion | X | | | X | |
| Paronychia | X | | | X | X |
| Tumor | X | X | X | X | X |
| Ingrown nail | X | | | X | X |
| Acropachy | | | | | X |
| Pain | X | X | | X | X |

A single onycholysis requires atraumatic nail plate removal to rule out a nail bed tumor (Fig. 23.20).

**NAIL MATRIX** Superficial or deep nail plate surface dystrophies (trachyonychia, fissure, longitudinal and transverse depression), longitudinal chromonychia (longitudinal melanonychia or erythronychia), nail matrix tumefaction, tumor, and pain may indicate a matrix origin.

Unilateral ingrowing nail and paronychia may be secondary to nail matrix or bony tumor.

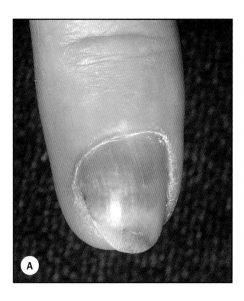
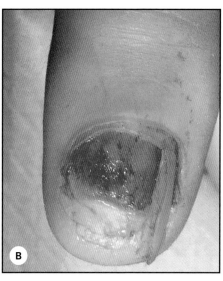

**FIGURE 23–20.** (A) Single onycholysis requires atraumatic nail plate removal; (B) nail plate section uncovers a pyogenic granuloma-like tumor, histology showing amelanotic melanoma Breslow thickness 2.4 mm.

**NAIL FOLDS** Chronic paronychia, pain, and nail fold skin alterations may indicate a nail fold origin.

As the inferior part of the proximal nail fold represents the most proximal part of the matrix, trachyonychia, transverse depressions (Beau's lines and longitudinal nail groove) may have a proximal nail fold origin.

Lateral nail fold tumors may also induce onycholysis or onychomadesis.

**NAIL PLATE** Superficial or deep chromonychia may indicate a nail plate origin (superficial or deep fungal chromonychia); in this case the nail plate itself is colored. Apparent nail plate coloration may be secondary to onycholysis (apparent chromonychia) pointing to a nail bed process (glomus tumor, pyogenic granuloma, felon, foreign body).

**BONY PHALANX** Acropachy, ingrowing nail, paronychia, onycholysis, nail bed or matrix tumor, and pain may be the symptoms of bone tumors and cysts, as well as of cartilaginous outgrowth.

**NAIL UNIT** It is not uncommon for inflammatory nail diseases or tumoral processes to have multiple anatomic localizations. On the other hand, it is not always possible to localize precisely the origin of a lesion. In these cases, a nail unit biopsy may be indicated. Laterolongitudinal biopsy or excision is often used when the pathology is lateralized.[21]

## Techniques[20]

We favor excisional biopsy when it is feasible. A larger nail unit sampling is preferred because histopathology may be challenging on a 3-mm punch; furthermore Breslow thickness measurement may be impaired if melanoma is diagnosed. Excision biopsy is also preferred because wound orientation and skin approximation warrant minimal scarring.

**PUNCH BIOPSIES** Punch biopsy is nonetheless useful; 3-mm nail bed or matrix punch biopsies leave a barely visible scar. No suturing is necessary when the punch diameter is ≤3 mm.

*PERIONYCHIUM* Proximal, lateral nail fold and the pulp may be easily punch-biopsied. Proximal nail fold sampling should be realized at least 5 mm proximal to the cuticle to avoid unsightly retraction.

*MATRIX* Except when the tumor has destroyed the nail plate and is clearly visible (e.g. pyogenic granuloma), we perform a proximal avulsion prior to a punch biopsy in this area. This allows direct visualization warranting a precise sampling.

The punch is rotated down to the bone; the specimen moving underneath the matrix epithelial level should be delicately held with the Adson forceps while sectioning its base.

*NAIL BED* The punch biopsy is realized after partial avulsion (Fig. 23.21) or nail plate lifting. The base of the specimen is always difficult to separate from the bony phalanx; it should be gently done with the 11-scalpel blade.

*BONE* Exostosis (osteochondroma) is a frequent toenail tumor that is often radiotransparent in its first few months of evolution. A punch biopsy is easily performed through the tumor when a digital X-ray is noncontributive.

*NAIL PLATE SAMPLING* Nail plate sampling is a useful tool to differentiate onychomycosis from other causes of nail plate pigmentation and subungueal hyperkeratosis (psoriasis), it is also helpful to localize the origin of a longitudinal melanonychia.

*NAIL NIPPER SAMPLING* We prefer the anvil-action nail nipper to sample distolateral nail plate specimens. This is possible when onycholysis is present. The nail nipper is introduced laterally beneath the nail plate, which is sampled when subungual hyperkeratosis is present. A distolateral triangular piece of nail plate (distally based) is taken as far proximally as possible.

**PUNCH SAMPLING** Nail plate punch sampling is very useful when a proximal white onychomycosis is suspected; anesthesia is advisable. The trephine is delicately rotated through the nail plate until it is transected, care being taken to avoid nail bed or matrix wounding during blade penetration. The specimen is meticulously separated from underlying nail tissues.

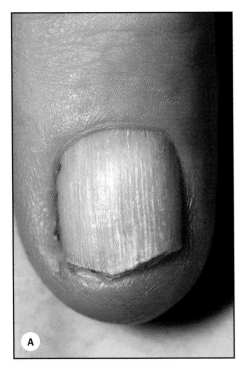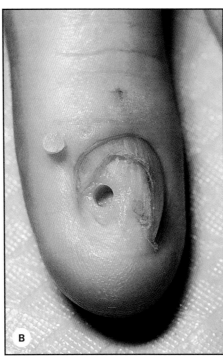

FIGURE 23–21. (A) Apparent leuconychia due to nail bed lichen planus; (B) nail plate section shows the nail bed, which is punch biopsied.

**SCALPEL BIOPSIES** The reader should refer to the excision section below.

# Excisions, Excisional Biopsies, and Destructive Techniques (Phenol, Cautery, Laser)

## Proximal nail fold

**CRESCENTIC EXCISION OF THE PROXIMAL NAIL FOLD** Small and distal lesions of the proximal nail fold may be biopsied/excised in crescent shape (Fig. 23.22). The proximal nail fold is separated from its nail plate attachment with an elevator. A crescent that is 3 to 5 mm in its maximum width can be safely excised. The incision is made with a 15-scalpel blade. Because the proximal nail fold has a triangular section, the blade and incision are oriented tangentially, the distal part of the blade pointing toward the distal nail bed. Healing by secondary intention takes place in 4 to 8 weeks.

**WEDGE EXCISIONS** Wedge excisions are used for proximal nail fold lesions that necessitate incisions that extend further than 5 mm proximal to the cuticle. Lesions 2 to 3 mm in width can be excised with a simple fusiform excision, whereas larger lesions will require unilateral or bilateral nail fold advancement flaps (see above).

## Lateral nail folds

Three millimeter large longitudinal biopsies/excisions may be realized parallel to the lateral nail sulcus. Small loss of substance of the lateral folds may be left to heal by secondary intention because local flaps would have to be taken from the pulp, interfering with finger sensibility.

## Pulp

**FUSIFORM EXCISIONS** Fusiform biopsies/excisions may be oriented transversally near the hyponychium or sagittally when localized in the ventral area.

**CRESCENT-SHAPED WEDGE EXCISION (DUBOIS' TECHNIQUE)**[22] This technique has been suggested to correct distal nail plate embedding when medical treatment (dorsoventral pulpar massaging, acrylic nail) is not successful. We have never had to use this procedure because the cases of distal nail plate embedding that we have seen were easily corrected with medical advices.

A fish-mouth incision is carried out 5 mm distal and parallel to the distal groove. A transversal fusiform excision 3 to 5 mm wide is performed. Undermining of the whole nail unit is realized over the bony phalanx. The defect is closed with 4-0 Vicryl rapide®.

## Matrix

**LONGITUDINAL MATRIX EXCISION**[23] (Fig. 23.23) Most authors recommend excising lesions with transversal incisions in the matrix area.[24] Unfortunately, nail matrix pigmentations and tumors at the origin of longitudinal melanonychia are longitudinally oriented so that transversal excision is not feasible. In fact, a 3-mm longitudinal melanoncyhia results in a rectangular pigmented macule that is 3 mm in the transversal axis and 5 mm in the sagittal axis. Even very small lesions cannot be easily excised with transversally oriented incisions. We have used longitudinal fusiform excisions in the matrix for 10 years without any significant postoperative nail dystrophy (slight focal, longitudinal nail plate thinning may be observed postoperatively).

The proximal nail matrix is exposed, a longitudinal elliptical excision of the lesion is done and incisions are done deep to the bone. It is possible to excise lesions up to 4 mm on the larger nails (thumbnail, big toenail); undermining is done for lesions larger than 3 mm. The smallest lesions (up to 2 mm) may be closed

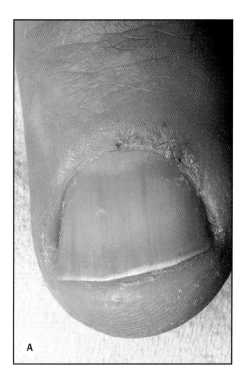
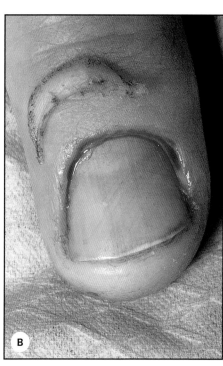

FIGURE 23-22. A crescent that is 3–5 mm at its maximum width can be safely excised.

without any undermining. Slightly larger lesions necessitate large undermining over the dorsal phalanx laterally and anteriorly; closure is then realized without tension when it is possible. If tension is excessive, a simple or double Johnson's flap is realized (see p. 289).[25]

Closure of the surgical defect is realized with absorbable suture material, the nail plate is positioned back and the proximal nail fold closed. This technique is most useful to excise lesions at the origin of longitudinal melanonychia that are less than 3 mm.

**TRANSVERSE MATRIX EXCISION** (Fig. 23.24) This technique is useful to biopsy large lesions or to expose subcutaneous tumors. After matrix exposure, a transversal incision is performed parallel to the distal border of the lunula. Subcutaneous glomus tumors may be excised through this incision. When a larger exposure is needed, the transversal incision may be prolonged by a sagittal incision to perform an A-T advancement flap (see p. 285). The wound is secured with 6-0 absorbable sutures.

**SHAVE EXCISION**[17,24,26] (Figs 23.25 and 23.26) Eckart Haneke[26] described the shave technique, which we use to sample wide pigmented bands that are considered benign. Reflection of the proximal nail fold and proximal nail plate hemi-avulsion give access to the matrix. A shallow vertical incision is made with an 11-blade to circumscribe the lesion to be sampled with 2-mm margins. The scalpel is held parallel to the nail matrix epithelium and the lesion is shaved with a tangential movement of the blade. A counterpressure applied over the patient's pulp with the help of an assistant facilitates hardening in the area.

*Modified shave technique*: because the shave technique is difficult to perform, an alternative is to dissect a very thin layer of tissue with the scalpel (superficial excision). The thinnest slice that it is possible to dissect with a hand scalpel reaches the level of the reticular dermis.

The tiny specimen should be transferred flat to a piece of cardboard, e.g. a piece from the cardboard suture packing. Superficial excisions of this type heal with minimal scarring, i.e. longitudinal erythronychia or superficial nail plate longitudinal thinning.

**SURGICAL MATRICECTOMY AND OTHER DESTRUCTIVE TECHNIQUES** Total nail matrix destruction is rarely needed to correct onychogryphosis.

*SURGICAL MATRICECTOMY* This surgical technique is difficult to perform and induces a longer walking impediment than the other procedures (phenolization, $CO_2$ laser photocoagulation and cauterization). Surgical matrix dissection should include the proximal and distal matrix, the lateral matrix horns, as well as the undersurface of the proximal nail fold.

The proximal nail plate is avulsed and the matrix exposed. The area to be excised is outlined with a shallow (2-mm deep) incision, and the epithelium is dissected from the distal part of the lunula to the matrix horns. The epithelium of the undersurface of the proximal nail fold is also removed. The proximal nail fold is positioned back in place after completion of surgery. Healing by secondary intention is obtained after 4 to 8 weeks.

*PHENOLIZATION* The phenol technique is the easiest method. Total nail avulsion is performed and the full-strength phenol applied meticulously over the entire matrix; this procedure should be repeated three to four times until surface blackening is observed, a total phenol application time of 60 seconds is necessary for adequately matrix destruction.

*CARBON DIOXIDE LASER PHOTOCOAGULATION* A carbon dioxide laser may be used in a defocused mode to vaporize the matrix epithelium after reflection of the proximal fold and proximal nail plate avulsion; care must be taken to treat the under

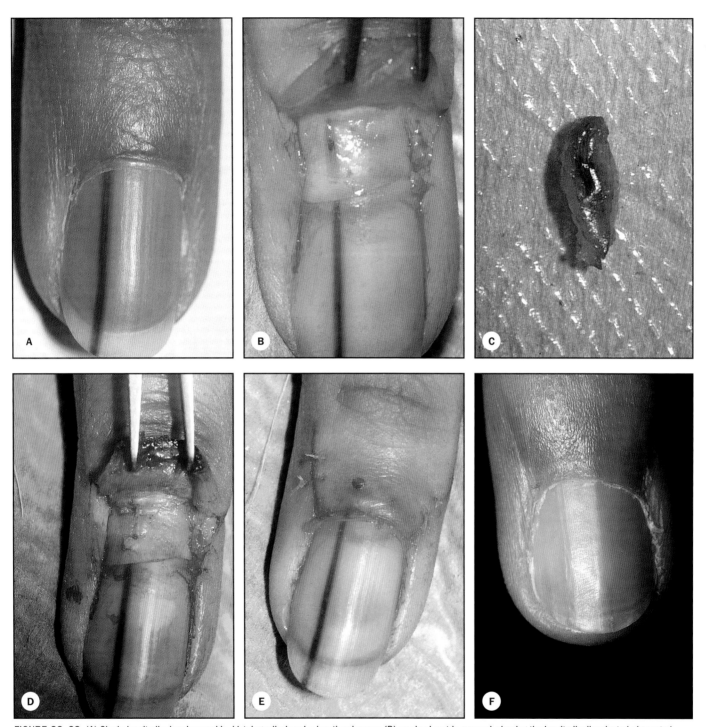

FIGURE 23–23. (A) Single longitudinal melanonychia, histology disclosed a junctional nevus; (B) proximal matrix exposed, showing the longitudinally oriented pigmented lesion; (C) longitudinally excised specimen; (D) the longitudinal wound sutured with 6-0 absorbable material; (E) the longitudinal wound is closed with absorbable material; (F) postoperative result showing slight longitudinal nail plate thinning.

surface of the proximal fold and the lateral horns. Healing takes place by secondary intention.

*CAUTERIZATION* Radiosurgery (Ellman surgitron®) and electrocautery are other alternatives. Specifically designed electrodes have been commercialized for this purpose (insulated matrix electrode set, ref H9, Ellman Corporation). Proximal nail plate avulsion is performed before electrosurgical coagulation of the matrix area,

lateral horns, and proximal nail fold undersurface. It is not necessary to open the proximal nail fold. Healing is by secondary intention.

## Nail bed

**LONGITUDINAL EXCISION** Fusiform longitudinal excision is used to biopsy or excise nail bed lesions. The nail plate is elevated

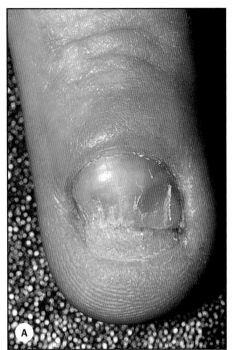 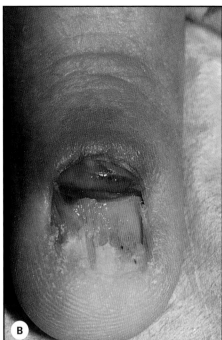 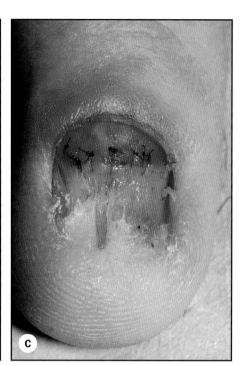

**FIGURE 23–24.** (A) Nail matrix tumor; (B) a fusiform biopsy performed after nail plate avulsion showing an orange tumor, histology diagnosed a giant cell tumor of the tendon sheath; (C) the wound is sutured with absorbable material.

or avulsed depending on the situation. A fusiform excision is performed deep to the bone; a simple excision can be realized if its width does not exceed 3 mm on the larger nails. As the nail bed dermis is firmly attached to the underlying bone without any subcutaneous interposition, its spontaneous mobility is minimal. Total nail bed and matrix undermining is necessary for the larger excisions. If closure is impossible or under tension, lateral contra-incisions in one of the two lateral nail sulci mobilize one or two flaps (see p. 285, Johnson's flap). The wound is approximated with a 5-0 absorbable suture material.

**SHAVE EXCISION** Superficial shave excision may be utilized to biopsy or excise benign superficial epidermal lesions such as onychopapillomas or to make a split thickness nail bed graft. The nail bed is exposed. The surface to be superficially excised is delimited by a shallow incision. The scalpel mounted with an 11-blade is oriented tangentially to be parallel to the nail bed surface. A progressive sliding movement excises the epithelium super-ficially. The excised material is placed on a piece of cardboard to avoid rolling up of the piece of tissue. The nail plate is positioned back in place and secured to the lateral folds by absorbable sutures. The nail bed graft should not include the deeper reticular dermis to avoid secondary scarring onycholysis.

### Hyponychium

Hyponychial lesions may be removed with an A to T flap (see p. 289, A-T advancement flap).

### Nail unit

#### LATEROLONGITUDINAL EXCISION AND SELECTIVE DESTRUCTIVE TECHNIQUES
*LATEROLONGITUDINAL EXCISION* (Fig. 23.27) This procedure is useful to biopsy[21] or remove lateral nail matrix

and/or nail bed tumors (epidermoid carcinomas, longitudinal melanonychia) or to sample the whole nail unit for dermato-pathologic examination. It is possible to remove 40 to 50% of the nail unit, i.e. 5 to 10 mm in the thumb or great toe.

The shape of the excision is that of an ellipse halved in its longitudinal axis, the straight side being on the nail plate side and the curvilinear part lying in the lateral nail sulcus or on the lateral nail fold. The incision lines are drawn before the surgery. The first incision, beginning 3 mm distal to the interphalangeal crease, is prolonged longitudinally, parallel to the lateral nail sulcus up to the pulp (3 mm distal to the distal groove). This incision transects the nail plate down to the phalangeal bone. Transection of the nail plate is done with a regular 15-blade that is progressively advanced in a sawing motion. The curvilinear side of the incision begins and ends at the same level as its straight side and curves to parallel the lateral nail sulcus (incision may be located in the lateral nail sulcus or in the lateral nail fold if its sampling is necessary). The wedge of tissue is removed over the bony phalanx, and great care should be taken to remove the lateral matrix horns. The smallest excisions (<3.5 mm) close easily without undermining. Undermining of the whole nail bed and matrix is done over the bony phalanx for larger excisions (more than one-third of the nail plate width). When closure is difficult, extending the incision up to the distal interphalangeal crease as well as soft tissue undermining of the pulpar aspect of the digit is easy and greatly facilitates the operation. This helps elevating a pulpar flap in the defect and facilitates its closure.

Suturing is realized with 4-0 (toenails) or 5-0 (fingernails) absorbable sutures. Reconstruction of the lateral nail fold is done with three stitches. A vertical mattress suture is first placed in the middle of the lateral nail fold; it is essential to obtain a slightly elevated nail fold. The suture is completed by two regular stitches, one at the level of the proximal nail fold (2 mm proximal to the cuticle) and the other at the level of the hyponychium.

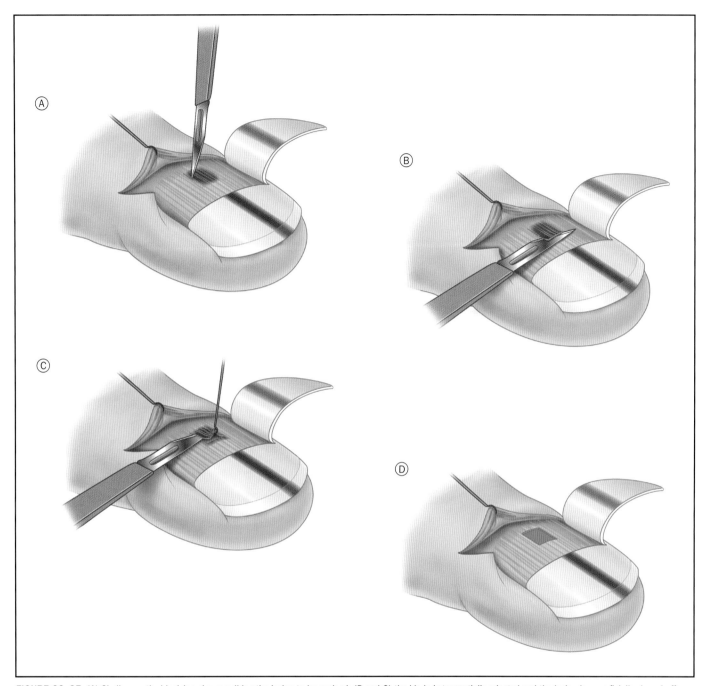

FIGURE 23–25. (A) Shallow vertical incision circumscribing the lesion to be excised; (B and C) the blade is tangentially oriented and the lesion is superficially shaved off; (D) the thinnest slice that can be made reaches the reticular dermis.

## Key Features

* The width of the excision cannot exceed 40% of the nail plate width
* Curettage of the nail matrix horns should be meticulous to avoid postoperative nail spicule growth
* Postoperative pain is always noticeable after this intervention; it should be anticipated and prevented. Adequate postoperative analgesia should be provided to the patient
* Postoperative nail aspect is very good; the rectitude of the normally rounded angle between the cuticle and the lateral nail fold is slightly noticeable

**SELECTIVE LATERAL NAIL UNIT DESTRUCTION** Selective nail unit destruction is used to correct all types of lateral ingrowing nails.

*SELECTIVE PHENOLIZATION* (see Fig. 23.13) Selective phenolization is our preferred method to correct lateral ingrown nails (juvenile type and pincer nail type). It is a simple technique with a high success rate (94.7%).[27]

The intervention begins with a unilateral or bilateral 3-mm lateral longitudinal avulsion (see longitudinal avulsions, p. 272). Although a cotton-tip applicator is recommended by most authors and may be used safely, we prefer the small 2-mm (fingernails) or

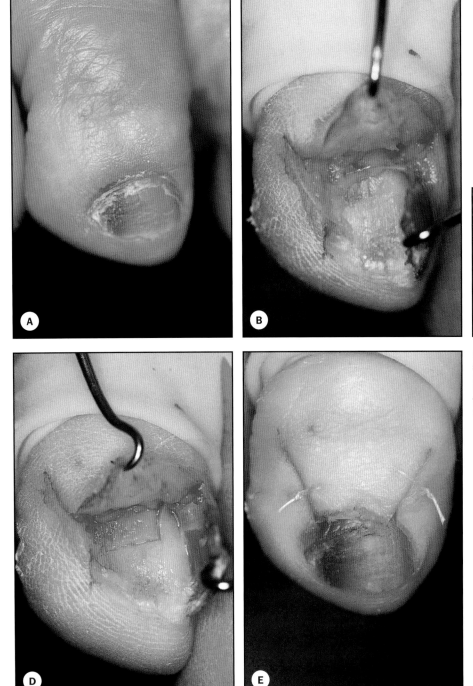

**FIGURE 23-26.** (A) Toenail longitudinal melanonychia suspected to be frictional; (B) nail matrix is exposed; (C) nail matrix specimen; (D) a shallow, vertical incision is made with an eleven blade to circumscribe the lesion that will be shaved; (E) nail fold is sutured with 5-0 absorbable material.

large 3-mm (toenails) curved elevator.[23] The lateral nail bed and matrix are carefully dried with a piece of gauze introduced along the lateral nail bed and under the proximal nail fold. This procedure, repeated from time to time during the operation, ensures a perfectly dried surgical field warranting phenol efficacy. The inferior (concave) side of the 3-mm large Lempert elevator is soaked in full-strength phenol (88%); any excess is absorbed on a piece of gauze. The tiny phenol layer covering the inferior part of the elevator is applied to the lateral matrix, ventral part of the proximal nail fold, and corresponding nail bed. When a pyogenic granuloma is associated, a drop of phenol is also applied over the granulation tissue. We generally repeat this procedure three to four times and massage these areas meticulously with phenol (until the epidermal layer slightly blackens). A total phenol application time of 60 seconds is necessary and sufficient. We take great care to treat the lateral horn(s) of the matrix(ces). Phenol is toxic to surrounding skin so care must be taken to avoid any exposure of the surrounding skin and nail tissue. We slightly rotate the digit on the same side as the phenol is applied to avoid any accidental spilling over any part of the matrix that is not to be treated.

The patients should be informed that a serous drainage can be observed for 4 to 6 weeks after a phenol matricectomy. Post-

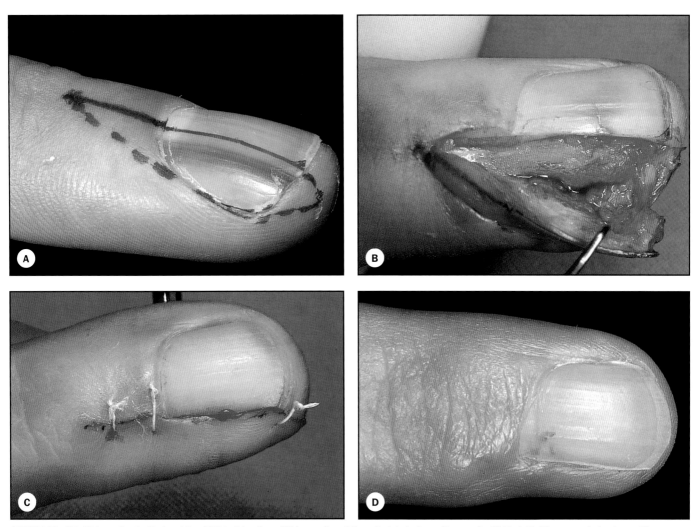

FIGURE 23–27. (A) Laterolongitudinal excision (LLE) incision lines; (B) transection of the nail plate is done with a regular 15 blade that is progressively advanced in a sawing motion and the wedge of tissue is removed over the bony phalanx; (C) suturing is realized with 5-0 absorbable sutures; (D) slight postoperative cuticular retraction.

operative pain is low (step 1 level of analgesia is recommended), as is walking impediment. Office work is possible on the next day and we recommend our patients to wear large shoes and avoid excessive walking for the first three postoperative weeks.

The recurrence rate of selective phenol matricectomy is low; it has been reported to be between 1.1%[27] and 3.9%.[28]

*OTHER TECHNIQUES* Carbon dioxide laser, electrosurgery, and radiosurgery (Ellman surgitron® and insulated matrix electrode set, ref H9, Ellman Corporation) may be used to selectively destroy lateral nail matrix and bed. These techniques are more difficult to perform, necessitate costly systems, and offer no advantages over phenolization.

*CENTROLONGITUDINAL EXCISION* Centrolongitudinal excision is a central sagittal excision that includes all the nail unit structures (proximal nail fold, matrix, and nail bed). This procedure was suggested[29] to perform a biopsy and/or appreciate the extent of malignant tumors. We have not found this technique useful because it leaves unsightly central scarring (split nail and dorsal pterygion); it can be advantageously replaced by other procedures.

*NAIL UNIT EN BLOC EXCISION* (Fig. 23.28) Nail unit excision may be used to remove malignant nail tumors or to sample the whole nail unit when a melanoma is expected.

The area to be excised is circumscribed by a shallow scalpel incision; this area is delimited laterally by the lateral nail sulci, proximally by a line standing 2 mm proximal to the cuticle, and distally by the distal groove standing proximal to the hyponychium. The proximal nail fold is reflected like a car cap by the means of two oblique incisions made at the angles of the proximal and lateral nail folds. The cuticular incision is utilized to dissect the most proximal part of the matrix constituted by the ventral part of the proximal nail fold. This dissection is quite difficult and goes proximal to the level of the insertion of the extensor tendon. The whole nail unit is then dissected over the phalangeal bone, from anteriorly and laterally. To avoid postoperative horn spike, it is mandatory to excise entirely the matrical horn. We routinely curette the lateral aspects of the distal phalanx base to avoid this potentially annoying complication.

A proximal nail fold flap is easily mobilized to cover the whole defect when localized at the 5th toenail. The defect is covered by a full-thickness skin graft that may be delayed for a couple weeks if waiting for dermatopathological results. When larger margins are

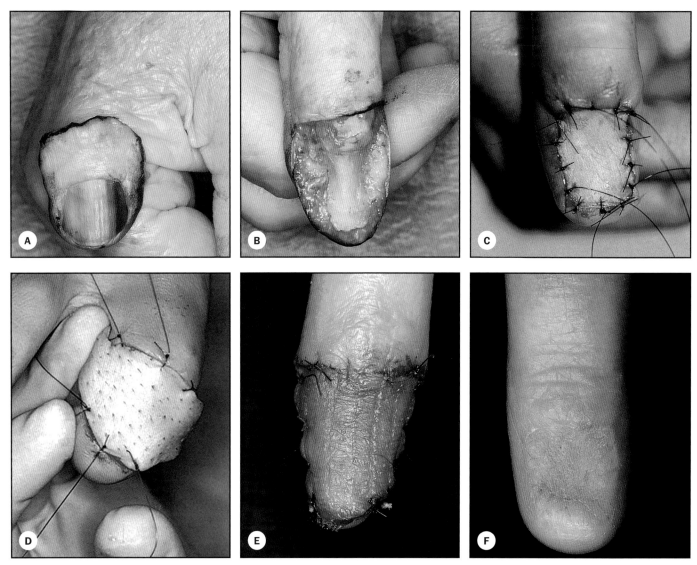

FIGURE 23–28. (A and B) Total nail unit 'en bloc excision' for a melanoma; (C) full thickness skin graft is in place; (D) tie-over dressing preparation; (E) FTSG at day 10; (F) postoperative result at 1 year.

necessary (secondary operations for melanoma in situ or spinous cell carcinoma), it is possible to circumscribe a larger excisional area (see Nail unit excision, p. 287).

*FLAPS* The lack of laxity of the nail unit is due to the absence of subcutaneous fat. This anatomical specificity explains the need to use flaps that help closure of nail unit surgical defects.

## Proximal nail fold (PNF)

Lesions of the PNF (mostly tumors) up to 3 mm in width may be excised by a crescentic nail fold removal. This technique does not necessitate any reconstruction. Healing is by secondary intention and is obtained after 6 to 8 weeks.

### ADVANCEMENT FLAPS

*WEDGE EXCISIONS* Small defects lying in the central PNF or at the junction of the lateral and proximal nail fold may be excised as wedges. The proximal nail plate is freed from its nail plate attachment by inserting the nail elevator under the PNF. Wedge excision of the lesion is then performed. In the case of a central PNF lesion, one or two relaxing incisions are made at the junction of the lateral and proximal nail folds. If the lesion is lying at the junction of one lateral nail fold with the proximal nail fold, a symmetric incision is then made at the opposite angle. Suturing of the primary defect is done with 5-0 absorbable sutures. The lateral secondary defect(s) are approximated. When complete cutaneous approximation is not feasible, the narrow secondary defects readily heal by secondary intention.

*SIMPLE ADVANCEMENT FLAP* In the 4th and 5th toes, where the nail bed is small, complete excision of the nail apparatus can be covered by simple advancement of the proximal nail fold. Two incisions are made on the nail fold up to the DIP joint. Excision is performed and closure is made by advancement of the proximal fold. Excessive tension can be relieved by raising the flap up to the proximal interphalangeal (PIP) joint. The two lateral incisions are extended laterally on the toe at the junction of the dorsal and volar skin. This flap is a variation of the bi-pedicular advancement flap described on the volar aspect of the finger.[30]

**TRANSPOSITION FLAPS**[31] Circular or quadrangular defects (up to 4 mm in diameter) lying proximal to the cuticle may be covered by a rhomboid transposition flap. The flap is raised from the skin lying in the proximal and lateral nail fold at the dorsal and ventral skin junction. The secondary defect may be left to heal by secondary intention or approximated when feasible.

**OTHERS** Larger lesions of the PNF are seen in avulsion or burn injuries. Many local flaps have been designed to reconstruct the proximal nail fold.[1] Rose also reported the use of a helix graft.[32] They are all adequate and their designs depend on the localization and extent of the defect.

One common problem with these flaps is the absence of adhesion of the undersurface of the flap to the nail plate, with secondary retraction. Shepard has proposed using a split-thickness nail bed graft on the undersurface to improve adhesion.[33]

### Lateral nail folds

The larger wounds are mostly seen in traumatology; they may also be secondary to a nail wall tumor excision. These defects are covered with larger pulpar flaps, the description of which[34,35] falls beyond the scope of this chapter. The flaps should be large enough to extend slightly over the nail plate in order to reconstruct the lateral nail fold.

### Pulp

**V-Y ADVANCEMENT FLAPS** Defects of the pulp lying close to the hyponychium may be covered by an island flap. A unilateral, longitudinal V-Y flap may be raised from the pulpar pad, or bilateral transversal symmetric island flaps may be mobilized from the skin lying at the junction of the dorsal and pulpar skin paralleling the lateral nail sulci. These flaps have been described in traumatology and fall beyond the scope of this chapter.[34,31,36]

### Nail bed and matrix

#### ADVANCEMENT FLAPS

*JOHNSON'S ADVANCEMENT FLAPS*[25] (Fig. 23.29) Simple, longitudinal fusiform excision of a nail bed is feasible when its width does not exceed 3 mm. Slightly larger lesions may be repaired by using the technique described by Johnson.

A relaxing incision is made longitudinally in one lateral nail sulcus. The entire nail bed and matrix are undermined over the phalangeal bone but left attached both proximally and distally to the hyponychial area. Sutures should be placed without tension. If it is necessary, a second relaxing incision is performed in the opposite lateral nail sulcus to gain a little more laxity. The primary defect is closed with 6-0 absorbable sutures. The secondary defects heal by secondary intention. This flap generally authorizes a 3.5- to 4.5-mm width excision on the thumb. The nail plate is positioned back and sutured after a lateral nail plate recut, which facilitates postoperative drainage.

**A-T ADVANCEMENT FLAP** We use the versatile A-T flap to close lunular (distal matrix, proximal nail bed) defects. The limbs

of the flaps curve with the lunula. The incisions that are lying in the semi circular lunular border are prolonged on both lateral sides to mobilize a bilateral advancing flap.

### Hyponychium

**A-T ADVANCEMENT FLAP**[37] (Fig. 23.30) Small lesions of the hyponychial area may heal by secondary intention. We found the A-T flap useful to reconstruct medium sized defects of this area. The A-T flap represents the shape of a triangular defect closed by advancing flaps from opposite sides of the triangle.

The nail plate is lifted to visualize the lesion excised in a triangular fashion, the base of the triangle sitting in the hyponychium and the two sides of the triangle in the nail bed. The incision lying in the hyponychial area is prolonged in both sides along the distal nail groove to mobilize a bilateral flap.

Undermining is done at the level of the subcutaneous fat on the pulpar aspect of the advancing flaps. The distal nail bed is undermined over the phalanx, mostly to facilitate suture placement. Depending on the location of the lesion, the base limbs may vary in length. The key suture is placed first; it closes the advancing edges of the two flaps together. The sides of the flaps are closed and a three-point closure is done at the end of the procedure.

### Nail unit

**SCHERNBERG'S TRANSLATION FLAP**[38] (Fig. 23.31) Central defects, up to 5 mm wide, may be repaired by a technique described by Schernberg and Amiel. The lesion is excised by a fusiform central or paracentral longitudinal excision including the nail plate, the nail bed, and the matrix. This excision extends proximally into the proximal nail fold and distally into the pulp. The larger half of the nail (when asymmetrical) is raised up and freed from its hyponychial attachment distally. The pulpar incision is prolonged laterally (3 mm from the lateral nail sulcus) on one of the lateral aspects of the digit up to the interphalangeal level at the junction of the dorsal and volar skin. The entire lateral nail fold is included in the flap when the pedicle is proximal. A constant artery, described by Flint,[19] irrigates this flap, which can be advanced and rotated so as to close the defect. The central defect is closed and the lateral one is partially left to heal by secondary intention. The Schernberg's flap leaves a central nail plate unsightly scar and should only be used in selected cases.

**BARAN AND BUREAU'S ROTATION FLAP**[39] This flap has been proposed to correct malalignment of the great toenail, whether congenital or acquired (usually secondary to nail bed scarring). When malaligment of the great toenail is associated with onycholysis, the missing or scarred nail bed should be grafted first with a nail bed split thickness graft. A crescent-shaped excision is performed, as in the Dubois procedure (see p. 277).[22] A Burrows' triangle is designed at one end of the incision, the side of which is indicated by the nail unit deviation. Burrows' triangle excision will authorize a nail unit rotation, making nail realignment feasible.

## Grafts

### Nail bed graft

Nail bed grafts are used to correct nail bed defects that cannot be repaired by the above-mentioned techniques.

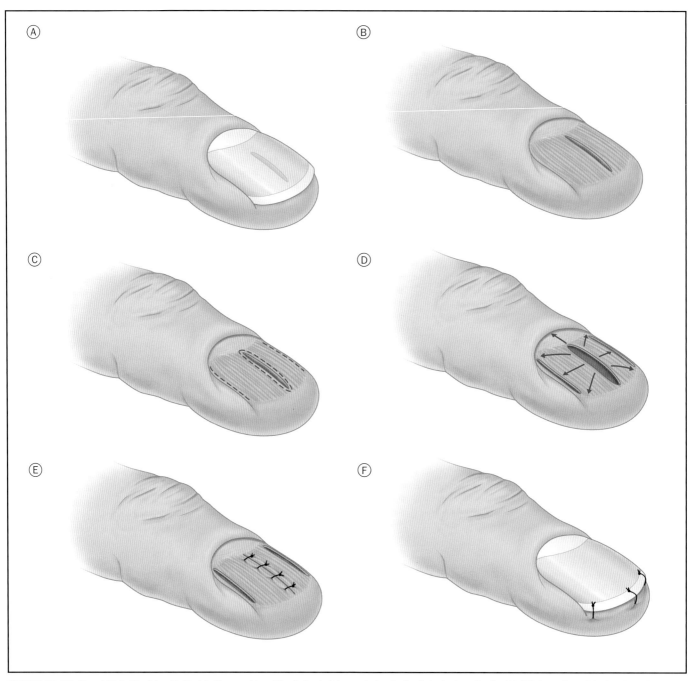

FIGURE 23–29. (A and B) Nail bed, longitudinal fusiform excision; (C) relaxing incision made longitudinally in the lateral nail sulci; (D) the entire nail bed and matrix are undermined over the phalangeal bone; (E) only the central nail bed wound is sutured; (F) nail plate is secured with 6-0 absorbable sutures.

Split-thickness nail bed grafts (STNBG), suggested by Shepard to correct post traumatic nail bed loss,[40] may also be used to reconstruct any significant nail bed epithelium defect that may be secondary to nail bed scarring or nail tumor excision.

The donor site is generally a great toenail bed, the nail plate of which is lifted up as a car cap and positioned back after the procedure. The split-thickness graft is harvested with a 15 blade held tangentially to the nail bed epithelium. The scalpel blade should be seen by transparency through the graft throughout the procedure to avoid unnecessary nail bed scarring pthat may result in postoperative onycholysis. As some contraction will occur, the graft should be slightly oversized.[33] The graft is sutured to its recipient site with untied (clear) 6-0 absorbable sutures and the nail plate is positioned back in place at the end of the procedure so as to mold the repair.

The following points issued from our experience and a literature review should be emphasized:
- Graft orientation is optional.[33]
- Split-thickness nail bed grafts are even successful on bone[33] and will gradually thicken with time.
- When the defect is small (1 cm²), the donor and the recipient sites may be on the same nail.

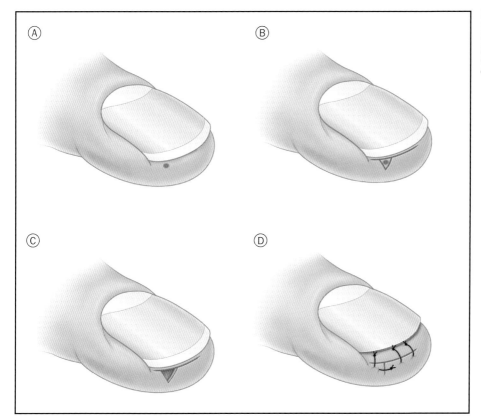

FIGURE 23–30. (A) Distal avulsion or nail plate lifting is necessary to visualize the lesion; (B) A-T flap design; (C) triangular lesion excision; hyponychial incisions are prolonged on both sides to mobilize the bilateral flap; (D) key suture is placed first; it closes the advancing edges of the two flaps together.

- Postoperative nail dystrophy is rare and mostly localized on the donor site; partial onycholysis may be observed.[41,42]

Full-thickness nail bed grafts[43] result in an unacceptable donor nail scarring, although they may be used in traumatology when an amputated finger or toenail is available as a donor.

## Matrix graft

A high failure rate and unacceptable donor nail scarring explain why nail matrix grafts have been abandoned.[44]

## Nail unit grafts

Shepard suggested en bloc nail unit grafts, including nail bed, matrix, and proximal nail fold to improve the matrix graft success rate. The full-thickness skin donor graft was placed directly over the bone of the recipient digit/toe.

Different teams reported interesting results obtained in traumatology. Shepard had a 50% success rate in eight cases;[33] we had two successes out of three cases, and Sellah reported good results in 11 out of 14 cases.[45] Nonetheless, this technique is hardly used because the donor nail unit has to be sacrificed and the quality of the results cannot be assured. Furthermore, we obtain very acceptable cosmetic results with the simple full-thickness skin grafts that we routinely use to reconstruct nail unit wound following nail tumor excisions.

## Skin graft (Fig. 23.28)

We have routinely used full-thickness skin grafts to repair complete nail unit defects for the past 12 years. Most of the time, nail unit removal is secondary to malignant nail tumor excision (melanoma, squamous cell carcinoma). These grafts protect the finger and preserve the distal phalanx when the nail unit has been removed. Although the aim of these grafts is not to replace or match any part of the nail unit, they are functional and offer an acceptable cosmetic presentation. Furthermore, full-thickness grafts often go unnoticed by a noninformed audience and are often forgotten by the patients themselves. However, patients can experience difficulty with precise handling, e.g. collar buttoning, reminding us of the role of the nail plate in fine manipulation.

From a functional point of view, our results show that most patients have normal interphalangeal motion, normal two-point test discrimination and are satisfied with the cosmetic result. We have had no nail spicule regrowth or tumor recurrence but 5 patients out of a series of 13 developed post-operative epidermal inclusion cysts.[46]

**TECHNIQUE** Draping of the donor as well as the recipient site is necessary. The technique of donor graft harvesting and placement is mostly the same as for any standard full-thickness skin graft.

*NAIL UNIT EXCISION* The incision lines are drawn first. The proximal incision line lies over the interphalangeal crease, whereas the distal line sits distal and parallel to the hyponychium (from 2 mm to 1 cm, depending on the excisional needs). A transverse incision is carried at this level down to the tip of the phalanx and prolonged laterally on both sides, paralleling the lateral nail folds. The lateral limits are guided by the excisional needs; they can be as close as 2 mm to the lateral nail sulci and extend 5 to 8 mm maximum ventrally. A transverse incision is then completed proximal to the nail matrix, usually over the distal interphalangeal

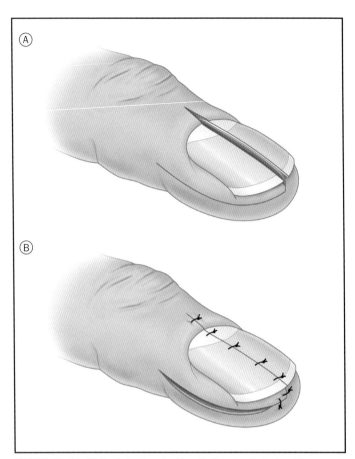

FIGURE 23–31. (A) The lesion is excised by a fusiform longitudinal excision; the pulpar incision is prolonged laterally on one of the lateral aspects of the digit; (B) the central defect is closed and the lateral one is partially left to heal by secondary intention.

joint crease. Care must be taken to prevent a distal extensor tendon injury. The lateral incisions merge with the end of the proximal one circumscribing the whole nail unit. Then, a distal to proximal sharp dissection of the nail bed and matrix is performed; great care must be taken to keep the scalpel blade in constant contact with the bone to ensure adequate excisional depth. No hemostasis is necessary.

*DONOR GRAFT SITE SELECTION* The criteria guiding donor area selection are: a minimal functional impairment, a maximal hiding of the donor site, as well as the proximity to the recipient site that will facilitate the surgery. A 4-cm² area of skin is needed; we have found the following donor sites useful: homolateral internal arms, legs or thighs; groin and gluteal folds.

*GRAFT HARVESTING* A humid gauze applied over the wound and cut to size will give a precise imprint of the surface to be excised. This imprint serves as a model to set the limits of the fusiform excision, which should have a 4 : 1 ratio in the internal arm. An injection of 10 to 20 mL saline into the dermis and subcutis before the incision helps maintain a clean dermohypodermal dissection that includes as few fat cells as possible. Tension caused by a Mosquito hemostat grasping the extremity of the excised side of the graft facilitates the procedure. The full-thickness skin

graft is harvested and the donor site is closed with subcutaneous absorbable sutures and Steri-strip® skin closure. The harvested graft is kept moist in refrigerated sterile saline.

*GRAFT PLACEMENT* The defatted full-thickness skin graft is placed directly over the deperiosted phalanx. We do not perform incisions over the graft. The graft is cut exactly to the shape of the defect and secured to the skin edges. The edges of the graft and the wound should be approximated as carefully as any side-to-side closure.[47] We generally use six to eight nonabsorbable stitches (Flexocrin® 4-0, Ethilon®), which are left long to fix the tie-over dressing that will be used. These stitches are placed at each angle and in the middle of each side of the square. Vicryl rapide® 5-0 stitches are placed in between the nonabsorbable sutures. An opened Adaptic® gauze is placed over the graft and covered by a humid, unfolded, compressed gauze. The long suture tails are tied over the Adaptic® and the gauze placed over the graft. This dressing is left untouched until it is removed on the sixth day, tied over suture are removed and a 15 minute chlorhexidine antiseptic soaking precedes adaptic dressing removal. A partial epidermal slough is not uncommon. It does not compromise the graft take but may take longer to heal completely. We have had one graft failure on the great toenail of an 80-year-old man, in whom nail unit removal was necessary for an invasive squamous cell carcinoma. Healing by secondary intention took place in 12 weeks.

### Nail unit transfer

Pedicled nail unit transfers, which were first described in the late 1970s, have mostly been abandoned. Microsurgical nail unit transfers may be used for nail unit reconstruction. A description of this technique is beyond the scope of this book but technical details can be found in a recent literature review.[48] However, this operation is rarely used because the donor nail unit has to be sacrificed and covered with a full-thickness graft. Furthermore, the cosmetic quality of the results cannot be fully guaranteed.

## REFERENCES

1. Dumontier C. L'Ongle. Paris: Elsevier; 2000
2. Krull EA, Zook EG, Baran R, Haneke E. Nail surgery: a text and atlas. Philadelphia: Lippincott, Williams & Wilkins, 2001
3. Hunfeld KP, Wichelhaus TA, Schafer V, Rittmeister M. [Evidence-based antibiotic prophylaxis in aseptic orthopedic surgery]. Orthopade 2003; 32 (12):1070–1077
4. Daly N. Fractures and dislocations of the digits. Clin Podiatr Med Surg 1996; 13 (2):309–326
5. Sylaidis P, Logan A. Digital blocks with adrenaline. An old dogma refuted. J Hand Surg [Br] 1998; 23 (1):17–19
6. Denkler K. A comprehensive review of epinephrine in the finger: to do or not to do. Plast Reconstr Surg 2001; 108 (1):114–124
7. Chiu DT. Transthecal digital block: flexor tendon sheath used for anesthetic infusion. J Hand Surg [Am] 1990;15 (3):471–477
8. Chevaleraud E, Ragot JM, Brunelle F, et al. [Local anesthesia of the finger through the flexor tendon sheath]. Ann Fr Anesth Reanim 1993; 12 (3):237–240
9. Cummings AJ, Tisol WB, Meyer LE. Modified transthecal digital block versus traditional digital block for anesthesia of the finger. J Hand Surg [Am] 2004; 29 (1):44–48
10. Salam GA. Regional anesthesia for office procedures: Part II. Extremity and inguinal area surgeries. Am Fam Physician 2004; 69 (4):896–900

11. Andrew M. Elizaga M. Ropivacaine. In: Andrew M, Elizaga M, eds. Wednesday morning conference, 26 March 1997. University of Washington, Department of Anesthesiology

12. Salem MZ. Simple finger tourniquet. Br Med J 1973; 2 (5869):779

13. Hixson FP, Shafiroff BB, Werner FW, Palmer AK. Digital tourniquets: a pressure study with clinical relevance. J Hand Surg [Am] 1986; 11 (6):865–868

14. Neumeister M, Danikas D, Wilhelmi BJ. Nail pathology. eMedicine, 2004. Online. Available: www.emedicine.com

15. Watcher MA, Wheeland RG. The role of topical agents in the healing of full-thickness wounds. J Dermatol Surg Oncol 1989; 15 (11):1188–1195

16. Scheinfeld N, Struach S, Ross B. Antibiotic prophylaxis guideline awareness and antibiotic prophylaxis use among New York State dermatologic surgeons. Dermatol Surg 2002; 28 (9):841–844

17. Abimelec P. Nail surgery made easy, can it be true? In: American Academy of Dermatology; March 1999, New Orleans

18. Dumontier C, Tilles G. Un bref rappel historique dermatologique et chirurgical de la pathologie unguéale. In: Dumontier C, ed. L'Ongle. Paris: Elsevier; 2000:3–10

19. Flint M. Some observations on the vascular supply of the nail bed and terminal segments of the fingers. Br J Plastic Surg 1955; 8:186–195

20. Rich P. Nail biopsy: indications and methods. Dermatol Surg 2001; 27 (3):229–234

21. de Berker DA. Lateral longitudinal nail biopsy. Australas J Dermatol 2001;42 (2):142–144

22. Dubois JP. [Treatment of ingrown nails]. Nouv Presse Med 1974; 3 (31):1938–1940

23. Abimelec P. Tricks and tips of nail surgery: nail symposium 344. In: American Academy of Dermatology Annual Meeting. March 1998; Orlando, FL

24. Zook EG, Baran R, Haneke E, Dawber RPR. Nail surgery and traumatic abnormalitiies. In: Baran R, Dawber RPR et al. eds Diseases of the nails and their management. Oxford: Blackwell Science; 2001:425–514

25. Johnson RK. Nailplasty. Plast Reconstr Surg 1971; 47 (3):275–276

26. Haneke E. The shave technique. In: Sixth meeting of the European Nail Society; 15 October 2003; Barcelona

27. Kimata Y, Uetake M, Tsukada S, Harii K. Follow-up study of patients treated for ingrown nails with the nail matrix phenolization method. Plast Reconstr Surg 1995; 95 (4):719–724

28. Mori H, Umeda T, Nishioka K et al. Ingrown nails: a comparison of the nail matrix phenolization method with the elevation of the nail bed-periosteal flap procedure. J Dermatol 1998; 25 (1):1–4

29. Siegle RJ, Swanson NA. Nail surgery: a review. J Dermatol Surg Oncol 1982; 8 (8):659–666

30. O'Brien B. Neurovascular pedicle transfers in the hand. Aust NZ J Surg 1965; 35:2–11

31. Lister G. The theory of the transposition flap and its practical application in the hand. Clin Plast Surg 1981; 8 (1):115–127

32. Rose EH. Nailplasty utilizing a free composite graft from the helical rim of the ear. Plast Reconstr Surg 1980; 66 (1):23–29

33. Shepard GH. Nail grafts for reconstruction. Hand Clin 1990; 6 (1):79–102; discussion 103

34. Lister G. Skin flaps. In: Green DP, Hotchkiss RN, Pederson WC, eds. Operative hand surgery. Edinburgh: Churchill Livingstone; 1998

35. Dumontier C, Legré R, Sautet A. [Perionychial reconstruction]. In: Dumontier C, ed. L'Ongle. Paris: Elsevier; 2000:97–105

36. Lister G. Local flaps to the hand. Hand Clin 1985; 1 (4):621–640

37. Abimelec P. Can everyone do nail surgery? In: American Academy of Dermatology; March 2000; San Francisco

38. Schernberg F, Amiel M. [Anatomo-clinical study of a complete nail flap]. Ann Chir Plast Esthet 1985;30 (2):127–131

39. Baran R, Bureau H, Sayag J. Congenital malalignment of the big toe nail. Clin Exp Dermatol 1979; 4 (3):359–360

40. Shepard GH. Treatment of nail bed avulsions with split-thickness nail bed grafts. J Hand Surg [Am] 1983; 8 (1):49–54

41. Pessa JE, Tsai TM, Li Y, Kleinert HE. The repair of nail deformities with the nonvascularized nail bed graft: indications and results. J Hand Surg [Am] 1990; 15 (3):466–470

42. Dumontier C, Nakache S, Abimelec P. [Treatment of post-traumatic nail bed deformities with split-thickness nail bed grafts]. Chir Main 2002; 21 (6):337–342

43. Saito H, Suzuki Y, Fujino K, Tajima T. Free nail bed graft for treatment of nail bed injuries of the hand. J Hand Surg [Am] 1983; 8 (2):171–178

44. McCash CR. Free nail grafting. Br J Plast Surg 1956; 8: 19–33

45. Sellah J, Andriamanday V, Rabaharisoa M, et al. [Composite nail transfer by the traditional method]. Chir Main 2000; 19 (1):56–62

46. Lazar A, Abimelec P, Dumontier C. Full thickness skin graft for nail unit reconstruction. J Hand Surg Br (in press)

47. Stegman S, Tromovitch T, Glogau R. Basics of dermatologic surgery. 1 edn. Chicago: Year Book; 1983

48. Endo T, Nakayama Y. Microtransfers for nail and fingertip replacement. Hand Clin 2002;18 (4): 615–622; discussion 623–624

# 24 Basic and Advanced Nail Surgery (Part 2: Indications and Complications)

Philippe Abimelec and Christian Dumontier

## INDICATIONS IN NAIL SURGERY

### Tumors

A very extensive range of tumors may be located in the nail unit. In our series of nail unit tumors – observed over the past 6 years – the most frequent were myxoid pseudocysts, warts, and fibromas, which represented about 40% of the total. These were followed in frequency by pyogenic granulomas, melanocytic nevi, glomus tumors, osteochondromas, onychopapillomas, keratoacanthomas, and onychomatricomas. Malignant tumors were not rare, squamous cell carcinomas and melanomas being equivalently represented in the range of 5%; chondromas, epidermal inclusion cysts, and giant-cell tumors of the tendon sheath were exceptional.

#### Benign epithelial tumors

**WARTS** Nail unit warts are notoriously difficult to treat and atypical warts should always be sampled to rule out squamous cell carcinoma. Children's warts most often disappear within a 2-year period and stubborn adult subungual warts respond to intra-lesional injections of bleomycin sulfate (0.3–0.6 mg/mL). In our view, electrosurgery or laser photocoagulation are seldom needed to treat subungual warts; cold steel surgery is not indicated.

**ONYCHOPAPILLOMA[1]** Onychopapilloma is a typical onycho-cytic tumor of the bed of the fingernail; the etiology is unknown. The lesion presents as a large (1–5 mm), monodactylous, longi-tudinal, pink–red band.[2] Splinter hemorrhages may be seen at the distal third of the lesion as well as a distal triangular onycholysis or a fissure. A filiform hyperkeratosis emerging from the hyponychium may sometimes be observed. Biopsy of atypical lesions is mandatory to rule out in situ squamous cell carcinoma. A shave biopsy is sufficient to ablate the lesion and offer histo-pathological examination; this should be performed along the lesion from the lunula to the hyponychium.

**EPIDERMAL/INCLUSION CYST** Epidermal inclusion cysts (Fig. 24.1) are the consequence of traumatic implantation of epidermis into the dermis or subcutaneous tissues. They can occur after a fingertip-penetrating trauma or a surgical procedure around the nail unit.[3] Periungual cutaneous cysts present as elastic, slowly enlarging subcutaneous tumors. Subungual epidermal cysts are most often asymptomatic and associated with fingernail clubbing, whereas bone cysts usually present as painful swelling of the terminal phalanx. Radiography is useful when it shows a localized zone of osteolysis. High-resolution MRI may be useful in selected cases.

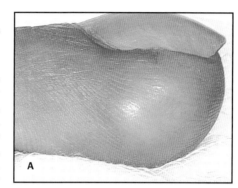
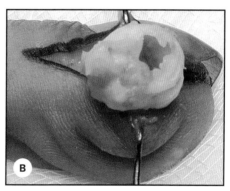

FIGURE 24–1. (A) Lateral nail fold tumefaction; (B) a lateral approach is chosen to expose the cyst.

A lateral approach is generally chosen to expose the tumor. The diagnosis becomes evident when the pearly epithelial lining and/or its characteristic content are visualized during the surgery.

Complete excision of the lesion, including its entire lining, is mandatory to avoid postoperative recurrence. In case of bony involvement, curettage of the distal phalanx until bleeding bone is found may promote healing.

**KERATOACANTHOMA** Distal digital keratoacanthoma (Fig. 24.2) presents as a painful, rapidly growing keratotic subungual tumor that is responsible for distal onycholysis.[4] Proximal lesions may present as a painful paronychia.[4] Radiographs demonstrate a well-defined cup-shaped area of phalangeal destruction. High-resolution MRI shows a large nodule with a homogenous signal and strong peripheral enhancement after intravenous gadolinium injection.[5] Subungeal keratoacanthoma seldom resolves spon-taneously and it is locally destructive. Squamous cell carcinoma is the main histological differential diagnosis. The diagnosis of distal keratoacanthoma should be based on the correlation of clinical, radiological and pathologic findings, a rapid growth being an essential criterion.[6]

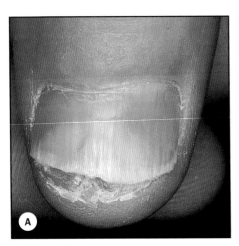

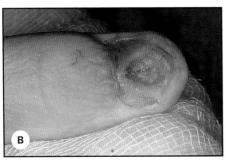

**FIGURE 24–2.** (A) Onycholysis due to distal digital keratoacanthoma; (B) the large defect secondary to the tumor excision will be responsible for a secondary onycholysis.

Complete surgical excision associated with bone curettage and histologic control of the margins is recommended. The tumor is most often located in the distal third of the nail unit. Nail plate lifting usually demonstrates the keratotic subungual mass, which is approached through a longitudinal nail bed incision; drainage of keratinous material is often spontaneous. The tumor should be carefully dissected from the surrounding tissues. The distal phalanx is often partially destructed by the tumor and bone curettage should be done carefully. Nail bed reconstruction is realized when feasible; Johnson's flap may be an option in the case of a moderately sized defect. Large loss of substance is left to heal by secondary intention. Secondary split thickness nail bed grafting is possible. Close follow-up is indicated to monitor local recurrences.

**ONYCHOMATRICOMA** Onychomatrichoma is a recently described fibroepithelial nail matrix tumor;[7] it is unique to the nail unit (Fig. 24.3). Onychomatrichomas can be unique or multiple, localized in the fingernails or more rarely on toenails. Onychomatricoma occurs in the sixth decade (mean age 51 years)[8] and presents as a partial or total longitudinal colored band (yellow, black, or white) associated with splinter hemorrhages and transverse nail plate over-curvature. Paronychia and tumefaction of the proximal nail fold may occur. The distal nail plate is greatly thickened. More rarely, this tumor may develop over the nail plate like a garlic glove fibroma.

After nail plate avulsion, the operative aspect is diagnostic. The proximal nail plate presents with multiple holes storing the filamentous digitations of the tumor that stands in the matrix area. Small tumors allow its superficial removal from the matrix without suturing; larger tumors require a deeper excision that will leave a

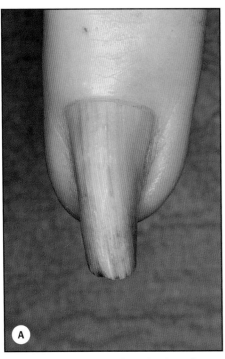

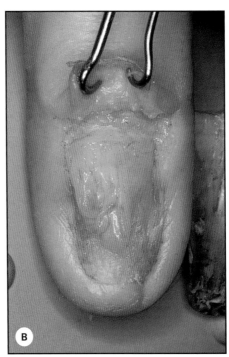

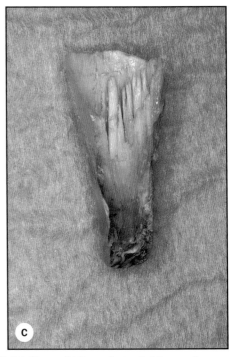

**FIGURE 24–3.** (A) Pincer nail associated revealing an onychomatricoma; (b) the matrix approach exposes the multidigitated tumor; (C) the proximal nail plate presents multiple holes storing the filamentous digitations of the tumor.

permanent onychoatrophy. Evolving lateral lesions require a lateral and longitudinal excision.

## Malignant epithelial tumors

### BOWEN'S DISEASE AND SQUAMOUS CELL CARCINOMA
Bowen's disease is a squamous cell carcinoma in situ; 3–5% of patients may develop an invasive tumor. Squamous cell carcinoma of the nail unit is linked to oncogenic subtypes of human papillomavirus associated with neoplasms of the anogenital tract.[9–11] There is often a long delay in diagnosis. Lesions are frequently monodactylous but polydactylous Bowen's disease has been reported.[11,12] The following clinical features have been associated with early evolving squamous carcinoma:[13,14]
- scaling and onycholysis that are disproportional to the verrucous changes
- periungual pigmented scaling
- lateral onycholysis with erosion of the nail bed or longitudinal melanonychia.

Other features of digital squamous cell carcinoma include periungual swelling and acropachy, hyperkeratotic tumors and plaques, crusts, nail plate dystrophy, and paronychia. An adequate biopsy specimen should be obtained to make the correct diagnosis. Multiple biopsies are often needed, and the suspected deepest part of the lesion should be sampled (ulceration, hyperkeratosis) because intraepidermal squamous cell carcinoma may be localized in some areas, whereas invasive squamous cell carcinoma may present in others. The main differential diagnoses are viral warts, infections,[15] and chronic inflammatory conditions.

The prognosis of squamous cell carcinoma is encouraging despite the frequent delay in diagnosis. Evolution is mostly local with a very low risk of distant metastasis.[16]

For most, Mohs' micrographic surgery is the treatment of choice but we have no experience with this technique.[17,18]

Early in situ squamous cell carcinoma can be treated with various destructive methods, none of which can provide adequate control of excisional margins, or complete histological examination of the specimen, which is the only way to ensure that the tumor is not invasive. In selected cases, and in experienced hands under close control, Bowen's disease of the nail unit may be treated with laser vaporization, cryotherapy, electrosurgery, or intralesional bleomycin injections (Abimelec, unpublished data). Imiquimod cream, which has been reported to be effective in a single observation, should be further evaluated before use.[19]

When Mohs' micrographic surgery is not feasible, we recommend 3-mm margins for in situ lesions; invasive squamous cell carcinoma should be resected with 5-mm margins (curettage and histopathology of the periosteum is always realized). Squamous cell carcinoma invading the bone requires amputation of the distal phalanx; sentinel node biopsy should be considered in these cases.[20] Total nail unit excision is most often needed; this is generally followed by a full-thickness graft. After surgery, patients should undergo regular follow-up.

## Soft tissue tumors

### FIBROUS TUMORS
Fibromas are benign tumors of the connective tissue. Acquired ungual fibrokeratoma (AFK), Koenen's tumors (KT), and dermatofibroma (DF) are the main forms that have been individualized.[21] Clinical and histological similarities argue for a single and identical pathologic process.[22] AFK may be post-traumatic; KT develops in nearly half of the patients with tuberous sclerosis, whereas DF appears spontaneously.[21]

Although the nail matrix is the most frequent location of these tumors, they may be localized on the periungual skin or – rarely – in the nail bed.

### MATRIX VENTRAL NAIL FOLD FIBROMAS
The elongated, conical, flesh-colored AFK tumor emerges from the undersurface of the proximal nail fold. It has been compared to a garlic clove, whereas DF tends to be spherical (pea shaped). These tumors may eventually grow within the nail plate. Matrix compression may induce nail plate thinning or a longitudinal groove.[21] KT are more often erythematous, polypoid, and digitated.

Matrix tumors are excised after matrix exposure and proximal avulsion; unilateral incision of the proximal nail fold (PNF) is indicated for small tumors. Proximal matrix is appended at the base of the matrix along the extensor tendon, simple excision is performed, and no suture is necessary. Great care should be taken to avoid extensor tendon injury. More distally located matrix lesions may require a longitudinal fusiform excision. The nail plate is positioned back and the PNF sutured. Postoperative disappearance of the nail plate caniliform depression is usual.

### PERIUNGUAL FIBROMAS
Periungual AFK appears as a keratotic papule/nodule with a peripheric collarette. Periungual DF looks similar but lacks the peripheral epidermal collarette.[21]

The preferred surgical technique depends on the size and anatomic location of the tumor (see Chapter 23):
- Proximal nail fold fibroma: Crescentic or wedge excision is often possible for small lesions; larger lesions require flaps or grafts.
- Lateral nail fold fibroma: Small lesions are left to heal by secondary intention; larger ones necessitate complex flaps.
- Pulpar fibroma: A fusiform transversal excision is realized, a fish-mouth incision, including nail unit lifting, helps to close the larger defects.

### NAIL BED FIBROMAS
These rare, pedicled tumors may be excised with a longitudinal excision technique; sessile tumors are deeply shaved, and onycholysis may result in this latter case.

## Vascular tumors

### PYOGENIC GRANULOMA
Pyogenic granuloma (PG) is a reactive process that occurs after dermal injury. Trauma, ingrown toenail, and medications promoting this complication (retinoid, protease inhibitor and anti-cancer drugs) are the most common causes of nail unit PGs. Early PGs fulfil criteria for granulation tissue. Fibrosis is present at later stages.

Periungual PG usually presents as a fleshy, ulcerated, sessile, papulonodule, which is often surrounded by an epidermal collarette. Location in the lateral nail fold of the great toe is generally associated with an ingrowing toenail.

Matrix PG has been associated with autoinduced chronic trauma, as has cast immobilization.[23] Nail bed PG (see Fig. 23.12) presents a reddish, macular discoloration seen through the nail plate and associated with onycholysis. Partial nail plate avulsion is mandatory to visualize, biopsy, and treat the lesion. Amelanotic malignant melanoma, ulcerated squamous cell carcinoma and other ulcerated tumors may be discussed; histopathology is always mandatory. Any provocative cause should be relieved (i.e. ingrown nail, retinoid). Shave/punch excision, which may be followed by slight electrodessication of the base, is curative; $CO_2$ laser may be used.

**GLOMUS TUMORS** Glomus tumors are rare. A recent review of 80 cases[24] shows that women are four times more frequently affected than men, the mean age of affected patients being 45 years. The vast majority of lesions were digital (94%), two out of three being located on the nail unit. Glomus tumors are characterized by intense, often pulsating, pain (96% of patients), which is exacerbated by the slightest contact and temperature change. A bluish-red macule may be visible either on the nail bed or the lunula in one out of two patients, and a longitudinal erythronychia or a distal fissure is suggestive; a bluish nail tumefaction or a localized nail plate destruction is rarely seen. Pin-point palpation (Love's sign[25]) exacerbates the pain in almost all patients, whereas the disappearance of pain after exsanguination of the limb and ischemia for about 1 minute (Hildreth's sign[26]) is observed in two-thirds of the cases. Love's sign and Hildreth's sign have a sensitivity of 100% and 71%, respectively, and both have an accuracy of 78%.[27] Cold sensitivity, which is present in about 50% of patients,[28] has a sensitivity and specificity of 100%.[27] Radiographs reveal a notch of the dorsal phalanx in about one out of five patients. MRI is a useful tool to visualize hidden tumors, multiple lesions, or postoperative recurrences.[5,29,30]

Complete surgical removal of the lesions is mandatory to avoid recurrences. Glomus tumors are small (mean diameter 3.5 mm, extremes 0.5–8 mm) and most often localized in the distal matrix (lunula).[24]

Two different approaches may be used:

1.  Transungual approach[31] (Fig. 24.4): We favor this approach, which we find easier. However, permanent nail scarring may be observed if the surgery is not performed meticulously according to the nail surgical principles.[32] The area where pin-point pain has been reproduced is localized with a skin marker before anesthesia. The nail matrix and nail bed approach is often necessary. This is realized by incising both sides of the proximal nail fold and completely avulsing the nail plate to obtain full exposure of the nail matrix and nail bed. Palpation can help to localize the lesion if a red macule is not visible; magnification is mandatory. Depending on the situation, incision of the nail bed and/or matrix may be longitudinal or transversal, and it should be long enough to expose the tumor without tension on the edges. Complete excision is performed, usually down to the periosteum. Closure with fine 6-0 sutures and nail plate repositioning is performed. With this technique, we had no permanent nail dystrophy in a series of about 25 cases. Bhaskaranand has proposed an elegant trick to better localize the tumor during surgery.[27] He places a tourniquet on the upper arm, without exsanguination or elevation, and places a digital tourniquet rolled over the finger. During surgery, he relieves the digital tourniquet. The soft tissues remain white and the glomus tumor becomes congested.
2.  Lateral approach[33] (see p. 274): The large incision that is necessary to expose adequately the subcutaneous nail bed and matrix is often responsible for postoperative scar hypersensitivity that may necessitate a specific treatment.[24]

After the surgery, patients are rapidly pain-free. Recurrence is the most frequent complication; it has been reported in 7 of the

80 cases of a series with a follow-up between 18 months and 5 years.[24] Multiple glomus tumors may be responsible for some of the surgical failures, which may be avoided by a preoperative MRI.

## Osteocartilaginous tumors

**SUBUNGUAL EXOSTOSIS (OSTEOCHONDROMA)[34]** Subungual exostosis (Fig. 24.5) is a benign reactive osteocartilaginous outgrowth, by far the most frequent cartilaginous tumor found in the distal phalanx. Biopsy of the lesion is easy and diagnostic in the case of evolving lesions that may be radiotransparent.[2]

Complete tumor removal, including its base of implantation into the phalangeal cortex, is required. Nail plate removal is necessary to explore the nail bed because the tumor always lies more proximally under the matrix than initially thought. We use either a nail bed approach or the fish mouth incision (see p. 278 and Fig. 24.5c) to lift the nail unit from the exostosis. Dissection is difficult because the tumor has usually thinned the nail bed and sometimes destroyed its distal part.[35,36] To avoid recurrences, it is important to completely excise the lesion, which may be adherent to the nail bed. When the cartilage cuff cannot be dissected from the bed it may be necessary to sacrifice some nail epithelium. 'En-bloc' resection is difficult because the phalanx cortices are usually hidden by the tumor. We prefer to remove as much as possible of the tumor with a bone chisel and then to excise its base with either a curette or a bone rongeur until we reach the spongiosous bone. We believe that it is safer to observe the spongiosous bone (i.e. remove the entire cortical bone) to be certain of a complete excision. This is necessary to avoid frequent recurrences in cases of partial removal. The incidence of postoperative recurrence is between 6 and 12%.[35,36] More aggressive resection may lead to unnecessary nail bed scarring and secondary onycholysis. Nonetheless, we feel that postoperative onycholysis is more often the consequence of tumoral nail bed destruction than surgical sequelae.

When surgical resection is responsible for a nail bed wound that cannot be repaired by simple approximation, healing by secondary intention is more appropriate than nail bed reconstruction with nail bed graft or flaps. The final postoperative follow-up of our patients has demonstrated that their nail unit returned to a normal aspect or presented a distal onycholysis associated with subungual hyperkeratosis.

**ENCHONDROMAS (CHONDROMAS)** Intraosseous enchondroma (Fig. 24.6) is a rare cartilaginous tumor in the distal phalanx.[37,38] Dermal tumors are exceptional. Enchondroma may be asymptomatic but usually presents as a pathological fracture. Large phalangeal tumors may be responsible for fingernail clubbing, paronychia, nail discoloration, longitudinal ridging, onycholysis, or a subungual tumor. When the lesion is revealed by a fracture, the cortical bone is so thin that bone fixation would be very difficult, and it is then safer to wait 1–2 months before tumor removal until healing is complete. Chondromas develop proximally into the phalanx; a lateral approach is indicated to preserve the nail bed. The cortical bone is usually very thin and can be cut with the blade. A small curette is useful to remove the blue–gray tumor, the texture of which is very soft. Complete removal of the tumor is mandatory; preoperative control (X-ray or fluoroscopic) may be needed. As the base of the phalanx is very thin, great care should be taken to avoid penetrating into the distal interphalangeal joint; bone grafting is superfluous. Remodeling of the phalanx shape may be required when the extremity has been distorted by the

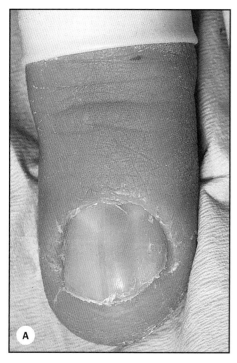
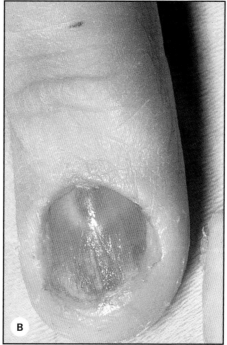
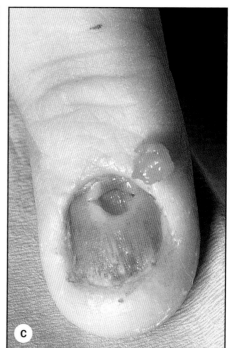

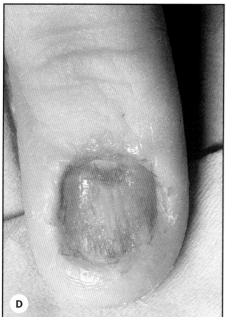
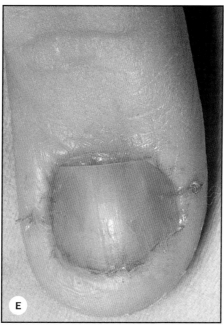

**FIGURE 24-4.** (A) Longitudinal erythronychia; (B) total nail plate avulsion expose the nail matrix tumor; (C) a transverse matrix incision exposes the subcutaneous tumor; (D) simple wound approximation with 6-0 absorbable sutures; (E) the nail plate is repositioned and sutured to the lateral nail fold.

slowly growing tumor. Phalangeal bone crushing is sometimes necessary to obtain adequate contouring.

**OSTEOID OSTEOMA** Osteoid osteoma rarely occurs in the distal phalanx; an 8% incidence has been reported.[39] Pain is the most common complaint (92%).[40] This is characteristically relieved by aspirin in 42% of individuals and pain relief frequently heralds radiographic changes. Swelling, clubbing, and nail thickening are the most common symptoms (75%).[40] Continuous tomography with thin continuous slices is the best imaging technique,[41] as standard radiographs may be nonspecific.[42]

Fish-mouth incision is the surgical approach of choice, (see p. 278) offering adequate phalangeal exposure. Bone grafting may be necessary.[42] Soft-tissue reduction has been suggested to avoid persistent digital swelling[43] when tumor removal is complete. The nail unit usually returns to its normal shape with time.[43]

## Melanocytic tumors

**LONGITUDINAL MELANONYCHIA** Longitudinal melanonychia (LM) presents as a tan, brownish, or black longitudinal stripe of the nail plate resulting from an increased melanin deposition.

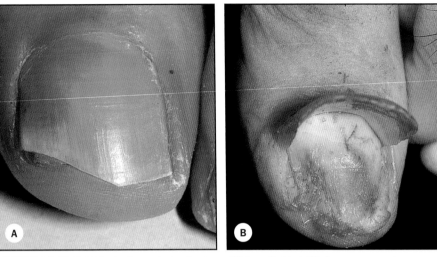
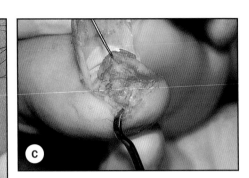
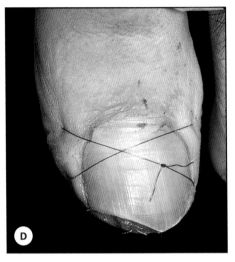

FIGURE 24-5. (A) Distolateral subungual osteochondroma; (B) the nail plate is lifted up as a car cap to expose the tumor; (C) tumor exposition; (D) the nail plate repositioned with an X stitch.

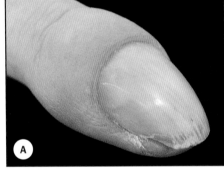
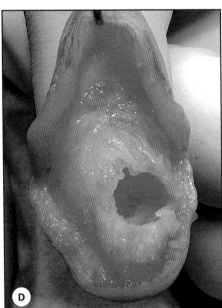
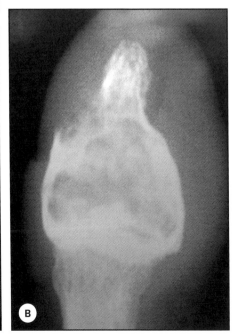
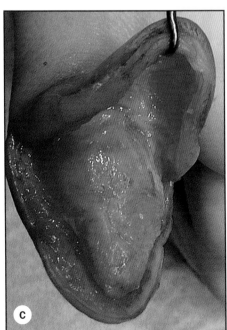

FIGURE 24-6. (A) Acropachy, clubbing and striated leukonychia; (B) X-ray showing the radiolucent defect; (C) the tumor is exposed by a fish-mouth incision; (D) the large tumor defect.

Pseudo LM resulting from nail bed pigmentation simulates this condition (i.e. splinter hemorrages, onychomycosis, foreign bodies). LM has numerous etiologies that can often be recognized by a careful medical history, clinical examination, and selected diagnostic tests. Because LM has been established to be an early sign of melanoma, a biopsy should be performed when its cause is not apparent.

In a recent study on 'idiopathic' single melanonychia in caucasian people, histopathology showed hypermelaninoses (i.e. melanocyte activation) in two-thirds of the patients, melanocytic nevus in 22%, lentigo simplex in 8% (increased number of single melanocytes), and melanoma in 5%.

We recommend the biopsy or excision of single LM with no clear etiology (onychomycosis, proximal nail fold rubbing, drug intake, etc.) or that fail to cure despite adequate treatment or preventive measures.

We differentiate small LM that can be entirely removed with good cosmetic results from large LM for which total excision may induce significant postoperative nail dystrophy on the following criteria:

- Small LM include central LM = 15% of the nail plate width (3 mm on the adult average thumb plus 0.5 mm margins on each side = 4 mm) or lateral LM = 30% of the nail plate width (6 mm on the adult average thumb plus 0.5 mm margins on each side = 7 mm).
- Large LM include central LM >15% or lateral of the nail plate width and lateral LM >30% of the nail plate width.

Although there is no way to differentiate accurately between a benign and a malignant LM, the ranking of the clinical signs of adult LM into intermediate- and higher-risk lesions is useful on practical grounds (Table 24.1). Histopathologic diagnosis of intra-epidermal (in situ) melanoma of the nail unit is difficult and it is always preferable to sample the whole lesion from the onset. A number of clinical signs have been associated with melanoma of the nail unit. We have classified clinical signs into intermediate and high risk, offering the possibility to artifically separate high risk LM from the larger subset of intermediate and lower risk lesions. Although there is no evidence to support this view, our experience shows that most of our adult patients presenting with LM with one of these high-risk signs have a melanoma.

A review of children's LM[44] has shown that 12.5% presented as totally black nail (two lentigo, three nevus). There are three main objectives for removing the lesion at the origin of an LM: (1) histopathologic confirmation of a nail unit melanoma as well as establishing the Breslow thickness and Clark's level; (2) histopathologic confirmation of a suspected benign LM (hypermelaninoses, lentigo simplex, melanocytic nevus) and removal of the lesion to avoid long-term follow-up, practitioner suspicions, and patient secondary anxiety; (3) clarifying a doubtful diagnosis.

We advise complete excision of LM when it is easily feasible without significant postoperative nail dystrophy.

### INTERMEDIATE-RISK LESIONS

- Central LM: Simple longitudinal fusiform excision (see p. 277) is our preferred method for smaller lesions. We perform either transversal matrix biopsy (see p. 278) or a shave excision (see p. 278) for larger lesions.
- Lateral LM: We recommend lateral longitudinal excision (see p. 279) of lateral LM. It is possible to remove 5–10 mm width in the thumb or great toe.

---

**TABLE 24–1.** Adult LM clinical signs ranking

| | INTERMEDIATE RISK | HIGH RISK |
|---|---|---|
| History | Personal or familial history of melanoma | |
| | Dysplastic nevus syndrome | |
| Age | Fifth decade or over | |
| Race | Dark skinned individuals | |
| Topography | Thumb, hallux, index finger | |
| | Dominant hand | |
| **Clinical presentation** | | |
| Color | Dark brown or black | Jet black color (Caucasian)[d] |
| | | Variegated colors (Caucasian)[c] |
| Width | LM ≥5 mm | Whole black nail[c] |
| Aspect | Atypical aspect compared to other bands in the same individual (multiple LM) | Multiple streaks of different hues (Caucasian) |
| | | Rectangular dots (dermoscopy) |
| | | Larger base width |
| | | Tumor[d] |
| Skin pigmentation | | Hutchinson's sign[a,c,d] |
| Nail plate | | Nail plate dystrophy[b,c] |
| Evolution | | No improvement despite adequate treatment |
| | | Rapid increase in size and growth rate of nail band[d] |

[a]Cutaneous periungueal true pigmentation is the absence of other recognized etiology.
[b]Onycholysis, fissure, destruction.
[c]This sign has been described or observed by one of the authors in association with a benign lesion in children.
[d]This sign has been described or observed by one of the authors in association with a benign lesion in adults.

*HIGH-RISK LESIONS* We recommend total excision of larger high-risk lesions; when the band is very large it means total nail unit excision from the onset. When the diagnosis of melanoma is highly probable, we do not close the wound and wait for histopathologic results before reoperation and reconstruction. When Hutchinson's sign extends far beyond the nail unit we excise the nail unit lesion and perform one or several distant punch biopsies.

*DIFFICULT CASES*

1. Longitudinal melanonychia in children: We recommend regular follow-up and removal of small (as defined above) LM as soon as it is possible to do this under local anesthesia, provided complete excision is secured from the onset. We remember the case of an 8-year-old Japanese girl whose excised LM demonstrated an incompletely removed junctional nevus. The lesion quickly recurred with extensive periungueal pigmentation over the PNF and the pulp requiring a large periungual skin excision that confirmed the benignity of the tumor. We counsel regular follow-up of large LM for which excision would require a surgery that will leave unnecessary scarring. We advise total excision of high-risk LM, especially when the lesion is rapidly widening and darkening. Nail unit melanoma is exceedingly rare but has been described in children.[45–48] As nail matrix biopsy can result in nail deformity, early and partial surgery can result in recurrence, and melanoma is rare in the pediatric age group, there is some controversy[49] as to whether this procedure should routinely be performed in children. Goettmann proposed that LM in children does not require diagnostic biopsy except for lesions that rapidly increase in width and in darkness of color.[44] Bukas reports two cases of dramatic longitudinal melanonychia in toddlers.[48]

2. Multiple LM (including multiple LM in darkly pigmented individuals): The follow-up of patients with multiple LM is always challenging because most of these individuals are dark skinned and are at increased risk of developing acral melanoma. We always look for any provocative cause, which we treat when feasible (drug intake, onychomycosis, etc.). We suggest regular follow-up and we sample any high-risk lesion. Nonetheless, it not rare to find dark-skinned individuals presenting multiple black nails (i.e. five toenails) or having multiple large LM with several streaks of different hues. In these difficult cases, evolution (rapid increase in size and growth rate of a single band) as well as comparison with other bands in the same individual (atypical aspect compared to other bands) plays an important role in deciding which band should be sampled.

**JUNCTIONAL NEVUS AND LENTIGO SIMPLEX** Melanocytic nevus of the nail apparatus is a benign neoplasm derived from melanocytes. Junctional nevus shows melanocytes arranged in nests at the dermoepidermal junction. Compound nevus shows melanocytes that are both present in nests at the dermoepidermal junction and in aggregates in the papillary dermis. Lentigo shows melanocyte hyperplasia; there is an increase in the number of melanocytes among basal onychocytes. There is no evidence to support the view that an acquired nail unit melanocytic nevus is at higher risk of malignant evolution than its skin counterpart. A recent study tends to show that acquired nevi on the soles, palms, and nail apparatus do not seem to be a risk factor for acral

melanoma in the Japanese population.[50] The incidence of nail unit melanocytic nevus within LM has been recorded to be 22% (22 of 100 adults and children with LM)[51] and 47.5% in children[44] (19 out of 40 children with LM).

The clinical aspects of nail matrix nevi (NMN) are often indistinguishable from those of malignant melanoma[51] (Fig. 24.7). NMN may be congenital or acquired. Among adults, NMN appear in the third decade. The thumb and the big toe are affected in nearly two-thirds of cases. NMN present as a single LM that is most often wide (mean width 4 mm, totally black nail in 12.5% of the patients). The color is dark brown in two-thirds of cases, sometimes with linear streaks of hyperpigmentation; a light brown color is noted in one-third of patients. Nail plate alterations, Hutchinson's sign, and gradual enlargement or fading are more rarely reported. A totally black nail was seen in 25% of children's NMN but was never present in adults.[51] The clinical differential diagnosis of NMN is that of LM. Because it is not possible to differentiate NMN from early evolving melanoma on clinical grounds, the recommendations and excision techniques proposed in the LM subchapter should be followed.

**BLUE NEVUS**[52,53] Nail unit blue nevus is a rare melanocytic proliferation of the nail unit that may present as a pigmented macule of the distal matrix; it may be associated with a longitudinal pigmented nail groove[54] (Fig. 24.8). Hyponychial and proximal nail fold blue tumors have been described,[39] as well as single case of malignant blue nevus.

Simple fusiform longitudinal excision or an A-T advancement flap may be indicated.

**MELANOMA** Life-threatening tumors such as melanomas need early recognition and appropriate treatment, which is not necessarily mutilating. Nail unit melanoma has a reported incidence of 0.75–3.5% of all melanomas in the White population;[55–57] this rises to 15–20% in the African–American population.[58]

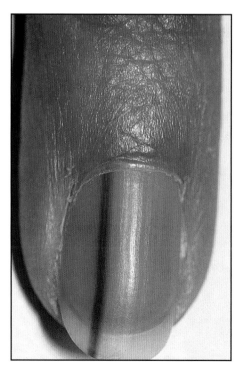

**FIGURE 24-7** Single longitudinal melanonychia; histology disclosed a junctional nevus.

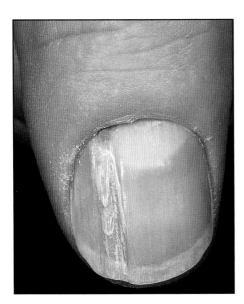

FIGURE 24–8 Lunular dark blue macule and longitudinal depression secondary to a blue nevus.

**TABLE 24–2.** Surgical margins of melanoma*

| STAGE | MARGIN |
| --- | --- |
| T1 (< 1.0 millimeter): | 1 centimeter (radial) |
| T2 (1.1–2.0 millimeters): | 1–2 centimeters, depending on location |
| T3 (2.1–4.0 millimeter): | 2 centimeters |
| T4 (> 4.0 millimeters): | 3 centimeters |

*Primary surgical closure wherever possible.

The prognosis of subungual melanomas is essentially related to their Breslow tumor thickness and Clark's level of invasion. Early diagnosis and surgical removal are necessary to improve the currently poor survival rates.

LM has been recognized as an early precursor of melanoma. Amelanotic melanoma accounts for between 11.7[59] and 22.8%[60] (21.7% in our personal series) of nail unit melanoma, the initial presentation of which lacks precision. We had the opportunity to observe six amelanotic melanomas that presented as: a violaceous pyogenic granuloma-like tumor of one lateral nail fold (Breslow thickness 2.7 mm), a longitudinal nail fissuration (Breslow thickness 0.1 mm), and a tumor growth destroying the nail plate (Breslow thickness 1.2 mm); three cases displayed onycholysis masking a pyogenic-like tumor growth (Breslow thicknesses 2.4 mm, 4 mm, and NA) (Fig. 24.9).

Initial assessment, staging, and follow-up are similar to that for melanomas of other skin sites. As there are no specific guidelines concerning the surgical treatment of nail unit melanoma, the recommended surgical guidelines on cutaneous sites based on

T staging (Table 24.2) apply. However, we feel that these recommendations should be adapted to localization and recent publications.[56]

For melanoma in situ, we take a 5 mm margin and advocate total nail unit excision to the underlying bone. The excision may be extended over the pulp when necessary and the phalanx shortened when necessary. The wound is covered by a full-thickness graft (see Fig. 23.30).

For invasive melanoma, amputation of the digit/toe is required. Studies have shown no benefit of proximal over distal amputations for nail unit melanoma.[61–63] Provided adequate excision of the lesion is performed, the level of amputation is chosen to obtain the best functional outcome (distal interphalangeal joint for the fingers, proximal interphalangeal or metatarsophalangeal joint for the toes). Although the study by Thomas[64] was not specific to nail unit melanomas, the results evidenced a significantly higher regional recurrence rate for high-risk melanoma (as defined by a tumor thickness of at least 2 mm) excised with 1 cm margins versus those for which a 3 cm margin was chosen, but a similar overall survival rate. Although there are no data to demonstrate any survival benefit in melanoma, sentinel node biopsy is proposed to our high-risk melanoma patients.[20] Therapeutic lymphadenectomy is advised when there is clinical evidence of metastatic disease in regional lymph nodes.

The delay in diagnosis is reflected in the relatively small number of patients diagnosed with stage I (TNM[20] classification) subungual melanoma (20%), as compared with cutaneous melanoma (80%).[57]

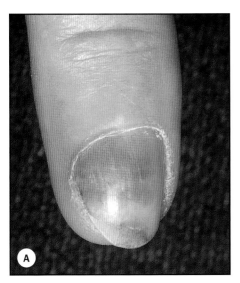

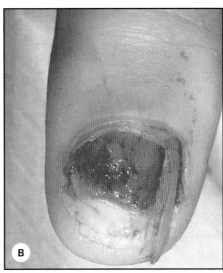

FIGURE 24-9. (A) Single onycholysis requires atraumatic nail plate removal; (B) nail plate section uncovers a pyogenic granuloma-like tumor, histology showing amelanotic melanoma Breslow thickness 2.4 mm.

The severe prognosis of melanoma is mostly the consequence of a late diagnosis. The frequency of failure of the first line physician to recognize the signs or to perform a biopsy from the correct site is the most important reason for this delay.[65] A late diagnosis may also relate to the patient not presenting early in the course of the disease.[65]

The prognosis of subungual melanoma depends mostly on its thickness; whereas previous reported series had poor 5-year survival rates[55,66–68] (16–60%), Breslow's thickness of the tumors was greater than 4 mm in most cases. Early evolving melanomas may be definitely cured after simple nonmutilating surgery. We have diagnosed 23 nail unit melanomas in the past 13 years, 10 of which were in situ (43.4%) and 13 of which were invasive, with an average Breslow thickness of 1.13 mm (0.1–2.7 mm). From these invasive melanomas, five were amelanotic (38.3%), reinforcing the need for early clinical recognition.

For these reasons, most single LM should be sampled to rule out subungual melanoma. Isolated onycholysis should be explored; nail plate sectioning is required and biopsy mandatory when a tumoral outgrowth is observed. Unexplained monodactylous nail lesions should be referred to an experienced dermatologist for further evaluation and biopsy.

## Pseudotumors

### Myxoid pseudocyst (ganglion, myxoid cyst)

Most authors believe that myxoid pseudocysts represent synovial joint herniation[69,70] associated with distal interphalangeal joint osteoarthritis. Periungual myxoid pseudocysts are easily recognized. Preoperative intra-articular injection of methylene blue dye generally identifies the cyst and its pedicle.[70,71] Periungual fingernail lesions are more frequently located on the radial fingers,[72,73] whereas toenail lesions are uncommon. Spontaneous discharge may lead to septic osteoarthritis. Subungual variants are not exceptional and may be coupled with the classical periungual type. They present as subungual tumors and may be associated with red lunula, and transverse nail plate over-curvature leading to an ingrowing nail.[74] The diagnosis is easily confirmed by high-resolution MRI.

Because the care of these lesions may be approached differently, we have presented the views of both the surgeon and the dermatologist.

**THE DERMATOLOGIST'S APPROACH** In our experience, the level of complications related to the treatment of myxoid pseudocyst is directly related to the aggressiveness of the technique, and hence to its success rate. Different medical treatments have been reported; cryotherapy, intralesional corticosteroid injection as well as injection of sclerosant[75], we have used the latter satisfactorily for 5 years.

Injection of sclerosant is our first choice: Local anesthesia is not mandatory. After meticulous skin prepping, the cyst is punctured and the jelly-like fluid evacuated. Compression on the lateral digit induces exsanguinations and a small amount of sodium tetradecyl sulfate 3% solution is injected into the cyst and the surrounding tissues (0.1 to 0.2 mL) with a 30-gauge needle. (In 1977, the French authorities labeled sodium tetradecyl sulfate 3% [Sotradecol®] as a treatment for mycoid pseudocysts as well as a vein sclerosant.) Local tissue necrosis and distal digital edema may be observed over the following days. Most patients are cured after

a single injection and very few need a second or third injection.[75] Patients have no postoperative pain or working impediment and we have not observed or heard of any significant complication. We do not use this technique when there is an open wound secondary to spontaneous discharge or in cases of vascular compromise (Raynaud's phenomenon, arteriopathy).

Minimally traumatic surgery[72] is our second preferred treatment if the sclerosant technique is contraindicated or failed to cure the patient. Our technique is similar to that described by de Berker.[70] We perform a preoperative methylene blue dye intra-articular opacification. The digit is positioned in 20° flexion and the needle introduced in the articular space through the volar joint crease. The solution is prepared with one tiny drop of methylene blue dye diluted with 1 cc of sterile saline solution; 0.1 or 0.2 cc are injected into the articular space. An L incision placed over the DIP exposes the blue-colored pseudocyst, which is meticulously dissected (Fig. 24.10). We place a 5-0 resorbable monofilament suture at the base of the cyst to enhance subcutaneous fibrosis obliterating the connection with the joint space. The articular space is not opened and the skin flap is closed. The postoperative course is mostly uneventful. de Berker reported a 94% cure rate for the fingernails; this fell to 57% for the toenails.

**THE SURGEON'S VIEW** Treatment is based on our 'knowledge' of the physiopathology. Surgical treatment is the only one that has been evaluated by large studies.[72,76] Since the recurrence rate of the surgical approach is reported to be between 10 and 20%[77–80] in most of the series, it is superior to the medical treatment in this regard.

Many surgical techniques have been proposed. We use a five-step technique:

1. 'En bloc excision' of the cyst and skin coverage in an elliptic fashion with respect to the underlying nail matrix. Simple excision of the cyst with skin suture at the end leads to a 25% recurrence rate.[78,79] de Berker reported a 3% recurrence rate in the finger after simple excision of the cyst and ligation of its base. However, he did not make a simple incision but designed a flap that he repositioned in place at the end of the procedure.[70] In the case of subungual myxoid pseudocysts, nail plate-lifting transverse matrix incision is necessary to approach and excise the lesion.
2. Opening of the joint between the extensor tendon and the collateral ligaments and excision of the osteophytes with a small curette.[81]
3. Large excision of the dorsal capsule from the collateral ligament to the extensor tendon.
4. Lavage to remove the synovial fluid and the debris.
5. Coverage of the skin loss of substance with either a rotation flap or a split-thickness skin graft. Many series consider skin excision and coverage as the most important factor to avoid recurrence.[69,78] We favor the graft because it seems to be less painful for the patient than rotational flaps that are always under tension.[82] It is also the only way to completely close the wound with a single technique. It also offers a way of reconstructing the proximal fold in cysts that extend distally. Unlike other authors,[81] we do not believe that skin graft or flaps can favor nail matrix injury and hence postoperative nail dystrophy.

Chaise reported a 1% recurrence rate[72] with the same technique. Other authors had less favorable results: A total of 17% of patients had a loss of extension (possibly due to the progression of

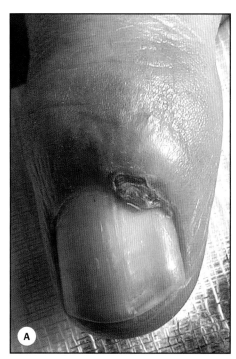

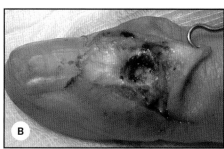

FIGURE 24-10.
(A and B) Pseudomyxoid cyst after methylene blue injection. The cyst lining and its articular connection are colored by the methylene blue.

colored 6-0 PDS® or 6-0 Vicryl®. Matrix exposure is often necessary.

At the end of the surgical procedure, a hole should be drilled in the nail plate to avoid hematoma and/or infection before replacing the nail plate in its original location. Replacing the nail plate has many advantages: It limits pain during dressing, protects and molds the repair, limits wound granulation, serves as a splint for phalangeal fractures, and increases pulp sensitivity. If the nail plate is absent, substitutes have been proposed but various dressings are usually cheaper.[85,87,88] We immobilize the finger with a large dressing and do not use complementary finger splints. Toenail surgery principles are similar but the higher frequency of infection makes antibiotic prescription mandatory. Infections are rare in the hand, even in case of an open fracture, and antibiotic prescription should be considered only on a case-by-case basis.[85,89]

### Subungual hematoma

Although unknown, the precise frequency is very high. Nail bed hematoma results from a crush injury that causes a blunt trauma to the nail bed; as the nail remains in place, blood collects under the nail, forming a hematoma, and hyperpressure causes excruciating pain. The thumb is the most commonly involved digit, followed by the index finger.[90] Small hematomas, i.e. involving no more than 25% of the visible nail plate, are usually not painful and do not require drainage, because they will be absorbed into the nail plate and evacuate with nail growth. Hematomas involving more than 25% of the nail plate should be drained to relieve pain and to avoid secondary infection or hyperkeratinization of the nail bed with secondary nonadherence.[90] Zook et al. have proposed a surgical exploration of the nail bed when the hematoma involves more than 25% of the visible nail plate.[85,88] However, this proposition is exaggerated because prospective studies have shown that: (1) less than 50% of patients have a lesion of 2–3 mm, i.e. amenable to sutures;[91] and (2) drainage of the hematoma, whatever its size and/or association with a phalangeal fracture, always cured patients without nail dystrophies.[89] To correctly evacuate the hematoma, trephination should be performed with one or two holes in the nail plate. Many techniques have been proposed but a red-hot paperclip remains the simplest and the most frequently used at the moment.[89,90] After piercing the hole(s), the hematoma should be evacuated with manual pressure, and the nail molded onto the nail bed to avoid recurrence. We usually fix the nail plate with one or two Steristrips®. Nail bed hematomas may only be removed if seen in the first 48 hours; antibiotics are not used.

### Subungual foreign bodies

One simple option is to lift the nail plate under anesthesia to remove the foreign body. For longitudinally oriented foreign bodies in patients who prefer not be anesthetized (mostly young children who need general anesthesia), it is possible to remove the foreign body with a #15 scalpel blade and to shave the nail plate above the foreign body. Once the nail plate is thin enough, the foreign body can easily be removed.[92] However, this technique leads to a groove in the nail plate that may take some weeks to disappear.

degenerative arthritis), there were two deep infections (which eventually required joint fusion), and 7% of patients developed a nail deformity that was not present preoperatively.[83] A prolonged edema interfering with PIP mobility is observed occasionally and acute septic arthritis requiring distal interphalangeal amputation has been reported (oral communication). The longitudinal nail plate canaliform depression that is most often present preoperatively always disappears after the intervention.[74]

## Traumatology

Finger injuries represent about 10% of all traumas and involve the nail one time out of four; crush injury is responsible for 50–80% of all nail lesions.[84,85] As nail bed and matrix are maintained between two rigid structures – the distal phalanx and the nail plate – a lesion means that, often, either the phalanx (about 50% of cases) or the nail plate is fractured.[84–86] Pulp and nail unit injuries are six times more frequent than isolated nail unit injuries.[85,86]

### Common principles of nail traumatology

The nail plate, often intact, hides the lesion and must be removed in almost all cases. All lesions must be repaired, using either non-

### Isolated nail plate avulsion

We think it is better to replace the nail plate in this rare injury after lavage and the drilling of one or two holes for drainage. The nail

plate may adhere temporarily and protect the nail bed. In the absence of associated lesions, the use of nail plate substitutes placed under anesthesia is probably useless.

### Nail bed injuries

These must be distinguished from matrix injuries because the therapeutic possibilities and potential sequelae are different. Inadequate initial management of nail bed injuries will lead to a loss of nail adherence (onycholysis).

### Simple injuries

These are linear wounds that require lavage without debridement because the nail bed is highly vascularized and not elastic enough for simple closure after debridement.[93] Wound closure will be performed using non-colored 6-0 sutures.[88] A few sutures are sufficient, as the nail plate that will be replaced at the end of the procedure will mold the repair. 'Normal' nails are observed in more than 90% of patients.

### Crush injuries

Basically, the treatment is similar, although removal of highly contused tissues may lead to loss of substance. Again, the dermatologist must be very economical and take advantage of two favorable circumstances: (1) the high vascularization of the nail; and (2) the possibility of healing as free graft of devascularized nail bed tissues.[88] Large wounds will be sutured using 6-0, and devascularized fragments will be replaced. Replacing the nail plate is mandatory to mold and maintain the fragments.[88,93]

### Associated phalangeal fractures

If the fracture is not displaced, which is the most frequent case, no complementary treatment is needed because the repositioned nail plate will serve as a splint. Displaced fractures must be reduced and stabilized with a K-wire or a needle according to size. Malunion is responsible for secondary nail dystrophies. Associated fractures lead to less satisfactory results.[86] Transversal nail bed wounds associated with fracture of the nail plate may be treated with a 20-mm needle passed through the nail plate and the nail bed on both sides of the fracture line. The suture is then wrapped around the needle, which acts as a tension band technique.[94]

Results
Results are good in 90% of the cases.[85,87,93] The more severe the lesion the worse the results obtained. Others have reported less satisfactory results with 30% of split nails, 9% of fragile nails, and 3% of distal onycholysis.[84]

### Nail bed loss of substance

These lesions carry the worst prognosis and represent about 15% of all nail lesions.[85] Two types of lesion should be described: if the nail bed is still adherent to the nail plate, this is a virtually ideal situation, and both the nail plate and nail bed should be replaced 'en bloc'. The nail bed will act as a free graft with an ideal tension. We have always had excellent results with this technique, like Shepard, who claimed 91% good results.[95] A lost nail bed fragment should be replaced because spontaneous healing always gives

unsatisfactory results. Many techniques have been described, but only three are still in use.

- A complete nail apparatus is available from an amputated finger. The nail bed must be used as a full-thickness nail bed graft as described by Saito.[96]
- If nail bed loss is distal and associated with a limited pulp injury, we recommend Foucher's technique, to treat both lesions at the same time. A V-Y pulp flap is designed with a de-epidermized distal part, and used to reconstruct the distal nail bed. In our experience, the nail plate always adheres over 75% of the nail surface.[97]
- If neither solution is possible, a split-thickness nail bed graft must be used.[98] In 1990, Shepard reported 84 split-thickness nail bed grafts.[95]

Only Ogunro has reported spontaneous healing without nail bed grafting under nail plate substitute, with 14 good results.[87] This limited experience raises the question of whether a nail bed adherent to the nail plate may be regenerated from the surrounding tissue.

### Nail matrix lesions

These must be distinguished from nail bed lesions because sequelae are more frequent and more severe, including split nails or absence of nail plate. When the proximal nail plate and matrix takes off the nail fold, results are usually good, as simple repositioning of the nail plate under the nail wall is sufficient.[88,98] Linear wounds must be sutured but results are usually less satisfactory than after nail bed wounds. In case of excessive tension, nail matrix flaps must be used; the nail matrix translation flap described by Johnson is sufficient for a 2–3-mm-wide loss of substance.[99] The nail matrix translation-advancement flap described by Schernberg is useful for a loss of substance of 4 to 5 mm in width[100] (see p. 285, Schernberg's translation flap).

In case of a loss of substance that cannot be closed with these techniques, free matrix grafts have always given disappointing results, whatever the technique, and microsurgical vascularized grafts must be considered.

### Distal amputations through the nail

When feasible, finger replantation is the best treatment option.[101] Nail bed dystrophies depend on the initial lesions and the quality of the revascularization.[102] Although fingertip replantation scores better than other techniques, it is far from being aesthetically perfect and frequently does not restore the appearance of the digit to normal.[103] Hyperesthesia and tenderness have been reported in up to 46% of cases of replantations and 18% of patients have had some residual nail deformity.[103,104] In another series, 9 replanted digits out of 27 have had a normal nail, 3 were slightly deformed, and 9 had a moderate deformity.[102] Technical details are beyond the scope of this chapter but are available elsewhere.[105] When microsurgical replantation is not possible, try – in the following order:

1. The reposition-graft technique: Nail apparatus and phalanx are replaced 'en bloc' and the pulp is reconstructed using a volar advancement flap.[106] Secondary nail dystrophies are frequent but the finger keeps its length and aesthetic and/or functional procedures may be used secondarily.[107] With the reposition-flap repair in two stages, Mantero reported 72% good results in 50 cases, but no details were available.[106]

The fingers were shorter by an average of 4.4 mm due to bone resorption from the distal fragment. Foucher, with a one-stage technique, reported 24% moderate hook-nail deformity, and all the fingernails were clawed in Dubert's series.[107,108] Time off work was twice as long as finger replantation and averaged 4 months in Dubert's series.

2. Finger shortening: This can be considered if the nail matrix is intact. The finger will be shorter but if the nail matrix still has a bony support, hook-nail deformity seems rare.[109]

3. Free pulp reposition: The first and only technique used initially, it seems that successes are less common than previously described.[110] Reported successful 'take' of this type of graft has been 75% when amputation is distal, at the level of the pulp, and 25% if it is at the level of the lunula.[112] Some technical improvements have been proposed to increase the success rate but large series are lacking.[112] Using ice and aluminum sheets, Hirase recently reported a 91% success rate.[101] In non-microsurgical replantation, Rose reported good results but there is some digital shortening[112] and deformed nails. With Hirase's cooling technique, 11 fingers survived completely and one developed partial necrosis (a survival rate of 90.9%). No details are given regarding nail regrowth or late bone resorption.[101]

### Nail fold lesions

These rare lesions may be responsible for cosmetic sequelae. Proximal nail wall lesions may be responsible for loss of the shinning of the nail plate. If the lesion goes beyond the nail plate, healing may lead to a pterygium that may limit nail growth. In case of loss of substance, local rotational flaps are usually sufficient.[113] To avoid a pterygium, some authors have proposed to use split-thickness skin graft at the deep part of the flap, while Shepard recommends split-thickness nail bed graft.[95] Our experience is limited but apparently these techniques give good results.

### Children's injuries

Basic principles are similar but the main problem is that some surgeons and many parents are reluctant to operate on young children. However, good results are usually observed after surgery and sequelae (pain and nail dystrophies) are frequently observed if surgical treatment has been inadequate or not used.[114]

## COMPLICATIONS AND SEQUELAE IN NAIL SURGERY AND THEIR TREATMENTS

All nail surgeries may have complications, which often depend on the type of procedure. In a general study of 78 patients, the complications of nail surgery included anesthetic allergy, infection, hematoma, nail deformity, pyogenic granuloma, inclusion cysts, persistent pain and swelling, and reflex sympathetic dystrophy.[115]

Nail surgery is delicate, requiring special training. Clumsiness and lack of experience or knowledge that may be responsible for inappropriate interventions cannot be regarded as complications. Some nail surgery procedures will necessarily result in nail sequelae that should be detailed with the patient preoperatively.

## Complications

### Pain and swelling

Pain and swelling are by far the most frequent complications after nail surgery. Pain management is explained above. Venous and lymphatic drainage of the nail is very efficient but swelling of the skin is frequent and mostly depends on the degree of the surgery. Meticulous handling of tissue, sutures without undue tension, postoperative elevation of the hand, non over-compressive bandage can help to prevent excessive swelling.

### Necrosis

Fingertip necrosis and toe necrosis have been reported after nail surgery when the tourniquet was left in place. Placing the entire glove or placing a clamp on the rolled glove are simple techniques to avoid this complication.[116]

Localized epidermal slough is usual after a full-thickness graft, its extent and frequency being somewhat greater on the toenails. Healing by secondary intention is generally obtained after a couple of weeks of standard wound care.

### Hematoma

Postoperative hematoma should be avoided; it is very painful and may be responsible for secondary infection. As no electrocautery is used during nail surgery, appropriate drainage is mandatory to avoid postoperative hematoma. Nail plate repositioning, nail plate holes or recuts (see p. 276), as well as compressive dressings to avoid dead space are simple and efficient techniques. Skin sutures should not be tied too strongly; it is useless and detrimental to place too many stitches.

### Infection

Most infections are the consequence of postoperative hematoma or tissue necrosis. They can be prevented by adequate drainage and by placing sutures without undue tension. Antibiotic prophylaxis is controversial (see p. 269, Preoperative assessment). We advise antibiotic prophylaxis for foot surgery and for patients whose mucous cyst has opened before the surgery. In cases where an infected nail requires surgery, it is preferable to culture the area and clear the infections with targeted antibiotics prior to surgery.

### Reflex sympathetic dystrophy

Although common after hand surgery or traumatic injury, reflex sympathetic dystrophy (RSD) has rarely been reported after nail procedures;[117] one case has been described after nail biopsy.[118] RSD is a complex and poorly understood condition evolving in three stages:

- The acute inflammatory stage includes a burning pain out of proportion to the extent of the injury, redness, swelling, increased sweating, coolness, and stiffness of the involved extremity. Paronychia resembling bacterial whitlow[119] and leukonychia[120] have been described at this stage.
- The inflammatory stage is followed by a dystrophic stage that begins after 1–3 months. The second stage is associated with increasing pain, pronounced stiffness, cyanosis, and radiographic evidence of patchy osteoporosis of the involved extremity.

• The third, atrophic, stage is characterized by skin and subcutaneous atrophy that may be disabling and last for years. Early recognition and treatment by an experienced team is essential to prevent disabling sequelae.[121] Analgesia, rest, sympathetic nerves blocks, and calcitonin injections are the mainstay of the treatment.

### Epidermal inclusion cysts

The incidence of postoperative inclusion cysts (Fig. 24.11A) has been reported to be 5.5%.[3] Prevention necessitates gentle mobilization of tissue when suturing or when using penetrating tools. See p. 291 for a treatment review.

### Nail spicules

Nail spicules (Fig. 24.11B) are seen after lateral matricectomies, lateral longitudinal excisions, or total nail unit removal. Some authors have reported that this complication was more frequent after phenol matricectomy than after a surgical one;[122] we do not share their experience.

To avoid spicule formation, it is mandatory to destroy the proximal nail matrix lying close to the junction of the volar and dorsal skin at the finger, and ventral to this junction at the toe. After a surgical matricectomy, lateral longitudinal excision or total nail unit removal, a meticulous curettage of the matrix horn to the bone is an essential step. Phenol matricectomy should be performed with the same elevator as the one that we use for partial avulsion, this instrument offering precise phenol application capability. Post phenol nail spicules are most often seen in the first three months after the surgery, evidenced by a proximal ingrowing nail that needs to be operated on at another time with the same method. Post surgical nail spicule generally occurs in the proximal nail sulcus or in the middle of the proximal nail fold. The treatment of this kind of spicule is always a technical challenge. We open the proximal nail fold unilaterally as explained for nail matrix exposition (see p. 276, nail matrix approach), the line of the incision being in line with the nail spicule. The incision is often extended laterally until the lateral horn of the matrix can be visualized. The nail spike is dissected meticulously to reach its base

at the matrix. We end the procedure by a delicate curettage of the base of the phalanx and suture back the PNF.

## Sequelae

### Nail matrix scarring

**DORSAL PTERYGION** Dorsal pterygion may be secondary to the surgical nail matrix scarring. Repositioning the nail plate has limited the incidence of postoperative pterygium in the surgery of glomus tumor.[80]

Pterygion repair may be attempted when its width is small. Nail plate avulsion exposes the matrix. Any proximal nail fold fusion is separated from the matrix and the scar is excised and sutured with 6-0 absorbable sutures. The volar surface of the proximal nail fold is grafted with a split-thickness nail bed graft according to Shepard[95] to avoid recurrence. The nail plate must be embedded in the sulcus to delineate the scarring tissues. Reparation may be imperfect and leave a smaller but noticeable midline nail split, about which the patient should be informed.

**LONGITUDINAL CHROMONYCHIA** Longitudinal chromonychia (erythronychia or leukonychia) may be secondary to a longitudinal or shave excision, a punch biopsy, or any limited (3 mm or less) nail matrix scarring.

**FOCAL NAIL THINNING** Focal nail plate thinning (Fig. 24.12) may be secondary to any nail matrix excision. Longitudinal nail biopsy leaves a slight longitudinal red nail plate flattening that is barely visible.

**BRITTLE NAIL** Brittle nail may be secondary to large nail matrix biopsy that was not adequately sutured.

**LONGITUDINAL NAIL FISSURE** Persistent longitudinal nail fissure (Fig. 24.13A) is secondary to longitudinal nail unit, matrix and/or nail bed excisions, and Schernberg's flap; these procedures should be avoided when feasible.

A limited nail matrix scarring (3 mm or less) will result in a temporary longitudinal fissure. This fissure is usually observed when

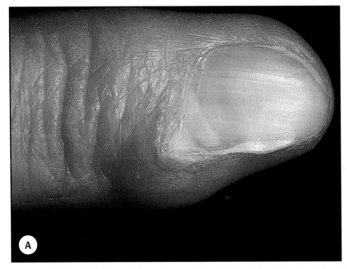
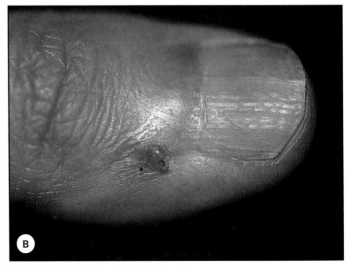

FIGURE 24–11. (A) Epidermoid inclusion cyst following lateral longitudinal excision; (B) nail spicule following lateral longitudinal excision.

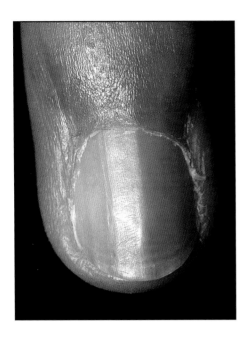

FIGURE 24–12. Postoperative result showing slight longitudinal nail plate thinning.

the nail regrows and will last for 4–6 months on fingernails and for 8–12 months on toenails. This longitudinal fissure will disappear being replaced by a permanent longitudinal chromonychia.

**DISTAL NAIL FRACTURE** This can be the consequence of nail matrix scarring secondary to an excision that was not sutured.

## Nail bed and hyponychial scarring

**ONYCHOLYSIS** Onycholysis (Fig. 24.13B) is the consequence of larger nail-bed loss, such as can occur after the removal of nail-bed or phalangeal tumors, e.g. an exostosis which can excessively thin the nail bed epithelium.

Scarring onycholysis may be repaired by a split thickness graft (see p. 286, nail bed grafts).

**VENTRAL PTERYGION** Hyponychial interventions may leave a painful ventral pterygion, the repair of which should be discussed on a case-by-case basis.

## Nail unit scarring

**SECONDARY MALPOSITION** Excessive lateral longitudinal excision has been reported to induce nail malposition.[123] Deviation of the distal nail towards the side of excision can be explained by two mechanisms. The matrix may become distorted by the unilateral loss of a ligamentous structure extending from the lateral ligament of the distal interphalangeal joint.[123] There may be a reduction of embedding of nail in the lateral nail fold on the operative side in spite of a thorough lateral nail fold reconstruction. This reduction may result in an unopposed inward force from the remaining nail fold.[123]

A Baran–Bureau rotation flap may be designed if the deviation is severe (see p. 285).

**ONYCHOATROPHY** Nail matricectomy will result in nail plate absence, also named onychoatrophy. The persistence of the nail bed will leave a thin layer of hard keratin that may be sufficient to position an acrylic nail plate. Nail matrix and nail unit removal may heal by secondary intention in small digits, providing the wound does not go down to the bone. The resulting scar will not be able to receive a false nail.

## Proximal nail fold scarring

**CUTICULAR RETRACTION AND CUTICULAR ASYMMETRY** This may be the consequence of a biopsy that is done too close to the cuticle. Biopsy or excision in this area should be performed

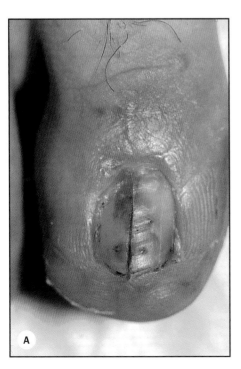

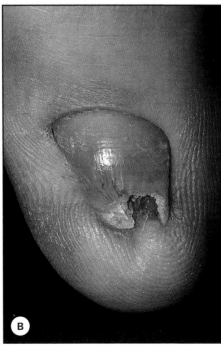

FIGURE 24–13. (A) Longitudinal fissure secondary to a Schernberg's flap; (B) onycholysis after osteochondroma removal.

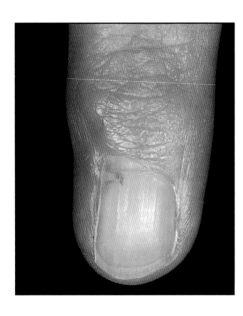

FIGURE 24-14. Slight postoperative cuticular retraction.

at least 5 mm proximal to the cuticle. Cuticular retraction (Fig. 24.14) or asymmetry may be corrected by 'en bloc' proximal cuticular resection.

**SUPERFICIAL NAIL PLATE ALTERATION** Because the inferior part of the proximal nail fold corresponds to the proximal matrix, any injury can induce a superficial nail plate alteration (localized trachyonychia).

# REFERENCES

1. Baran R, Perrin C. Longitudinal erythronychia with distal subungual keratosis: onychopapilloma of the nail bed and Bowen's disease. Br J Dermatol 2000; 143 (1):132–135
2. Abimelec P, Grußendorf-Conen EI. Tumors of hair and nails. In: Hordinsky MK, Sawaya M, eds. Atlas of hair and nails. 1st edn. Philadelphia: Churchill Livingstone; 2000:141–150
3. Wadhams PS, McDonald JF, Jenkin WM. Epidermal inclusion cysts as a complication of nail surgery. J Am Podiatr Med Assoc 1990; 80 (11):610–612
4. Baran R, Goettmann S. Distal digital keratoacanthoma: a report of 12 cases and a review of the literature. Br J Dermatol 1998; 139 (3):512–515
5. Drape JL, Idy-Peretti I, Goettmann S, et al. Subungual glomus tumors: evaluation with MR imaging. Radiology 1995; 195 (2):507–515
6. Baran R, Mikhail G, Costini B, et al. Distal digital keratoacanthoma: two cases with a review of the literature. Dermatol Surg 2001; 27 (6):575–579
7. Haneke E, Franken J. Onychomatricoma. Dermatol Surg Dermatol Surg 1995; 21 (11):984–987
8. Perrin C, Goettmann S, Baran R. Onychomatricoma: clinical and histopathologic findings in 12 cases. J Am Acad Dermatol 1998; 39(4 Pt 1):560–564
9. Moy RL, Eliezri YD, Nuovo GJ, et al. Human papillomavirus type 16 DNA in periungual squamous cell carcinomas. JAMA 1989; 261 (18):2669–2673
10. Theunis A, Andre J, Noel JC. Evaluation of the role of genital human papillomavirus in the pathogenesis of ungual squamous cell carcinoma. Dermatology 1999; 198 (2):206–208
11. McGrae JD, Jr., Greer CE, Manos MM. Multiple Bowen's disease of the fingers associated with human papilloma virus type 16. Int J Dermatol 1993; 32 (2):104–107
12. Koch A, Schonlebe J, Haroske G, et al. Polydactylous Bowen's disease. J Eur Acad Dermatol Venereol 2003; 17 (2):213–215

13. Baran R, Dupre A, Sayag J, et al. [Bowen disease of the nail apparatus. Report of 5 cases and review of the 20 cases of the literature (author's transl)]. Ann Dermatol Venereol 1979; 106 (3):227–233
14. Sau P, McMarlin SL, Sperling LC, Katz R. Bowen's disease of the nail bed and periungual area: a clinicopathologic analysis of seven cases. Arch Dermatol 1994; 130 (2):204–209
15. Bizzle PG. Subungal squamous cell carcinoma of the thumb masked by infection. Orthopedics 1992; 15 (11):1350–1352
16. Lai CS, Lin SD, Tsai CW, Chou CK. Squamous cell carcinoma of the nail bed. Cutis 1996; 57 (5):341–345
17. de Berker D, Dahl MG, Malcolm AJ, Lawrence CM. Micrographic surgery for subungual squamous cell carcinoma. Br J Plast Surg 1996; 49 (6):414–419
18. Zaiac MN, Weiss E. Moh's micrographic surgery of the nail unit and squamous cell carcinoma. Dermatol Surg 2001; 27 (3):246–251
19. Laffitte E, Saurat JH. [Recurrent Bowen's disease of the nail: treatment by topical imiquimod (Aldara)]. Ann Dermatol Venereol 2003; 130 (2 Pt 1):211–213
20. Wagner JD, Evdokimow DZ, Weisberger E, et al. Sentinel node biopsy for high-risk nonmelanoma cutaneous malignancy. Arch Dermatol 2004; 140 (1):75–79
21. Baran R, Perrin C, Baudet J, Requena L. Clinical and histological patterns of dermatofibromas of the nail apparatus. Clin Exp Dermatol 1994; 19 (1):31–35
22. Baran R, Haneke E. Fibrous and fibroepithelial tumors. In: Krull EA, Zook EG, Baran R, Haneke E, eds. Nail surgery: a text and atlas. Philadelphia: Lippincott Williams & Wilkins; 2001:214–223
23. Tosti A, Piraccini BM, Camacho-Martinez F. Onychomadesis and pyogenic granuloma following cast immobilization. Arch Dermatol 2001; 137 (2):231–232
24. Dailiana Z, Pajardi G, Le Viet D, Foucher G. Les tumeurs glomiques de la main – à propos d'une série de 80 patients. In: Dumontier C, ed. L'Ongle. Paris: Elsevier; 2000:201–205
25. Love JG. Glomus tumors; diagnostic and treatment. Mayo Clin Proc 1944; 19:113–116
26. Hildreth DH. The ischemia for glomus tumours: a new diagnostic test. Rev Surg 1970; 27:147–148
27. Bhaskaranand K, Navadgi BC. Glomus tumour of the hand. J Hand Surg Br 2002; 27B (3):229–231
28. Ozdemir O, Coskunol E, Ozalp T, Ozaksar K. [Glomus tumors of the finger: a report on 60 cases]. Acta Orthop Traumatol Turc 2003; 37 (3):244–248
29. Dupuis P, Pigeau I, Ebelin M, Barbato B, Lemerle JP. [The contribution of MRI in the study of glomus tumors]. Ann Chir Main Memb Super 1994; 13 (5):358–362
30. Theumann NH, Goettmann S, Le Viet D, et al. Recurrent Glomus Tumors of Fingertips: MR imaging evaluation. Radiology 2002; 223 (1):143–151
31. Heim U, Hanggi W. Subungual glomus tumors. Value of the direct dorsal approach. Ann Chir Main 1985; 4 (1):51–54
32. Tada H, Hirayma T, Takemitsu Y. Prevention of postoperative nail deformity after subungual glomus resection. J Hand Surg [Am] 1994; 19 (3):500–503
33. Gandon F, Legaillard P, Brueton R, et al. Forty eight glomus tumors of the hand. Retrospective study and four years follow up. Ann Hand Surg 1992; 11:401–405
34. Dumontier CA, Abimelec P. Nail unit enchondromas and osteochondromas: a surgical approach. Dermatol Surg 2001; 27 (3):274–279
35. Matthewson MH. Subungual exostoses of the fingers. Are they really uncommon? Br J Dermatol 1978; 98 (2):187–189
36. Landon GC, Johnson KA, Dahlin DC. Subungual exostoses. J Bone Joint Surg Am 1979; 61 (2):256–259
37. Takigawa K. Chondroma of the bones of the hand. A review of 110 cases. J Bone Joint Surg Am 1971; 53 (8):1591–1600
38. Floyd WE IIIrd, Troum S. Benign cartilaginous lesions of the upper extremity. Hand Clin 1995; 11 (2):119–132
39. Baran R, Haneke E, Drape JL, Zook EG. Tumours of the nail appratus and adjacent tissue. In: Baran R, Dawber RPR, de Berker DAR, et al., eds. Diseases of the nails and their management. Oxford: Blackwell Science; 2001:515–630

40. Zook EG. Osteoid osteomas. In: Krull EA, Zook EG, Baran R, Haneke E, eds. Nail surgery. A text and atlas. Philadelphia: Lippincott Williams & Wilkins; 2001:293–295

41. Drape JL. Nail unit anatomy and imaging with high resolution magnetic resolution imaging. Paris: Paris XI; 1997

42. Foucher G, Lemarechal P, Citron N, Merle M. Osteoid osteoma of the distal phalanx: a report of four cases and review of the literature. J Hand Surg Br 1987; 12B (3):382–386

43. Bowen CV, Dzus AK, Hardy DA. Osteoid osteomata of the distal phalanx. J Hand Surg [Br] 1987; 12 (3):387–390

44. Goettmann-Bonvallot S, Andre J, Belaich S. Longitudinal melanonychia in children: a clinical and histopathologic study of 40 cases. J Am Acad Dermatol 1999; 41 (1):17–22

45. Kato T, Usuba Y, Takematsu H, et al. A rapidly growing pigmented nail streak resulting in diffuse melanosis of the nail. A possible sign of subungual melanoma in situ. Cancer 1989; 64 (10):2191–2197

46. Durrani AJ, Moir GC, Diaz-Cano SJ, Cerio R. Malignant melanoma in an 8-year-old Caribbean girl: diagnostic criteria and utility of sentinel lymph node biopsy. Br J Dermatol 2003; 148 (3):569–572

47. Kiryu H. Malignant melanoma in situ arising in the nail unit of a child. J Dermatol 1998; 25 (1):41–44

48. Buka R, Friedman KA, Phelps RG, et al. Childhood longitudinal melanonychia: case reports and review of the literature. Mt Sinai J Med 2001; 68 (4–5):331–335

49. Leaute-Labreze C, Bioulac-Sage P, Taieb A. Longitudinal melanonychia in children. A study of eight cases. Arch Dermatol 1996; 132 (2):167–169 [published erratum appears in Arch Dermatol 1996; 132 (9):1127]

50. Rokuhara S, Saida T, Oguchi M, et al. Number of acquired melanocytic nevi in patients with melanoma and control subjects in Japan: nevus count is a significant risk factor for nonacral melanoma but not for acral melanoma. J Am Acad Dermatol 2004; 50 (5):695–700

51. Tosti A, Baran R, Piraccini BM, et al. Nail matrix nevi: a clinical and histopathologic study of twenty-two patients. J Am Acad Dermatol 1996; 34 (5):765–771

52. Vidal S, Sanz A, Hernandez B, et al. Subungual blue naevus [letter]. Br J Dermatol 1997; 137 (6):1023–1025

53. Causeret AS, Skowron F, Viallard AM, et al. Subungual blue nevus. J Am Acad Dermatol 2003; 49 (2):310–312

54. Moulonguet-Michau I, Abimelec P. Subungual blue nevus: two cases. Ann Derm Syph 2004; 131.

55. Blessing K, Kernohan NM, Park KG. Subungual malignant melanoma: clinicopathological features of 100 cases. Histopathology 1991; 19 (5):425–429

56. Moehrle M, Metzger S, Schippert W, et al. 'Functional' surgery in subungual melanoma. Dermatol Surg 2003; 29 (4):366–374

57. Levit EK, Kagen MH, Scher RK, et al. The ABC rule for clinical detection of subungual melanoma. J Am Acad Dermatol 2000; 42(2 Pt 1):269–274

58. Oropezza R. Melanoma in special sites. In: Andrade SL, Gumpert GL, Popkin G, Reese TD, eds. Cancer of the skin. Philadelphia: Saunders; 1976:974–987

59. Kato T, Suetake T, Sugiyama Y, et al. Epidemiology and prognosis of subungual melanoma in 34 Japanese patients. Br J Dermatol 1996; 134 (3):383–387

60. Banfield CC, Redburn JC, Dawber RP. The incidence and prognosis of nail apparatus melanoma. A retrospective study of 105 patients in four English regions. Br J Dermatol 1998; 139 (2):276–279

61. O'Leary JA, Berend KR, Johnson JL, et al. Subungual melanoma. A review of 93 cases with identification of prognostic variables. Clin Orthop 2000; 378:206–212

62. Brochez L, Verhaeghe E, Sales F, et al. Current guidelines in melanoma treatment. Dermatology 2000; 200:160–166

63. Wagner JD, Gordon MS, Chuang T-Y, Coleman JI. Current therapy of cutaneous melanoma. Plast Reconstr Surg 2000; 105:1774–1799

64. Thomas JM, Newton-Bishop J, A'Hern R, et al. Excision margins in high-risk malignant melanoma. N Engl J Med 2004; 350 (8):757–766

65. Dawber RP, Colver GB. The spectrum of malignant melanoma of the nail apparatus. Semin Dermatol 1991; 10 (1):82–87

66. Rigby HS, Briggs JC. Subungual melanoma: a clinico-pathological study of 24 cases. Br J Plast Surg 1992; 45 (4):275–278

67. Paul E, Kleiner H, Bodeker RH. [Epidemiology and prognosis of subungual melanoma]. Hautarzt 1992; 43 (5):286–290

68. Park KG, Blessing K, Kernohan NM. Surgical aspects of subungual malignant melanomas. The Scottish Melanoma Group. Ann Surg 1992; 216 (6):692–695

69. Kleinert HE, Kutz JE, Fishman JH, McCraw LH. Etiology and treatment of the so-called mucous cyst of the finger. J Bone Joint Surg Am 1972; 54 (7):1455–1458

70. de Berker DA, Lawrence CM. Treatment of myxoid cysts. Dermatol Surg 2001; 27 (3):296–299

71. Jayson MI. Articular hypertension, valves and juxta-arterial cysts. Proc R Soc Med 1973; 66 (4):392

72. Chaise F, Gaisne E, Friol JP, Bellemere P. [Mucoid cysts of the distal interphalangeal joints of the fingers. Apropos of a prospective series (100 cases)]. Ann Chir Main Memb Super 1994; 13 (3):184–189

73. Brown RE, Zook EG, Russell RC, et al. Fingernail deformities secondary to ganglions of the distal interphalangeal joint (mucous cysts). Plast Reconstr Surg 1991; 87 (4):718–725

74. de Berker D, Goettman S, Baran R. Subungual myxoid cysts: clinical manifestations and response to therapy. J Am Acad Dermatol 2002; 46 (3):394–398

75. Audebert C. Treatment of mucoid cysts of fingers and toes by injection of sclerosant. Dermatol Clin 1989; 7 (1):179–181

76. Angelides AC. Ganglions of the hand and wrist. In: Green DP, ed. Operative hand surgery. Edinburgh: Churchill Livingstone; 1988:2290–2291

77. Isaacson NH, McCarthy DD. Recurring myxomatous cutaneous cysts. Surgery 1954; 35:621–623

78. Crawford RJ, Gupta A, Risitano G, Burke FD. Mucous cyst of the distal interphalangeal joint: treatment by simple excision or excision and rotation flap. J Hand Surg [Br] 1990; 15 (1):113–114

79. Dodge LD, Brown RL, Niebauer JJ, McCarroll HR, Jr. The treatment of mucous cysts: long-term follow-up in sixty-two cases. J Hand Surg [Am] 1984; 9 (6):901–904

80. Gross RE. Recurring myxomatous cutaneous cysts of the fingers and toes. Surg Gynecol Obstet 1937; 65:289–302

81. Kasdan ML, Stallings SP, Leis VM, Wolens D. Outcome of surgically treated mucous cysts of the hand. J Hand Surg Usa 1994; 19 (3):504–507

82. Constant E, Royer JR, Pollard RJ, et al. Mucous cysts of the fingers. Plast Reconstr Surg 1969; 43 (3):241–246

83. Fritz GR, Stern PJ, Dickey M. Complications following mucous cyst excision. J Hand Surg [Br] 1997; 22 (2):222–225

84. O'Shaughnessy M, McCann J, O'Connor TP, Condon KC. Nail re-growth in fingertip injuries. Ir Med J 1990; 83 (4):136–137

85. Zook EG, Guy RJ, Russell RC. A study of nail bed injuries: causes, treatment, and prognosis. J Hand Surg [Am] 1984; 9 (2):247–252

86. Guy RJ. The etiologies and mechanisms of nail bed injuries. Hand Clin 1990; 6 (1):9–19; discussion 21.

87. Ogunro EO. External fixation of injured nail bed with the INRO surgical nail splint. J Hand Surg [Am] 1989; 14(2 Pt 1):236–241

88. Zook EG. The perionychium: anatomy, physiology, and care of injuries. Clin Plast Surg 1981; 8 (1):21–31

89. Seaberg DC, Angelos WJ, Paris PM. Treatment of subungual hematomas with nail trephination: a prospective study. Am J Emerg Med 1991; 9 (3):209–210

90. Ranjan A. Subungual haematoma. J Indian Med Assoc 1979; 72 (8):187–188

91. Simon RR, Wolgin M. Subungual hematoma: association with occult laceration requiring repair. Am J Emerg Med 1987; 5 (4):302–304

92. Schwartz GR, Schwen SA. Subungual splinter removal. Am J Emerg Med 1997; 15:330–331

93. Ashbell TS, Kleinert HE, Putcha SM, Kutz JE. The deformed finger nail, a frequent result of failure to repair nail bed injuries. J Trauma 1967; 7 (2):177–190

94. Foucher G, Merle M, van Genechten F, Denuit P. [Ungual synthesis]. Ann Chir Main 1984; 3 (2):168–169

95. Shepard GH. Nail grafts for reconstruction. Hand Clin 1990; 6 (1):79–102; discussion 103

96. Saito H, Suzuki Y, Fujino K, Tajima T. Free nail bed graft for treatment of nail bed injuries of the hand. J Hand Surg [Am] 1983; 8 (2):171–178

97. Dumontier C, Tilquin B, Lenoble E, Foucher G. [Reconstruction of distal loss of substance in the nail-bed by a de-epithelialized flap from the digital pulp]. Ann Chir Plast Esthet 1992; 37 (5):553–559

98. Shepard GH. Treatment of nail bed avulsions with split-thickness nail bed grafts. J Hand Surg [Am] 1983; 8 (1):49–54

99. Johnson RK. Nailplasty. Plast Reconstr Surg 1971; 47 (3):275–276

100. Schernberg F, Amiel M. [Anatomo-clinical study of a complete nail flap]. Ann Chir Plast Esthet 1985; 30 (2):127–131

101. Hirase Y. Salvage of fingertip amputated at nail level: new surgical principles and treatment. Ann Plast Surg 1997; 38:151–157

102. Nishi G, Shibata Y, Tago K, et al. Nail regeneration in digits replanted after amputation through the distal phalanx. J Hand Surg [Am] 1996; 21 (2):229–233

103. Elliot D, Sood MK, Flemming AFS, Swain B. A comparison of replantation and terminalization after distal finger amputation. J Hand Surg Br 1997; 22B:523–529

104. Kim WK, Lim JH, Han SK. Fingertip replantations: clinical evaluation of 135 digits. Plast Reconstr Surg 1996; 98 (3):470–476

105. Dumontier C. Distal replantation, nail bed, and nail problems in musicians. Hand Clin 2003; 19 (2):259–272, vi

106. Mantero R, Bertolotti P. Fingertip replantation and cross-finger flaps. Ann Chir 1985; 29:1019–1023

107. Dubert T, Houimli S, Valenti P, Dinh A. Very distal finger amputations: replantation or 'reposition-flap' repair? J Hand Surg [Br] 1997; 22 (3):353–358

108. Foucher G, Braga Da Silva J, Boulas J. ['Reposition-flap' technique in amputation of the finger tip. Apropos of a series of 21 cases]. Ann Chir Plast Esthet 1992; 37 (4):438–442

109. Kumar VP, Satku K. Treatment and prevention of 'hook nail' deformity with anatomic correlation. J Hand Surg USA 1993; 18 (4):617–620

110. Beasley RW. Reconstruction of amputated fingertips. Plast Reconstr Surg 1969; 44 (4):349–352

111. Schiller C. Nail replacement in finger tip injuries. Plast Reconstr Surg 1957; 19:521–530

112. Rose EH. Small flap coverage of hand and digit defects. Clin Plast Surg 1989; 16 (3):427–442

113. Rosenthal EA. Treatment of fingertip and nail bed injuries. Orthop Clin North Am 1983; 14 (4):675–697

114. Ardouin T, Poirier P, Rogez JM. [Fingertips and nailbed injuries in children. Apropos of 241 cases]. Rev Chir Orthop Reparatrice Appar Mot 1997; 83 (4):330–334

115. Moossavi M, Scher RK. Complications of nail surgery: a review of the literature. Dermatol Surg 2001; 27 (3):225–228

116. Haas F, Moshammer H, Schwarzl F. [Iatrogenic necrosis of the large toe after tourniquet placement – clinical course and reconstruction]. Chirurg 1999; 70 (5):608–610

117. Roca B, Climent A, Costa N. [Reflex sympathetic dystrophy after nail surgery]. Ann Med Interna 2000; 17 (9):506

118. Ingram GJ, Scher RK, Lally EV. Reflex sympathetic dystrophy following nail biopsy. J Am Acad Dermatol 1987; 16(1 Pt 2): 253–256

119. Tosti A, Baran R, Peluso AM, et al. Reflex sympathetic dystrophy with prominent involvement of the nail apparatus. J Am Acad Dermatol 1993; 29(5 Pt 2):865–868

120. Vanhooteghem O, Andre J, Halkin V, Song M. Leuconychia in reflex sympathetic dystrophy: a chance association? [letter]. Br J Dermatol 1998; 139 (2):355–356

121. Zyluk A. The sequelae of reflex sympathetic dystrophy. J Hand Surg [Br] 2001; 26 (2):151–154

122. Leshin B, Whitaker DC. Carbon dioxide laser matricectomy. J Dermatol Surg Oncol 1988; 14 (6):608–611

123. de Berker DA, Baran R. Acquired malalignment: a complication of lateral longitudinal nail biopsy. Acta Derm Venereol 1998; 78 (6):468–470

# 25 Glossary

**agnail:**[1] Hangnail; hard spicules at the edge of the nail.

**anonychia:** Absence of nail plate or nail unit.

**brachyonychia:**[2] Short nails.

**chromonychia:** Color changes appearing in the nail unit.

**clubbing:** Increase of the ungual–phalangeal angle greater than or equal to 180°; usually accompanied by fibrovascular hyperplasia of the more proximal nail unit (see Chapter 15).

**defluvium unguium:**[1] Nail shedding starting at the base and extending forward; onychomadesis.

**dolichonychia:**[2] Quotient between length and width of nail is greater than 1 ± 0.1; seen in Ehlers–Danlos syndrome and Marfan syndrome.

**eggshell nails:**[3] Hapalonychia developing a transparent bluish-white hue.

**elkonyxis:**[4] Loss of nail substance (more than pitting); oval, 2 to 3 mm.

**eponychium:** Most distal horny extension of the proximal nail fold cuticle.

**fragilitas unguium:**[1] Brittle nails.

**hapalonychia:**[1] Soft nails.

**heloma:**[5] Corn.

**hyponychium:** Area of the nail unit distal to the nail bed having a granular layer (the only part of the nail unit normally having a granular layer).

**koilonychia:** Spooning of the nail plate (see Chapter 15).

**leukonychia:** Whitening of the nail plate (either apparent or real) (see Chapter 15).

**lunula:** Half-moon; distal part (often visible) of the nail matrix.

**macronychia:** Unusually large nail often wider than normal.

**median nail dystrophy:**[1] Dystrophia mediana canaliformis; median canal or split in the nail plate, often idiopathic; usually thumbnails.

**micronychia:** Small nail often shorter or narrower than normal.

**nail apparatus:** Nail plate, nail folds, nail matrix, nail bed, hyponychium (nail plate and surrounding and underlying soft structures extending from the proximal nail matrix region distally).

**nail bed:** Supporting structure of the nail plate extending from the nail matrix distally to the hyponychium.

**nail field:**[6] Earliest anatomic sign of the nail, occurring at about 9 weeks of fetal development.

**nail folds:** Two lateral, one proximal; outline and support the nail unit and guide the growth of the nail plate.

**nail matrix:** Producer of the nail plate extending from under the proximal nail fold distally to the nail bed.

**nail plate:** Horny, keratinized portion of the dorsal nail unit; usually extending from the proximal matrix region distally.

**nail unit:** Same as nail apparatus.

**onychalgia:** Nail unit pain.

**onychia:** Inflammation somewhere in the nail unit.

**onychin:**[3] Antiquated term, substance similar to keratin making up the nail plate.

**onychoclavus:**[4] Subungual corn.

**onychocryptosis:**[4] Ingrown nail.

**onychogryphosis:** Ram's horn nail; hypertrophy of the nail plate, often hornlike, probably resulting from trauma. One side of nail seems to grow faster than the other, often curving the nail plate away from the site of trauma.

**onychoheterotopia:** Abnormally placed nail on the digits as the result of displaced matrix material.

**onycholysis:** Distal separation of the nail plate from underlying hyponychium and nail bed.

**onychomadesis:** Proximal separation of the nail plate from the matrix-nail bed area.

**onychomycosis:** Fungal infection of the nail unit.

**onychophagia:**[1] Nail biting.

**onychophosis:**[5] Localized or diffuse hyperkeratosis of varying degree that develops on the lateral or proximal nail folds, in the space between the nail folds and the nail plate, or even subungually. Common in elderly patients in the first and fifth toes, and is due to repeated trauma.

**onychoptosis:** Loss of the nail plate.

**onychorrhexis:** Longitudinal striations of the nail plate, usually superficial.

**onychoschizia:** Superficial splitting of the nail plate (layering), usually beginning distally.

**onychotillomania:** Tearing, picking, destroying nails by some method.

**pachyonychia:** Thickening of nail plate, often the entire plate.

**panaritium:**[1] Abscess at the side or base of the nail (whtilow).

**paronychia:** Inflammation or infection of the nail folds.

**periungual:** Around the nail. One should not use paronychial as a synonym.

**pincer (trumpet) nails:** Abnormally narrow, curved nails often caused by lateral pressure on the nail unit (as when shoes are too tight). Can occur idiopathically in fingernails.

**platonychia:**[1] Increased nail curvature in the long axis.

**polyonychia:** More than one nail on a digit.

**pterygium:** Scarring of the proximal nail fold region involving the matrix.

**pterygium inversus unguium:** Fusing (scarring) of the distal nail plate to the underlying hyponychium and nail bed.

**retronychia:**[7] Acute onychomadesis.

**Rosenau's depressions:**[4] Depression, erosion, or excavation of the nail surface.

**scleronychia:**[7] Hard nails.

**tinea unguium:** Infection of the nail unit by a dermatophyte.

**trachyonychia:**[2] Rough nails.

**unguis incarnatus:** Ingrown nail.

**usure des angles:**[1] Wearing away of nails usually from scratching.

## REFERENCES

1. Samman PD. The nails in disease. 2nd edn. Springfield, IL: Charles C Thomas; 1972
2. Baran R. Diseases of the nail and their management. Oxford: Blackwell Scientific; 1984
3. Pardo-Castello V. Diseases of the nails. 2nd edn. Springfield, IL: Charles C Thomas; 1947
4. DeNicola P. Nail diseases in internal medicine. Springfield, IL: Charles C Thomas; 1974
5. Cohen, PR, Scher RK. Geriatric nail disorders: diagnosis and treatment. J Am Acad Dermatol 1992; 26:521
6. Zaias N. The nail in health and disease. New York: SP Medical and Scientific Books; 1980
7. Baran R, Dawber RPR, deBerker DAR, et al. Diseases of the nails and their management. 3rd edn. Oxford: Blackwell; 2001

# Index

# C